Skin Disease
Diagnosis and Treatment

Second edition

Commissioning Editor: *Sue Hodgson/Shuet-Kei Cheung*
Project Development Manager: *Hilary Hewitt*
Project Manager: *Glenys Norquay*
Illustration Manager: *Mick Ruddy*
Design Manager: *Jayne Jones*
Illustrator: *Debbie Maizels*

Skin Disease
Diagnosis and Treatment

Second edition

Thomas P Habif MD
Adjunct Professor of Medicine (Dermatology)
Dartmouth Medical School
Hanover, NH
USA

James L Campbell Jr MD MS
Adjunct Assistant Professor of Medicine
(Dermatology)
Dartmouth Medical School
Hanover, NH
USA

James GH Dinulos MD
Assistant Professor of Medicine and Pediatrics
(Dermatology)
Dartmouth Medical School
Hanover, NH
USA

M Shane Chapman MD
Assistant Professor of Medicine (Dermatology)
Dartmouth Medical School
Hanover, NH
USA

Kathryn A Zug MD
Associate Professor of Medicine (Dermatology)
Dartmouth Medical School
Hanover, NH
USA

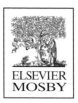
ELSEVIER
MOSBY

Philadelphia Edinburgh London New York Oxford St Louis Sydney Toronto 2005

ELSEVIER
MOSBY

An affiliate of Elsevier Inc

© 2001, Mosby Inc.
© 2005, Elsevier Inc. All rights reserved.

First published 2001
Second edition 2005

ISBN-13: 978–0–323–02753–3
ISBN-10: 0–323–02753–9

British Library Cataloguing in Publication Data
A catalogue record for this book is available from the British Library

Library of Congress Cataloging in Publication Data
A catalog record for this book is available from the Library of Congress

---

Notice

Medical knowledge is constantly changing. Standard safety precautions must be followed, but as new research and clinical experience broaden our knowledge, changes in treatment and drug therapy may become necessary or appropriate. Readers are advised to check the most current product information provided by the manufacturer of each drug to be administered to verify the recommended dose, the method and duration of administration, and contraindications. It is the responsibility of the practitioner, relying on experience and knowledge of the patient, to determine dosages and the best treatment for each individual patient. Neither the Publisher nor the authors assume any liability for any injury and/or damage to persons or property arising from this publication.

The Publisher

Printed in China

Last digit is the print number: 9   8   7   6   5   4   3

Working together to grow
libraries in developing countries
www.elsevier.com | www.bookaid.org | www.sabre.org

ELSEVIER   BOOK AID International   Sabre Foundation

The Publisher's policy is to use paper manufactured from sustainable forests

Contents

Preface

∙∙∙

Changes in health care delivery require an increasing level of sophistication among primary care providers in all medical disciplines. Dermatology is no exception, since 10% of all outpatient medical visits to primary care physicians are for dermatologic problems.

This book was designed as a field guide for the diagnosis and management of common dermatologic conditions. Content is meant to be current, concise, and consistent rather than all-inclusive. Photographs were chosen to illustrate key diagnostic features of specific conditions. Color-coded figures represent statistical maps showing the likely distribution of skin lesions.

With this second edition, we refine our goal of a field guide for the identification and management of common dermatologic conditions. We would like to thank those who provided invaluable feedback that has allowed us to improve and evolve in our endeavour.

The content remains concise rather than all-inclusive and has been updated to remain current. Diagnoses are presented with clinical images and color-coded distribution maps of skin lesions. The formulary contains the latest in over-the-counter and prescription therapeutics.

We trust that this edition will find its way to an easily reached area of your medical library.

Thomas P Habif
James L Campbell Jr
M Shane Chapman
James GH Dinulos
Kathryn A Zug

1 Topical Therapy

Basic Principles of Treatment

Maintaining the Skin Barrier
- The skin assists in fluid homeostasis and protects against infections, toxins and harmful effects of ultraviolet radiation.
- The outermost layer of the epidermis, the stratum corneum provides this protection though an impermeable barrier made up of fatty acids, cholesterol, and ceramides cemented between tight-knit protein-rich cornified cells.
- One goal of topical or systemic dermatologic therapy is to restore and maintain the essential functions of the skin barrier.

Skin Cleansing
- For most individuals, full body daily bathing is not necessary for healthy skin.
- Patients should use mild soaps and cleansers such as Cetaphil, Dove, Keri, or Oil of Olay, and avoid excessive use of exfoliating scrubs, washcloths and brushes.
- Soaps with fragrances and antibacterial agents can be irritating.
- Patients should avoid washing with very hot water.

Skin Moisturization
- Immediately after washing, the skin should be patted dry and moisturized with an emollient.
- The principle difference between emollients is the ratio of oil and water. For most emollients, petrolatum is the "oil" base and water is added to produce creams and lotions. Some solutions and lotions have alcohol bases.
- Pure petrolatum effectively maintains skin moisture and acts as a barrier to skin irritants and is the least irritating emollient.
- Thick emollients such as petrolatum feel "greasy" and can block follicular and eccrine openings, producing acne and miliaria in rare cases.
- Lotions spread easily on to the skin, although they do not moisturize and protect as well as thicker creams and petrolatum.
- In some patients, preservatives in creams and lotions cause skin irritation and allergic contact dermatitis.
- Patients with sensitive skin should apply fragrance-free lotions.
- Many creams and lotions have "anti-aging" additives such as vitamin A, C and E, but their efficacy is not proven.
- Sun protection factor is added to many creams and lotions and is an effective method to slow skin aging.
- Triceram cream is a formulation of ceramides normally found in the stratum corneum and is thought to be an effective emollient.
- Keratolytic emollients containing glycolic acids (lactic acid, salicylic acid) and urea are useful to gently exfoliate the skin.
- Sarna lotion (camphor and menthol) and Pramosone (pramoxine) are examples of lotions with additives to decrease itch.
- Patients should check with their physician for specific skin care recommendations.

Examples of Lubricating Creams and Lotions
In addition to those named here, many other effective products are available.

Thicker Creams and Ointments
- Vaseline petroleum jelly
- Aquaphor ointment
- Eucerin cream

Lighter Creams

- Acid Mantle
- Cetaphil cream
- DML cream
- Moisturel cream
- Nutraplus cream

Lighter Lotions

- Cetaphil lotion
- DML lotion
- Nutraderm lotion
- Curel lotion
- Aveeno lotion

Topical Formulations

- Two main factors determine the effectiveness of a topical medication: the drug and the vehicle.
- For any given topical drug to be effective, it must be administered in an adequate concentration and delivered to the skin with an appropriate formulation.
- Vehicles not only assist in drug delivery, but they also have therapeutic properties.
- Powders are drying and are effective in moist intertriginous areas. They are vehicles for many antifungal agents.
- Like powder, water can dry weepy rashes and it can be effective in removing scale and treating widespread skin disease (oatmeal bath, tar bath).
- Ointments are greasy water-in-oil emulsions and are helpful to deliver medications to dry skin. Ointments increase the potency of a compound when compared to the cream formulations (e.g. Elocon ointment is more potent than Elocon cream).
- Creams are oil-in-water emulsions. They can be cooling and are not as occlusive as ointments.
- Pastes are ointments with 20–50% powder (zinc oxide, starch). They are more drying than ointments and are less greasy.
- Solutions and lotions are clear or milky white liquids that evaporate on the skin and thus can be drying. They are effective to deliver drugs to hairy areas such as the scalp, arms and legs. Patients can experience stinging when used on open wet areas or on mucus membranes.
- Gels are clear and greaseless. They dry skin on contact, leaving a thin film. They are effective for acne and skin disease in hairy areas. Foams are similarly greaseless.

Topical Application and Dosing

- Medications should be gently massaged into the skin in one thin layer. Thicker applications do not increase skin penetration.
- One gram of cream covers an area 10×10 cm and ointments spread slightly further.
- The fingertip unit (FTU) is another method to assess how much cream to dispense and apply. A fingertip unit is the amount of ointment expressed from a tube with a 5-mm diameter nozzle and applied from the distal skin crease to the tip of the index finger. In an adult, 1 fingertip unit weighs approximately 0.5 g. The number of fingertip units required to cover specific body areas is illustrated in Appendix C.
- Dosing frequency varies with the medication, but most dermatology medications are applied once to twice per day.
- The ability of a medication to penetrate the skin varies according to the anatomic site (mucous membranes > scrotum > eyelids > face > torso > extremities > palms and soles).
- Conditions producing skin breakdown allow increased drug penetration. As the epidermal barrier function improves, less percutaneous absorption occurs.
- Medications placed under occlusive dressings or body suits are more readily absorbed into the skin.

Wet Dressings

- Wet dressings, or compresses, are a valuable aid in the treatment of exudative (wet) skin diseases.

1. Obtain a clean, soft cloth such as bed sheeting or shirt material. The cloth need not be new or sterilized.
2. Fold the cloth and cut to fit an area slightly larger than the area to be treated.
3. Wet the folded dressings by immersing them in the solution, and wring them out to the point of sopping wet (neither running nor just damp).
4. Place the wet dressings on the affected area. Do not pour solution on a wet dressing to keep it wet because this practice increases the concentration of the solution and may cause irritation. Remove the dressing and replace it with a new one.
5. Leave the dressings in place for 30 minutes. Dressings may be used two to four times a day or continuously. Discontinue the use of wet dressings when the skin becomes dry. Excessive drying causes cracking and fissures.

- The temperature of the compress solution should be cool when an anti-inflammatory effect is desired and tepid when the purpose is to debride an infected, crusted lesion.
- A wet dressing should not be covered with a towel or plastic. These items inhibit evaporation, promote maceration, and increase skin temperature, which facilitates bacterial growth.

Benefits of Wet Dressings

- Inflammation suppression—the evaporative cooling causes the constriction of superficial vessels, thereby decreasing erythema and the production of serum. Wet dressings soothe acute inflammatory processes such as acute poison ivy.
- Wound debridement—the dressing macerates vesicles and crust, helping debride these materials when the dressing is removed.
- Drying—repeated cycles of wetting and drying promote drying of weeping wet lesions.

Pediatric considerations

- Infants have a markedly increased body surface area compared to body mass, placing them at risk for systemic side effects and toxicity from topically applied medications.
- Premature infants have compromised epidermal permeability barriers, allowing percutaneous absorption and systemic toxicity from medications and even benign substances such as soaps and cleaning solutions.
- Infants under warming lights and post-mature infants often have dry, flaky skin with fissures and benefit from application of bland ointments and creams.

Topical Corticosteroids

Description

- Hydrocortisone was first introduced in 1952, and since then topical corticosteroids have been the principal medications used to treat inflammatory dermatosis. Over time, they have proven to be safe and effective when used properly. In dermatology, topical corticosteroids are used for their anti-inflammatory properties.

Generic vs Brand Names

- Many generic topical corticosteroid formulations are available and provide substantial financial savings for patients.
- Despite these savings, generic formulations can differ significantly from their brand-name counterparts with respect to their anti-inflammatory potency and preservative content.

Corticosteroid Potency: Groups I–VII

- Topical corticosteroids are organized in seven groups, based on their anti-inflammatory activity (group I are the strongest; group VII are the weakest; see Appendix F: Dermatologic Formulary).
- Throughout the book, topical corticosteroids are referred to by group number.

Choosing the Appropriate Strength

- The success or failure of therapy depends largely on selecting a topical corticosteroid of the correct strength.
- A few essential factors to consider include diagnosis, location, age, and financial resources of the patient.
- Certain rashes such as nummular eczema and discoid lupus erythematosis require group I or II corticosteroids for adequate control. Seborrheic dermatitis is extremely responsive to group V-VII corticosteroids.
- Dermatitis on the eyelids should be treated with group V-VII corticosteroids. Palms and soles require group I-III corticosteroids because the thick skin lessens efficacy.

- Patients who do not show adequate response after 2 weeks of therapy should be re-evaluated.
- By convention, topical corticosteroids are lightly massaged into the skin twice daily.
- Concentrations reflect relative strength for a particular corticosteroid (triamcinolone 0.025%, 0.05%, 0.1%) and cannot be used to compare strengths between corticosteroids. For example, clobetasol propionate 0.05% is much more potent than 1% hydrocortisone.
- Some corticosteroids are referred to as "fluorinated" because a fluorine atom has been added to increase potency.
- Fluorinated topical corticosteroids cause atrophy, telangiectasia, and striae more readily than non-fluorinated corticosteroids.

Prescribing Topical Corticosteroids

Dosing Schedules

- These are general guidelines; specific instructions and limitations must be established for each patient.

Superpotent Topical Corticosteroids (Group I)

- Patients should not use more than 45-60 g of cream or ointment per week.
- Cyclic dosing, such as corticosteroid application for 2 weeks, followed by 1 week of rest, can limit side effects.
- Patients must be prescribed limited amounts of these superpotent corticosteroids and have close monitoring.
- Difficult-to-treat inflammatory diseases such as plaque psoriasis and hand eczema respond most effectively when a group I topical corticosteroid is applied twice a day for 2 weeks, followed by 1 week of rest. This schedule is repeated until the condition is well controlled.

Group II–VII Topical Corticosteroids

- Group II–VI topical corticosteroids should be applied twice each day.
- Adequate response should be seen in 2-6 weeks.
- Prescribing a weak group VII topical corticosteroid (hydrocortisone) for an

intense inflammatory condition is a common mistake and should be avoided.

Methods of Application (Simple and Occlusive)

Simple
- A simple application refers to massaging a topical corticosteroid thinly into the skin without the aid of an occlusive dressing.
- Washing is not necessary before each application.
- Different skin surfaces vary in their ability to absorb topical corticosteroids.
- Eyelid dermatitis responds quickly to group VI or VII steroids. Higher-potency corticosteroids should be avoided in this area.
- The skin on the palms and soles is thick, requiring group I–III corticosteroids.
- Intertriginous areas (e.g. axilla, groin, perineum, and the inframammary region) respond quickly to group V–VII corticosteroids because the moisture and occlusion increase percutaneous absorption.
- Topical corticosteroids are absorbed readily in inflamed skin, resulting in a rapid initial response.

Occlusive
- Occlusive dressings (e.g. Saran Wrap) hydrate the stratum corneum and allow for enhanced corticosteroid absorption, allowing for use of lower strength corticosteroids.
- Lengthy application of an occlusive dressing can produce superficial skin infection (usually *Staphylococcus aureus*) and/or inflamed hair follicles. If pustules develop, topical (Bactroban) or systemic antistaphylococcal antibiotics (Keflex 500 mg two to three times daily for 7–10 days) should be administered.
- Occlusive dressings can be used during the day for periods up to 2 hours or 8 hours during sleep. Simple applications can be alternated with applications assisted by an occlusive dressing.

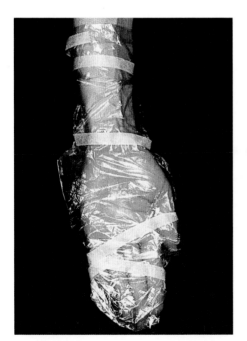

Occlusion of the hand. A plastic bag is pulled on and pressed against the skin to expel air. Tape is wound snugly around the bag.

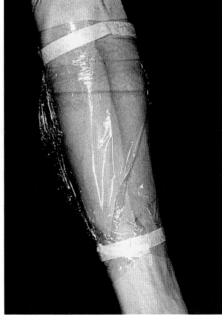

Occlusion of the arm. A plastic sheet (e.g. Saran Wrap) is wound around the extremity and secured at both ends with tape. A plastic bag with the bottom cut out may be used as a sleeve and held in place with tape or an Ace bandage.

Method of Occlusion

■ The area should be cleaned with mild soap and water. Antibacterial soaps are unnecessary.

■ The topical corticosteroid is gently rubbed into the lesions, and the entire area is covered with plastic (e.g. Saran Wrap, Handi-Wrap, plastic bags, or gloves).

■ The dressing is secured with tape so that it is close to the skin and the ends are sealed. An airtight dressing is not necessary. The plastic may be held in place with an Ace bandage or a sock.

■ The best results are obtained if the dressing remains in place for at least 2 hours. Many patients find that bedtime is the most convenient time to wear an occlusive dressing.

■ More medicine is applied shortly after the dressing is removed and while the skin is still moist.

■ Vinyl exercise suits (sauna suits) are effective to occlude large body surface areas.

Systemic Absorption

■ With proper use of corticosteroids, systemic effects are rare.

■ Persistent, unsupervised use of topical corticosteroids over wide areas can result in significant systemic absorption.

Steroid–Antibiotic Mixtures

■ Some products contain a combination of antibiotics and corticosteroids.

■ The majority of corticosteroid-responsive skin diseases can be managed successfully without topical antibiotics, making these combination products unnecessary.

■ Neomycin is a common cause of allergic contact dermatitis, and should be avoided.

■ Antifungal–corticosteroid combinations (Mycolog, Lotrisone) are expensive and have limited uses. The topical corticosteroid betamethasone diproprionate found in Lotrisone is too strong for intertriginous areas and can cause permanent striae.

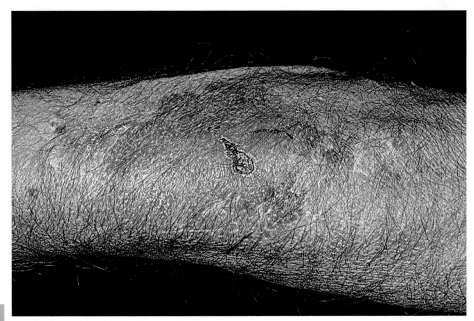

Steroid atrophy. Long-term application of clobetasol, a group I topical steroid, caused dermal atrophy and skin fragility. Bleeding and skin tearing occurred with the slightest trauma.

Adverse Reactions

■ Topical corticosteroids have the
  following potential side effects:
  - Allergic contact dermatitis
  - Burning, itching, irritation, dryness
    (largely due to the vehicle)
  - Hypertrichosis
  - Hypopigmentation
  - Miliaria and folliculitis
  - Skin breakdown
  - Glaucoma, cataracts
  - Rebound phenomenon (i.e. psoriasis
    becomes worse after treatment is
    stopped)
  - Rosacea, perioral dermatitis, acne
  - Skin atrophy with telangiectasia,
    stellate pseudo-scars (arms), purpura,
    striae
  - Skin blanching from acute
    vasoconstriction
  - Systemic absorption
  - Tinea incognito, impetigo incognito,
    scabies incognito

Pediatric Considerations

- Topical corticosteroids have
  been used in children for over
  40 years and have a proven
  track record for safety, when
  used correctly.
- Many parents have concerns
  about topical steroids. Parents
  should be educated about
  potential side effects and
  shown how to apply topical
  steroids correctly.
- Infants are more susceptible to
  systemic side effects due to
  their increased ratio of body
  surface to weight. Systemic side
  effects such as hypothalamic–
  pituitary axis suppression can
  occur with long-term use or
  when the skin barrier is
  compromised (acute dermatitis,
  premature infants).

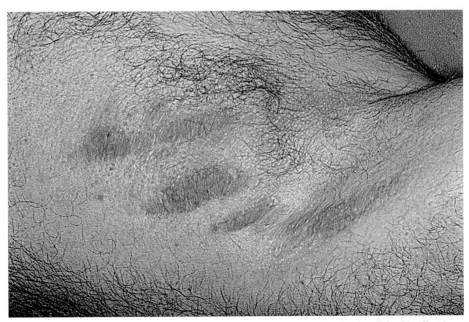

Striae. Long-term application of a group V topical steroid to the axillae produced striae. This side effect is irreversible.

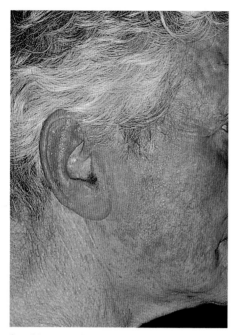

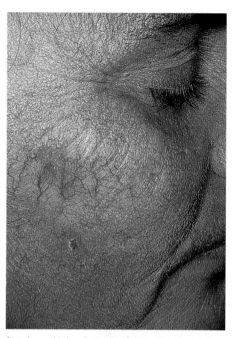

Steroid rosacea. Numerous papules and pustules appeared on the face after stopping application of a group II topical steroid. The topical steroid had been applied daily for 12 weeks.

Atrophy and telangiectasia after continual use of a group II topical steroid for 6 months. The atrophy may improve after the topical steroid is discontinued, but the telangiectasia often persists.

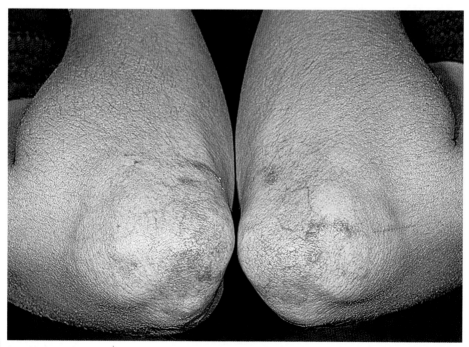

Steroid atrophy. Atrophy with prominence of the underlying veins and hypopigmentation after the use of a superpotent steroid applied daily for 3 months to treat psoriasis. Note that small plaques of psoriasis persist. Atrophy improves after topical steroids are discontinued, but some hypopigmentation may persist.

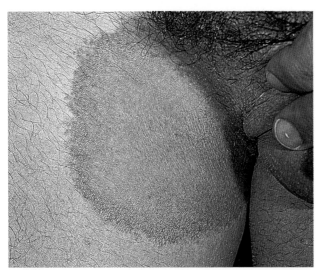

Typical presentation of tinea of the groin before treatment. A fungal infection of this type typically has a sharp, scaly border and shows little tendency to spread.

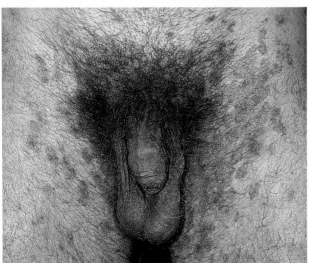

Tinea incognito. Bizarre pattern of wide-spread inflammation created by applying a group II topical steroid twice daily for 3 weeks to an eruption similar to that in the photograph above. A potassium hydroxide preparation showed numerous fungi.

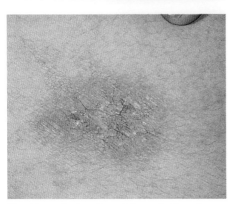

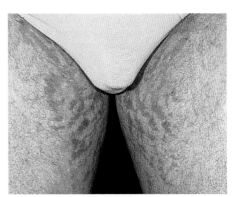

Steroid atrophy. Long-term daily application of clobetasol, a group I topical steroid, caused epidermal and dermal atrophy with telangiectasia. Veins can be seen through the thinned skin.

Striae of the groin after long-term use of group V topical steroids for pruritus. These changes are irreversible.

2 Eczema

Acute Eczematous Inflammation

Description

■ Acute eczematous inflammation is characterized clinically by erythema, edema, and vesiculation. Weeping or oozing of acute lesions is typical. Pruritus is often severe.

History

■ There are multiple causes of acute eczema. They include allergic contact hypersensitivity to specific plant allergens such as poison ivy, oak, or sumac and other allergens

■ Nickel, topical medicaments such as bacitracin, neomycin, and benzocaine fragrances, preservatives in personal care products and rubber additives are also common causes of acute eczematous inflammation. Irritant dermatitis is common after repeated water, solvent or detergent exposure.

■ In an "id reaction" acute eczema with vesicles occurs at a distant site (e.g. the hands) from an active fungal infection (e.g. the feet).

■ Stasis dermatitis, scabies, irritant reactions, and dyshidrotic and atopic eczema may present as an acute eczematous inflammation.

Skin Findings

■ Findings include erythema, edema, vesiculation, and weeping. Inflammation can be moderate to intense. Tiny, clear, fluid-filled vesicles are seen on the skin surface. Bullae may develop.

Laboratory

■ Patch testing to evaluate for delayed-type hypersensitivity should be considered if the distribution suggests a contact exposure, if the problem is recurrent or refractory to therapy, or if there is known occupational, hobby or other exposure to cutaneous allergens.

■ Consider mineral oil preparation to evaluate for scabies, especially in eczema of new or recent onset. Consider scraping scale for potassium hydroxide examination to evaluate for dermatophyte fungus infection. Blood tests are almost never helpful in the evaluation of acute eczema.

Course and Prognosis

■ If the provoking factors can be avoided, the eruption improves over 7–10 days, with clearing usually by 3 weeks.

■ Excoriation predisposes to infection and causes serum, crust, and purulent material to accumulate. Excoriation can result in secondary staphylococcal infection, and aggravation and prolongation of the dermatitis.

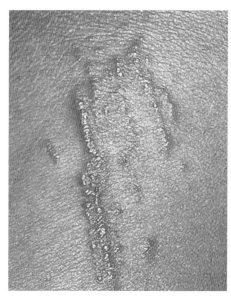

Acute eczema. Vesicles are present in a linear distribution, suggesting contact dermatitis.

Management

- Cool wet dressings and topical steroid creams allow vasoconstriction and suppress inflammation and itching. A clean cloth is soaked in cool water or Burrow's solution and then placed on affected areas for 30 minutes. Then an appropriate topical steroid cream (group II or III) is applied and rubbed in well.
- Oral corticosteroids are reserved for severe or generalized acute eczema. The dosage is approximately 1 mg/kg/day initially, tapering over 3 weeks. Too short a course may result in recurrence and rebound of the dermatitis.
- Oral antihistamines such as diphenhydramine (Benadryl) and hydroxyzine (Atarax) can relieve itching, and their sedative effect may promote better sleep.
- If secondary infection is suspected, an anti-*Staphylococcus aureus* antibiotic (e.g. cephalexin, dicloxacillin) is administered for 10–14 days.

Pearls

- Acute eczema may be confused with acute infections such as cellulitis; the often marked itching associated with acute eczema should help distinguish them.
- Repeated bouts of acute eczema on the face, exposed hands or arms suggests a contact allergic problem, which should be evaluated by patch testing.
- Remove all the patient's topicals (lotions, topical over-the-counter medicaments, anti-itch preparations) and treat with topical steroids only, or with bland emollients—keep the skin care and exposures minimal and simple.
- Elevation of the legs, if they are affected, is helpful in decreasing dependent edema and dermatitis.

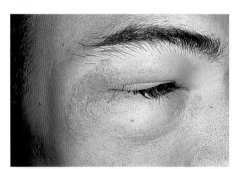

Acute inflammation causes swelling, oozing, and crusting.

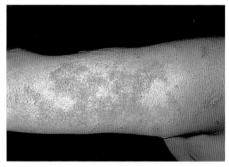

Vesicles are characteristic of the acute phase of eczematous inflammation. Itching is often intense.

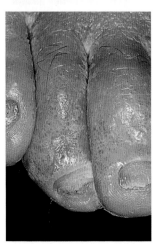

Acute eczematous inflammation. Vesicles and intense itching are the hallmark of acute eczema. This patient was allergic to chemicals in shoes.

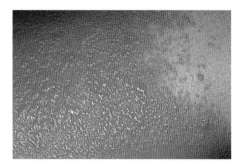

Acute eczema. Poison ivy may cause intense acute eczematous inflammation. Vesicles and blisters form on a red base. The blisters may coalesce and become very large. The itching is unbearable and is best controlled with cold wet dressings.

Rhus Dermatitis (Poison Ivy, Poison Oak, Poison Sumac)

Description

- Poison ivy, oak, and sumac (plants of the Anacardiacea family) and *Toxicodendron* genus are the most common causes of allergic contact dermatitis in the United States; this problematic prototype of contact dermatitis is rarely reported in Europe, though related plants grow in Southeast Asia, Central America and South America.
- Oleoresin (lipid-soluble portion) contains a mixture of highly allergenic catechol chemicals called "urushiols". Urushiol is derived from the Japanese word for sap, *urushi*.

History

- Contact with the plant's leaf, stem, or root, even in autumn and winter, results in a pruritic bullous eruption within 8-72 hours of exposure in a previously sensitized individual and 12-21 days for an individual who has not yet been sensitized (primary sensitization).
- Primary sensitization can result from exposure to the allergenic plant. This process requires an intact immune system. After an individual has become allergic (sensitized), repeat exposure will cause the rash to occur more promptly (a process called elicitation).
- About half of American adults develop the rash if they are exposed; 30-40% require prolonged exposure to produce the dermatitis.
- About 10-15% of Americans will not become sensitized.

Skin Findings

- Clinical findings vary with the quantity of oleoresin that contacts the skin, with the pattern of contact, individual susceptibility and regional variations in skin reactivity.
- Findings include pruritic, edematous, linear erythematous streaks, usually with vesicles and large bullae on exposed skin.
- Airborne particulate matter from burning the plant can result in intense, pruritic facial erythema and marked edema; the eyelids can be dramatically swollen.
- Trauma to the skin from the plant may leave a temporary black mark on the skin—a clue to exposure and a result of dried and oxidized urushiol allergen.

Course and Prognosis

- The itchy eruption lasts for 10 days to as long as 3 weeks.
- Short courses of oral corticosteroids (such as dose packs) are inadequate and may result in a rebound phenomenon with prompt blistering when discontinued.
- The rash resolves completely without scarring.
- Impetigo or cellulitis may occur from scratching and secondary bacterial infection (usually *Staphylococcus aureus*).
- Short-term disability and time lost from work are significant occupational problems associated with this contact dermatitis, especially among firefighters, foresters, landscapers, and woodsmen.

Discussion

- Poison ivy is not spread by blister fluid, and is not spread from person to person.
- The allergenic oleoresin can be spread by contaminated clothing, garden tools, or animals.
- Cross-reacting allergens from other plants of the Anacardiacea family include mango peel, the oil of raw cashew nut shells, Japanese lacquer, and ginkgo fruit pulp. Individuals sensitized to poison ivy may also react after exposure to these related plants.
- Poison ivy grows as a shrub or climbing vine. In the USA, Eastern poison oak is typically found in the southeast, while Western poison oak grows typically on the west coast, in the form of a small shrub or tree. Poison sumac prefers a moist location, and is common in peat bogs and wetlands of the eastern US and south-eastern Canada.

Management

- The skin should be washed with soap to inactivate and remove allergic oleoresin, thereby preventing further skin penetration and contamination. Washing is most effective if done within 15 minutes of exposure.
- Exposed clothing and tools should be cleansed with soapy water.
- Short, cool tub baths, with or without colloidal oatmeal (Aveeno), are soothing for itching and swelling.
- Calamine lotion controls itching, but prolonged use can lead to excessive drying.
- Oral antihistamines hydroxyzine and diphenhydramine may control itching. They are sedating and may be best used at night to reduce night-time scratching, to promote rest, and offer relief from the stress of intense itch which often interferes with sleep.
- Cool wet dressings made with tap water or Burrow's solution are highly effective during the acute blistering stage. They are applied for 15–30 minutes several times a day for 1–4 days until blistering and severe itching are controlled. Tap-water cool wet dressings are very useful for severe facial or eyelid edema.
- A medium-potency topical steroid (group II–V) should be generously applied after the wet dressing. If the peri-orbital skin is involved, a weaker topical steroid (group VI–VII) is advised for a specified limited duration (twice daily for 7 days).
- The newer immunomodulatory topical therapies, pimecrolimus and tacrolimus (Elidel and Protopic) are not advised for acute allergic contact dermatitis to poison ivy, given their cost, the amount often required, and delay of efficacy compared to topical steroids.
- A course of oral corticosteroids for severe, widespread inflammation is started at 0.75–1 mg/kg/day every morning and is slowly tapered over 3 weeks.

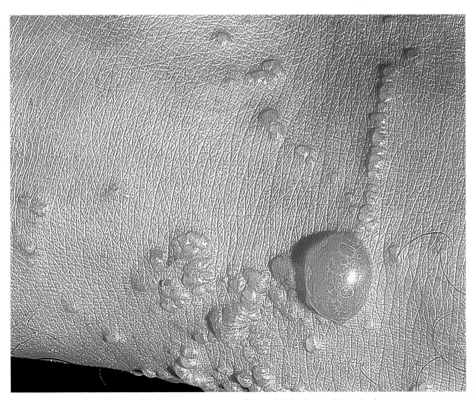

Classic presentation of poison ivy. Vesicles appear in a linear distribution and vary in size.

- A barrier cream, Ivy Block, contains quaternium bentonite that can be successful in preventing the dermatitis, or reducing the severity of reactions. However, it is essential that it be applied prior to anticipated exposure.
- Poison ivy oleoresin in capsules and an injectable form for hyposensitization have been removed from the market as a result of side effects and incomplete efficacy. There are no means available currently for desensitization to poison ivy.

Pearls

- The classic presentation of poisonous plant contact dermatitis is varying sized vesicles and bullae appearing in a linear distribution on exposed skin.
- Generally repeated exposure over short periods of time (i.e. the summer months) results in increasingly severe bouts of the dermatitis.

- Oral ingestion of raw or incompletely roasted cashews can cause an "internal–external" reaction—a sudden erythematous pruritic dermatitis in a characteristic distribution on the buttocks, upper inner thighs and periaxillary skin in individuals sensitized to urushiol.
- Poison ivy, oak or sumac can involve wide areas. The decision to use oral or topical steroids depends on the severity of the symptoms, the age of the patient, and potential for short-term adverse reactions anticipated through review of the medical history.
- Short courses of low-dose systemic corticosteroids are inadequate treatment for severe, generalized cases of poison ivy.

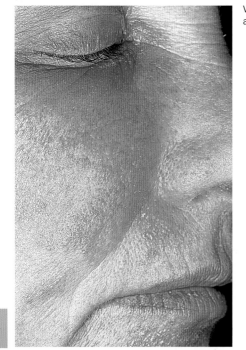

Vesicles disappear, and erythema and scaling appear as the acute phase ends. Itching is less intense.

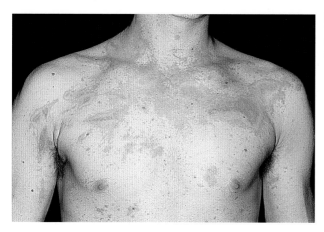

Poison ivy can involve wide areas. The decision to use oral or topical steroids depends on the severity of the symptoms.

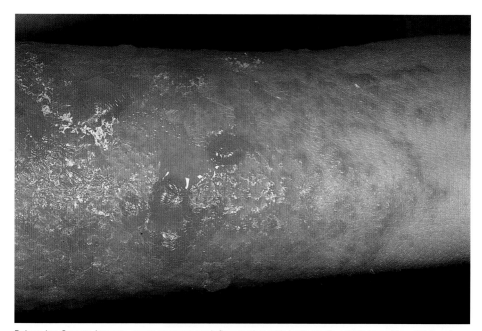

Poison ivy. Severe, intense, acute eczematous inflammation with large confluent blisters. Many blisters have ruptured. The serum that leaks onto the skin does not spread poison ivy. Cool wet compresses applied for 30 minutes several times a day would help control the inflammation.

Subacute Eczematous Inflammation (Subacute Eczema)

Description

■ This eczematous inflammation consists of itchy, red, and scaling patches, papules and plaques in various configurations.

History

■ This condition may evolve from acute (vesicular) eczema.

■ This is the most common clinical manifestation of atopic dermatitis.

■ Patients complain of dermatitis that has been present over 1 week.

■ Itching is variable; it can be moderate to severe, or rather mild.

■ The condition resolves without scarring when provoking or contributing aggravating factors are removed. It may require treatment to resolve.

■ Excoriation and repeated exposure to aggravating conditions (water, detergents, irritants, or other common irritant or allergic offenders) convert this condition to a chronic process.

Skin Findings

■ Erythema and scaling occur in various patterns.

■ Often there are indistinct borders.

■ Redness may be faint or intense.

Etiology and Clinical Presentation

■ Contact allergy, contact irritation, atopic dermatitis, stasis dermatitis, nummular eczema, fingertip eczema, and fungal infections are dermatoses that may present as subacute eczema.

■ If there is not a strong atopic history, search for new cutaneous irritant or allergen exposures. Stress can aggravate and contribute to this problem but is not a common sole cause.

Treatment

Steroids and Other Non-steroid Topical Prescription Therapies

■ Group II–V steroid creams twice a day with or without plastic occlusion are administered. Occlusion hastens resolution while increasing absorption of topical steroid. Duration of occlusion should be specified, limited and supervised.

■ Steroid ointments can be applied twice a day without occlusion.

■ Non-steroid topical immune modulators tacrolimus (Protopic ointment 0.1, 0.03%) and pimecrolimus (Elidel cream 1%) can be applied twice daily to affected skin and are especially useful in subacute eczema of the face or peri-orbital eyelid skin. They may initially cause some stinging or burning of the skin which subsides in a few days. These therapies are useful for chronic

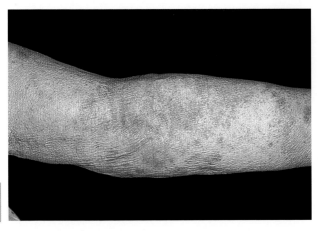

Erythema and scaling with indistinct borders are characteristic. Vesicles may never appear. This is often the initial presentation in the winter in atopic patients.

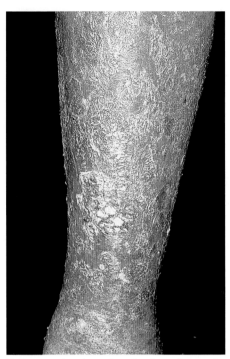

Erythema and scale can be extensive and suggest a diagnosis of psoriasis. Psoriatic plaques often have distinct borders.

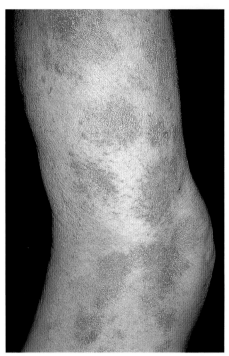

The configuration of subacute inflammation varies. Plaques may be patchy or confluent, round or diffuse.

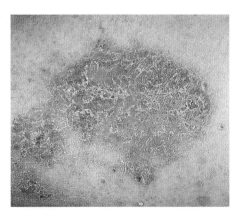

This plaque is dense and covered with scale. The borders are somewhat distinct. Differentiation from psoriasis in this case would be difficult. The history and types of plaques in other areas may be needed to confirm a diagnosis.

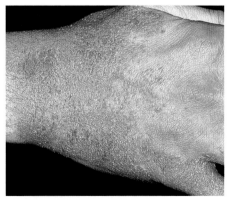

Atopic dermatitis. The back of the hands is a common site to find subacute irritant dermatitis.

management of subacute eczema in atopic patients.

■ Tar ointments and creams (many over-the-counter preparations) provide an alternative for steroid-resistant lesions and are moderately effective in some patients.

■ Wet dressings should be avoided because they cause excessive dryness.

Moisturizers

■ Moisturizers are an essential part of daily therapy.

■ Moisturizers work best when applied a few hours after topical steroids.

■ Application should continue for days or weeks after the inflammation has cleared.

■ Frequent application is encouraged.

■ Moisturizers are most effective when rubbed in well and applied directly after the skin is patted dry following a shower.

■ Creams with simple formulations lacking the most common allergy-associated ingredients (e.g. Aveeno, Cetaphil, DML, Acid Mantle) are better than lotions. Plain petroleum jelly is an excellent moisturizer and has the advantage of being plain, without allergenic additives or irritating ingredients. Greasiness limits patient acceptability.

■ Infrequent washing with bar-type mild soap (e.g. Dove, Cetaphil, Keri, Purpose, Basis) is also helpful.

Antibiotics

■ Antibiotics (e.g. cephalexin, dicloxacillin) are used for secondary bacterial infections (usually *Staphylococcus aureus*).

Pearls

■ Subacute eczema is a clinical manifestation of ongoing inflammation. Attention to cutaneous exposures of irritants, allergens, and the patient's overall skin care regimen is vital to addressing cause and aggravating factors.

■ Consider a potassium hydroxide exam of scale to rule out dermatophyte infection.

■ Ask about the patient's occupation, house duties and hobbies as they may contribute to ongoing skin irritation or allergy. Gloves serve as a useful protective barrier if repeated exposure to water, irritants, or allergens is occurring. Vinyl gloves are a good choice because they do not contain common rubber-related allergens (gloves can be ordered online from http://www.allerderm.com).

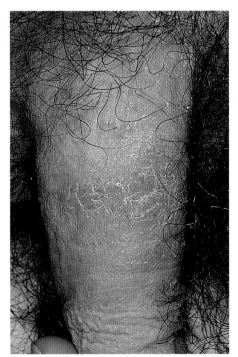

Subacute eczematous inflammation is characterized by erythema and scaling. There are no blisters. An allergic reaction to neomycin ointment produced this eruption.

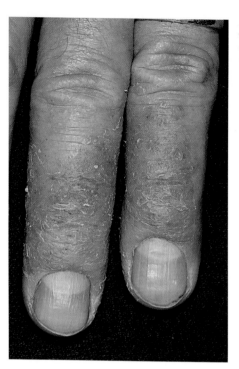

Subacute eczema of the fingers is common in people who have repeated exposure to moisture. New mothers who wash and clean are at a high risk for irritant eczema.

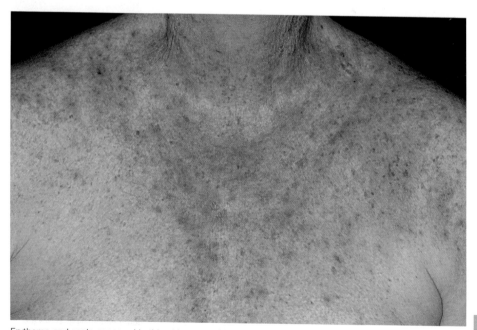

Erythema and scale appeared in this older man with dry skin. Scratching made the eruption worse. This pattern is commonly seen during the winter.

Chronic Eczematous Inflammation

Description
■ Affected skin is inflamed, red, scaling, and thickened (lichenified).

History
■ There is moderate to intense, prolonged itching.
■ Scratching and rubbing become habitual and may be done subconsciously.
■ The disease becomes self-perpetuating.
■ Scratching leads to thick skin, which itches even more.

Skin Findings
■ Intense itching can lead to excoriations.
■ Inflamed, itchy skin thickens, and surface skin markings become more prominent.
■ Thick plaques with deep parallel skin markings appear (lichenification).
■ Sites commonly involved are those easily reached or creased areas.
■ Common locations are the back of the neck, popliteal fossae, ankles, eyelids, and anogenital skin.
■ Hyperpigmentation or hypopigmentation can occur on affected skin.

Etiology and Clinical Presentation
■ Atopic dermatitis, chronic allergic or irritant contact dermatitis, habitual scratching, lichen simplex chronicus, chapped and fissured feet, nummular eczema, asteatotic eczema, fingertip eczema, hyperkeratotic eczema are possible etiologies.
■ The evolution of this process is the result of a chronic process.

Treatment
■ Chronic eczematous inflammation is often resistant to treatment; the key to success is breaking the itch–scratch cycle through treatment and removal of the cause or sources of aggravation.
■ A cool wet dressing on the affected skin for 20 minutes will help soothe and diminish itch; it can be very helpful for the night-time itch urge.

Topical Steroids
■ Group I or II creams or ointments applied twice a day can be effective.

■ Group II–V steroids are used with plastic occlusion for 2–8 hours.
■ Intralesional injections (e.g. Kenalog 10 mg/ml) are very effective; resistant plaques are reinjected at 3–4 week intervals.
■ Steroid-impregnated tape (e.g. Cordran tape) should be left on for 12 hours.

Pearls
■ Chronic rubbing or scratching is at least part of the problem—address it and aim to diminish it.
■ Ointments penetrate lichenified skin well and are generally more effective than creams on lichenified skin.
■ Consider and evaluate for contact irritants and allergens. Simplify the skin regimen: i.e. mild soaps, bland emollients (petrolatum, Aquaphor, Aveeno) only.
■ Protopic ointment (tacrolimus) can be helpful for involved lichenified chronic eczema on the face.

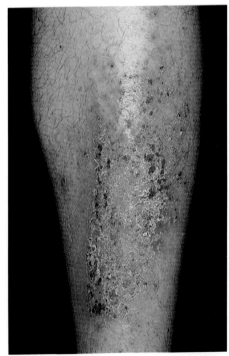

Weeks of scratching and rubbing with the heel has caused skin thickening. The chronically inflamed and excoriated skin has become infected. Crust and purulent material cleared after a course of Cephadroxil 500 mg twice daily for 5 days.

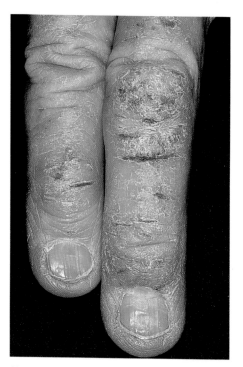

Chronic eczematous inflammation. The skin is dry, cracked, and scaling. Excoriation has caused skin thickening.

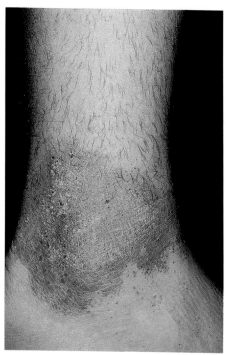

The isolated plaque is thick with accentuation of skin lines. Scratching for weeks produces this picture.

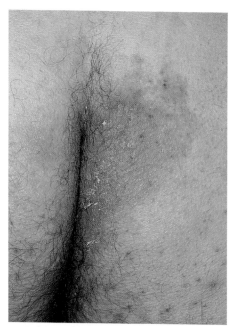

Itching about the anal area is common. Long-term scratching caused thickening of the skin and accentuation of the skin lines.

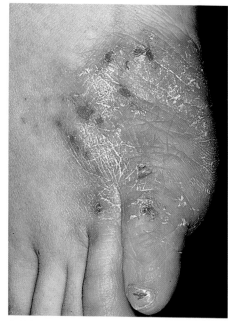

Rubbing and scratching has thickened the skin. This exacerbates and perpetuates the chronic inflammation.

Lichen Simplex Chronicus

Description
- A localized plaque of chronic eczematous inflammation is created by habitual rubbing and scratching.
- The affected skin is frequently located on the wrists, ankles, anogenital skin, and back of the neck.

History
- This condition is more common in adults but may be seen in atopic children.

Skin Findings
- Findings include a sharply demarcated, deeply violaceous colored or red scaly plaque with prominent skin lines (lichenification).
- Although this is a chronic eczematous disease, acute changes of vesiculation and weeping may result from sudden allergy to topical treatments.
- Moist scaling, serum, crust, and pustules signal secondary infection.
- Nodules, usually smaller than 1 cm and scattered randomly in the scalp, occur in patients who frequently pick at the scalp.
- The areas most commonly affected are conveniently reached; these areas include the outer portion of the lower legs, wrists and ankles, posterior neck, scalp, upper eyelids, the fold behind the ear, scrotum, vulva, and anal skin.

Laboratory
- A potassium hydroxide scraping should be considered to look for tinea. Tinea infection can mimic lichen simplex chronicus.
- A contact allergy may cause, lead to or complicate lichen simplex chronicus. Patch testing to identify the role of allergens can be helpful.

Course and Prognosis
- A typical plaque stays localized and shows little tendency to enlarge with time. Once established, the plaque does not usually increase in size.

Treatment
- Stress may play a role in some individuals and should be acknowledged and addressed.
- The patient should understand that the rash does not resolve until even minor scratching and rubbing are stopped.
- Scratching frequently takes place during sleep, and the affected area may have to be covered.
- Treatment consists of a 5-minute water soak followed by the application of a topical steroid with medium-to-high potency in an ointment base.
- The treatment of the anal area, genitalia, or fold behind the ear does not require the administration of potent topical steroids; rather, these areas should be treated with low potency topical steroids in an ointment base.
- For scalp lesions, a group I or group II steroid gel such as fluocinonide (Lidex) or a solution such as clobetasol (Cormax scalp solution) is applied twice each day.
- Moist, secondarily infected areas respond to oral antibiotics and a topical steroid lotion.
- Grenz ray (superficial x-ray therapy) can be helpful, but has limited availability.
- Nodules caused by picking at the scalp may be very resistant to treatment, requiring monthly intralesional injections with triamcinolone acetonide (Kenalog 5-10 mg/ml).

Discussion
- This condition was once referred to as "localized neurodermatitis".
- The patient derives great pleasure from scratching to relieve the inflamed site.

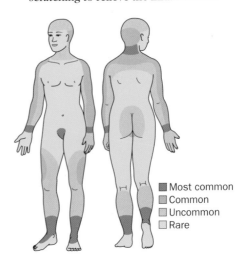

Most common
Common
Uncommon
Rare

Loss of pleasurable sensation or continued subconscious habitual scratching may explain why this eruption frequently recurs.

- Lichen simplex chronicus affecting the genitalia or anus can be a very chronic, difficult problem causing considerable distress and frustration.

Pearls

- The occipital scalp is possibly the most common target for anxiety-induced scratching. Very thick plaques may form that are difficult to manage, and sometimes they become infected.
- Though stress does not cause this condition, it most definitely contributes

to aggravating and perpetuating it. Ask about stress, address the role it can play, and seek avenues for stress reduction.

- Night-time itching can be diminished with this routine: oral antihistamines such as diphenhydramine (Benadryl) or hydroxyzine (Atarax), followed by a 20-minute cold tap-water wet dressing, followed by application of a topical steroid to the affected skin.
- Consider patch testing for lichen simplex chronicus affecting the periorbital skin, the dorsal hands or feet, or the anogenital skin.
- Compliance is important to resolution of this problem. Take time and be specific in the explanation of your goals and treatment.

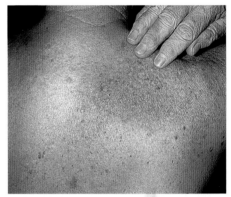

The upper back is another target for repetitive scratching and excoriation. Linear white scars that are evidence of a habit that has existed for months or years should be sought.

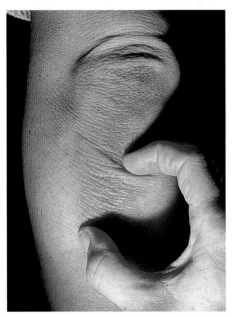

The classic presentation. Skin lines are markedly accentuated. Itching becomes more intense as the plaque thickens and a vicious cycle continues.

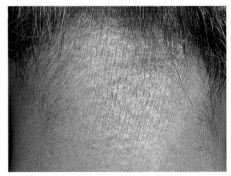

The occipital lower scalp is possibly the most common target for anxiety-induced scratching. Very thick, difficult-to-manage plaques may form and sometimes become infected. Psoriasis can present with similar features. Short courses of oral antibiotics are sometimes the appropriate initial treatment before potent topical steroids are started.

Hand Eczema

Description

■ Hand eczema is a common, often chronic problem with multiple causative and contributing factors.

■ Hand eczema can be categorized as follows: irritant; keratolysis exfoliativa; atopic; fingertip; allergic; hyperkeratotic; nummular; pompholyx (dyshidrosis); lichen simplex chronicus, and "id reaction". Each of these types of hand eczema is covered separately elsewhere in this book.

■ Irritant hand eczema is most common, followed by atopic hand eczema.

■ Allergic contact dermatitis accounts for perhaps 10–25% of hand eczema.

History

■ Women are affected more often than men.

■ Occupational risks include irritant chemical exposure, frequent wet work, chronic friction, and work with sensitizing (allergenic) chemicals.

Exogenous Factors

■ Irritants include chemical irritants (such as solvents, detergents, alkalis and acids), friction, cold air, and low humidity.

■ Allergens include occupational and non-occupational sources of allergen exposure. Immediate type I allergy can involve reactions to latex and food proteins, and the more common delayed-type IV allergy can involve reactions to rubber additives, nickel, medicaments (bacitracin, neomycin and hydrocortisone) and commonly found chemical ingredients in personal care products (such as preservatives, fragrance, sunscreen, and other additives). Ingested allergens (e.g. nickel) may play a role.

■ Infection can involve "id reactions", including hand eczema as a reaction to a distant focus of fungal ("dermatophytid") or bacterial ("bacterid") infection.

Endogenous Factors

■ Atopic diathesis (hay fever, asthma, atopic eczema) is often a predisposing factor, and may contribute to susceptibility for the disease, and chronicity of the problem, despite appropriate treatment and care measures.

Skin Findings

■ The entire skin should be examined for clues and contributing factors and for exclusion of other dermatoses (i.e. psoriasis).

■ This condition is variable; acute, subacute, and chronic eczematous changes may be seen. Although there is no reliable association between clinical pattern and etiology, the following findings may prove useful:

● Xerosis, erythema, burning more than itching on dorsal or volar hands: irritant factors should be suspected.

● Nummular eczema, dorsal hands and fingers: allergy, irritation, or atopy can play a role: occasionally, contact urticaria (type I allergy) is the culprit.

● Recurrent crops of intensely pruritic vesicles on lateral fingers and palms: pompholyx, otherwise called dyshidrotic eczema, should be suspected.

● Fingertip eczema (dryness, splitting, tenderness, no itch): an irritant, an endogenous factor (atopy during the winter), or frictional eczema should be suspected.

● Erythema, scaling, itching, in "apron" (base of the fingers) area of palm: atopy should be suspected.

Non-skin Findings

■ Atopic patients may have a personal or family history of atopy, including eczema in childhood, hay fever, or asthma.

Course and Prognosis

■ If exposures to irritants and allergens can be identified and avoided early in the course, the prognosis is often good for complete recovery.

■ Continued or longstanding exposure to irritants and allergens can result in chronic dermatitis.

■ Avoidance and appropriate care often improve the condition, but

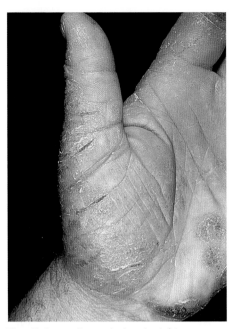

The skin is very dry, cracked, and painful. Longstanding hand eczema may be a continuous cycle of acute (vesicle), subacute (redness and scaling), and chronic (very dry, cracked) inflammation.

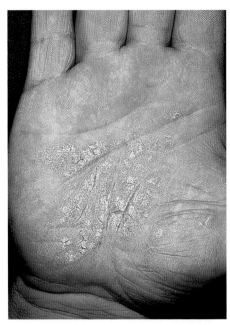

Dry, thick, fissured hyperkeratotic eczematous plaques are difficult to treat. They last for months or years and may be impossible to distinguish from psoriasis.

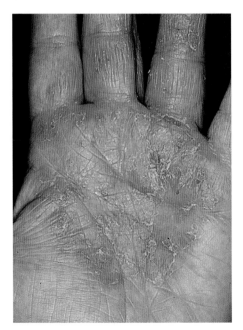

Irritant hand eczema occurred in this woman who cleaned without glove protection. Scratching prolongs the disease.

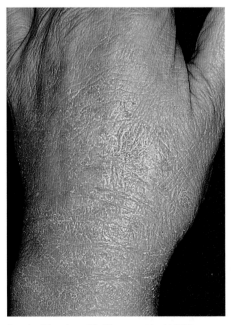

Constant hand washing has perpetuated this chronic eczematous dermatitis on the back of the hands. The eruption cleared rapidly when a group IV topical steroid and plastic occlusion was applied at bedtime for 7 days.

some patients may not resolve it entirely.

Treatment

- Treatment involves the identification and avoidance of irritants such as frequent hand washing and water exposure, soaps, detergents, and solvents. Chronic frictional trauma is also an irritant that can result in persistent dermatitis.
- Protective measures (e.g. vinyl gloves for wet or chemical work) can be taken.
- Topical corticosteroids with medium-to-high potency (groups II–IV) are administered twice daily. Ointments are preferred to creams. Occlusion with plastic to increase penetration should be considered. It is preferable to refrain from superpotent (group I) agents unless the dermatitis is severe. Topical steroids for hand dermatitis are most effective when used intermittently, rather than chronic management.
- For severe dermatitis, a superpotent topical corticosteroid is applied after wet dressings containing Burrow's solution, twice a day for the initial 3–5 days of treatment, followed by the application of a medium-potency topical corticosteroid twice a day for several weeks.
- The following should be considered: topical tar hand soaks with Balnetar oil, two or three capfuls diluted in a basin of water for 15–30 minutes twice a day, followed by the application of topical corticosteroid.
- Systemic steroids (prednisone 0.75–1 mg/kg/day with tapering over a 3 week course) may occasionally be required to bring a severe acute inflammation under control.
- Most patients improve with avoidance of irritants, treatment with topical corticosteroids, and frequent lubrication.
- If allergy is suspected (hand edema, vesiculation, itching, and particularly dorsal hand or fingertip eczema) patch testing should be done to evaluate for contributing or causal allergens. Relevant occupational allergens should be included in the tested materials.
- The patient should be referred to a dermatologist in chronic unresponsive cases. Other treatments that may be considered include topical psoralen ultraviolet A treatment, and Grenz ray therapy. In disabling cases, management with weekly low-dose methotrexate (5–15 mg weekly), or oral low-dose daily cyclosporin is reasonable.

Discussion

- Chronic, cyclic vesicular hand dermatitis (pompholyx) represents a most difficult management problem.
- Patch testing to occupational and environmental allergens should be considered if hand eczema does not improve or resolve with simple measures.

Pearls

- Referral to a dermatologist for evaluation and patch testing is warranted when hand eczema does not resolve after a trial of sensitive skin care, including daily emollient use, protective use of gloves for frequent wet or chemical work, and a few weeks' course of topical steroid treatment.
- Psoriasis on the palms can mimic eczema. If there is sharp demarcation of plaques on the palms, with silvery or yellowish chronic scaling and symmetrical involvement, a diagnosis of palmar psoriasis should be considered.
- Causal or contributing factors to hand eczema are not well identified unless the clinician seeks to know how and what the hands are exposed to: the occupation, household duties, hobbies, and hand care should be explored in detail. Though new routines or exposures can lead to a new case of hand eczema, chronic exposures may also be ones that lead to allergy.

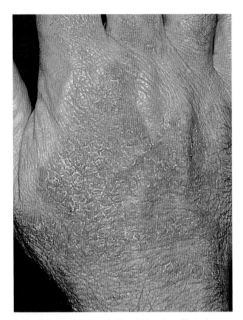

Scratching has caused skin thickening. Chronic plaques of eczema may look like psoriasis. Plaques of psoriasis tend to have well defined borders. The borders in this eczematous plaque are ill defined and indistinct.

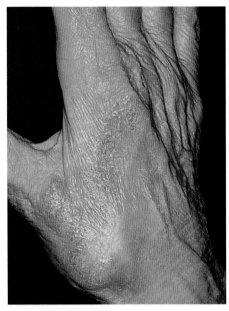

Irritant contact dermatitis was caused by exposure to cleaning solutions. The rash persisted with scratching. The potassium hydroxide preparation was negative for fungi. Psoriasis may have a similar appearance, and even a biopsy may not be able to differentiate the two diseases.

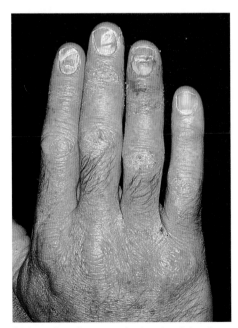

Adult atopic patients may develop chronic hand eczema, especially on the back of the hands. The chronic inflammation has caused the nails to be distorted. Tinea of the back of the hand would have a more sharply defined border.

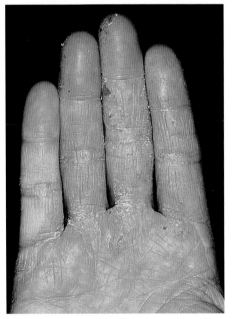

Irritant hand dermatitis on the palmar surface of the fingers is difficult to treat and tends to be chronic. Intermittent topical steroids, constant moisturizing, and protection with gloves are the mainstays of treatment.

Asteatotic Eczema

Description

- A distinctive clinical pattern of eczematous dermatitis that is caused by excessive dryness and chapping of the skin. This is also referred to as eczema craquele.

History

- Asteatotic eczema is a form of subacute eczematous dermatitis that tends to be chronic and low grade with wintertime seasonal flares, due to low humidity.
- Men and women are equally affected.
- It is more common in patients with the atopic diathesis (see section on atopic dermatitis), especially in later life.
- Most patients have a history of previous similar flares.
- The prevalence peaks in late winter and improves in summer, especially in colder, drier climates.
- Any cutaneous site may be affected, although the lower legs are most commonly involved.
- Early on, affected individuals often note that their skin looks and feels dry.
- With progression, itch, with increasing inflammation, becomes the most prominent symptom.
- Burning and stinging occur in advanced cases with fissures and crusting.

Skin Findings

- The clinical picture is that of subacute eczematous dermatitis.
- Xerosis with accentuated skin markings are constant features from the onset.
- Inflammation is at first subtle but becomes more pronounced over time.
- Faint, poorly defined erythema progresses to fiery red, acute eczematous papules that coalesce into broad plaques.
- Vesicles are not typically seen, although excoriations are nearly universal.
- Dry, thin desquamation progresses toward a pattern termed eczema craquelé, with thin superficial fissures reminiscent of the cracked finish on porcelain or of a dried river bed.
- The skin is very dry, cracked, and fissured. The skin may be painful.

- With progression, the eczema develops acute features with weeping, crusting, and intense erythema.

Non-skin Findings

- Fever is unusual and suggests cellulitis.

Laboratory

- The clinical picture is distinctive enough that skin biopsy is rarely needed to establish the diagnosis.
- Skin biopsy confirms epidermal spongiosis with dermal inflammation and often secondary impetiginization.

Course and Prognosis

- Seasonal recurrence during the winter months should be expected.
- Mild seasonal flares with itching and xerosis tends to improve with warmer weather seasonal change and repetitive skin lubrication.
- Active subacute inflammation generally responds with topical medium-potency corticosteroid ointments and also improves with the season.
- A severe localized flare with acute features such as weeping and crusting also responds to individualized topical therapy as outlined later.
- Severe flares should be treated aggressively because they may become generalized.

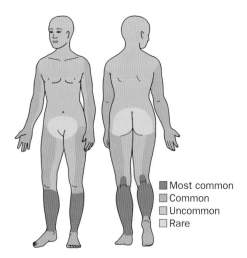

Most common
Common
Uncommon
Rare

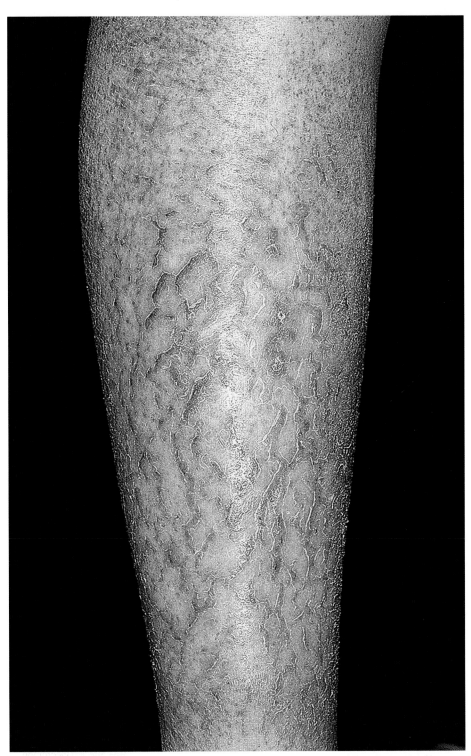

The skin is very dry, cracked, and fissured. This pattern evolved in an atopic patient who continued to wash excessively dry skin. The skin may be painful.

Discussion

- The differential diagnosis includes other subacute eczematous dermatoses such as stasis dermatitis, irritant contact dermatitis, atopic dermatitis, allergic contact dermatitis, and cellulitis.
- More than one dermatosis may be present. The second dermatosis may mask or exacerbate the primary eczematous process.
- Irritant and allergic contact dermatitis may develop as a result of the patient's own efforts at self-treatment.
- The patient should be asked about what he or she has been applying to the involved areas.
- Stasis dermatitis occurs, commonly on the lower legs, in older patients. There is usually a history of vascular insufficiency and leg edema and the presence of hemosiderin staining of the skin.

Management

- Therapy is determined by the stage (acute, subacute or chronic) of the asteatotic eczema and the degree of inflammation.
- For xerosis, therapy consists of sensitive skin measures, namely the limited use of mild soap and the liberal use of emollients.
- Petrolatum offers a preservative-free choice as a lubricant, although patient compliance may be difficult.
- Moisturizers containing lactic acid, urea, or glycolic acid may also be useful.
- Early inflammation is best treated topically with a medium-potency corticosteroid, preferably in an ointment base.
- Therapy should be continued until the erythema and scaling resolve.
- Liberal use of emollients should then be continued as a prophylaxis against recurrence. Bland, fragrance free emollients are best.
- Localized flares with acute eczematous features of weeping and crusting should be treated first as acute eczema.
- Patients require close follow-up during this stage because localized flares may become generalized.
- Referral to a dermatologist should be considered for the management of recurring acute flares and an evaluation for possible allergic contact dermatitis.
- Wet dressings with Burrow's solution along with a medium-potency topical corticosteroid in a cream base are helpful for débridement and reducing inflammation.
- Oral antibiotics may be indicated for secondary impetiginization, indicated by honey colored sticky crusts.
- Once the weeping, induration, and crusting improve, the wet dressings should be stopped to avoid excessive drying of the involved areas.
- A medium-potency topical corticosteroid ointment (group II or group IV) should be continued until the redness and scaling resolve, approximately 2–3 weeks.
- Thereafter, sensitive skin care, including emollients, are helpful in limiting recurrence.
- Systemic steroid therapy is rarely indicated for asteatotic eczema.

Pearls

- Affected skin often appears like cracked porcelain early on. This stage often responds very nicely and promptly to routine use of emollients and removal of any irritating soaps or other irritants (i.e. winter swim programs in pools treated with bromine or chlorine).
- The patient should be asked what he or she is doing to treat the dermatitis and what skin care regimen is used.
- Home remedies might include household bleach, astringents, hot water, shake lotions, and other potential irritants that may be exacerbating the condition.
- Neomycin, corticosteroids, and preservatives in various medicaments are potential sources of allergens.
- Referral to a dermatologist should be considered for patients with refractory dermatitis.

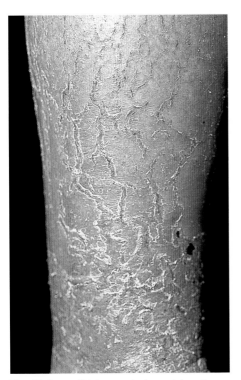

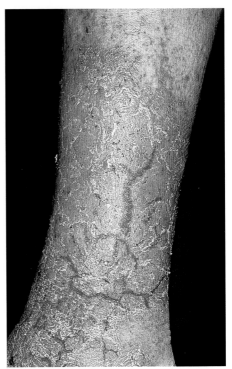

The skin has split into a cracked porcelain pattern that is the hallmark of asteatotic eczema.

Asteatotic eczema. Severe longstanding inflammation. There are large, deep fissures and secondary infection.

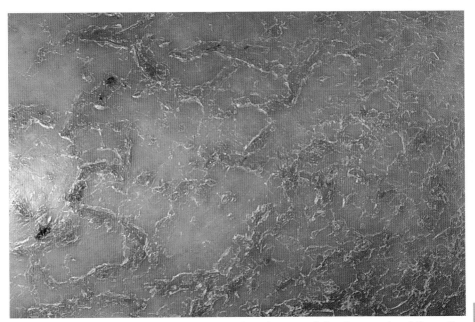

Serum oozes from the fissures and dries into linear and annular crusts. Subacute eczematous inflammation surrounds the fissures.

Chapped, Fissured Feet

Description

- Findings include scaling, erythema, and tender fissuring of the plantar feet.
- The tendency for severe chapping is age related; it is most common in prepubertal children but can occur in adults.

History

- Chapped, fissured feet are most common in early autumn, when the weather becomes cold and heavy socks and impermeable shoes or boots are worn.
- Symptoms include soreness and pain.
- The mean age of onset is 7 years; the mean age of remission is 14 years.

Skin Findings

- The skin on the plantar feet—especially the weight-bearing skin of the toes and metatarsal regions—is dry, erythematous, scaly, and fissured. Fissuring may be deep and very tender.
- Chapping may extend to the sides of the toes.
- Eventually, the entire sole may be involved.

Discussion

- Atopy is suspected in these patients, but this is not well accepted.

Differential Diagnosis

- Tinea pedis infection
- Allergic contact dermatitis
- Psoriasis

Treatment

- The feet should be kept dry; prolonged time in moist, occlusive shoes should be avoided.
- A thick emollient ointment (Aquaphor, petrolatum, Cetaphil or Aveeno cream) should be applied several times each day.
- If the condition is pruritic, topical steroids provide some relief. Group II or III topical steroid ointments are applied twice a day, preferably with plastic-wrap occlusion at bedtime, for 2-3 weeks.
- A 15-minute soak with tar oil (Balnetar) is followed by the application of a lubricating ointment or topical corticosteroid.
- Preventative measures include changing into light leather shoes after the removal of wet boots, alternating footwear to allow complete drying, and changing cotton socks frequently if moist.

Pearls

- Symmetric involvement of the soles. Inflammation may be confined to just part of the soles.
- Atopic dermatitis in children occurs mainly on the dorsal toes. Children with chapped, fissured feet complain of soreness and pain.
- Cracks and fissures appear in cases of long duration. Pain becomes more intense than itching.
- The key to improvement lies in frequent heavy moisturization of the skin, and prompt removal of moist footwear.

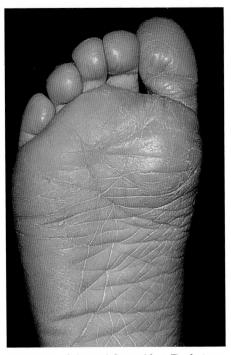

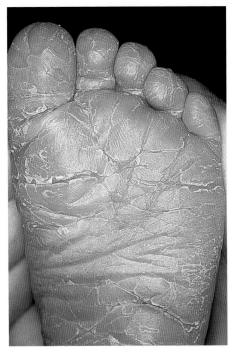

Early stages of chapped, fissured feet. The feet are dry, smooth, and red.

Cracks and fissures appear in cases of long duration. Pain becomes more intense than itching.

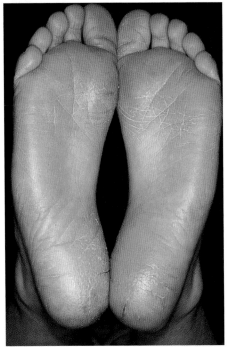

Chapped, fissured feet begin with erythema and scale on the toes and heels. Later the entire sole becomes dry and the heels and toes crack.

Allergic Contact Dermatitis

Description

■ Allergic contact dermatitis is a delayed-type hypersensitivity reaction caused by skin contact with an allergen. Allergic contact dermatitis is eczematous dermatitis.

■ Sensitization is required and allergy is specific to a particular chemical; allergens typically have low molecular weights, are lipid soluble, and are reactive chemicals.

■ Poison ivy, poison oak and poison sumac dermatitis are prototypes of allergic contact dermatitis.

■ Common causes of allergic contact dermatitis include metals such as nickel and chromate; rubber additives in gloves and shoes (carbamates, thiurams, mercaptobenzathiazole); preservatives or other additives in products such as skin lotions, sunscreens and other cosmetics and toiletries (quaternium-15, imidazolidinyl urea, diazolidinyl urea, methylchloroisothiazolinone); fragrances and fragrance additives; dyes; formaldehyde and related chemicals; nail polish additives; and topical medicaments (e.g. bacitracin, neomycin, hydrocortisone).

History

■ Initial exposure and primary sensitization result in clinical inflammation generally 14–21 days after exposure. Exposure to a chemical is required for allergy to develop.

■ The time required for a previously sensitized person to develop clinically apparent inflammation is about 12–48 hours but may vary from 8 hours to 120 hours—the rash is delayed somewhat from the contact. The rash can last as long as 3 weeks after one exposure.

■ Allergy to products (e.g. cosmetics, topical treatments, occupation-related allergens) or other exposures can occur even when there is a history of prolonged use without difficulty. The rash is recurrent if the exposure is recurrent; since many products have the same or chemically related ingredients, changing topical products often does not result in resolution of the eczematous rash.

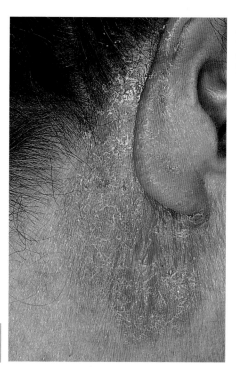

Neosporin was used to treat seborrheic dermatitis of the posterior ear. Allergy to neomycin is common. Patients think skin infection is common, and use topical antibiotics as first-line treatment for many inflammatory skin diseases.

- Some patients develop multiple contact allergies.
- Careful history should include date of dermatitis onset, possible relationship to work (i.e. whether the condition improves during the weekend or prolonged vacations), type and specifics of contact to work exposures, hobby and home exposures, and type of skin care products used.
- Some allergy-causing substances are photoallergens; sunlight together with the chemical are required for the allergic reaction to occur.
- Individuals sensitized to topical medications or other allergens may develop generalized eczematous inflammation if those medications or chemically related substances are ingested (internal–external reaction). For example, a patient may be sensitized to topical diphenhydramine in a cream, and then react with a generalized rash to oral diphenhydramine.

Skin Findings

- The intensity of the eczema depends on the individual's degree of sensitivity, concentration of the allergen, and quantity of antigen exposure.
- Allergic contact dermatitis is characterized by vesicles, edema, redness and, often, extreme pruritus. Strong allergens such as poison ivy result in bullae.
- Dermatitis distribution is usually first confined to the area of direct exposure. If exposure is chronic, allergic dermatitis may spread beyond the areas of direct contact.
- Itch and swelling are key components of the history and can be a tip-off to allergy. Burning is more often typical of irritant dermatitis.
- Dermatitis caused by plants is often distributed in linear streaks.
- Allergy to a topical product used on the face may manifest as a pruritic patchy erythema, asymmetrically distributed. Involvement of the face rarely manifests with vesicles.
- Strong sensitizers such as poison ivy may produce intense inflammation despite low concentration or exposure; weak sensitizers may cause only pruritic erythema.
- The hands, forearms, and face are the most common sites of allergic contact dermatitis. Allergic contact dermatitis may affect very limited skin sites such as the eyelids, dorsal hands, and lips, the tops of the feet, or genitalia.
- Airborne particulate matter (e.g. burning poison ivy) can lead to dermatitis of the face (including the eyelids and postauricular skin), the neck, and other exposed skin surfaces.
- Photoallergic contact dermatitis typically affects the exposed skin of the face, neck, forearms, and dorsal hands; there is usually submental, upper eyelid, and postauricular sparing.

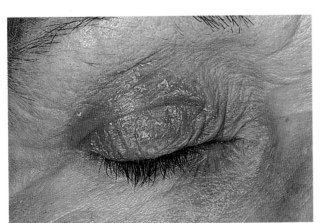

Subacute inflammation of the upper lid was caused by make-up and perpetuated by rubbing. Atopic dermatitis produces a similar picture.

- Most occupational allergic contact dermatitis affects the hands; the face and eyelids may be affected if there is an airborne allergen, or indirect hand-to-face transfer of the allergen.

Laboratory

- Patch testing is performed by physicians trained in the technique and is indicated for people with persistent or recurrent dermatitis despite appropriate topical therapy.
- Patch testing should be performed to a broad panel of screening allergens, items of occupational or avocational relevance, and personal care products. Some important allergens may be missed by patch testing with a small panel of allergens or not testing occupationally relevant allergens.
- The availability of much needed and useful diagnostic patch test allergens is presently limited in the United States.
- Proper patch testing technique requires three visits; one to apply allergen chemicals in proper concentration; another to remove the tests, read and grade the results; and the last for a final, delayed reading. Omitting the delayed reading will result in missed identification of allergens.
- Photopatch testing should also be performed in patients with photodistributed dermatitis.

Differential Diagnosis

- Irritant contact dermatitis (patch testing is not performed for irritant-type dermatitis; the clinical findings can be indistinguishable clinically, especially on affected hands)
- Atopic dermatitis (distribution can be helpful; atopic patients can and do develop contact allergies)
- Cellulitis (swelling and erythema can be similar, but cellulitis usually is painful, without itch)
- Connective tissue disease (persistent eyelid erythema; clues are no itch of affected skin, and possible cuticle hypertrophy in dermatomyositis)
- Rosacea (distribution of erythema, flushing, and burning are helpful)

Treatment

- Avoidance of the allergenic substance is essential to recovery.
- Identification of the allergen(s) is essential. If the cause is not obvious—which typically it is not—treatment should be started, and further evaluation and patch testing should be planned. Physicians and patients are poor predictors of a patient's specific allergies.
- Begin topical treatment by simplifying what is applied to the skin, and using a topical corticosteroid. Discontinue all moisturizers, lotions and topicals, except plain petrolatum, if needed, for dryness. To treat the dermatitis, advise a topical corticosteroid ointment twice a day for 2-3 weeks.
- Choice of corticosteroid potency is based on the body site affected: low potency for the face; medium potency for the arms, legs, and trunk; and high potency for the hands and feet.
- When possible, corticosteroid ointment, rather than cream, should be prescribed because additives in creams may be allergenic.
- The patient's skin regimen should be simplified to avoid further possible allergen exposure. No other topical products (except plain petrolatum or the prescribed corticosteroid) should be used during treatment. Hydrocortisone is best avoided since cases of contact allergy can occur, and other alternatives (desonide) are available.
- For severe or generalized allergic contact dermatitis, a 3-week tapering course of oral corticosteroids is appropriate. This should not be relied on repeatedly.
- Some allergens (such as hair-dye chemicals and glues) can penetrate rubber gloves, so glove protection may not be adequate.
- Some allergens, such as nickel and chromate, are associated with chronic dermatitis, despite avoidance.
- Time should be spent on patient education, detailing potential sources of exposure.
- Once an allergen is determined by diagnostic patch testing, reviewing

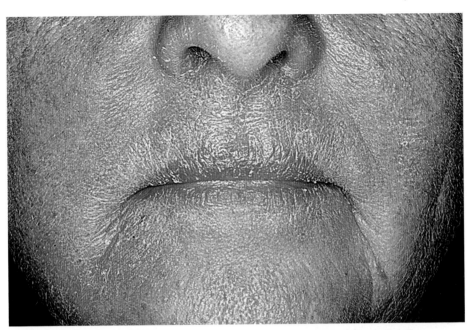

Contact dermatitis to a preservative in a lip balm caused subacute eczematous inflammation. The inflammation intensified when the balm was used twice daily as a treatment for the inflammation.

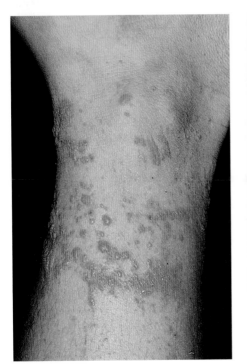

The classic presentation of poison ivy with vesicles, blisters, and linear lesions.

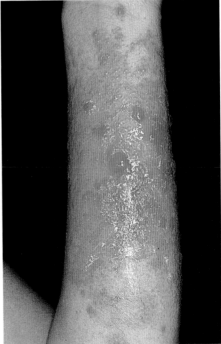

Vesicles become confluent and form blisters. Blisters rupture and ooze serum. Patients must understand that the serum does not contain the poison chemical and cannot spread the disease. Cold wet dressings applied several times a day will provide rapid control and relief.

allergen exposure lists in depth, educating patients about avoidance of the allergen and potentially related substances, and providing suitable alternatives is vital to a good outcome.

Pearls

- Allergy can develop after years of exposure to products and medications; new exposures also can cause allergic contact dermatitis.
- Consider patch testing in a patient with recurrent hand and facial dermatitis.
- Always ask about occupation and exposures; there may be both irritant and

allergic factors of importance. Some occupations with a higher risk of allergic contact dermatitis include hairdressing and dentistry, and those employed as health care workers, florists, and machinists.

- Other factors may contribute to an eczematous dermatitis (atopic dermatitis, stasis dermatitis) and contact allergy may aggravate these conditions substantially. Consider patch testing in a patient with a history of dermatitis whose problem is flaring or poorly controlled.

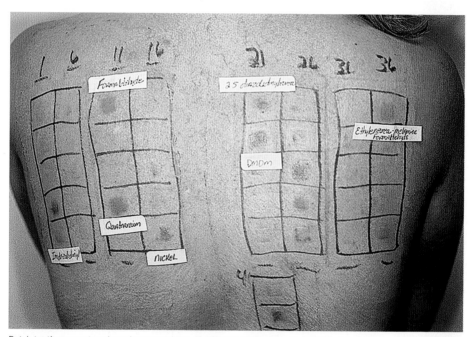

Patch testing experts rely on large numbers of different antigens to investigate for allergic contact dermatitis.

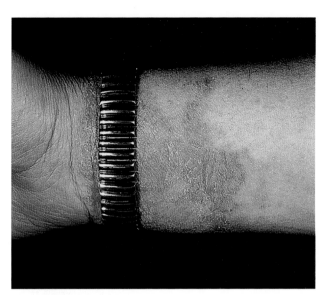

Allergic contact dermatitis to nickel.

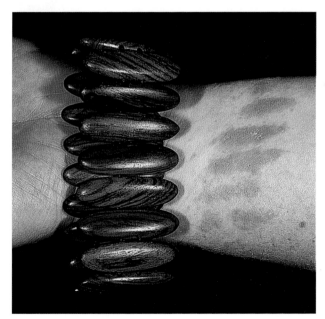

Allergic contact dermatitis to lacquer.

Irritant Contact Dermatitis

Description

- Irritant contact dermatitis is an eczematous dermatitis often caused by repeated exposure to mild irritants such as water, soaps, heat, and friction. Strong irritants include acids, alkalis, and wet cement; these chemicals can result in the acute lesions of chemical burns. Chronic exposure to mild irritants is the more common problem resulting in eczematous changes.
- The intensity of the inflammation is usually related to the concentration of irritant and the exposure time. Mild irritants cause dryness, fissuring, and erythema; strong irritant chemicals may produce an immediate reaction characterized by burning, erythema, edema, and possibly ulceration of the skin.
- About 80% of cases of contact dermatitis involve irritant contact dermatitis.
- In contrast to allergic contact dermatitis, irritant contact dermatitis is non-specific and does not require sensitization.

History

- A background of atopy (hay fever, asthma, or eczema) predisposes to an increased susceptibility to skin irritation. Susceptibility to an irritant is individual and can be variable.
- Irritant contact dermatitis is the most common type of occupational skin disease, accounting for 80% of cases.
- Employment duties and household duties, including child care and hobbies, are critical parts of the history. Jobs characterized by repeated wet work, such as food service, health care, child care, and hairstyling predispose the patient to irritant contact dermatitis.
- Common irritants include detergents, acids, alkaline chemicals, oils, organic solvents, oxidants, reducing agents, and water.
- Coarse fibers, such as particulate fiberglass, or wood dust can cause irritant contact dermatitis.
- Exposure may occur from direct contact or the airborne route.
- Examples of irritants that can cause an airborne irritant contact dermatitis include fiberglass, formaldehyde, epoxy resins, industrial solvents, glutaraldehyde, and sawdust.
- Repeated friction and mechanical irritation can result in chronic irritant contact dermatitis.
- Irritant eczematous dermatitis may occur with continuous exposure to mild irritants. Once the irritation threshold is reached, persistent dermatitis may result from less exposure to mild irritants.
- Low environmental humidity reduces the threshold for irritation.
- Continuous exposure to moisture and wet–dry cycles in areas such as the hands, the diaper area, or the skin around a colostomy, may eventually cause eczematous inflammation.
- An irritant dermatitis may become complicated by allergy as the number of applied topical remedies increases and damaged skin allows better penetration of allergens.
- Atopic individuals are predisposed to irritant contact dermatitis and often have prolonged dermatitis that is more difficult to manage.

Skin Findings

- The hands are most often affected. Both dorsal and palmar surfaces can be affected. The eyelids are another irritant prone site. Chronic lip lickers will develop an irritant dermatitis from repeated wet–dry cycles.
- Erythema, dryness, painful cracking or fissuring, and scaling are typical. Vesicles may be present, but typically are not.
- Symptoms of tenderness and burning are common. Often burning predominates over itch.
- Acute irritant dermatitis may show juicy papules and/or vesicles on an erythematous patchy background, with weeping and edema.
- Persistent, chronic irritant dermatitis is characterized by lichenification, patches of erythema, fissures, excoriations, and scaling.
- A hyperkeratotic form characterized by repeated scaling, cracking, and low-grade erythema may result from repeated mechanical trauma, such as paper handling.
- Open skin may burn on contact with topical products that are otherwise usually tolerated.

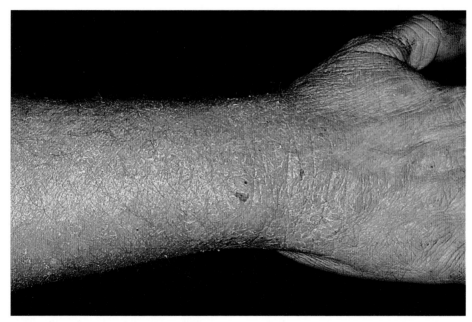

Irritant contact dermatitis. This diesel mechanic developed irritant eczema. It cleared when he was on vacation. Topical steroids provided relief but the rash re-appeared on exposure to oil. Patch testing was negative. Protection provided little relief and the patient had to find a different profession.

Laboratory

- A potassium hydroxide examination may be performed to exclude tinea infection.
- Patch testing should be performed to evaluate the role of allergic contact dermatitis if the history suggests it (i.e. exposure to allergens) or if the condition is refractory or persistent despite treatment and preventive measures. Patch testing is usually performed with a ready-to-use screening series of 24 patches (e.g. the TRUE Test; http://www.truetest.com).
- Skin biopsy, which is rarely performed, shows spongiosis, dermal edema, and an inflammatory infiltrate of predominantly lymphocytes.

Differential Diagnosis

- Allergic contact dermatitis (vesicles and itch are often more common in allergic contact dermatitis than in irritant contact dermatitis)
- Atopic dermatitis
- Tinea infection

Treatment

- Early diagnosis, treatment, and preventive measures can prevent the development of a chronic irritant dermatitis.
- The avoidance of or decreased exposure to cutaneous irritants is critical for recovery of an effective skin barrier.
- The number of wet-and-dry cycles resulting from activities, such as repeated hand washing, should be decreased.
- Cotton gloves under vinyl gloves may allow for a decreased frequency of hand washing for wet work (gloves can be ordered online at http://www.allerderm.com).
- The mildest cleanser possible (Cetaphil, Dove, Aquanil) should be used and, when appropriate, no cleanser should be used.
- Appropriate protective gloves should be worn for specific solvent or chemical exposure.
- When the patient's occupation is deemed relevant, Material Safety Data Sheets are consulted for exposure and protection information.
- Frequent application of a bland emollient such as Vaseline or Aquaphor to affected skin is essential.
- For irritant hand dermatitis, a medium-potency or high-potency topical steroid ointment applied twice a day for several weeks can be helpful in reducing erythema, itching, swelling, and tenderness.

Pearls

- Vesicles are not a typical finding in irritant contact dermatitis, unless there has been exposure to strong irritants. Subacute or chronic eczema are the most characteristic clinical findings of irritant contact dermatitis.
- Stopping the cycle of repeated exposure to low level irritants (such as water, soaps and detergents, repeated frictional contact) is essential to recovery. Repairing the skin barrier takes time and effort—irritants need to be avoided and a bland emollient needs to be applied frequently.
- Irritant and allergic contact dermatitis can be impossible to distinguish clinically; if the condition remains chronic or persistent despite appropriate care and protective measures, patch testing is indicated to evaluate the contributing role of delayed-type hypersensitivity (type IV allergy).

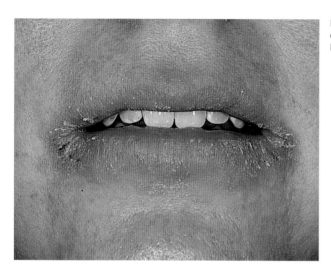

Lip licking causes dryness and chapping. Eczema will develop if licking is continued.

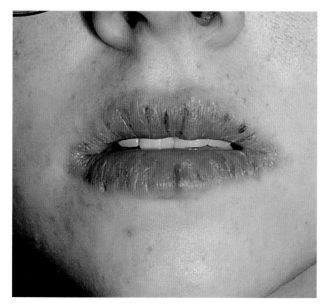

Lip licking for several weeks resulted in severe chapping with painful fissures.

Fingertip Eczema

Description

- This common form of eczema is limited to the fingertips.
- One finger or several fingers can be affected.
- Itch is limited or is absent often.
- Tenderness and burning are common.

History

- Usually fingertip eczema is a recurring winter problem, but it may occur all year round.
- It is uncommon in children and occurs most frequently in adults.

Etiology

- Atopy may be a predisposing factor.
- Irritant chemicals or frictional contact may play a role. Repeated frictional contact with paper handling has been implicated as an aggravating factor.
- A less frequent etiology is allergic contact dermatitis to plants, resins, and glues.
- Occupational and hobby-related allergens, heat, repeated water exposure, repeated wet-and-dry cycles, and friction should be considered.

Skin Findings

- Dry, scaling, pink, and fissured fingertips characterize fingertip eczema.
- Peeling reveals red tender skin.
- The tips are very dry, smooth, red and fragile. The inflammation tends to be chronic.
- Vesiculation is not typically seen.
- The process stops before the distal interphalangeal joint is reached.

Course and Prognosis

- The condition may last for months or years and can be very resistant to treatment.
- Precipitating factors are often not easily or consistently avoided.
- Inflammation may start on the fingertips but may slowly spread to involve the fingers and palms.

Discussion and Differential Diagnosis

- Contact allergy and psoriasis should be ruled out. Look carefully for other signs and sites of psoriasis to exclude this diagnosis.
- An uncommon presentation of contact allergy should be considered in handlers of tulip bulbs, florists, and dentists, or others who work with acrylate-type adhesives.
- An allergy to artificial nails should also be considered.
- If the nail is separated from the nail bed (onycholysis), candidal infection should be considered.

Management

- Management involves the avoidance of repeated wet-and-dry cycles, irritating detergents or solvents, heat, and friction.
- The condition should be managed as a subacute or chronic eczema; irritants should be avoided, and affected areas must be lubricated frequently.
- A bland emollient such as Vaseline should be applied frequently.
- A lactic acid cream (Lac-Hydrin or Amlactin 12% cream) may be helpful.
- Medium-potency topical steroids, with or without occlusion, give temporary relief.
- Cotton gloves and heavy moisturizers at night can help control this highly resistant form of eczema.
- Tar creams such as Fototar or MG 217 applied twice each day may be tried if other measures fail.

Pearls

- Cyanoacrylate glue (Crazy glue) is often used to seal the fissured painful fingertip cracks; contact allergy to this chemical is uncommon but is possible.
- Protection of the hands and affected skin by repeated application of petrolatum and use of cotton gloves can be very helpful.
- Decreasing irritation from repeated hand washing and decreasing exposure to other irritants is a cornerstone of treatment. Household gloves should be used for wet work and cleaning duties.
- Patch test the patient where occupational exposures to glues, adhesives, resins, or plants (including florists, dental hygienists and dentists) may be relevant, despite a lack of history of contact with "new" exposures.

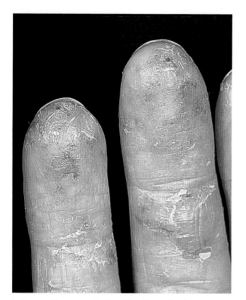

Inflammation may start on the fingertips but eventually may slowly spread to involve the fingers and palms.

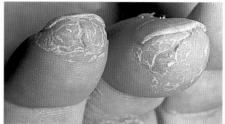

Patients protect these deep, painful cracks with bandage strips. They wear cotton gloves and heavy moisturizers to bed in an attempt to control this highly resistant form of eczema.

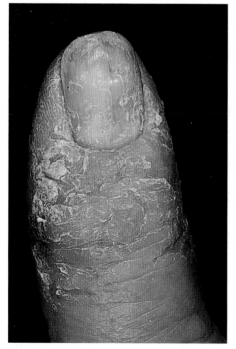

Fingertip eczema is a chronic form of irritant eczema. It is difficult to treat.

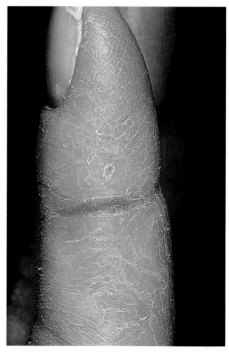

Dry skin is a constant feature of fingertip eczema. Here a deep fissure has appeared in a skin crease.

Keratolysis Exfoliativa

Description

■ Keratolysis exfoliativa is a common, chronic, asymptomatic, non-inflammatory, symmetric peeling of the palms and soles. The cause is unknown.

History

■ Keratolysis exfoliativa occurs most commonly during the summer.
■ It is often associated with sweaty palms and soles.
■ Some people have repeated episodes, and others experience this phenomenon only once.

Skin Findings

■ Scaling starts simultaneously from several points on the palms or soles with 2-3 mm of round scale that appears to have originated from a ruptured vesicle; however, vesicles are not seen.

■ The scales continue to peel and extend peripherally, forming larger, roughly circular areas that resemble ringworm, and the central area becomes slightly red and—in a few cases—tender.
■ Scaling borders may coalesce.

Course

■ This condition resolves in 1-3 weeks but may recur.

Treatment

■ No therapy other than lubrication is required.

Pearls

■ This condition improves with moisturization and generally resolves with age.
■ It is worthwhile to do a potassium hydroxide exam to exclude tinea infection.

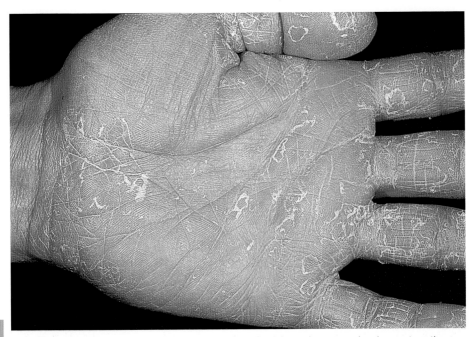

Spontaneous peeling of the palms is common and unexplained. It may be seasonal and asymptomatic. Moisturizers are usually sufficient, and the process resolves with age.

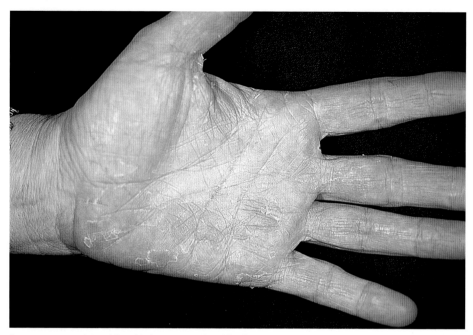

Some cases persist and the skin becomes red and fragile.

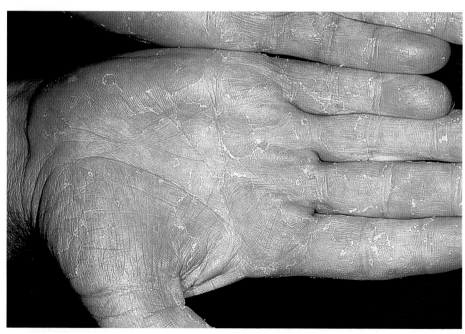

Longstanding cases may not respond to treatment and may be misdiagnosed as tinea.

Nummular Eczema

Description
- Nummular eczema is a form of eczema characterized by often generalized, exceedingly pruritic, round (coin-shaped) lesions of eczematous inflammation.

History
- Adults are most often affected. Men are more commonly affected than women.
- The onset is usually gradual, with no clear precipitant, and usually no history of eczema.
- Nummular eczema often begins with a few isolated lesions on the legs; with time, multiple lesions occur, seemingly without any particular distribution.
- Lesions often resolve or improve after the administration of topical corticosteroids, only to recur in the same area after corticosteroid withdrawal.

Skin Findings
- Sharply demarcated, scaling, round eczematous plaques appear on the trunk and extremities.
- Weeping of lesions and vesiculation can characterize flares.
- Secondary infection may result in disease flares.
- A yellow honey-colored crust indicates secondary impetiginization.

Laboratory
- Patch testing reveals a relevant positive result in a quarter to a third of cases.
- A culture of the lesion may reveal *Staphylococcus aureus*. Antibacterial treatment usually helps, but does not often resolve the problem.

Differential Diagnosis
- Psoriasis (often more obviously symmetric and geographic with silvery scales)
- Tinea infection (central healing and peripheral scaling; potassium hydroxide exam is helpful for differentiation)
- Cutaneous T cell lymphoma on the lower legs (may be confused with nummular eczema; a skin biopsy can exclude this diagnosis)

Course and Prognosis
- This is one of the most difficult forms of eczema to treat.
- The course is variable and unpredictable; this condition may be chronic relapsing for years.
- Once lesions are established, they tend to remain the same size and recur on previously affected skin.

Treatment
- See the sections Subacute Eczematous Inflammation or Chronic Eczematous Inflammation.
- Patch testing should be considered in refractory cases.
- Discontinue any unnecessary routine topical moisturizing products, over the counter oral medications, or dietary supplements and herbal preparations for at least 3–4 months.

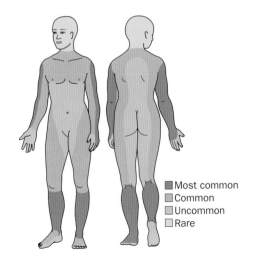

- Most common
- Common
- Uncommon
- Rare

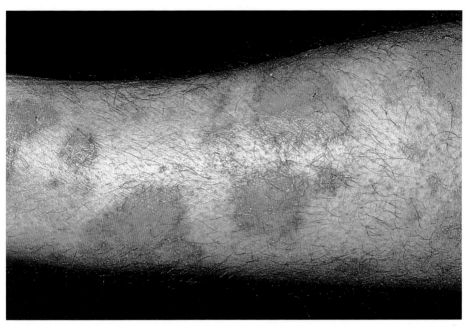

Nummular eczema may look like ringworm or psoriasis. The borders of ringworm and psoriasis are usually sharply defined. The lesions' borders are indistinct in this case of nummular eczema.

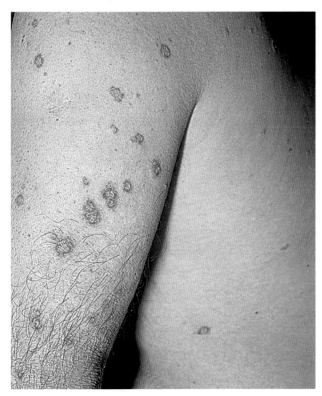

The most common areas are the dorsa of the hands, the lower legs, the upper extremities (shown here), and the trunk. Men are most commonly affected.

- Active tinea pedis should be sought; tinea is treated with antifungal agents if it is present, since occasionally, generalized nummular eczema may be an "id reaction" to a distant site of tinea infection.
- The use of topical steroids with medium-to-high potency and bland emollients (Aquaphor, Eucerin, and Vaseline) should be aggressive.
- A topical steroid is applied to affected skin twice a day for 2–3 weeks. It is best to treat a week or so longer than deemed necessary to resolve the lesion.
- The efficacy of topical steroid is increased by using occlusion with plastic wrap or a sauna suit, by hydrating the skin with a bath before medication application, or by using both techniques.
- A secondary infection is treated with systemic antistaphylococcal antibiotics (e.g. dicloxacillin 250 mg four times a day; cephalexin 250 mg four times a day).
- Antihistamines can be prescribed for itching.
- Systemic corticosteroids should be avoided for long-term management.
- Refractory cases should be referred to a dermatologist.

- Light therapy can help resolve lesions when topical treatments have failed. Narrow band ultraviolet B, and broad-band ultraviolet B are the best choices for light therapy; psoralen plus ultraviolet A can be used if ultraviolet B therapy fails.

Discussion
- The cause is unknown. Changes in soap or detergent usually make no difference.
- Lesions last for months and years and, unlike other forms of eczema, they are treatment resistant.

Pearls
- Topical allergens such as fragrance and medicaments (Bacitracin, Neosporin, hydrocortisone) may drive some cases of nummular dermatitis. Affected patients should be counseled against using them at all.
- Lesions may be acute with exudate and crusts or chronic with erythema and scale. Itching is of variable intensity, but typically is quite aggravating.
- Sunlight or ultraviolet B therapy can be very helpful in what is usually a treatment-refractory condition.

Nummular eczema. Lesions may be acute with exudate and crusts, or chronic with erythema and scale. Itching is of variable intensity.

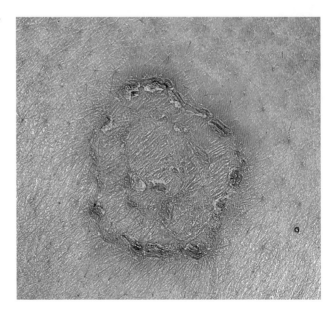

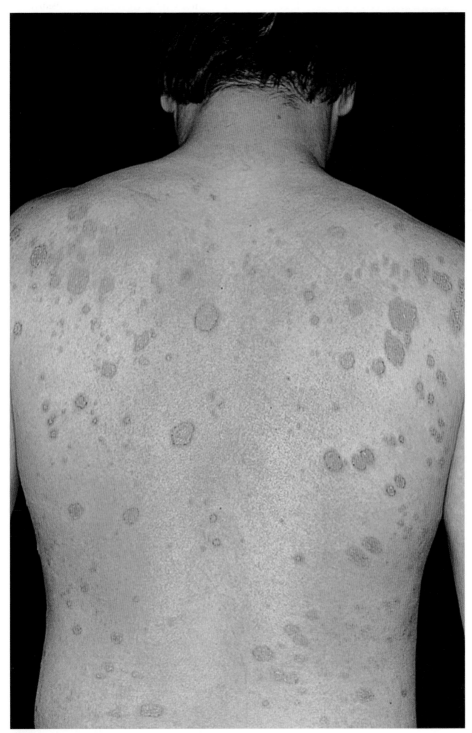

Nummular eczema. Coin-shaped lesions appear as vesicles and papules that enlarge and become confluent. They are 1–5 cm in diameter and are often confused with fungal infections.

Pompholyx

Description

- Pompholyx is also referred to as dyshidrosis or dyshidrotic eczema.
- As much as 20-25% of hand eczema may be characterized as pompholyx.
- It is a distinctive, chronic relapsing, vesicular eczematous dermatitis of unknown etiology.
- Pompholyx is characterized by sudden eruptions of usually highly pruritic, symmetric vesicles on the palms, lateral fingers, and/or plantar feet.

History

- Affected patients frequently have an atopic background (personal or family history of asthma, hay fever, or atopic eczema).
- Moderate or severe itching typically precedes a flare or recurrent eruption.
- Hyperhidrosis (increased sweating) often aggravates or accompanies this condition.
- Peak incidence is in the early 20s for women and mid-40s for men.

Skin Findings

- Vesicles are 1-5 mm in diameter, are monomorphic, deep seated, filled with clear fluid, and resemble tapioca. Vesicles erupt suddenly and symmetrically on the palms or lateral fingers or on the plantar feet.
- Rings of scale and peeling follow the eruption as itch diminishes.
- Depending on the phase of the disease, the clinician may see only brown spots. When the acute process ends, the skin peels, revealing a red cracked base with brown spots. The brown spots are sites of previous vesiculation.

Course and Prognosis

- Vesicles resolve slowly over 1-3 weeks.
- Chronic eczematous changes with erythema, scaling, and lichenification may follow.
- Waves of symmetrically distributed vesiculation can recur indefinitely.
- For unknown reasons, the chronic recurring eruption sometimes ceases with time.

Differential Diagnosis

- Pustular psoriasis of the palms and soles (pain more than itch is often the chief complaint)
- Id reaction (resulting from a distant focus of tinea infection)
- Inflammatory tinea (potassium hydroxide exam is positive)
- Acute allergic contact dermatitis
- Bullous pemphigoid (may be hemorrhagic)
- Cutaneous T cell lymphoma (rarely)

Management

- The initial treatment consists of cold wet dressings twice a day with either tap water or Burrow's solution, followed by the application of a medium-potency or high-potency steroid cream (group I–III).
- Prednisone 0.5–1 mg/kg/day tapered over 1–2 weeks is prescribed.
- Tacrolimus ointment (Protopic 0.1%) rotating with a topical medium-strength corticosteroid (group II–III) twice daily for cycles of 3–4 weeks can provide some relief.
- Corticosteroids should not be relied on for repeated or chronic treatment.
- Oral antihistamines can alleviate pruritus.
- Topical hand psoralen plus ultraviolet A is a treatment option for frequent, refractory eruptions.
- In individuals allergic to nickel, attempts to control pompholyx with elimination diets (such as a nickel-

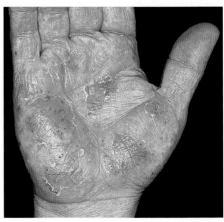

The acute process ends as the skin peels, revealing a red cracked base with brown spots. The brown spots are sites of previous vesiculation.

reduced diet) may be worth a trial in difficult cases. The administration of disulfiram (Antabuse 200 mg/day for 8 weeks) may be helpful in patients with nickel sensitivity and pompholyx hand dermatitis.

- If distant focus of tinea is identified with a positive potassium hydroxide test, treat that focus with aggressive topical antifungal medication (econazole or terbinafine cream every day for 3 weeks) or a short course of oral antifungal medication (terbinafine or itraconazole) of appropriate duration and dose for the site of infection.
- Moderating or eliminating stress can be helpful and is anecdotally curative for some people.
- For chronic or severe disabling dyshidrotic eczema a dermatologist should be consulted.
- If avoidance of allergens implicated by patch testing does not result in improvement and the condition remains disabling, further therapies include tap water iontophoresis, intradermal botulinum toxin (100–160 international units), low-dose weekly methotrexate, azathioprine (100–150 mg/day to gain control, then maintenance of 50–100 mg/day) and low-dose external beam radiation therapy.

Discussion

- The causes of this recurrent, sometimes disabling, dermatitis is unknown; provoking factors seem heterogeneous. Since eliciting factors are numerous, this cutaneous sign is non-specific, and the sources identified above need exploration in each individual. The role of atopy, occupational and/or other contact chemicals, and distant tinea infection should be considered.
- Systemic contact allergens may play a role, since some individuals with positive patch tests show vesicular reactions on the hands when challenged orally with nickel, cobalt, or chromium.
- Contact allergy is as common in dyshidrotic eczema as in other forms of hand eczema. Allergens positive on patch testing most commonly include nickel,

chromate, colophony, fragrance, balsam or peru, rubber-related mercaptobenzathiazole and thiuram mix, and paraphenylenediamine.
- Some relationships with stress and smoking have been postulated but these have been poorly studied.

Pearls

- The term "dyshidrosis" is a misnomer—the sweat glands are uninvolved and are not dysfunctional. However, most affected patients do have hyperhidrosis that seems to aggravate the condition, and complain of aggravation from protective glove occlusion and sweating.
- Occupations associated with contact allergy as a possible cause or aggravating factor for dyshidrotic eczema include those in the construction industry, the service industry (including food and money handling, e.g. cashiers), health-related occupations, hairdressing, metallurgy, chemical, and textile industries.
- Search for distant sources of tinea, especially on the feet when the hands are involved. Treat the tinea infection, if found, with either a short course of oral antifungal medication or with aggressive topical antifungal medication.
- This condition can be very frustrating given the chronic relapsing nature. Establishing a good therapeutic relationship is vital, and then assessing the risks and benefits of more aggressive treatment strategies is crucial.

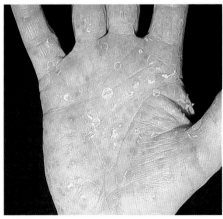

Pustular psoriasis. Differentiation from dyshidrotic eczema is sometimes impossible.

Prurigo Nodularis

Description
- Prurigo may be considered an idiopathic, papular or nodular form of lichen simplex chronicus.
- In prurigo nodularis, there are very pruritic firm papules and nodules on easily accessed skin. Lesions are secondary to repeated, localized scratching and picking.

History
- The onset is usually gradual and occurs in the setting of pruritus.
- Prurigo nodularis occurs primarily in adults.
- Stress is often anecdotally implicated.
- Individuals with atopy and diabetes may be predisposed.
- Affected patients may be compulsive "pickers."

Skin Findings
- A few to numerous dull, erythematous or hyperpigmented nodules are randomly distributed. Extensor arms and legs are typically affected; the lumbosacral area, nape of the neck, and dorsal hands are reachable areas that are typically involved.
- Lesions are created by repeated rubbing, picking and scratching.
- The small papules and nodules are red or brown, hard, and often dome-shaped with a smooth, crusted, or warty surface.
- Often there are clues to a chronic process—hypopigmented scars or postinflammatory hyperpigmentation on skin accessible to repeated scratching and picking.

Laboratory
- Skin biopsy is rarely necessary but may help confirm the diagnosis when in question. Histology shows chronic inflammation and marked epidermal hyperplasia.
- In generalized prurigo of recent onset (less than 1 year) systemic causes of pruritus should be evaluated and excluded.

Differential Diagnosis
- Causes of generalized pruritus should be excluded in recent and generalized cases; these include chronic renal disease, drug reactions, hypothyroidism, occult liver disease (including hepatitis C), infection with the human immunodeficiency virus, occult malignancy (including solid-organ metastatic disease and leukemia or lymphoma).
- Uncommon mimics of prurigo lesions have been reported and include dermatitis herpetiformis, nodular scabies, metastatic cancerous lesions, Langerhans cell histiocytosis, and atypical lymphoproliferative diseases.

Course and Prognosis
- Prurigo nodularis is often resistant to treatment and lasts for years.
- Cessation of itching, digging, and scratching is critical to lesion resolution and successful treatment.

Treatment
- Medium-potency or high-potency topical corticosteroids (groups II–IV) can be used with plastic-wrap occlusion to enhance penetration and provide a barrier to scratching.
- Corticosteroid-impregnated tape (Cordran) applied to lesions every day. The covering and occlusion of lesions provides a barrier from the trauma from repeated scratching, while medicating the underlying skin.

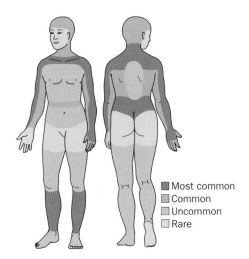

■ Most common
□ Common
□ Uncommon
□ Rare

- Topical superpotent steroids can be applied twice a day to individual lesions for several weeks.
- Intralesional steroid injections (Kenalog 5-10 mg/ml) can be given and repeated every 4-6 weeks if needed. Hypopigmentation in dark skin may occur from such treatment.
- Pramoxine with hydrocortisone (Pramosone ointment) or Sarna lotion may help relieve intense pruritus.
- Light therapy with ultraviolet B, narrow-band ultraviolet B, or psoralen plus ultraviolet A can be considered for severe, generalized cases.
- Cryotherapy is sometimes successful.
- Excision of individual nodules is rarely performed but is sometimes required.

Discussion

- Complaints of pruritus vary. Few patients claim there is no itching. Scratching is habitual; for most, pruritus is intense.
- Stress is commonly a factor in perpetuating the problem and seems to relate clinically to recurrence or flares.

Pearls

- Do not shy away from discussing stress and anxiety. In some cases it will be very relevant. Exploring the impact of these important contributors can provide much needed relief and support.
- Providing an alternative "something" to apply can be useful as well—try a bland

emollient such as A&D ointment, zinc oxide ointment, Aquaphor, or petrolatum.
- Intralesional steroid injections and cryotherapy are very effective, and are probably the quickest methods for resolving individual lesions.
- Selective serotonin reuptake inhibitors may be helpful.

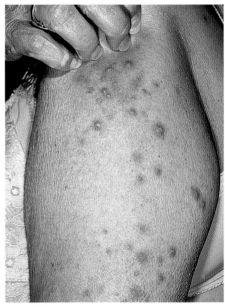

Thick, hard nodules are typically found on the extensor surfaces of the arms and legs. Chronic picking causes them.

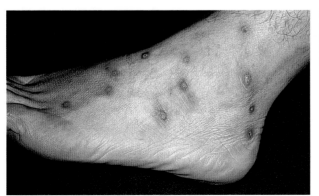

Lesions measure 0.5–1 cm and are red to dark brown. They persist, are difficult to treat, and recur if habitual picking is not controlled.

Stasis Dermatitis

Description

- Stasis dermatitis is an eczematous dermatitis of the legs, associated with edema, varicosed and dilated veins, and hyperpigmentation.
- Stasis dermatitis is a chronic problem and commonly relapses.

History

- There is often a prior history of deep venous thrombosis, surgery, trauma or ulceration.
- There is often a family history or personal history of varicose veins.
- The patient complains of heaviness or aching in the leg that is aggravated by prolonged standing or walking.
- The legs are swollen at the end of the day.
- Dermatitis and itching is a common finding, and can be chronic.

Skin Findings

- Dilated and tortuous veins are frequently present on the affected leg. These should be looked for with the patient in a standing position.
- Subacute and chronic eczematous dermatitis appears on the lower legs or surrounding a venous ulcer.
- The dermatitis is obvious and is associated with dry, fissured, erythematous skin.
- The dermatitis can become generalized ("id reaction") if the condition persists.
- Edema, brown discoloration (hemosiderosis), erosion, or ulceration are common findings.

- Pruritus is troublesome to the patient; excoriation can potentiate secondary infection.
- White scars on the medial calf indicate previous ulceration. They may have an atrophic, stellate appearance (atrophy blanche).
- Stasis papillomatosis (elephantiasis nostra) and verrucous hyperplasia are found in chronically congested limbs, occurring with local lymphatic disturbances such as chronic venous insufficiency, primary lymphedema (Milroy's disease), trauma, and recurrent erysipelas.
- Secondary infection with *Staphylococcus aureus* (impetiginized) is common, especially in excoriated skin.

Laboratory

- If indicated, the veins are studied with color duplex ultrasonography.
- An ankle brachial index is obtained to check for arterial disease; results of less than 0.8 indicate significant arterial disease.
- In patients with a strong family history or personal history of multiple deep vein thrombosis, the clotting cascade (protein S, protein C, activated protein C resistance, factor V Leiden, cryofibrinogens, and homocysteine level) should be checked.

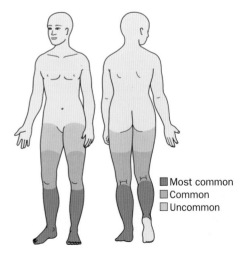

Most common
Common
Uncommon

Treatment

- Cool water dressings are applied for 10-20 minutes twice a day for acute exudative inflammation.
- Group II-V topical steroids are applied twice a day (cream if acute, and ointment if chronic) for 2-3 weeks.
- Domeboro dressings and a course of oral antibiotic (e.g. dicloxacillin, cephalexin) are administered if there is indication of infection.
- For generalized dermatitis (id reaction) an oral steroid is administered with a 3-week taper.
- Oral antihistamines (e.g. hydroxyzine) 10-25 mg every 4-6 hours as needed may help control itching.

- Lubrication with bland emollients can help alleviate dryness. More Vaseline-like bases are preferable to lotions, such as plain petrolatum, Aquaphor, Aveeno, Cetaphil cream. Popular moisturizers contain fragrance and preservative ingredients that may contribute to the development of an aggravating contact allergy. Simplify topicals.
- Compression (20-30 mmHg) is accomplished with stockings (e.g. Venosan, Sigvaris, or Jobst or Ace wraps).
- More aggressive compression (30-40 mmHg at the ankle) may be required.
- Superficial venous incompetence may benefit from vein stripping or sclerotherapy.

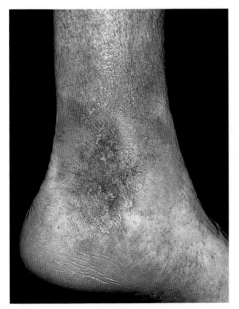

Subacute eczema with erythema and scale are present over a wide area. Inflammation had been present for several weeks. Cefadroxil 500 mg twice a day for 5 days was followed by application of a group V topical steroid ointment applied twice a day for two weeks. Moisturizers and compression stockings were used to prevent recurrence.

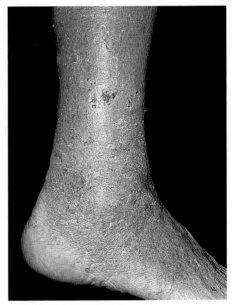

Erythema and scale have extended onto the foot and involve most of the lower leg. A group III topical steroid ointment used for two weeks cleared this eruption.

57

Differential Diagnosis

- Contact dermatitis (especially neomycin, bacitracin, fragrances, preservatives in popular moisturizing lotions, and hydrocortisone; allergic contact dermatitis is commonly associated with stasis dermatitis)
- Cellulitis (sudden pain and increased swelling are clues)
- Tinea corporis (a potassium hydroxide exam of the scale is helpful; especially if there is a moccasin distribution of erythema and scaling on the plantar feet, or onychomycosis)

Pearls

- A careful history often indicates that irritants or potential allergy-causing contactants are being applied by the patient with the intention of healing the skin.
- Simplify the topical management.
- Elevation and compression with graded stockings are mainstays of treatment.
- Topical steroids are very useful for the inflammatory or dermatitis component.
- Patients are often fearful of topical steroids; encourage proper application of topical steroids and use them in ointment base. The patient needs to apply enough, to rub them in well, and to do so for 2–3 weeks for acutely eczematous stasis dermatitis.
- If a patient is not agile enough or strong enough to put on compression hose, an Ace wrap can be used successfully to reduce edema. This is applied shortly after rising in the morning.

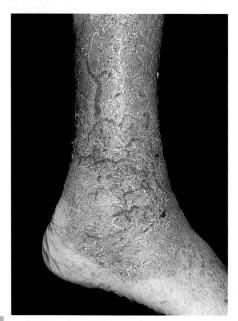

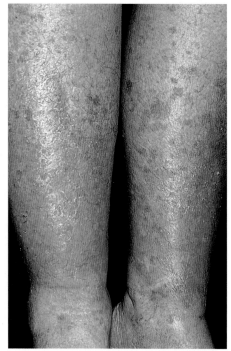

Infection or irritation from washing can precipitate severe acute exacerbations of stasis dermatitis. The deep fissures are infected.

Inflammation has been present for months. The skin is thickened from itching. Both legs are swollen.

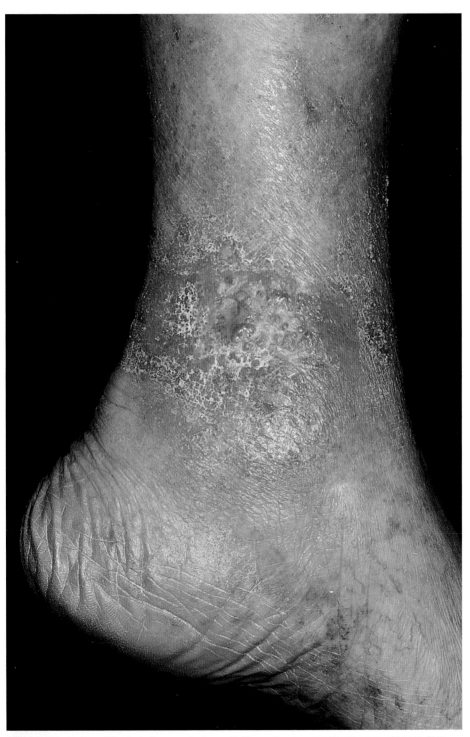

Recurrent stasis dermatitis. Periodic exacerbations of inflammation are common in areas of stasis. This patient has had recurrent inflammation for years. White sclerotic skin over the ankle is evidence of healed stasis ulcers.

Venous Leg Ulcers

Description

- A venous leg ulcer is a chronic non-healing ulcer typically located on the medial aspect of the lower leg in association with chronic venous insufficiency.

History

- Venous leg ulcers often occur in middle-aged and elderly people.
- About 20% of those affected develop ulceration by age 40; 13% do so by age 30.
- They are more common in women than in men.
- Ulcer formation often occurs suddenly, often after slight trauma.
- Preceding leg injury, phlebitis, obesity, and deep vein thrombosis are also important risk factors.
- Severe pain may indicate other pathologic conditions (e.g. infection or arterial disease).
- Healing is slow, taking weeks or months—even with proper care.
- Venous leg ulcers can be a chronic, recurrent, life-long problem.
- Ulcers may be asymptomatic or mildly tender; they do not typically cause severe pain.

Skin Findings

- Ulcers are typically located in the region of the medial malleolus. They are flat, have sharp or slightly sloping borders, and are typically shallow with a covering of granulation tissue.
- Edema, usually pitting, is common; it improves at night with elevation of the legs.
- Chronic edema, trauma, infection, and inflammation lead to subcutaneous tissue fibrosis where the skin has a firm, non-pitting "woody" quality.
- Ultimately, there is loss of subcutaneous tissue and a decrease in the lower leg circumference.
- Patients complain of aching and swollen legs; the pain is worse with standing and better in the morning.

- Ulcers may be asymptomatic or mildly tender; they do not typically cause severe pain.
- Advanced disease is represented by an "inverted bottle leg"; when the proximal leg swells, the lower leg shrinks.
- Vein varicosities are often prominent.
- The patient may have secondary eczematous dermatitis (stasis dermatitis),
- There is often hyperpigmentation, from either chronic inflammation or capillary leakage, and hemosiderin deposition in the skin of the lower legs.
- The ulcer remains small or may enlarge rapidly without any further trauma.
- Removing crust and debris reveals a moist base with granulation tissue.
- Ulcers are replaced with ivory-white atrophic sclerotic scars (atrophy blanche).

Laboratory

- Color duplex ultrasonography identifies the presence and source of significant venous reflux, an ankle: brachial index is useful in assessing concomitant arterial peripheral vascular disease (the ratio is discussed in the section on Stasis Dermatitis)
- Chronic lesions are biopsied to rule out cancer (basal cell or squamous cell carcinomas), and for tissue culture. A biopsy should be performed if the wound persists > 3 months.
- Cultures are not usually helpful; ulcers are often colonized, not infected.
- If infection is a concern a biopsy should be done and the tissue submitted for bacterial identification and quantification.

Differential Diagnosis

- Most leg ulcers are caused by venous disease. However, the differential diagnosis includes:
  - Arterial ulcers
  - Neuropathic ulcers (secondary to diabetes)
  - Infectious ulcers
  - Neoplastic ulcers
  - Metabolic causes
  - Pyoderma gangrenosum
  - Antiphospholipid syndrome or other coagulation disorder
  - Other clotting disorders

Treatment

Control of Chronic Venous Insufficiency

- Proper leg compression can avert recurrence and worsening of the problem.
- Elevation of the legs above the heart level for 30 minutes three to four times daily and at night.
- Compression is achieved with Ace wraps, graded compression stockings, or external pneumatic compression devices.
- Multi-layer compression bandages are associated with faster healing rates than single-layer bandage systems.
- Unna boots (bandages impregnated with zinc oxide) are also helpful; apply and replace them weekly until the ulcer has resolved.

- The routine use of systemic antibiotics does not increase healing rates.
- Group III–V topical steroids are used (for 7–14 days) for stasis dermatitis.
- Heavy moisturizers (e.g. Aquaphor, petrolatum, Aveeno cream) protect the skin and help resolve dermatitis.
- Neomycin-containing antibiotics, which may sensitize the skin, should be avoided. Other common contact allergens include preservatives in moisturizing lotions, hydrocortisone, and bacitracin. Avoid these if possible.
- Pentoxifylline (Trental) 400 mg three times a day increases fibrinolytic activity and may reduce lipodermatosclerosis.

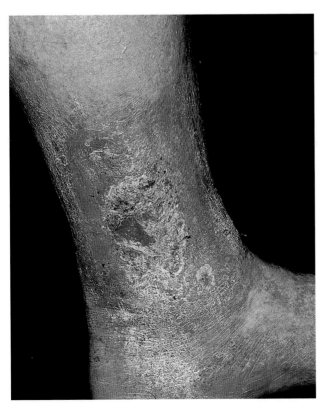

The skin is diffusely red, thickened, and bound down by fibrosis. Ulceration occurs with the slightest trauma.

Ulcer Therapy

- The crust and exudate are surgically or mechanically debrided.
- Proteolytic enzymes have little benefit in debriding.
- The application of occlusive film promotes rapid healing by suppressing crust formation and enhancing epidermal migration.
- Metronidazole gel (MetroGel) applied before dressing helps decrease odor.
- A variety of synthetic dressings are now available.
- Hydrocolloid dressings (e.g. DuoDerm CGF) are effective and easy to use as the initial treatment.
- The type of dressing should be changed if healing is slow.
- Exudative and draining ulcers are treated with an absorbant dressing of the calcium alginate group.
- Continuous wet saline dressings can debride the crust in deep ulcers and promote granulation tissue.
- Signs of malnutrition (e.g. a low serum albumin level) should be noted and corrected.
- Aspirin 300 mg/day may improve healing.
- Vitamin and mineral supplementation should be considered. This includes ascorbic acid (1–2 g daily), zinc sulfate (220 mg three times a day), and vitamin E (200 mg twice a day).
- Skin grafting should be considered for difficult cases; it is most successful when applied to granulation tissue free of exudate and when edema has been controlled.

- Artificially engineered skin-tissue equivalents (e.g. Apligraft, Dermagraft, Graftskin) are available and should be considered for refractory ulcers.
- Stanozolol has fibrinolytic activity, and can be effective in reducing pain and induration in lipodermatosclerosis, but the healing rate is not affected.

When to Refer

- Refer a patient with a large ulcer size, or for an ulcer of long duration. Refer a patient when ulcer size does not decrease after 1–3 months of therapy.

Pearls

- Make every effort to have your patient understand the importance of good compression measures, such as the daily use of compression stockings. Though difficult at first, often the relief is so great with repeated use that graded compression stockings (Jobst, Sigvaris 30–40 mmHg at the ankle) are embraced by the patient. These stockings promote more rapid healing and dramatically reduce recurrence.
- An unna boot is a relatively simple therapy which can provide relief from pain and swelling while healing the ulceration.
- Elevation of the affected leg is an important measure—a patient who must stand all day long may not be able to heal an ulcer. Time off work may be required for healing.
- Venous ulceration can have a major impact on work productivity and quality of life.

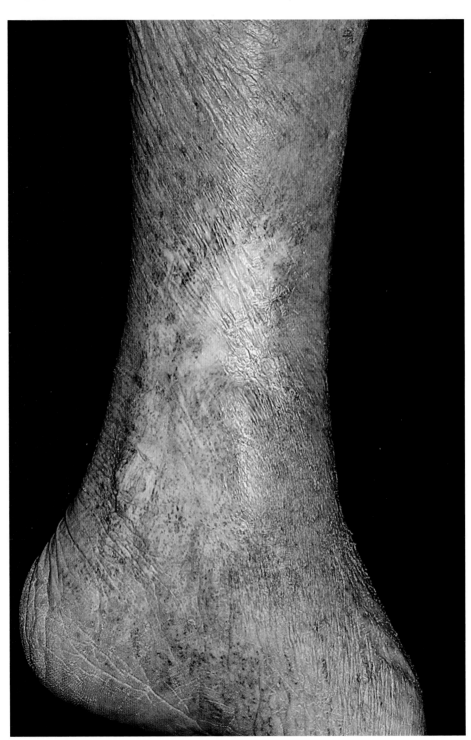

Stasis ulcers. Ulcers heal with a smooth ivory-colored surface. The surrounding skin is permanently stained brown from leaking blood vessels (hemosiderosis) and post-inflammatory hyperpigmentation.

Atopic Dermatitis

Description
- Atopic dermatitis is an eczematous eruption that is distressingly pruritic, recurrent, often flexural, and symmetric.
- Atopic dermatitis generally begins early in life and is characterized by periods of remission and exacerbation. The distribution of affected skin varies with age.

Major Criteria (Four Required for Diagnosis)
- Pruritus
- Young age at onset
- Typical morphology and distribution
- Flexural lichenification and linearity in adults; facial and extensor involvement in infants
- Chronic or chronic and relapsing course
- Personal or family history or atopy (asthma, allergic rhinoconjunctivitis, atopic dermatitis)

Minor (or Less Specific) Features
- Xerosis
- Ichthyosis
- Palmar hyperlinearity
- Keratosis pilaris
- Immediate type I skin test responses
- Dermatitis of the hands and feet
- Cheilitis
- Nipple eczema
- Increased susceptibility to cutaneous infections
- Perifollicular accentuation

History
- The incidence is 7–24 per 1000, and seems to be on the rise; most common in children.
- About 70% of patients have a family history of one or more of the following: asthma, hay fever, or eczematous dermatitis.
- Aggravating factors include contact irritants and allergens, perspiration, excessive heat, rough fibers (such as wool), tight clothing, cool dry air with no humidity, and emotional stress.

- The role of dust mite and food allergies in cases of severe infantile atopic eczema is controversial.
- Atopic dermatitis becomes less severe in most children when they reach their teenage years. Most children outgrow atopic dermatitis, but some develop chronic relapsing disease, especially of the eyelid and hand, and retroauricular dermatitis.
- Atopic dermatitis seems to result from a vicious cycle of dermatitis associated with elevated T cell activation, hyperstimulatory Langerhans cells, defective cell-mediated immunity, and over-production of immunoglobulin by B cells.

Skin Findings
- Atopic inflammation often begins abruptly with erythema and severe pruritus.
- Typical lesions are red pruritic papules, patches of erythema, and scaling.
- Acute lesions may be oozing and vesicular; subacute lesions are scaly and crusted; and chronic lesions are often dull red, lichenified, and very pruritic.
- Dermatitis distribution varies according to age.

Infantile Phase (2 Months to 2 Years)
- Atopic dermatitis appears on the cheeks, perioral area and scalp
- The extensor tops of the feet and the elbows are often involved
- The lesions are often exudative and weeping

Childhood Phase (2–12 Years)
- Flexural involvement (antecubital and popliteal fossae, neck, wrists, and ankles) is typical
- Scratching and chronicity lead to lichenification

Adult Phase (12 Years to Adult)
- Flexural involvement is common
- Hand dermatitis may be the only manifestation
- Dermatitis of the upper eyelid is another frequent finding
- Atopic dermatitis can be diffuse and patchy on the body

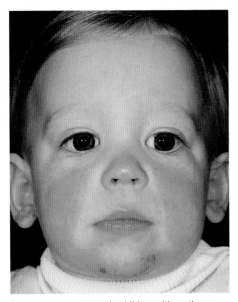

A common appearance in children with erythema and scaling confined to the cheeks and sparing the perioral and paranasal area.

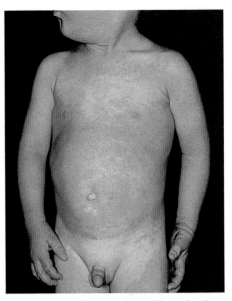

Generalized infantile atopic dermatitis sparing the diaper area, which keeps the skin hydrated and protected from scratching.

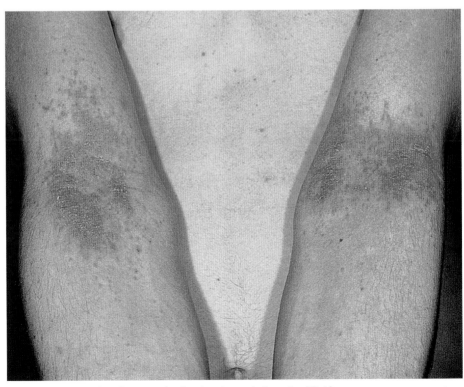

Classic appearance of confluent papules forming plaques in the antecubital fossa.

- Associated findings are dry skin, ichthyosis vulgaris, and keratosis pilaris

Complications
- Lesions are frequently colonized with *Staphylococcus aureus*; secondary infection resulting in another flare of dermatitis or persistence is common.
- Increased susceptibility to viral infections (herpes simplex, molluscum contagiosum, cutaneous fungal infections) is frequent.
- Hypopigmentation and hyperpigmentation may result from previous inflammation.
- Emotional and behavior problems may be frequent in children affected by moderate to severe disease.

Non-skin Findings
Often, there is a personal or family history of asthma, hay fever, or seasonal rhinitis.

Laboratory
- Laboratory studies are not routinely indicated or performed.
- Culture and sensitivity testing of crusted or oozing lesions is performed if bacterial superinfection is suspected.
- Elevated immunoglobulin E levels (> 200 International Units/ml) occur in approximately 80–90% of patients.
- The incidence of eosinophilia correlates roughly with disease activity.
- Routine allergy testing, dietary testing, and environmental or dietary manipulation are often not productive.
- Patch testing should be considered if the pattern of dermatitis changes, or the condition becomes more refractory to treatment.
- Children with severe atopic dermatitis may have food allergies. Evaluation and elimination of suspected foods under medical supervision can be helpful in some cases. Food allergy is rarely a problem for adults with atopic eczema.

Differential Diagnosis
- Contact dermatitis (irritant or allergic types)
- Nummular eczema and seborrheic dermatitis
- Scabies (consider in new-onset eczematous disease)
- Cutaneous T cell lymphoma (consider especially in adults with refractory disease)
- Tinea infections (potassium hydroxide exam of scale is helpful)
- Uncommon: congenital disorders, metabolic disorders (zinc deficiency), immune deficiency disorders (Wiskott–Aldrich syndrome, hyperimmunoglobulinemia E syndrome, severe combined immunodeficiency, Netherton syndrome)

Treatment
- Inflammation and infection should be controlled or eliminated.
- Topical corticosteroids of appropriate strength for the patient's age and the affected area are applied twice daily to inflamed skin for 10–21 days.
- Topical immune modulators: tacrolimus (Protopic) ointment 0.03% for children aged 2–15 years and 0.03% and 0.1% for adults, or pimecrolimus (Elidel) cream 1% twice daily for short-term and intermittent long-term therapy are effective topical immune modulators. Their use can avoid the adverse effects associated with chronic topical steroids. They are especially helpful for atopic dermatitis of the face, eyelids, or areas of limited involvement.
- Oral antibiotics such as dicloxacillin and cephalexin (Keflex) are administered for secondary infection. Topical Mupirocin (Bactroban) cream twice daily for 5 days may be helpful if infection is limited.
- For acute lesions and severe flares, wet dressings with Burrow's solution is applied for 20 minutes two or three times a day, followed by the application of a topical steroid.
- If lesions suddenly become exquisitely tender with small ulcerations, consider herpes simplex infection complicating atopic eczema (eczema herpeticum).
- The skin barrier should be restored and preserved.
- Bland emollients, such as Vaseline petroleum, should be used. A plain, thick,

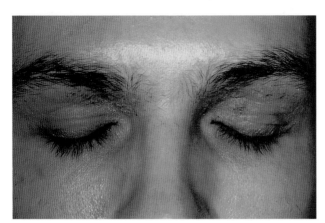

Atopic dermatitis of the upper eyelids, an area that is often rubbed with the back of the hand.

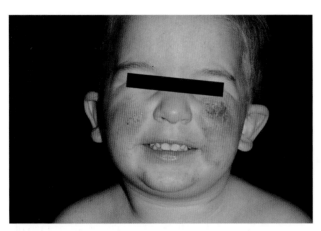

Erythema and scale on the cheeks is one of the most common presentations for atopic dermatitis in infants. Crusting suggests infection with *staphylococci*.

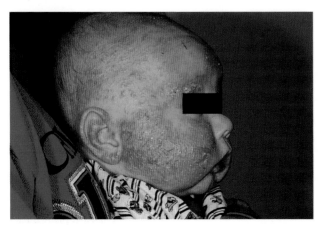

The mother was afraid to use topical steroids. Washing and scratching caused the inflammation to spread over a wide area. Antistaphylococcal oral antibiotics followed by application of a group VI topical steroid ointment cleared the eczema. Pimecrolimus cream (Elidel) was used to prevent recurrence.

greasy moisturizer (Vaseline, Aquaphor, Aveeno, Vanicream) without fragrances or common sensitizing preservatives is ideal, and is preferable to commonly available lotions or creams.

■ Aggravating factors must be eliminated or controlled.

■ Excessive sweating, which is irritating to the skin should be avoided.

■ Soft, light cotton clothing is best; wool or other coarse fibers are to be avoided.

■ The environment should be cool and well ventilated.

■ Stress reduction techniques may be helpful.

■ Pruritus must be controlled.

■ Oral antihistamines with sedative effects are helpful (such as diphenhydramine (Benadryl), hydroxyzine (Atarax), and doxepin) especially at night to allow more restful sleep.

■ A dermatologist should be consulted for the management of severe, refractory disease.

Severe Atopic Dermatitis

■ A *short* course of oral corticosteroids can break the cycle of inflammation.

■ Tacrolimus ointment (Protopic) or pimecrolimus cream (Elidel) are both effective when applied twice a day, but may not work as fast as topical steroids.

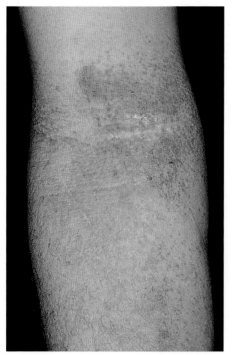

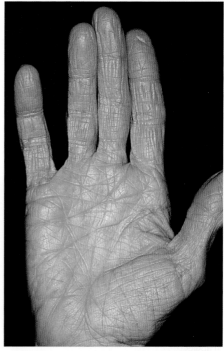

Papules and lichenification are characteristic of atopic dermatitis. Scratching has extended the eruption beyond the antecubital fossa.

Accentuation of the skin creases on the palms (hyperlinear creases) are a distinctive sign of the atopic diathesis.

- Consider hospitalization for rest, environmental control, and stress reduction, and wet dressings two times a day followed by the application of a medium-potency topical steroid.
- A medium-potency topical steroid with vinyl-suit occlusion can be applied for 2 hours twice a day for 1–2 weeks.
- Ultraviolet light therapy includes broad- or narrow-band ultraviolet B, and psoralen plus ultraviolet A.
- Other immunomodulating therapeutic options for severe refractory atopic eczema include oral cyclosporin, azathioprine, low-dose methotrexate, and interferon gamma.

Pearls

- Control aggravating external environmental factors.
- Win patient compliance by support, empathy and good listening. Schedule follow-up visits— even if just for support.
- Be specific with your treatment recommendations.

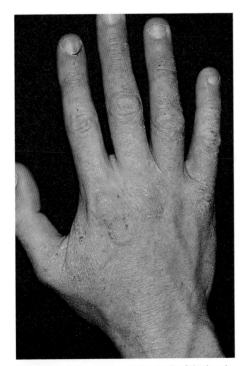

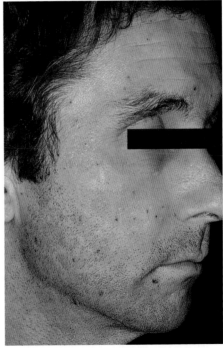

Eczematous inflammation on the back of the hands in adults is a common presentation of atopic dermatitis. Atopic people are more likely to develop inflammation when exposed to irritants and repeated cycles of wetting and drying.

Atopic dermatitis may be chronic and debilitating. Inflammation has persisted for months with constant rubbing and scratching. Low-grade infection interferes with treatment.

Autosomal Dominant Ichthyosis Vulgaris

Description
- Dominant ichthyosis vulgaris is a disorder of keratinization characterized by dry, rectangular scales resembling a cracked pavement; these scales appear most prominently on the extensor extremities.
- It is associated with the atopic diathesis in 50% of cases.

History
- The onset is in early to middle childhood.
- The condition may improve with age or may persist throughout life.
- The scales are more noticeable and often pruritic in the winter, when the humidity is low.
- Ichthyosis vulgaris is autosomal dominant; 1 in 300 have the disorder.
- It may be confused clinically with X-linked ichthyosis.

Skin Findings
- Findings are often mild.
- Dry, small, rectangular scales appear on the extensor extremities.
- The lower extremities, particularly the anterior shins, are often more noticeably affected.
- Affected skin has the appearance of cracked pavement or fish scales.
- This condition characteristically spares the flexor surfaces.
- It is usually asymptomatic but may become pruritic or chapped in the winter.
- Palmar creases may be accentuated.
- Keratosis pilaris may also be present.
- Scaling rarely involves the entire cutaneous surface.
- Scaling of the skin results from the retention of scale rather than increased proliferation.
- The condition may result from a defect in the synthesis of epidermal proteins, profilaggrin and filaggrin.

Laboratory
- No tests are routinely indicated, unless there is a question of X-linked ichthyosis.
- Skin biopsy is rarely performed; when performed, it shows in a subset of patients a decreased or an absent granular layer.

Differential Diagnosis
- Dry skin
- Acquired ichthyosis (more sudden and later onset, generalized, as a manifestation of systemic disease—that is, infection with the immunodeficiency virus, malignancy, drugs, autoimmune disease, and in bone marrow transplant patients with a history of chronic graft-versus-host disease)
- X-linked ichthyosis (affected males have deficient steroid sulfatase activity; large scales are a dirty brown color; flexures may be involved, although usually spared; a fluorescence in situ hybridization test is performed on fibroblasts, keratinocytes and lymphocytes, and is a sensitive test for X-linked ichthyosis)

Treatment
- Ichthyosis vulgaris often improves with age; infrequently, it resolves completely.
- Increased environmental humidity and warmth often result in resolution or improvement.
- Regular application of moisturizing cream or lotion decreases pruritus and improves skin appearance.
- The optimal time for applying moisturizer is immediately after bathing and hydrating the skin.
- Emollients containing lactic acid, urea, or alpha-hydroxy acids are helpful for treating severe dryness and scaling.
- Ammonium lactate 12% (Lac-Hydrin,

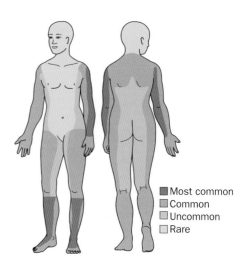

Most common
Common
Uncommon
Rare

Amlactin) lotion or cream is very effective when applied daily.

Pearls

■ Clues to the differential diagnosis of X-linked ichthyosis include

cryptorchidism in affected patients, and a birth history of delayed labor. Half of affected males and female carriers develop comma-shaped corneal opacities.

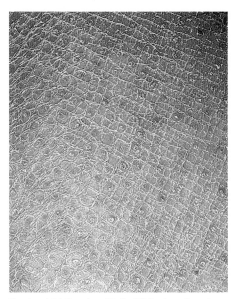

Dominant ichthyosis vulgaris. White, translucent quadrangular squares on the extensor aspects of the arms and legs. This form is significantly associated with atopy.

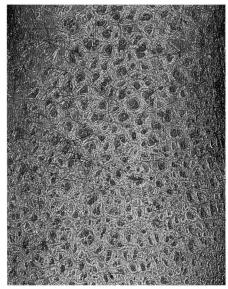

Sex-linked ichthyosis vulgaris. Patients have dry skin in the summer months that evolves into large, brown, quadrangular scales during the dry winter months.

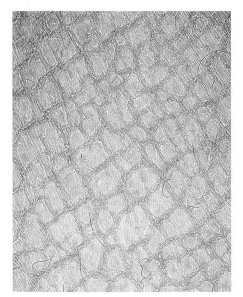

Dominant ichthyosis is a disorder of keratinization characterized by the development of dry, rectangular scales. The skin on this patient's lower leg shows features of ichthyosis and asteatotic eczema.

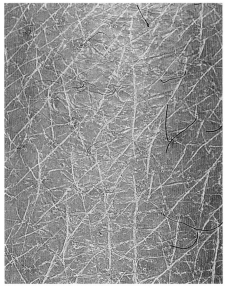

This patient has severe dry skin that has cracked and resembles ichthyosis.

Keratosis Pilaris

Description
- Keratosis pilaris consists of rough, monomorphic, tiny, follicle-based scaling papules most commonly on the posterolateral aspects of the upper arms but occasionally more widespread, including the anterior and lateral thighs and the buttocks.
- It results from mild follicular plugging and perifollicular inflammation.

History
- Keratosis pilaris is very common in young children, peaking in adolescence.
- It is probably more common in atopic individuals.
- It is usually asymptomatic but may be somewhat pruritic.
- Treatment is often sought for a troubling cosmetic appearance.
- The unusual adult diffuse pattern persists indefinitely.

Skin Findings
- Small, pinpoint follicular papules, and occasionally pustules, remain in the same areas for years.
- A red halo appears at the periphery of the keratotic papule.
- The skin feels rough, like sandpaper.
- Lesions most commonly appear on the posterolateral upper arms and anterior and lateral thighs. Occasionally, the condition is generalized and appears on the trunk, extensor arms and legs.

Laboratory
- No laboratory tests are necessary.

Differential Diagnosis
- Acne (facial lesions may be confused with it; uniform small size and association with dry skin and chapping differentiate keratosis pilaris from pustular acne)

Treatment
- Many patients seek treatment for cosmesis, since most often the lesions are asymptomatic.
- Keratosis pilaris often improves or resolves by adulthood.

- Scratching, wearing tight-fitting clothing, or undergoing treatment with abrasive washes or gritty scrubs may aggravate the condition.
- Tretinoin (Retin-A) may induce temporary improvement, but irritation is usually unacceptable.
- Lac-Hydrin cream 12% or lotion 12% twice a day can reduce roughness and improve appearance.
- Low-potency topical steroids may be used in limited courses to temporarily reduce the redness but should not be used on a long-term basis.
- The recognition of keratosis pilaris helps avoid inappropriate treatment.

Pearls
- Keratosis pilaris is common on the face of children and is frequently confused with acne.
- Treatment is often desired because of the visible typical location of keratosis pilaris

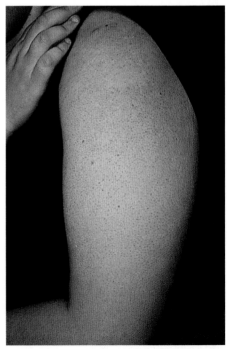

The upper arm is the most common site to find keratosis pilaris. This is an unusually extensive eruption.

on the extensor upper arms and thighs. Otherwise, the condition is generally asymptomatic.

■ Use of an emollient daily can lessen the appearance and inflammation of keratosis pilaris, which can be especially apparent during winter months.

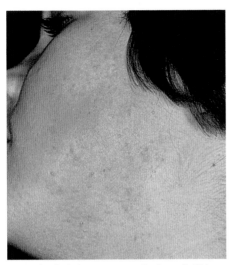

Keratosis pilaris is common on the face of children and is frequently confused with acne.

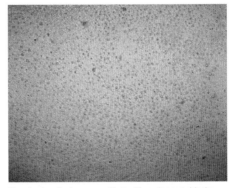

Keratosis pilaris presenting with a deep red halo tends to be widespread and lasts into adulthood.

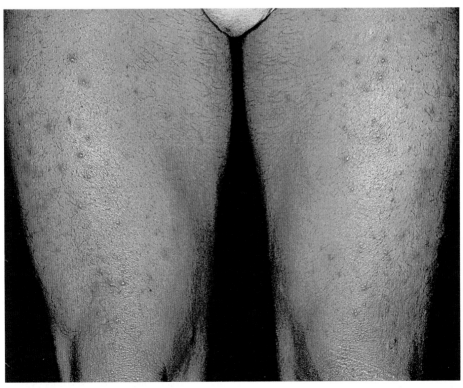

Infected lesions in a uniform distribution. Typical bacterial folliculitis has a haphazard distribution.

Pityriasis Alba

Description

■ Asymptomatic, hypopigmented, slightly elevated, fine, scaling patches with indistinct borders, typically on the lateral cheeks.

■ Pityriasis alba affects the lateral cheeks, lateral upper arms, and thighs; it occurs more frequently in young children and usually resolves by early adulthood.

History

■ Pityriasis alba is asymptomatic.

■ Children and young adults are affected.

■ There is no history of prior rash, trauma, or inflammation.

■ Affected individuals are often atopic.

■ Loss of pigment is often more noticeable and distressing in darkly pigmented people.

Skin Findings

■ The white macules are round to oval and vary in size; they are generally 2-4 cm in diameter.

■ A fine surface scale may be seen on close inspection.

■ Lesions are most common on the lateral cheeks, lateral upper arms, and thighs.

■ The condition is more obvious in the summer, and in darker skin types, when affected skin does not tan.

Laboratory

■ A potassium hydroxide examination of the fine scale is negative.

Differential Diagnosis

■ Eczematous dermatitis

■ Tinea versicolor (rare on the face)

■ Vitiligo (more sharply demarcated, often over joints, symmetric, and more widespread)

■ Chemical leukoderma

Treatment

■ Usually no treatment is recommended, as the problem is benign and self resolving. Emollient use every day may be helpful.

■ The patient should be reassured that the loss of pigment is not permanent.

■ Hypopigmentation usually fades with time.

■ Hydrocortisone cream or ointment 1% applied for a limited time (a few weeks) on affected skin may help the patients who are most distressed by the pigment irregularity.

Pearls

■ Hypopigmented round spots are a common occurrence on the faces of atopic children.

■ The superficial hypopigmented plaques become scaly and inflamed as the dry winter months progress.

■ Reassurance is the best and most benign treatment.

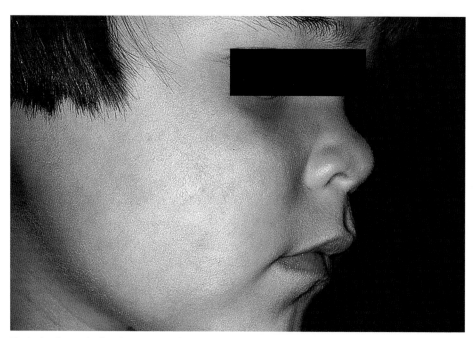

Pityriasis alba on the face is a common finding. Parents are concerned about the cosmetic appearance. They are reassured when informed that the white spots will disappear in time.

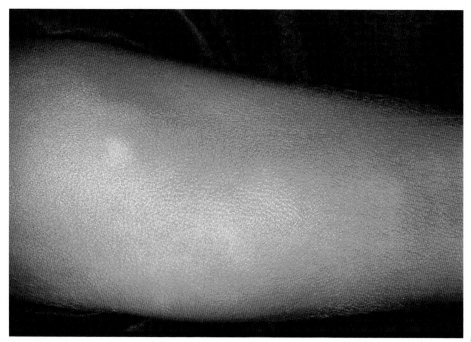

Pityriasis alba. Loss of pigment on the arms is often misdiagnosed as tinea versicolor or vitiligo. Both tinea versicolor and pityriasis alba present with fine scale. A potassium hydroxide examination shows clusters of budding cells and hyphae with tinea versicolor. Tinea versicolor rarely involves the face.

3 Urticaria

Acute Urticaria (Hives)

Description
- Urticaria or hives is divided into acute and chronic forms, which is based on the duration of the hives.
- Acute urticaria is a variably pruritic, common, distinctive reaction pattern.
- Acute urticaria, by definition, lasts for less than 6 weeks while chronic urticaria lasts more than 6 weeks.
- Transient, edematous, red plaques vary in size and shape. Individual lesions last less than 24 hours.

History
- Acute urticaria may occur at any age.
- It is more common in atopic individuals.
- The etiology is undetermined in some cases.
- Histamine release by allergens (e.g. drugs, foods, pollens) is mediated by immunoglobulin E.
- Hives are notoriously pruritic.
- The pruritus is milder in deeper forms of hives (angioedema).

Skin Findings
- The plaques are pink to flesh-colored, non-pitting, and edematous.
- The lesions may be uniformly red, pink or flesh-colored, or surrounded by a white or red halo.
- The lesions vary in size and are round or oval; when confluent, they become polycyclic.
- The plaques change size and shape by peripheral extension, migrate and regress.
- This is a dynamic process; new lesions evolve as old ones resolve.
- Rarely, bullae or purpuric lesions appear with intense swelling.
- The distribution is usually generalized and haphazard.
- Linear lesions suggest dermagraphism (physical urticaria).

Laboratory
- There are no routine studies for diagnosis.
- Biopsy is usually not needed for diagnosis of acute hives, but can be used to evaluate for urticarial vasculitis.

Differential Diagnosis
- Urticaria vasculitis (painful lesions lasting more than 24 hours and resolving with purpuric changes)
- Drug eruption
- Viral exanthem
- Bites (papular urticaria)
- Bullous pemphigoid in an elderly patient
- Hereditary angioedema

Treatment
- All suspected triggers (drugs, food and drink, inhalents) should be discontinued.
- Antihistamines are typically administered initially; this includes type 1 histamine receptor antagonists (H_1 blockers) such as hydroxyzine 10–25 mg every 4–6 hours. Non-sedating H_1 blockers do not work as well, but they are useful for the daytime hours (prevent somnolence); these include loratadine (Claritin 10 mg), cetirizine (Zyrtec 5 mg, 10 mg) and fexofenadine (Allegra 60 mg, 180 mg).
- Prednisone (e.g. 60 mg for 2 days, 40 mg for 5 days, and then 20 mg for 7 days) can be given periodically and may work in people whose condition is difficult to control with antihistamines.
- Epinephrine (adrenaline) is administered for extensive, severe cases.
- Generally, keeping the patient cool physically and emotionally is advisable.
- Cool, soothing baths (e.g. with Aveeno) can be suggested.
- Hot showers should be avoided as they only worsen the pruritus afterwards.
- Topical steroids are generally not effective.

Pearls

- Lesions occur on any skin surface, including the palms and soles. These lesions may have a clear center, and the surrounding skin is diffusely red and less swollen.

- The etiology may not be discovered in all cases.
- By definition, acute urticaria resolves within 6 weeks, with or without treatment.

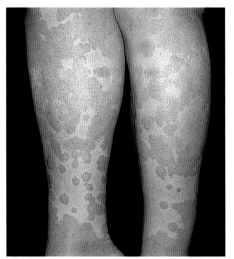

Circumscribed, raised, edematous, red plaques involve the superficial portion of the dermis. The itch varies in intensity. Lesions vary from a few to numerous and vary in configuration.

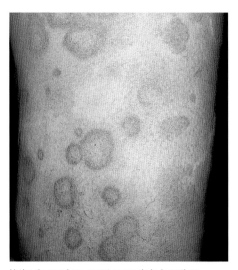

Urticaria resolves spontaneously in less than 14 days in most patients. It persists for months and sometimes years in about 5% of patients. These lesions have a clear center, and the surrounding skin is diffusely red and less swollen.

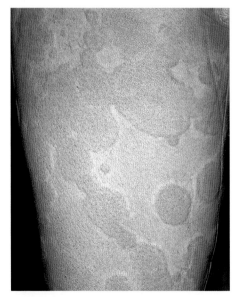

Lesions occur on any skin surface, including the palms and soles. They appear in many forms and last 12–24 hours. The most characteristic presentation is a red, raised plaque surrounded by a faint white halo. When confluent, they become polycyclic.

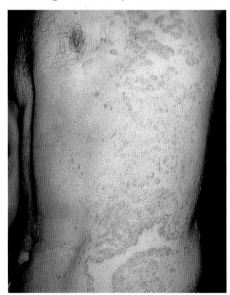

Plaques have become confluent on the trunk.

Chronic Urticaria (Hives)

Description
- Chronic urticaria is defined as urticaria or whealing of the skin for more than 6 weeks.

History
- The cause is discovered in only 5–20% of cases.
- People of all ages the world over are affected, but the highest incidence is in young adults.
- Chronic urticaria is usually easily diagnosed but presents a major problem in treatment and management.
- The course of the disease is unpredictable, and can last months or years.
- Patients should be evaluated for the five *I*s:
  - Ingestants (common): foods, additives, and drugs such as antibiotics or other drugs that are relatively new to the patient
  - Inhalants: dust, feather, pollen
  - Injectants: drugs, stings, bites
  - Infections: bacterial, viral, fungal, parasitic
  - Internal diseases: such as chronic infections, thyroid disease, lupus erythematosus

Skin Findings
- These are pink to red, figurate and annular, edematous, migrating wheals or plaques.
- Lesions vary in size from just millimeters to areas that can cover an entire hand.
- These plaques can be coalescing and polycyclic and change in size and shape over time.
- Individual lesions resolve within 24 hours, while new lesions appear.

Laboratory
- If the cause is unclear after routine history and physical examination, laboratory tests are rarely helpful.
- Tests to consider include a complete blood count, sinus x-rays to evaluate for sinusitis, dental x-rays to evaluate for an occult dental abscess, rapid streptococcal test or pharyngeal culture, and a thyroid-stimulating hormone and thyroid microsomal antibody test for autoimmune thyroid disease.

Differential Diagnosis
- Physical urticaria
- Erythema multiforme
- Urticarial vasculitis
- Bullous pemphigoid

Treatment
- Antihistamines are prescribed initially.
- Hydroxyzine 10–25 mg can be administered every 4 hours, up to 100 mg every 4 hours as needed. Hydroxyzine causes sedation.
- Non-sedating antihistamines should be considered for daytime use. These include desloratadine (Clarinex 5 mg), cetirizine (Zyrtec 5 mg, 10 mg), and fexofenadine (Allegra 60 mg, 180 mg).
- Histamine receptor type 1 antagonists (H_1 blockers) may be combined with type 2 antagonists (H_2 blockers) such as cimetidine 400 mg twice daily or ranitidine 150 mg twice daily.
- Oral steroids are a second line of treatment for hives; however, their use for chronic urticaria is controversial and sometimes detrimental.

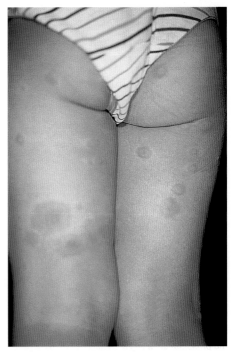

Urticaria is common, occurring in up to 25–50% of the population. People of all ages are affected, but the highest incidence is in young adults.

■ Empiric antibiotic therapy may be tried if an occult infection, such as a tooth abscess, is suspected.

■ Despite aggressive therapy many cases of chronic urticaria persist indefinitely.

Pearls

■ Individual urticarial lesions are recurrent, migratory and pruritic, but tend to resolve in a 24-hour period, while new lesions appear.

■ Urticarial vasculitis is a systemic disease that may be related to lupus erythematosus, which mimics chronic urticaria, but differs in that it leaves purpuric patches. Diagnosis is made via biopsy.

■ Early bullous pemphigoid may present with urticarial plaques, prior to bullae formation.

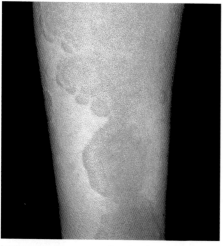

Lesions may become confluent and sometimes cover an entire extremity.

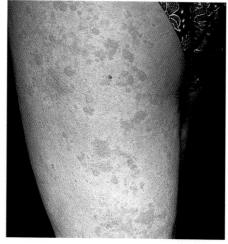

A portion of the border may be reabsorbed, giving the appearance of incomplete rings. A variation in color is usually present in superficial hives. Thicker plaques have a uniform color.

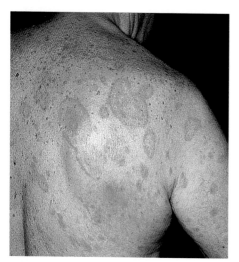

The presentation is highly variable. Here, the lesions resemble the targets of erythema multiforme.

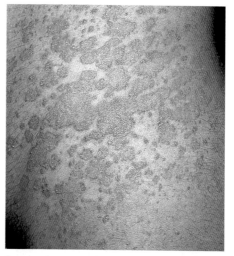

Some patients with extensive involvement have systemic symptoms such as shortness of breath, wheezing, nausea, abdominal pain, diarrhea, and headache.

Physical Urticaria

Description
- Physical urticaria is a brief attack of urticaria or hives induced by physical stimuli such as scratching, pressure, vibration, heat, cold, and ultraviolet light.

History
- The major distinguishing feature is that these eruptions are brief and usually self-limited.
- Most of these attacks of urticaria last 1–6 hours.
- Dermatographism is the most common physical urticaria. In this case, hives are produced by rubbing and stroking the skin. This entity can be triggered by viral infection, by antibiotic therapy, or emotional upset, although the cause is usually not determined.
- Pressure urticaria occurs 4–6 hours after a pressure stimulus and may last from 8–72 hours. Deep burning, or painful swelling occurs. The hands, feet, trunk, buttocks, lips, and face are commonly affected. Lesions are induced by standing, by walking, by wearing tight garments, or sitting on a hard surface for long time. This condition can be disabling for those performing manual labor.
- Cholinergic urticaria is a variant of hives that begins within 1–20 minutes of overheating from exercise, exposure to heat, or emotional stress. It may last for minutes to hours. This condition presents in people aged 10–30 years of age and tends to be chronic.
- Cold urticaria occurs with a sudden drop in air temperature or exposure to cold water. This condition often begins after infection, drug therapy, or emotional stress. The age of onset is 18–25 years and can be chronic.
- In solar urticaria, hives occur minutes after exposure to the ultraviolet light and disappear in about 1 hour. Several different wavelengths of ultraviolet light cause solar urticaria. In most, this condition is persistent.

Skin Findings
- Pruritic, linear wheals after rubbing or scratching define dermatographism.
- Repeated deep swelling at sites of prolonged pressure is a clue to the diagnosis of pressure urticaria.
- Annular, papular hive lesions, 2–4 mm in diameter, surrounded by extensive red flare are characteristic of cholinergic urticaria.
- Cold and solar urticaria are similar in clinical appearance to other forms of urticaria and are generally diagnosed by history.

Tests
The diagnosis is usually suspected by the clinical examination and history, and confirmed by one of several simple office tests.
- For dermatographism or physical urticaria, a tongue blade drawn firmly across the arm or back produces a linear wheal within 1–3 minutes.
- In pressure urticaria, testing with localized pressure points can usually confirm the diagnosis.
- In cholinergic urticaria, the patient runs in place or uses an exercise bicycle for 10–15 minutes. Then the patient is observed for up to 1 hour to detect typical papular hives.
- In cold urticaria, hives are induced with an ice pack or an ice cube held against the skin for 1–5 minutes.
- In solar urticaria, phototesting with ultraviolet A, ultraviolet B, and visible light identifies the wavelengths that produces the hives.

Differential Diagnosis
- Polymorphous light eruption and lupus erythematosus can be confused with solar urticaria. Although controversial, some think all three of these entities might be related.

Treatment
- In dermographism, treatment is often unnecessary. Symptomatic dermographism is treated with antihistamines (e.g. hydroxyzine); low dosages (10–25 mg every 4 hours) provide adequate relief. The conditions

of many patients are controlled for long periods with very low doses of hydroxyzine. Long-acting, non-sedating antihistamines can also be effective.

■ In cholinergic urticaria, strenuous exercise is limited. Hydroxyzine (10–50 mg) can be taken 1 hour before exercise.

■ In cold urticaria, the patient should be protected from sudden decreases in temperature. Cyproheptadine (Periactin) is effective but sedating. The dosage is adjusted to control symptoms.

■ In solar urticaria, antihistamines can be employed, but sunscreens and vigorous sun avoidance should be recommended. For some patients, small, incremental increases in ultraviolet light may be helpful.

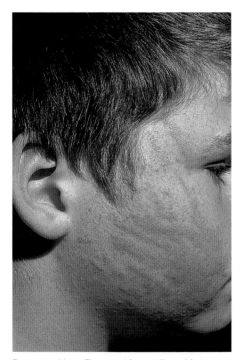

Dermographism. The onset is usually sudden; young patients are affected most commonly. The degree of response varies. Young patients may be highly reactive for months and then appear to be in remission, only to have symptoms recur.

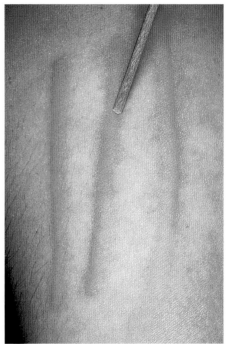

Dermographism is the most common form of physical urticaria. Scratching produces a linear wheal that fades in 15 to 60 minutes. Itching is mild to intense. The skin should be stroked in any patient who complains that scratching creates itching and swelling.

Angioedema

Description
■ Angioedema is an acute or chronic hive-like swelling in the subcutaneous tissue of the skin and mucosa.

History
■ Hives and angioedema commonly occur simultaneously.
■ The deeper reaction (angioedema) produces a more diffuse swelling.
■ Itching is usually absent, but burning and painful swelling are typical.
■ The lips, palms, soles, limbs, trunk, and genitalia are most commonly affected.
■ Involvement of the gastrointestinal and respiratory tracts produces dysphagia, dyspnea, colicky abdominal pain, and attacks of vomiting and diarrhea.
■ There are two forms of the disease: acute and chronic.
■ In acute angioedema, there is a severe allergic type 1 immediate hypersensitivity immunoglobulin E-mediated reaction. The disease is usually self-limited.
■ Identification and removal of the offending agent (e.g. drugs, contrast dyes) is usually curative. Most of these acute attacks resolve within 24–48 hours.
■ The etiology of most cases of chronic angioedema is unknown. The condition is most common in 40–50-year-old women. The pattern of recurrence is unpredictable, and episodes can occur for 5 or more years.
■ Late-onset, recurrent angioedema may indicate an acquired deficiency of C1q esterase inhibitor.
■ Two types of acquired angioedema are described. One form is associated with malignancy (usually B cell lineage); the other is defined by the presence of an autoantibody directed against the C1 inhibitor molecule. Both are very rare.

Skin Symptoms
■ The reaction is similar to that of hives, but there is also deeper edema (swelling) of the subcutaneous tissues of the skin and mucosa. The clinical appearance tends to be more dramatic than hives and can cause disfigurement to the point where the patient is unrecognizable.

Laboratory
■ Thyroid microsomal and thyroglobulin antibodies are present in some patients with chronic angioedema.
■ Patients with acquired C1-inhibitor deficiency have low levels or absence of functional C1-inhibitor activity, and low levels of CH_{50}, C1q, C1, C4, and C2.

Treatment
■ Acute severe attacks are treated with epinephrine (adrenaline) and high dosages of antihistamines.
■ EpiPen or EpiPen Jr is prescribed for patients who experience severe reactions.
■ Affected patients should wear a medical alert bracelet that identifies the diagnosis.
■ For chronic disease, antihistamines such as hydroxyzine can be used.
■ Systemic corticosteroids may be required for suppression.
■ The use of levothyroxine should be considered if patients are hypothyroid.

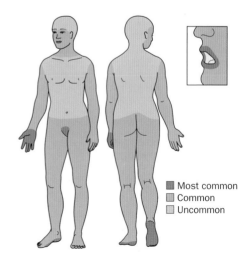

■ Most common
■ Common
□ Uncommon

Pearls

- Angioedema affects the face, lips, palms, soles, or a portion of an extremity. It may become confluent and cover wide areas. The color is uniform, whereas hives are generalized and may vary in color.

- Angioedema is a hive-like swelling cause by increased vascular permeability in the subcutaneous tissue of the skin and mucosa. Hives and angioedema may occur simultaneously.

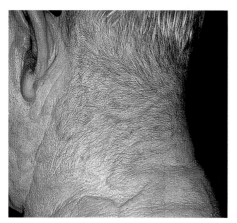

Angioedema affects the face, lips, palms, soles, or a portion of an extremity. It may become confluent and cover wide areas. The color is uniform. Hives vary in color.

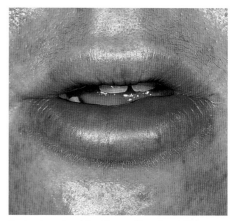

Angioedema is a hive-like swelling caused by increased vascular permeability in the subcutaneous tissue of the skin and mucosa. Hives and angioedema may occur simultaneously. Itching is usually absent. Symptoms consist of burning and painful swelling.

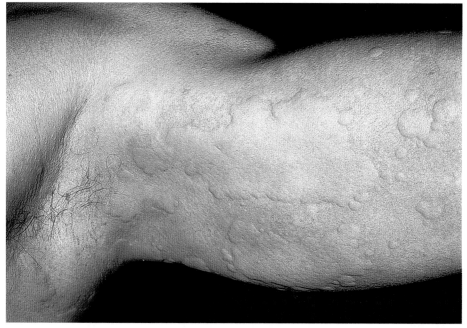

Angioedema. Urticarial plaques are confluent and cover wide areas.

Mastocytosis (Urticaria Pigmentosa)

Description
- Mastocytosis or urticaria pigmentosa is a rare disease in which the skin is excessively infiltrated by mast cells.
- There are several clinical presentations; the pediatric cutaneous or urticaria pigmentosa form is the most common.
- Other variants of cutaneous mastocytosis and mast cell disease include telangiectasia macularis eruptiva perstans, solitary mastocytoma, and diffuse cutaneous mastocytosis.
- There are more severe systemic variants of mast cell disease (including mast cell leukemia) but these are rare.

History
- The incidence is 1 in 1000 to 1 in 8000 live births.
- Mastocytosis is usually confined to the skin in young children.
- Adults are more likely to develop systemic forms of mast cell disease.
- The cause is unknown; familial occurrence is rare.
- The onset occurs between birth and 2 years in 55% of cases.
- Typically, the condition improves gradually and usually clears spontaneously by puberty.
- Mast cell disease that begins after age 10 usually persists for life.
- When this disease is systemic, the gastrointestinal tract and the skeletal system are most commonly involved and there can be an associated mast cell leukemia.
- When large numbers of mast cell lesions are present, pruritus can be severe and difficult to treat.

Skin Findings
- There are two main types: localized and generalized.
- The most common presentation is pediatric-onset localized cutaneous disease.
- Findings consist of reddish-brown, slightly elevated, non-blanchable macules and patches, averaging 0.5–1.5 cm in diameter.
- Patches may occur in small groups or be generalized on the trunk.
- The patches are often dismissed as variations of pigmentation or café-au-lait macules.
- A larger, nodular and solitary lesion is called a mastocytoma.
- Erythema and blisters (often after scratching) are common in the first 2 years of life.
- Stroking any lesion induces intense erythema and a wheal response; this is termed Darier's sign. Such a reaction is the hallmark of urticaria pigmentosa, but can also be seen in leukemia cutis.

Laboratory
- A skin biopsy can be very helpful, but special stains are required.
- Metachromatic stains, such as Giemsa and toluidine blue, stain cytoplasmic mast cell granules deep blue, which is characteristic.
- Sparse numbers of mast cells are normally present in skin, but significantly increased numbers of mast cells around vessels are diagnostic.
- Quantitation of urinary N-methylimidazoleacetic acid (a major metabolite of histamine) and other metabolites are used as a measure of systemic disease.

Differential Diagnosis
- Urticaria
- Dermatographism
- Bites
- Café-au-lait spots
- Congenital pigment abnormalities

Treatment
- Topical steroids, often under occlusion, are useful for limited areas.
- Recognition helps parents limit unintentional scratching and trauma of the lesions.
- In children, more generalized disease is treated with antihistamines and oral cromolyn.

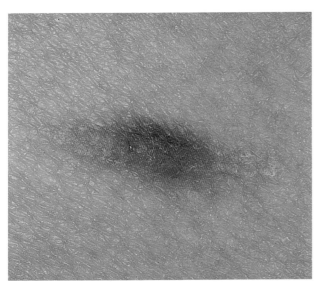

A single small brown macule was stroked with the wood end of a cotton-tipped applicator. Intense erythema occurred in about one minute. This was rapidly followed by intense swelling and itching.

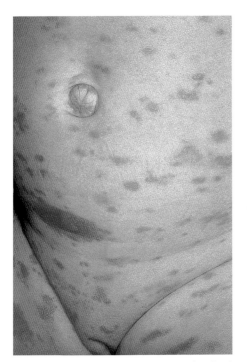

A few to many slightly elevated plaques, colored red to brown, typically occur between birth and 2 years of age. The trunk is the most common site.

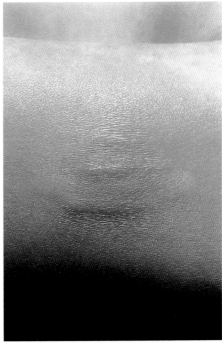

Stroking a lesion produces a wheal surrounded by intense erythema (Darier's sign). The reaction occurs within minutes.

■ Systemic disease is managed in a stepwise manner.
- Antihistamine H_1 blockers for flushing and pruritus
- Antihistamine H_2 blockers or proton-pump inhibitors for gastrointestinal manifestations
- Oral cromolyn sodium can be helpful for diarrhea and abdominal pain
- Non-steroidal antiinflammatory agents can be used for severe flushing; they block mast cell biosynthesis of prostaglandin D_2

■ Photochemotherapy with psoralen plus ultraviolet A can be useful in extensive cases.
■ Avoidance of mast cell stimulators such as morphine, codeine, dextromethorphan.

Pearls
■ Stroking a lesion produces a wheal surrounded by intense erythema (Darier's sign) within minutes. This sign is the hallmark of urticaria pigmentosa.

PEDIATRIC CONSIDERATIONS
- Most cases of urticaria pigmentosa occur in the neonate and infant. Parents need reassurance that this is not a life-threatening problem, and it often resolves later in life.
- Multiple, reddish-brown, slightly elevated macules and patches typically occur between birth and 2 years of age. The trunk is the most common site.
- Parents must know about potential mast cell degranulators or triggers and avoid them whenever possible. Non-immunologic mast cell degranulators are shown in the table opposite.
- Children with urticaria pigmentosa may be at increased risk of anaphylaxis after insect stings. The parents should carry an epinephrine (adrenaline) pen (EpiPen Jr) and should ensure that their children wear a medical alert bracelet.

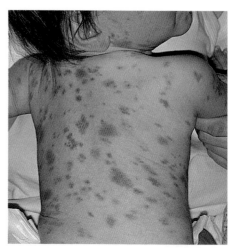

Urticaria pigmentosa. Lesions vary in size and number. Many patients present with just a few brown macules that may be misinterpreted as café-au-lait spots. Other patients have many large lesions. These patients are unstable and may have many episodes of severe itching.

Non-Immunologic Mast Cell Degranulators

Venoms (snakes, insect stings)

Aspirin and other non-steroidal anti-inflammatory drugs

Iodine-containing radiocontrast media

Narcotics (codeine, morphine)

Polymyxin B

Dextran

Jellyfish stings

Neuromuscular blocking agents (used in general anesthesia)

Sympathomimetics (amphetamines, ephedrine, dextromethorphan)

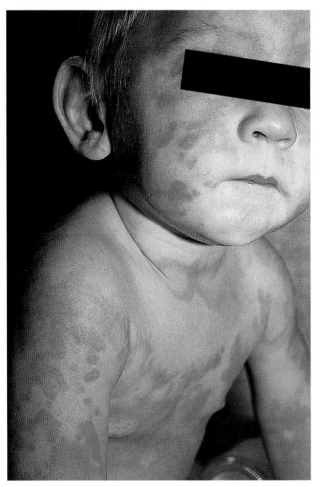

Urticaria pigmentosa. Lesions tend to be larger in children than adults. Lesions in children are more hyperpigmented than erythematous. The trunk is the most commonly affected area. Involvement of the face and scalp does occur. Vesicles and blisters may form on lesions in children. These blisters are tense and may become hemorrhagic, but they heal without scarring. The tendency to form blisters resolves after age 3.

Pruritic Urticarial Papules and Plaques of Pregnancy

Description
- Pruritic urticarial papules and plaques of pregnancy is the most common gestational dermatosis.
- It is characterized by intensely pruritic papules and urticarial plaques that start on the abdomen and within striae late in the third trimester.

History
- The average age of onset is 25 years (range 16–40 years).
- The incidence is 1 in 160 pregnancies.
- About 40% of cases involve primigravidas, 30% involve women who are pregnant for the second time, and about 15% involve women who are pregnant for the third time.
- Most cases begin late in the third trimester, but they can occur in the first or second trimester. Postpartum onset (3–5 days) is very rare.
- The mean duration is 6 weeks, but the rash is usually not severe for more than 1–3 weeks.
- Recurrence with future pregnancies is unusual.

Skin Findings
- The problem begins on the abdomen in 90% of patients.
- In those with striae, the problem most often presents in or around the striae.
- The rash spreads in a few days in a symmetric fashion to involve the buttocks, upper and lower extremities, chest, and back. The hands, feet, palms, soles, and face are usually not involved.
- Itching is moderate to intense; excoriations are rarely seen.
- Lesions begin as red papules that are often surrounded by a pale halo.
- They quickly increase in number and may become confluent, forming edematous urticarial plaques. Blisters do not occur.

Laboratory
- Biopsy reveals a slight to moderate perivascular infiltrate of mononuclear cells, some eosinophils, and variable epidermal spongiosis.
- There are no laboratory abnormalities; the results of direct immunofluorescence of lesional and perilesional skin are negative. This separates the disease from herpes gestationis, which would show positive direct immunofluorescence with immunoglobulin G and C3 at the basement membrane zone.

Course and Prognosis
- There are no associated complications during pregnancy and delivery.
- Recurrences in subsequent pregnancies are unusual.
- Infants do not develop the eruption.
- If vesicles and bullae develop, direct immunofluorescence should be performed to evaluate for herpes gestationis.

Discussion
- Congenital abnormalities are absent or are unrelated to this disease.
- Unlike acute urticaria, the eruption remains fixed and increases in intensity, clearing in most cases before or within 1 week of delivery.

Treatment
- Treatment is supportive. The expectant mother can be assured that the pruritus will quickly terminate before or after delivery.

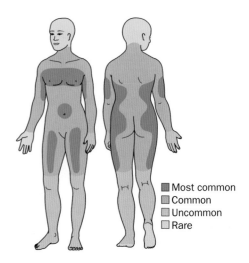

Most common
Common
Uncommon
Rare

- Itching can be relieved with group II–V topical steroids, with cool, wet dressings, antipruritic lotions (Sarna lotion), and antihistamines.

- Prednisone 30–40 mg per day may be required if the pruritus becomes intolerable, but this is rarely needed.

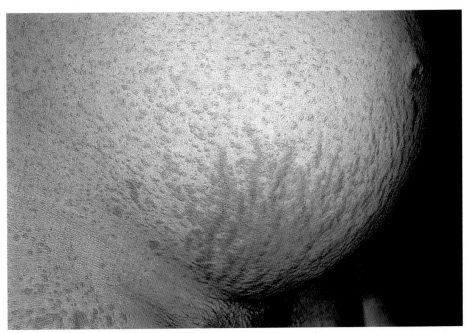

Lesions begin as red papules surrounded by a narrow, pale halo. They increase in number and become more confluent. Unlike urticaria, these lesions remain fixed and may not disappear until after delivery.

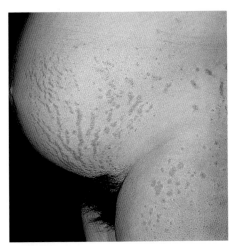

The abdomen is often the initial site of involvement. Initial lesions may be confined to striae.

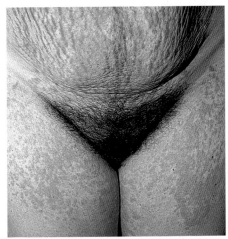

Lesions spread in a symmetric fashion to involve the buttocks, legs, arms, and back of the hands. The face is not involved.

4 Acne, Rosacea and Related Disorders

Acne

Description

- Acne is a papular or pustular eruption, involving the face, chest, and back.

History

- Acne is common in the teenage years, but may persist well into adulthood.
- Plugged sebaceous pores, increased sebum production, and *Propionibacterium acnes* are thought to promote acne.
- There are several variants of acne.
  - Steroid acne (a comedonal and pustular acne on the chest 2–5 weeks after a steroid has been taken)
  - Neonatal acne (acne at birth)
  - Infantile acne (during infancy)
  - Acne necrotica (itchy acne of the scalp)
  - Acne excoriée (acne that has been manipulated by the patient, leaving erosions and scars)
- Fatty foods cause obesity, not acne.

Skin Findings

- Acne lesions are divided into inflammatory and noninflammatory lesions.
- Non-inflammatory lesions consist of open comedones (blackheads) and closed comedones (whiteheads).
- Inflammatory lesions are characterized by the presence of papules, pustules, and nodules (cysts).
- Papules are smaller than 5 mm in diameter.
- Pustules have a visible central core of purulent material.
- Nodules are larger than 5 mm in diameter. They may become suppurative (cysts) or hemorrhagic.
- Recurring rupture and reepithelialization of cysts lead to epithelial-lined sinus tracks, often accompanied by disfiguring scars.

Non-Skin Findings

- Patients with androgen excess can develop signs of virilism (thinning of scalp hair, hirsutism) and precocious puberty.
- Rarely, acne occurs in association with fever and bone and joint problems (acne fulminans).
- Significant psychosocial issues may be present including depression, anxiety and social withdrawal.

Laboratory and Biopsy

- Laboratory evaluation is indicated for female patients with persistent acne and evidence of a hyperandrogenic state (facial hair, muscle hypertrophy, irregular menses).
- Tests include measurements for testosterone, follicle-stimulating hormone, luteinizing hormone, and dehydroepiandrosterone sulfate.
- Bacterial and fungal cultures can be done to rule out infectious folliculitis.

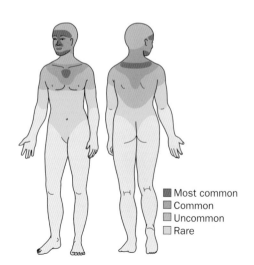

- Most common
- Common
- Uncommon
- Rare

Differential Diagnosis

- Rosacea (flushing and blushing but no comedones)
- Bacterial (gram negative) and yeast folliculitis (not typical on the face)
- Keratosis pilaris (location more typical on the extensor upper arms)

Course and Prognosis

- Men have more severe disease than women; men are less likely to seek early medical treatment.
- Androgens can aggravate acne. It is important to ask about use of anabolic steroids, especially in athletes.
- The propensity to form scars varies from patient to patient.
- The redness and pigmentation after resolution of acne lesions may take many months to fade.
- Many women notice premenstrual flares.
- Areas where the skin is rubbed, such as under the hat or under a chin strap, may have accentuated acne.
- Acne occurs with variable severity. Sometimes only comedones appear; at other times, cystic lesions predominate.
- Acne usually begins between ages 10 years and 15 years and lasts for 5–10 years.
- Children who require oral medications at an early age tend to have a more severe course.
- Women over the age of 25 are a special problem in the treatment of acne. They tend to have long-term low-grade acne.

Treatment

- Therapy should take into account medical and psychosocial issues.
- A program can be established in three visits for most patients.
- It takes at least 2 months for most topical medications to show their full effect, so patience must be exercised.
- Most treatment is continual and prolonged, since it is control—not cure— that is most often achieved.
- A patient's propensity to scar should be determined. Patients who show evidence of scarring may be given a 2-month trial of topical therapy and oral antibiotics.

- Isotretinoin (Accutane, Amnesteen, Sotret) can be considered if there is no substantial improvement. Patients with nodulocystic acne may be started on isotretinoin as initial therapy.
- Treatment should be aggressive; scarring should not be allowed.
- A framework that helps in acne therapy is to think about the disease as oily skin, blocked pores, and inflamed pores.

Oily Skin

- Washing with warm water (not scrubbing) is useful; excessive washing interferes with most treatment programs.
- Hair conditioners and oils should be avoided.
- Low-dose isotretinoin is useful for patients with very oily skin. Dermatologists have various treatment schedules for this use.
- If cosmetics are used, they should be oil free and water based.
- Patients should not pick or pop their acne lesions.

Non-Inflamed Blocked Pores (Comedones—Blackheads and Whiteheads)

- Agents that induce continuous mild drying and peeling are used. These agents are used alone or combined with tretinoin and related drugs.

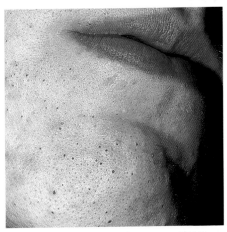

Open comedones (blackheads). Impacted sebum and cellular debris distend the follicular orifice.

- Prescription and over-the-counter products used for this purpose contain sulfur, salicylic acid, resorcinol, and benzoyl peroxide.
- Some examples of benzoyl peroxide preparations are Benzac AC 2.5%, 5%, 10%, Benzagel 5%, 10%, Brevoxyl 4%, 8%, and Triaz 3%, 6% or 9%. Many of these preparations are available as a wash (Brevoxyl Creamy wash 4%, 8% and Triaz wash 4%, 6%, 9%).
- Azelaic acid (Finaca cream) is comedolytic and antibacterial.
- Tretinoin and related drugs are comedolytic. Tretinoin (Retin-A) is available in several preparations. Retin-A solution (0.05%) is the most irritating. Retin-A gel (0.025%, 0.01%) is drying and is for oily skin. Retin-A cream (0.1%, 0.05%, 0.025%) is lubricating and is best for dry skin. Retin-A micro (0.04, 0.1%), Avita cream (0.025%), and Renova cream (0.02%, 0.05%) are less irritating formulations of tretinoin. Adapalene (Differin) 0.1% gel, cream, pads, or solution may be less irritating. Adapalene does not cause the heightened sensitivity to sunlight found with tretinoin and tazarotene. Tretinoin causes photosensitivity and increased burning tendency even when applied at bedtime.
- Tazarotene (Tazarac 0.05%, 0.1% gel and cream) is a strong and effective comedolytic. Using the cream formulation or having the patient use the gel formulation and wash it off at increasing intervals (short contact therapy) are methods to lessen irritation. It carries a pregnancy category X warning.
- Facial peels (glycolic acid, salicylic acid) are sometimes used to free blocked pores.

Inflamed Pores (Papules and Pustules)
- Many patients have a combination of comedones, papules, and pustules.
- Tretinoin or related drugs plus a benzoyl peroxide preparation are administered for comedones, papules, and pustules. Tretinoin is applied at bedtime and the benzoyl peroxide in the morning.
- Topical antibiotics, or benzoyl peroxide, or a combination of both (e.g. Benzaclin, Duac) plus sulfacetamide with or without sulfur are administered for papules and pustules. One preparation is applied in the morning and the other in the evening.
- Topical antibiotics can be prescribed initially or as adjunctive therapy after the patient's condition has adapted to tretinoin, to benzoyl peroxide, or both agents.
- Topical antibiotics include clindamycin (Clindagel, Cleocin T lotion, Clindets pads), erythromycin (A/T/S, EryDerm, Erygel, Erycette pads, Staticin, T-Stat pads), 3% erythromycin with 5% benzoyl peroxide (Benzamycin) and 1% clindamycin with 5% benzoyl peroxide (Benzaclin, Duac).
- Sulfacetamide-containing and sulfur-containing products (e.g. Sulfacet-R, AVAR cream or gel, Plexion TS) can be administered. Klaron lotion contains sulfacetamide. Specify tinted or tint free when prescribing Sulfacet-R (generic preparations tend to be too thin). Sulfacetamide and sulfur washes (e.g. AVAR, Plexion, Rosanil, Clenia) are effective and convenient.
- With oral antibiotics better clinical results and a lower rate of relapse are achieved by starting at higher dosages and tapering only after control is achieved.

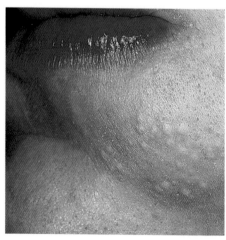

Closed comedones (whiteheads). Tiny white, dome-shaped papules have a very small follicular orifice.

- Typical starting dosages are tetracycline 500 mg twice a day; erythromycin 1 gm/day in divided doses; doxycycline 100 mg twice a day; and minocycline 100 mg twice a day.
- Antibiotics must be taken for weeks to be effective and are used for months to achieve maximal benefit.
- Available scientific and pharmacokinetic data do not support the hypothesis that antibiotics (with the exception of rifampin) lower the contraceptive efficacy of oral contraceptives.

Inflamed Nodules and Cysts (Nodulocystic Acne)

- Isotretinoin (Accutane, Amnesteen, Sotret) is very effective.
- A steroid (triamcinolone 2.5 mg/ml) can be injected into individual cysts. Caution is advised given the potential for atrophy.

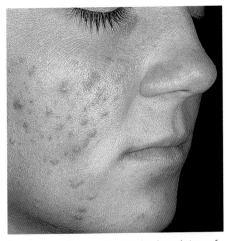

Papular acne. Red papules may be the only type of lesion. Topical medications and oral antibiotics are usually effective for control.

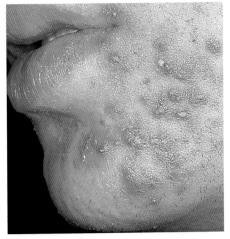

Pustular acne. The classic inflamed acne lesion. Scarring is possible. Topical medications and oral antibiotics are the treatments of first choice. Patients who have the potential to scar and in whom conventional treatment fails are candidates for isotretinoin.

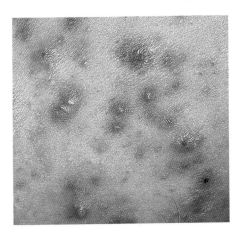

Cystic acne. Cysts are deeper in the skin than papules and pustules. They have the potential to extend and destroy surrounding follicular structures that result in scarring.

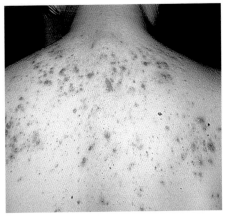

Cystic acne. The face, chest, and back are frequently involved. Some patients heal with extensive keloidal or atrophic scars. Cystic acne resists conventional topical medications and oral antibiotics. Isotretinoin is often required for control.

- Oral prednisone is sometimes used as initial therapy for very severe acne.
- In female patients, oral contraceptives (e.g. Ortho Tri-Cyclen, Yasmin, Alesse) can be beneficial.
- Spironolactone should be considered for women, especially in those not able to take an oral contraceptive, and for women who have relapsed after a course of isotretinoin. The dose is 50 mg twice daily. Some women require higher doses (up to 100 mg twice daily). Spironolactone may be taken with oral contraceptives. Pregnancy should be avoided.

Changes in Pigment and Scarring

- For scarring, referral to a dermatologic surgeon is advisable only after the acne is quiescent for at least 1 year. This allows for maximal normal healing before any invasive procedure.
- Red macules fade with time and are not true scars.
- Some patients, especially if they have dark complexions, develop light and/or dark macules that take many months or years to resolve, and which are permanent in some patients.
- Scars may be raised and thick (keloid) or depressed (ice-pick scars).
- Treatments for pigment changes include hydroquinone, tretinoin, azelaic acid, chemical peeling, and laser resurfacing.
- Treatment for acne scars include excision, laser, dermabrasion, chemical peeling, and injection with "fillers" (collagen, fat). Intralesional steroid (Kenalog) 2.5–10 mg/ml injections and application of silicone gel sheeting can be helpful for thick scars.

When to Refer

- Patients with the possibility of an underlying endocrine abnormality should be evaluated in consultation with a dermatologist and an endocrinologist.
- Patients with scarring acne, or acne that fails to respond to conventional treatment should be referred to a dermatologist.

Pediatric Considerations

- Neonates and infants can develop acne. Topical medicine is usually sufficient to control the acne, however, if recalcitrant inflammatory lesions or scarring are present, oral erythromycin or isotretinoin may be required.
- Tetracycline, doxycycline and minocycline should not be used in children less than age 12 years to avoid staining permanent teeth.

Pearls

- Combination therapy is essential to successful management of acne.
- Set realistic expectations with patients on the first visit, but be encouraging, and let patients know that acne therapy is extremely effective when used consistently and appropriately.

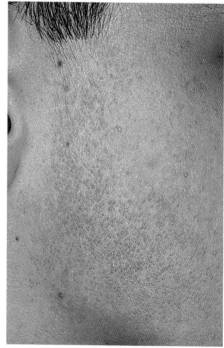

Parents often think that keratosis pilaris on the cheeks is acne. These pinpoint papules last for months or years (see p. 72).

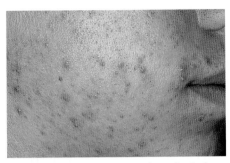

Papulopustular acne of moderate intensity. Oral antibiotics, sulfacetamide, and sulfur applied every day and 5% benzoyl peroxide applied every day were used as initial treatment. Rapid control was achieved after 8 weeks of treatment. Tretinoin gel was then substituted for sulfacetamide.

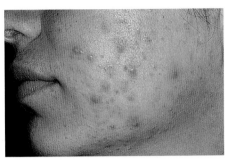

Cystic acne did not respond to oral antibiotic or topical medication and isotretinoin was prescribed.

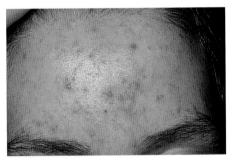

Papulopustular and comedone acne. Tretinoin gel applied every day and a combination of benzoyl peroxide and clindamycin (Benzaclin, Duac) applied every day were used as initial treatment.

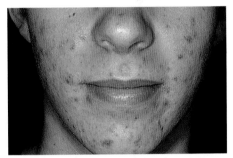

Papulopustular acne of moderate intensity. Oral antibiotics were refused. A combination of benzoyl peroxide and clindamycin (Benzaclin, Duac) applied at bedtime and sulfacetamide and sulfur were applied every morning.

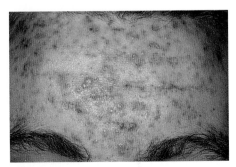

Acne can evolve quickly and scar. Parents do not understand this and often seek advice when the damage is already done.

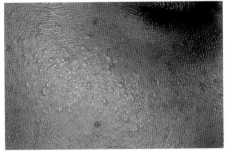

Milia are microcysts that are often misdiagnosed as closed comedone acne. They respond poorly to topical retinoids. Incision with an #11 surgical blade, followed by application of pressure by a comedone extractor removes the tiny amount of material.

Perioral Dermatitis

Description

■ Perioral dermatitis is a distinctive scaly papular eruption around the mouth, nose, and eyes that occurs almost exclusively in women.

History

■ The eruption may start around the mouth but may also involve the perinasal and periocular regions.
■ This condition is asymptomatic, or somewhat itchy.
■ Patients may have tried topical steroids, which cause temporary improvement but may contribute to refractory progressions.
■ Perioral dermatitis typically occurs in young women and can occur in children.
■ Isolation of a *Fusobacterium* suggests a bacterial etiology.
■ The routine use of moisturizers and fluorinated products may be a cause.

Skin Findings

■ Pinpoint papules and pustules on a red and scaling base are confined to the chin and nasolabial folds.
■ There is a clear zone around the vermilion border.
■ Pustules on the cheeks adjacent to the nostrils are common.
■ Sometimes, perioral dermatitis remains confined to the perinasal area. Sometimes, it occurs lateral to the eyes.
■ Children often have periocular and perinasal lesions.

Differential Diagnosis

■ Acne
■ Seborrheic dermatitis
■ Atopic (eczematous) dermatitis
■ Impetigo

Course and Prognosis

■ There are varying degrees of involvement.
■ A persistent eruption continues for months.
■ With oral treatment, most problems clear in 2 weeks.
■ Relapse is common.
■ Patients are retreated with renewed activity and sometimes long-term maintenance is required.

Treatment

■ Topical treatment involves twice daily use of 1% metronidazole cream (MetroGel), sodium sulfacetamide 10% plus sulfur 5% (Sulfacet-R), clindamycin (Cleocin T pads, solution, and lotion) or erythromycin 2% solution (A/T/S) or gel (Emgel), pimecrolimus cream 1% (Elidel), and tacrolimus 0.03%, 0.1% ointment (Protopic). Oral antibiotics are used if a 4-6-week course of topical treatment fails.
■ Tetracycline (500 mg twice a day), erythromycin (500 mg twice a day), doxycycline (100 mg twice a day), or minocycline (100 mg twice a day) is given for a 2-4-week course. The condition of many patients responds to lower doses.
■ Once the condition is resolved, the antibiotic is stopped or tapered over 4-5 weeks.

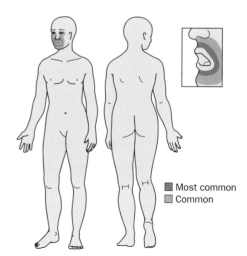

■ Most common
■ Common

Pearls

- The patient should consider limiting the use of moisturizers.
- Warn patients that prolonged use of topical steroids on the face worsens this disease.
- Discontinuing topical steroids will cause the disease to flare, but this is necessary to cure the disease.

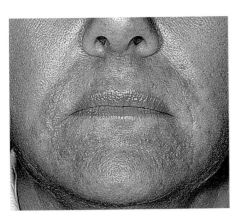

Group V topical steroids were used for months. The eruption flared each time they were discontinued.

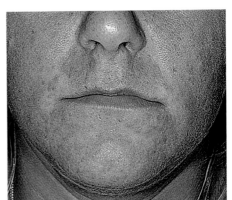

A classic case with the typical distribution. Pinpoint papules and pustules are located about the mouth, nasolabial folds and chin.

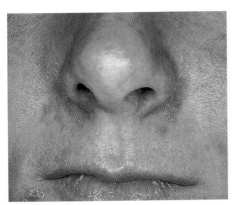

Pinpoint pustules next to the nostrils may be the first sign or only manifestation of the disease.

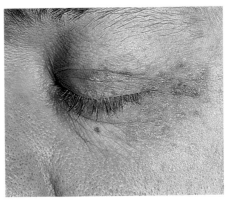

Pinpoint papules and pustules similar to those seen next to the nostrils are sometimes seen lateral to the eyes.

Rosacea (Acne Rosacea)

Description
- Rosacea is a common facial eruption characterized by redness, telangiectasia, flushing, blushing (vascular component) and papules and pustules (inflammatory component).

History
- Patients are usually over age 30.
- Rosacea can occur in children.
- The cause is unknown.

Skin Findings
- Eruptions appear on the forehead, cheeks, and nose and about the eyes.
- Erythema and/or telangiectasias are present.
- Usually, there are fewer than ten papules and pustules at any one time.
- Severe cases have numerous pustules, telangiectasia, diffuse erythema, oily skin, and edema (cheeks and nose).
- Chronic, deep inflammation of the nose leads to an irreversible skin thickening called rhinophyma. This is more common in men.
- Uncommonly, rosacea papules can involve the scalp, the torso, and the arms and legs.

Non-skin Findings
- Ocular symptoms include mild conjunctivitis with soreness, grittiness, and lacrimation.
- Ocular signs include conjunctival hyperemia, telangiectasia of the lid, blepharitis, superficial punctate keratopathy, chalazion, corneal vascularization and infiltrate, and corneal vascularization and thinning.

Laboratory and Biopsy
- The diagnosis usually is made with clinical exam. Tests are unnecessary.
- If lesions are atypical, bacterial culture is obtained to rule out folliculitis.
- If there is scaling, a potassium hydroxide test is performed to rule out tinea.
- A biopsy can be considered to rule out lupus.

Differential Diagnosis
- Acne (no comedones in rosacea)
- Pustular tinea
- Perioral dermatitis
- Infectious folliculitis (staphylococcal, gram negative acne)
- Lupus erythematosus

Course and Prognosis
- Rosacea is exacerbated by ingestion of hot foods and drinks, ingestion of alcohol (red wine) or heat and sun exposure.
- The condition is chronic (years) with episodes of activity followed by quiescence.

Treatment
- The patient should avoid hot food and drinks, spicy foods, red wine, and sunlight.
- Green-based cosmetic foundations will mask the redness.
- Sunscreens are recommended.
- The pustular component is treated topically or systemically.
- For topical treatment, metronidazole (MetroGel, MetroCream, MetroLotion, Noritate) and sulfacetamide plus sulfur lotion (e.g. AVAR, Sulfacet-R, Plexion TS, Rosac) are the most effective. Sulfacet-R is especially useful for oily skin; it is

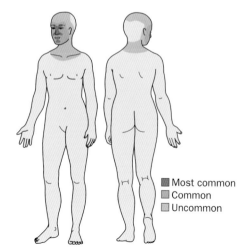

Most common
Common
Uncommon

available tinted or tint free. AVAR is available as a cream or gel. A special green formulation of AVAR cream and gel masks red skin. Rosac Clindamycin (Clindagel, Cleocin T solution, pads, or lotion) and erythromycin (Erycette pads, Emgel, T-Stat lotion or pads) are less effective.

■ Systemic therapy is more effective. Tetracycline (500 mg twice a day), erythromycin (500 mg twice a day), doxycycline (100 mg twice a day), or minocycline (100 mg twice a day) in a 2–4-week course usually controls the pustules. In many patients, this condition then responds to lower doses.

■ Bactrim DS twice a day or metronidazole 250 mg/day may be used for resistant cases.

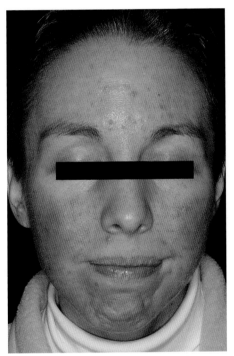

Active rosacea with pustules on the central forehead, cheeks and chin. Erythema is intense. Oral antibiotics and topical sulfacetamide with sulfur provided rapid control.

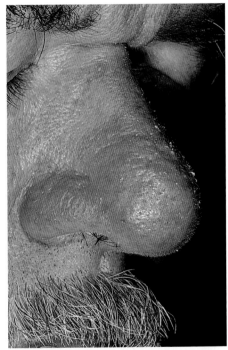

Deep erythema of the nose is highly characteristic of rosacea. Long-term treatment with oral antibiotics is often required. Drying topical therapy with sulfacetamide and sulfur is effective.

- Ocular symptoms are treated with systemic antibiotics.
- Medication is stopped or tapered after the condition resolves.
- The response after therapy is unpredictable.
- Recurring disease is retreated; then medication is tapered to the minimum dosage that provides adequate control.
- For chronic relapsing cases or failure to respond, isotretinoin (Accutane) 0.5 mg/kg/day for 20 weeks should be considered.
- Rhinophyma is treated with electrosurgery, carbon dioxide laser surgery, and plastic surgery.

Pearls

- Rarely, rosacea can present with granulomatous lesions (granulomatous rosacea) and mimic lupus or sarcoidosis.
- Patients can develop persistent facial edema called solid facial edema.

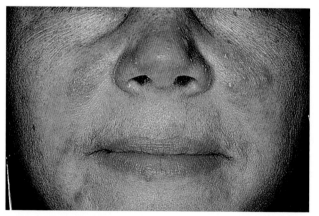

Acne and rosacea may coexist. Erythema of the nose is characteristic of rosacea. Pustules on the cheeks occur with rosacea and acne.

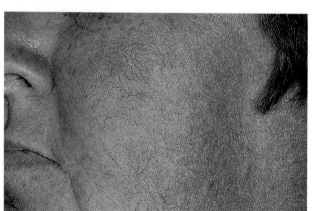

Erythema and telangiectasia may be the only sign of rosacea. The diagnosis may be difficult to establish because these same changes appear in some light-complexioned people. These changes respond poorly to topical or oral medication.

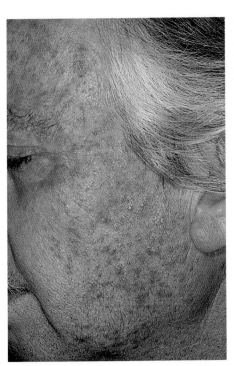

Steroid rosacea occurs when a patient who has used long-term continuous topical steroid therapy stops using the cream. There is a rapid and intense flare with papules and pustules. Application of the offending medication is resumed and re-establishes the vicious cycle.

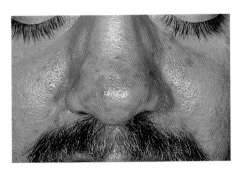

Papules and pustules on the nose are treated initially with oral antibiotics. Topical treatment should start at the same time as treatment with either sulfacetamide and sulfur, or metronidazole.

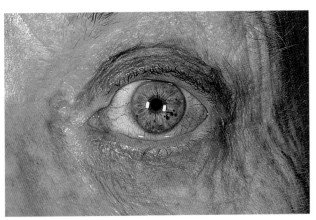

Ocular complications often occur in patients with rosacea. The diagnosis should be considered when a patient's eyes have one or more of the following signs and symptoms: watery or bloodshot appearance, foreign body sensation, burning or stinging, dryness, itching, light sensitivity, blurred vision, telangiectases of the conjunctiva and lid margin, or lid and periocular erythema. Blepharitis, conjunctivitis, and irregularity of the eyelid margins also may occur.

Hidradenitis Suppurativa

Description

■ Hidradenitis suppurativa is a chronic suppurative and scarring disease occurring in the axillae, in the anogenital regions, and under the female breast.

History

■ Hidradenitis suppurativa is more common in females.
■ It presents with a painful "boil."
■ It usually does not appear until after puberty. Most cases appear in the second and third decades of life.
■ There is clustering in families.
■ Sebum excretion is not an important factor, and this may explain the unsatisfactory therapeutic effect of conventional acne treatment and retinoids.

Skin Findings

■ The hallmark is the double comedone (a blackhead with two or more surface openings).
■ Sinus tracts are common.
■ Extensive, deep, dermal inflammation results in large, painful abscesses.
■ At involved sites there are cord-like bands of scar tissue.

Laboratory

■ Biopsy shows follicular occlusion by keratinous material, folliculitis, and secondary destruction of the skin adnexa (apocrine glands) and subcutis.

Differential Diagnosis

■ Acne
■ Furuncle or carbuncle

Course and Prognosis

■ It is worse in obese people.
■ The disease is progressive and self-perpetuating.
■ There is great variation among patients in the clinical severity.

Treatment

■ Large fluctuant cysts are incised and drained.
■ Intralesional triamcinolone acetonide (Kenalog) 2.5–10 mg/ml is administered for smaller cysts.
■ Weight loss can sometimes be helpful.
■ Long-term oral antibiotics are a mainstay of treatment. Agents include tetracycline (500 mg twice a day), erythromycin (500 mg twice a day), doxycycline (100 mg twice a day), and minocycline (100 mg twice a day). Lower dosages are tried for maintenance.
■ Second-line antibiotics include trimethoprim–sulfamethoxazole Bactrim DS (one by mouth twice a day), metronidazole (375 mg twice a day), and clindamycin (150 mg twice a day).
■ Oral contraceptives are sometimes helpful, especially with premenstrual flares.
■ Isotretinoin (1 mg/kg/day for 20 weeks) is effective in selected cases (best in early non-scarred sinus tract lesions).
■ Surgical excision is often the only solution.
■ Local opening of the sinus tract can be helpful.
■ Laser hair removal may be of benefit.
■ Powder (e.g. Zeasorb) and topical antiperspirants (e.g. Xerac) reduce friction.

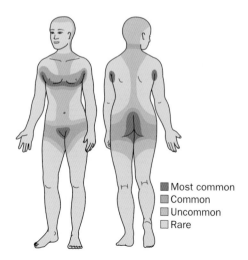

■ Most common
■ Common
■ Uncommon
□ Rare

Pearls

- This condition can be seen in prepubertal children—even those who are not obese.

- Early disease can present with very small tender pustules in the groin and axillae
- Suspect hidradenitis when women complain of "boils in the groin".

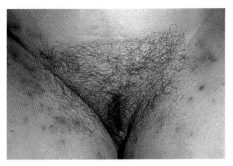

Hidradenitis should be suspected when a patient complains of boils in the groin. Comedones, which are markers for this disease, should be carefully sought.

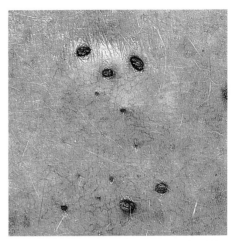

Double and triple comedones are blackheads with two or more surface openings that communicate under the skin. They are a hallmark of hidradenitis. The axillae, the area under the breast, the groin, and the buttock area should be examined for markers of the disease.

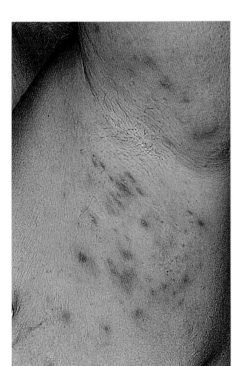

Hidradenitis of the axillae. Cysts were present for months and were eventually controlled with long-term oral antibiotics.

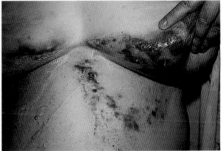

Hidradenitis may occur under the breasts. This is a particularly severe case with confluent cysts.

Hyperhidrosis

Definition

- The term hyperhidrosis is used to describe excessive sweat production.
- Hyperhidrosis is common and can involve localized or widespread areas of skin.

History

- Hyperhidrosis can be classified according to anatomic location (axillary, palmar, plantar), underlying stimulus (emotional, thermal, drug, toxin), or neural origin (cortical, hypothalamic, medullary, spinal, axonal).
- Sweating at night can be caused by a number of underlying systemic conditions (e.g. Hodgkin's lymphoma).
- Exercise and emotional stress are the most common causes of hyperhidrosis.
- Careful history is important to determine the underlying cause of hyperhidrosis.

Skin Findings

- Chronic effects of excessive skin moisture include dry, flaky skin with cracks and fissures.
- Patients with excessively moist skin are susceptible to bacterial overgrowth (pitted keratolysis) and yeast infection.
- Patients with pitted keratolysis develop small superficial pits on the soles, associated with intense foot odor.

Non-skin Findings

- Non-skin findings are dependent upon the underlying cause of hyperhidrosis.

Laboratory and Biopsy

- Sweat turns black when combined with iodine and starch (starch to iodine reaction). The three methods described below use the starch–iodine reaction to semiquantify sweat production.
  - Iodinated starch powder (0.5–1 g of iodine crystals to 500 g of soluble starch, stored in an airtight bottle) applied directly to the skin.
  - Iodine solution applied to the skin and dried followed by a light dusting of starch powder.
  - Iodine-impregnated paper (made by exposing 100 sheets of iodine paper to 1 g iodine crystals for 1 week in an airtight container) exposed to a sweaty skin surface (paper–iodine technique).
- Laboratory evaluation for underlying medical conditions should be directed by history and physical examination.

Differential Diagnosis

- The following conditions may induce hyperhidrosis
  - Infections (febrile illnesses, tuberculosis)
  - Metabolic/endocrine (hyperthyroidism, diabetes mellitus, obesity, carcinoid syndrome)
  - Vasomotor (Raynaud's phenomenon)
  - Neurologic (Parkinson's disease, postencephalitis)
  - Neoplasia (lymphoma)
- Many drugs can induce hyperhidrosis as a side effect (insulin, caffeine)
- Toxins such as mercury and arsenic can produce hyperhidrosis

Course and Prognosis

- Hyperhidrosis is socially and occupationally debilitating for patients.
- Treatment of underlying systemic conditions improves hyperhidrosis.

Treatment

- Topical application of 6% (Xerac) or 20% (Drysol) aluminum chloride hexahydrate under occlusion, at night for 3–4 nights, and then as needed is helpful for most patients. Mild skin irritation is a common side effect.
- Tap water iontophoresis (Drionic, General Medical Co., Department DM-8, 1935 Armacost Avenue, Los Angeles, CA 900025) given daily for 15–30 minutes and then two or three times a week, can be an effective method to control palmoplantar hyperhidrosis.
- Oral glycopyrrolate can diminish sweating in some patients, but can cause anticholinergic side effects.
- Botulinum toxin inhibits release of acetylcholine and is a very effective method to suppress sweating. Injections

are painful, and may require a topical anesthetic or nerve block for palmar hyperhidrosis. The axillae do not require anesthesia.

■ Cervical–thoracic and lumbar sympathectomy are other effective methods to control palmoplantar hyperhidrosis.

■ Local surgical ablation has been used to treat axillary hyperhidrosis.

Pediatric Considerations

● Emotional hyperhidrosis begins around puberty and improves with time.

● Boys and girls are affected equally, although girls more readily seek medical attention.

Psoriasis and Other Papulosquamous Diseases

Psoriasis

Description
- A common, chronic, inflammatory, papulosquamous disease of unknown etiology due to abnormal T lymphocyte function/communication.
- Skin, nails and joints are affected.
- There are several distinct clinical forms.
- The common presentation is chronic scaly plaques involving the elbows, knees, and scalp.

History
- Prevalence estimated at 1–3% of the population.
- Etiology is multifactorial and not completely understood.
- There are known inherited genetic factors with several documented environmental triggers.
- Men and women are equally affected, siblings and offspring are at increased risk of developing psoriasis.
- Onset at any age, though early onset implies a less stable, more severe clinical course.
- Age of onset peaks during 20s and again in late 50s.
- Once expressed, psoriasis is likely to follow a relentless, waxing and waning course.
- Extent and severity of disease varies widely.
- Environmental factors, including treatment, influence the course and severity.
- Factors which may exacerbate psoriasis include human immunodeficiency virus infection, physical trauma (Koebner phenomenon), infections (Streptococcus and Candida), drugs (lithium, beta-blockers, antimalarials, and corticosteroid withdrawal), and winter season.

- The degree of pruritus varies.
- The psychosocial impact can be severe.
- One-third of patients have nail involvement.
- Psoriatic arthritis (rheumatoid factor negative) is found in 5–8 % of the psoriatic population. Onset may precede, accompany, or follow skin manifestations.

Skin Findings
Plaque Psoriasis
- The most common presentation begins as red, sharply defined, scaling papules that coalesce to form stable round to oval plaques.
- It typically involves extensor extremities (elbows and knees), scalp, and sacrum.
- It usually spares the palms, soles, and face.
- The deep rich red color is a characteristic feature that remains constant.
- The scale is adherent, silvery white and reveals bleeding points when removed (the Auspitz sign).

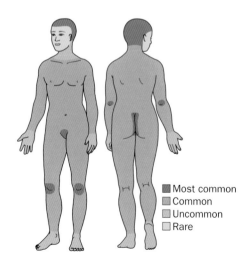

Most common
Common
Uncommon
Rare

- Scale may become extremely dense, especially on the scalp.

Guttate Psoriasis

- This is an unstable form, associated with sudden appearance of innumerable monomorphic psoriasiform papules on the trunk.
- It is often associated with group A streptococcal pharyngitis, viral infections and—less often—with systemic steroid withdrawal.

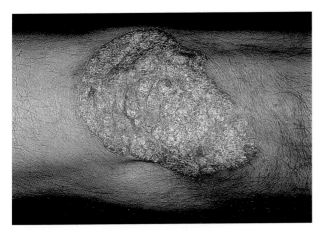

Plaque psoriasis. The classic presentation. The thick red plaques have a sharply defined border and an adherent silvery scale.

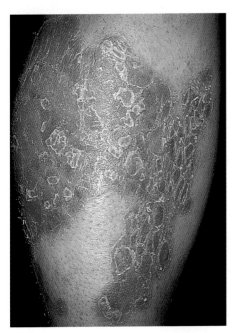

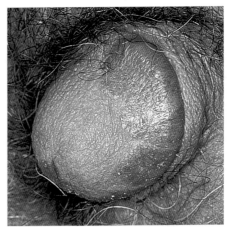

Plaque psoriasis. Plaques may become red and inflamed. Inflamed plaques need to be treated carefully with topical medication. All topical medications except topical steroids can aggravate these active lesions.

Plaque psoriasis. A fixed red plaque with a sharp border on the glans is a common presentation for psoriasis. It may be the only cutaneous lesion. The plaques often last for months and years. Topical steroids provide temporary relief but should not be used constantly. Most other topical medications are too irritating. Patients should be reassured that this disease is not contagious. Patients often misinterpret this disease as a yeast infection.

Localized Pustular Psoriasis (Palmoplantar Pustulosis)

- This chronic recurrent form has been associated with tobacco use.
- Small sterile pustules evolve from a red base on palms and soles.
- Pustules do not rupture but turn dark brown and scaly as they reach the surface; they are often quite painful
- Nail involvement is common.

Inverse (Intertriginous) Psoriasis

- An uncommon form occurring in flexural or intertriginous areas, often in the groin and under the breasts.
- There are smooth, red and sharply defined plaques with a macerated surface.
- Superimposed candidal infections are seen more commonly in diabetic patients and with topical steroid use.

Generalized Pustular Psoriasis

- An uncommon, severe form requiring immediate medical attention.
- It may be associated with fever and tenderness.
- It may be drug related.
- Sterile pustules are regional or generalized, and often occur in waves.

Erythrodermic Psoriasis

- This uncommon severe form requires immediate medical attention.
- There is total body redness with chills and skin pain.
- It may be drug related.

Nail Disease

- Clinical findings vary and are related to the specific areas of nail matrix involvement.
- Pitting, onycholysis (separation of nail from nail bed), subungual debris, oil drop sign, and nail dystrophy may occur.
- Nail findings offer supporting evidence of the diagnosis when skin changes are equivocal or absent.

Joint Disease

- Several distinct clinical patterns, which are rheumatoid factor negative.
- The asymmetric oligoarticular form is the most common, affecting 70% of those with arthritis.
- The distal interphalangeal type affects 10%, with nail changes.
- Symmetric polyarthritis is similar to rheumatoid arthritis.
- The mutilating type affects 5%; it has early onset.
- The spinal type affects 20% and is debilitating.

Laboratory

- Punch biopsy shows acanthosis (thickening of epidermis) with regular elongation of the rete, hyperkeratosis with retention of nuclei in stratum

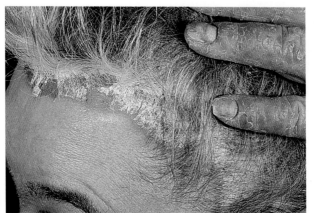

Scalp psoriasis. Dense scale covering a part or the entire scalp surface is highly characteristic of psoriasis. The scalps of all patients with psoriasis should be examined.

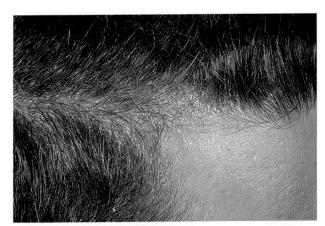

Scalp psoriasis. Sometimes it is impossible to distinguish between scalp psoriasis and seborrheic dermatitis. The ears and faces of patients with seborrheic dermatitis are often involved.

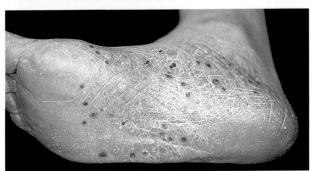

Pustular psoriasis of the soles. Extensive involvement is painful. Systemic medication is sometimes required.

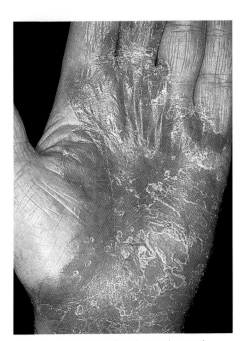

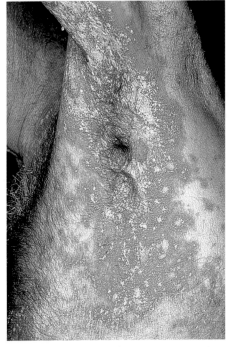

Psoriasis of the palms. This deep red, smooth plaque is painful.

Pustular psoriasis. This rare form of psoriasis can be extensive and serious. It responds to cyclosporine, methotrexate or acetritin.

corneum (parakeratosis), hypogranulosis, and neutrophils high in the epidermis (Munro microabscesses).
- In guttate psoriasis confirm streptococcal pharyngitis with an antistreptolysin-O titer or throat culture.
- In inverse psoriasis perform a potassium hydroxide exam to rule out *Candida.*
- In severe recalcitrant cases, evaluate for infection with human immunodeficiency virus.

Differential Diagnosis
- Seborrheic dermatitis (involves the face more often than psoriasis, but is not mutually exclusive on the scalp)
- Eczema (dyshidrotic hand/foot eczema; more vesicular than pustular)
- Tinea capitis (onychomycosis should be excluded with a potassium hydroxide exam)
- Candidiasis (not mutually exclusive, and may be superimposed on inverse psoriasis; a potassium hydroxide exam should be performed)
- Pityriasis rosea (look for herald patch, collarette of scale, or Christmas-tree distribution.)
- Acute generalized exanthematous pustulosis

Treatment
- The three categories of treatment—topical therapy, phototherapy or systemic therapy—may be combined or alternated.

Topical Therapy
Topical Tar Preparations
- These are available in lotions, ointments, and shampoos.
- They are relatively inexpensive, and may be compounded with topical steroids.
- They may cause irritation, odor, and staining of clothing.
- Calcipotriol (Dovonex) is a vitamin D_3 analogue in a cream, ointment, and scalp solution which can be applied every day or twice daily as tolerated in amounts up to 100 g per week.
- Confine medication to the plaques.

- Side effects are mild/transient local irritation and erythema.

Topical Steroids (Group I–V)
- Topical steroids (Group I–V) give fast but temporary relief.
- Use Group I–V topical steroids (applied at a different time of day) to control irritation.
- Optimum results may be obtained when calcipotriol is applied twice daily during the week, and the topical steroid is applied twice daily at weekends.
- These are the best agents for reducing inflammation and itching (e.g. intertriginous disease).
- Treat few, small, chronic plaques with intralesional steroid (Kenalog 10 mg/ml); use caution to avoid atrophy.
- Steroids become less effective with continued use.
- Side effects include atrophy and telangiectasia with long-term use.
- Best used in cycles e.g. twice daily for 7–14 days with a break of 7–14 days.

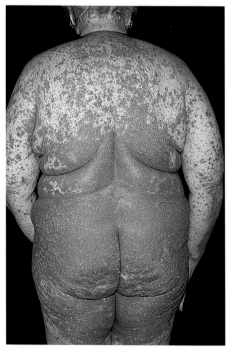

Erythrodermic psoriasis. Generalized intense inflammation can occur and often requires systemic medications for control.

- Anthralin (Drithocreme 0.1%, 0.25%, 0.5%, 0.1% HP; Micanol 1% cream) is useful for chronic extensor surface plaques and for the scalp.
  - Use a short contact method—apply and wash off in 20 minutes.
  - Leave medication on for longer if tolerated.
  - Confine medication to the plaque.
  - Side effects include irritation and staining.
- Tazarotene (Tazorac) gel or cream (0.05%, 0.1%)
  - Use topically once per night.
  - Confine medication to the plaque.
  - Apply steroids (groups I–V) once per day to control irritation and use less frequently once irritation is controlled.
  - A side effect is severe irritation.

Topical Scalp Treatment
- The scalp is difficult to treat. The goal is to provide symptomatic and/or cosmetic relief.
- Scale should be removed first to facilitate penetration of medicine.
- Superficial scale can be removed with salicylic acid or tar shampoos.

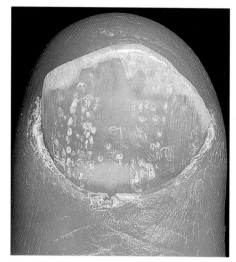

Psoriasis pitting. Foci of inflammation of the proximal nail matrix results in the accumulation of parakeratotic cells on the nail surface. These are shed as the nail grows out, leaving depressions or pits, in the nail surface.

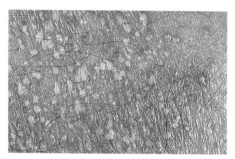

Pustular psoriasis.

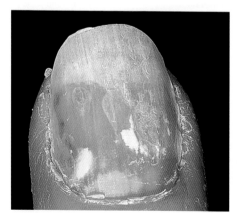

Psoriasis oil spot lesion. Accumulation of parakeratotic debris and serum under the nail produces a yellow–brown stain under the nail.

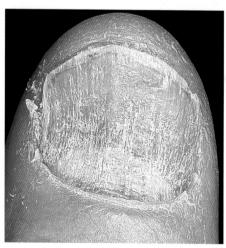

Psoriasis nail deformity. Inflammation of the proximal nail matrix causes surface deformity of the nail plate.

- Diffuse scalp psoriasis removed with Derma-Smoothe oil (apply to entire scalp at bedtime, cover with a shower cap and wash out the following morning). Repeat for 5–10 days. This treatment removes scale and controls inflammation.
- Baker's P&S (phenol, sodium chloride, and liquid paraffin) should be applied at bedtime and washed out in the morning.
- Hot olive oil turbans and manual scale debridement might work for very thick scale.
- Steroid gels (Lidex, Temovate, Topicort) or steroid foams (Olux, Luxiq) penetrate through hair and into scale.
- Smaller plaques can be treated with intralesional steroid (5–10 mg/mL Kenalog).

Topical Nail Treatment
- Nails are difficult to treat so the physician's goal is to provide symptomatic/cosmetic relief.
- Topical calcipotriene solution, clobetasol solution and tazarotene gel may be helpful if applied to the posterior nail fold area; this requires months of treatment.

- Intralesional Kenalog is painful to administer but often provides temporary improvement.

Phototherapy
Ultraviolet B
- This is a very effective treatment; ultraviolet light may be used in combination with topical treatment. A minority of patients do not respond, while others get worse.
- Ultraviolet B is typically given 3–5 times per week.
- Tar or lubricants enhance its effectiveness.
- Steroid use diminishes the length of remission.
- Side effects are burning, premature skin aging, and skin cancer.
- Narrow-band form is more effective than broad-band, but is less widely available.
- Excimer laser (308 nm) is similar to and possibly more effective than the narrow-

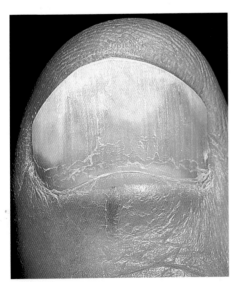

Psoriatic onycholysis. Psoriatic inflammation of the skin at the fingertip causes distal nail plate separation. The picture can be identical to that seen with traumatic onycholysis.

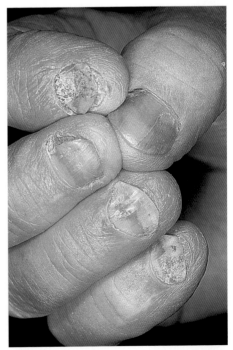

Psoriasis onycholysis and nail deformity. Inflammation of various parts of the nail matrix produces a bizarre pattern of nail deformity. Clinical differentiation from onychomycosis is sometime difficult.

band form, though it is not widely available.

Psoralen plus Ultraviolet A

- Psoralen plus ultraviolet A needs to be given three times a week until the skin is clear, and then it is tapered off.
- Patients take photosensitizing psoralen 1.5–2 hours prior to exposure.

- This is an effective method of controlling but not curing psoriasis.
- Indications are for symptomatic control of severe, recalcitrant, disabling, plaque psoriasis.
- Side effects include gastrointestinal intolerance of drug, sunburning, photo-damaged skin, cataracts, and increased skin cancer risk.

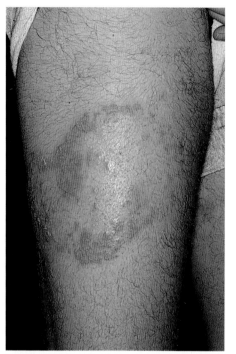

Psoriatic plaques typically clear in the center and then improve at the periphery.

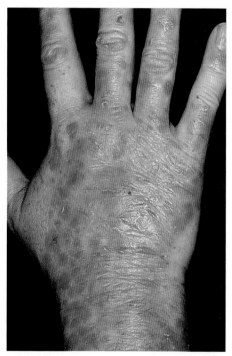

Inflammatory plaque psoriasis may be painful. This active disease failed to respond to topical steroids and methotrexate was started.

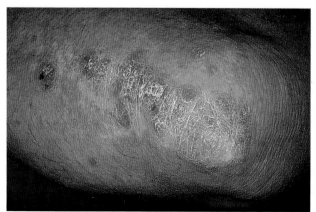

This plaque has partially responded to clobetasol cream. Topical steroids usually do not clear a plaque completely and the disease typically returns after topical application is stopped.

Systemic Therapy

■ Patients with psoriasis involving more than 20% of the body surface or who are very uncomfortable should consider systemic therapy. Systemic therapy is complicated and best managed by a dermatologist.

Rotational Therapy

■ A rotational approach to therapy minimizes long-term toxic effects from any one therapy and allows effective long-term management.

Methotrexate

■ Methotrexate is effective in unstable erythrodermic, generalized pustular psoriasis and extensive chronic plaque disease.
■ It is effective for psoriatic arthritis.
■ It can be given orally, intramuscularly or subcutaneously.
■ Work up to a dose of 12.5–22.5 mg weekly.
■ Give folic acid 1 mg daily, but not on the methotrexate day.
■ Close follow-up is needed; monitor complete blood cell count, liver function, and liver biopsy should be performed periodically.
■ Beware of drug interactions with salicylates, many non-steroidal antiinflammatory agents, trimethoprim–sulfamethoxazole, penicillins, and others.

■ Side effects include nausea, anorexia, fatigue, oral ulcerations, leukopenia, and thrombocytopenia, hepatic fibrosis or cirrhosis. Caution in the elderly or patients with any renal insufficiency.

Cyclosporine (Neoral)

■ Cyclosporine is best for severe inflammatory psoriasis (best used for acute control).
■ Dosage is 2.5–5.0 mg/kg/day.
■ Taper dosage after control is achieved.
■ Close monitoring of blood pressure is needed, as well as complete blood count, creatinine, magnesium and cholesterol/triglyceride levels.
■ Decrease dose if creatinine increases by 30% from baseline.
■ Beware of drug interactions.
■ Side effects include hypertension and nephrotoxicity.

Acitretin (Soriatane)

■ Highly effective for generalized pustular and erythrodermic psoriasis, and moderately effective for palmoplantar psoriasis.
■ Useful in combination with psoralen plus ultraviolet A and ultraviolet B.
■ Start at 10–25 mg/day as a single dose.
■ Side effects are similar to those of isotretinoin, which limits treatment for many patients; they include teratogenicity, dry skin, sticky skin, myalgias, arthralgias, pseudotumor cerebri, depression, hair loss, hepatitis, pancreatitis, increased cholesterol/triglycerides.

Chronic inflammation of the palms is a difficult diagnostic problem. Psoriasis and eczema may have a similar appearance. Both are difficult to treat.

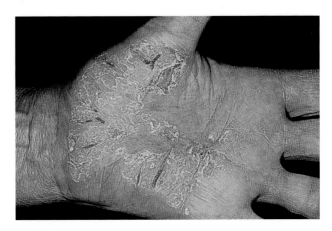

Biologicals

- Our increasing knowledge of T cell physiology and cell interactions have enabled the re-engineering of specific human proteins involved in T cell function.
- These new forms of immunomodulatory therapy interact with specific molecular targets in T cell-mediated inflammatory processes and exert an antiinflammatory effect.
- Efalizumab (Raptiva) is a humanized immunoglobulin G monoclonal antibody specific to LFA-1, which interferes with T cell trafficking into the skin. It is given subcutaneously.
- Alefacept (Amevive) is a fusion protein analog of LFA-3, the ligand for the T cell CD2 receptor which, when administered intramuscularly, competitively inhibits LFA-3/CD2 interaction and reduces circulating T cell subsets involved in psoriasis.
- Infliximab (Remicade) is a chimeric monoclonal antibody, given intravenously, which binds and blocks the proinflammatory effect of tumour necrosis factor-alpha.
- Etanercept (Enbrel) is a recombinant soluble tumour necrosis factor-α receptor fused to the Fc portion of a human immunoglobulin G molecule. It is given subcutaneously. The agent binds soluble tumor necrosis factor-α, thus blocking its proinflammatory effect. Etanercept is approved for the treatment of psoriatic arthritis and psoriasis.

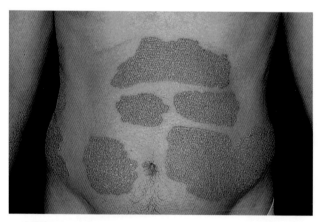

Chronic plaque psoriasis may be asymptomatic. This patient was not uncomfortable and became discouraged with topical treatments. He was satisfied with using just moisturizers.

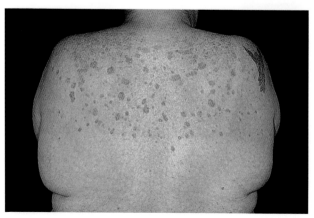

Sunlight is an effective treatment, but sunburn can initiate a psoriatic flare.

Seborrheic Dermatitis

Description
- Seborrheic dermatitis is a common, chronic, inflammatory papulosquamous disease.
- It has been proposed that *Pityrosporum* yeast is the cause.

History
- All ages can be affected.
- It has greater severity and is more difficult to control in patients with neurologic disease (e.g. head trauma, spinal cord injury, Parkinson's disease, stroke) or patients with human immunodeficiency virus infection.

Skin Findings
- The papules are moist, transparent to yellow, greasy and scaling, among coalescing red patches and plaques.
- May be diffuse, though usually favors areas where the concentration of sebaceous glands is maximal: the scalp margins, central face and presternal areas.
- Characteristic locations are the eyebrows, the base of eyelashes, nasolabial folds and paranasal skin, and external ear canals.
- May affect flexural skin including the postauricular, inguinal, and inframammary folds as well as the anogenital area.
- Scale adherent to the eyelashes and lid margins with variable amounts of erythema is characteristic of seborrheic blepharitis.

Laboratory
- Skin biopsy is not usually necessary
- Fungal culture and potassium hydroxide examination are indicated for atypical or resistant cases of scalp or facial scaling.

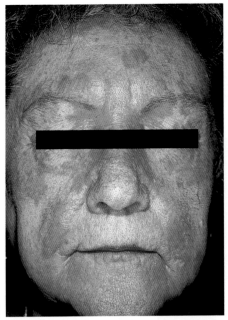

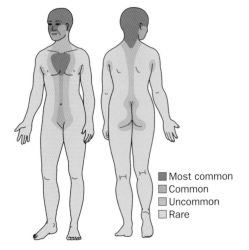

Most common
Common
Uncommon
Rare

116

Erythema and scaling may be extensive and extend beyond the nasolabial folds.

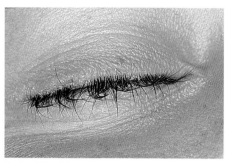

Scale of the lid margins occurs more often in children. The scales may irritate the conjunctiva.

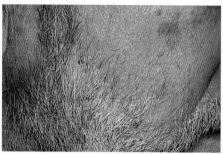

Patients with a propensity to develop seborrheic dermatitis will develop erythema and scale if they grow a beard. The disease will clear if the hair is shaved.

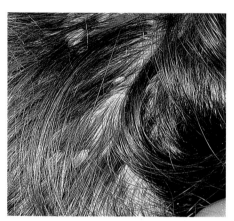

Dense patches of quadrangular scale occur in children. The scale adheres to the hair.

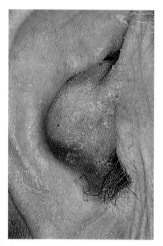

Seborrheic dermatitis of the ears usually requires group V topical steroids for control. The disease may be persistent and resistant to treatment.

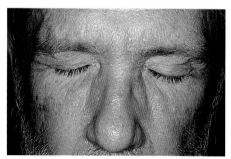

Active disease in all of the characteristic areas. The inflammation cleared with ciclopirox lotion (Loprox).

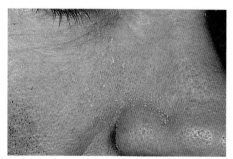

A classic presentation for seborrheic dermatitis. Ketoconazole cream failed. A 7-day course of a group V topical steroid was effective. The patient was warned not to use topical steroids continuously on the face.

Pediatric Considerations

- Yellow, greasy adherent scale on the vertex of the scalp (cradle cap) with minimal underlying redness.
- Scale may accumulate, becoming thick and adherent over much of the scalp.
- Diaper area and axillary skin may become involved, often with redness that is more obvious than scaling.
- Secondary bacterial and candidal infection can occur.
- Infantile seborrheic dermatitis is easy to diagnose. Infants who do not respond to standard treatment measures can rarely have an underlying systemic illness such as Langerhans cell histiocytosis or zinc deficiency.
- Infantile seborrheic dermatitis is usually a self-limited condition often not requiring treatment. Usually gentle removal of scale and a low-strength corticosteroid are sufficient to control infantile seborrheic dermatitis.
- Referral to a dermatologist is indicated for infants with severe recalcitrant seborrheic dermatitis or with widespread disease.

Differential Diagnosis

- Tinea of the face (tends to have annular plaques; potassium hydroxide examination is confirmatory)
- Cutaneous lupus (often flares with sun exposure; skin biopsy supports the diagnosis)
- Rosacea, an acneiform disorder (may coexist with seborrheic dermatitis or flare from topical steroid use)
- Psoriasis (may overlap with seborrheic dermatitis, especially on the scalp and in fold areas)
- Pemphigus foliaceous (confirmed by skin biopsy with immunofluorescence)

Treatment

- Adults tends to have a chronic course with remissions and exacerbations.
- Flares are precipitated by stress, fatigue, and seasonal climate change.
- Mild to moderate facial seborrheic dermatitis may respond well to topical antifungal creams, such as ketoconazole (Nizoral), or gels such as ciclopirox (Loprox).
- Daily facial washing with antidandruff shampoo or soaps containing zinc pyrithione (ZNP) or selenium sulfide (Selsun) or sulfacetamide/sulfur (Rosanil) diluted with water is also effective.
- Group VI or VII topical steroid creams or lotions (hydrocortisone or desonide) applied twice daily for several days may be required periodically for control.
- Off-label use of Protopic 0.1% ointment or Elidel 1% cream applied daily are effective long-term alternatives to topical steroids.
- Mild to moderate scalp involvement is best managed with frequent and extended shampooing with antidandruff shampoos.
- Effective formulations may contain ketoconazole (Nizoral), ciclopirox (Loprox), coal tar (Tarsum, T-Gel), salicylic acid (T-Sal), selenium sulfide (Selsun), and zinc pyrithione (Head and Shoulders).
- Sulfacetamide foam is an effective alternative (Ovace foam). This is applied at bedtime for several days and may be repeated as needed.
- Dense, thick, adherent scale is removed by applying warm mineral or olive oil to the scalp and washing several hours later.
- At bedtime apply 10% liquor carbonis detergens (LCD) in Nivea oil or Derma-Smoothe FS lotion (peanut oil, mineral oil, fluocinolone acetonide 0.01%) to the scalp and wash out in the morning. Wetting the scalp prior to application and using a shower cap will help penetration.
- Severe cases may require oral antifungal therapy to eradicate *Pityrosporum ovale*.
- Antifungal therapy includes ketoconazole 200 mg every day, or fluconazole 150 mg every day, or itraconazole 200 mg every day, for 1 or 2 weeks.

- Brief use of oral corticosteroids may be considered.
- Oral antistaphylococcal antibiotics (dicloxacillin, cephalexin) should be used for secondary infection with heavy serum and crusting.
- Blepharitis may be suppressed by lid massage and frequent washing with zinc or tar-containing antidandruff shampoos.

Pearls

- If scaling is not improving, assess the frequency and duration of treatment. Most shampoos will work well if used often enough and left on for long enough.

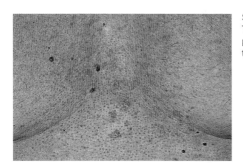

Seborrheic dermatitis occurs on the presternal area. This eruption was controlled with ZNP bar soap (2% pyrithione zinc) and periodic treatment with a group V topical steroid.

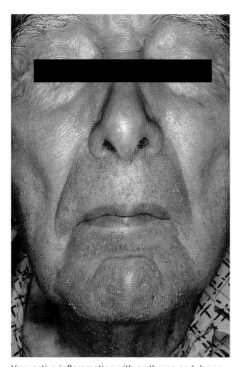

Very active inflammation with erythema and dense scale. Inflammation of this intensity usually responds to ciclopirox lotion (Loprox) or ketoconazole (Nizoral cream).

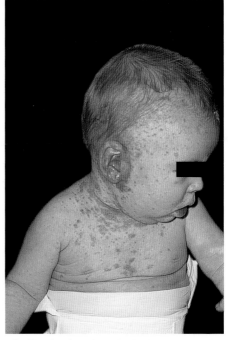

Infantile seborrheic dermatitis begins on the scalp (cradle cap). There are well-defined red to salmon colored plaques covered with greasy scale. They may descend to involve the face, trunk and diaper area. Itching is minimal. Atopic dermatitis itches.

119

Grover's Disease (Transient Acantholytic Dermatosis)

Description
■ An uncommon, acquired, self-limited, acantholytic disorder of unknown etiology.
■ Despite the name, the eruption often persists for several months to years.
■ Itching is intermittent, mild to severe, localized to lesions, and exacerbated by heat or sweating.

History
■ Typically Caucasian men over 40 years of age.
■ The male to female ratio is 3 to 1.
■ Itching may precede the appearance of lesions, though it usually coincides.
■ There is often a history of heat exposure, such as a hot tub or sauna, or summer onset.

Skin Findings
■ The keratotic papules are red to brown, measuring 1–3 mm, and they are often excoriated, and not exclusively follicle based.
■ Regional distribution on the chest, the lower rib cage, upper back, and lumbar areas.
■ May spread to the lateral neck, shoulders and upper thighs.
■ Lesions resolve with postinflammatory hyperpigmentation or hypopigmentation.

Laboratory
■ Skin biopsy reveals acantholysis (separation of cells in the epidermis) and dyskeratosis (changes in epidermal cells) such as that seen in Darier's disease.
■ Spongiosis (fluid in the epidermis) and hyperkeratosis are commonly seen.
■ Immunofluorescence is negative.

Differential Diagnosis
■ Hot tub folliculitis (similar sudden onset but usually resolves spontaneously in 7–10 days)
■ Candidiasis (this usually extends into intertriginous areas; potassium hydroxide examination confirms the diagnosis)
■ Dermatitis herpetiformis (scalp, elbows and knees; characteristic immunofluorescence findings)
■ Drug eruptions and viral exanthems (more common and less persistent than Grover's disease; history and skin biopsy are helpful)
■ Pityriasis rosea (similar distribution though there is usually a preceding herald patch)
■ Miliaria rubra (heat rash; resolves within 1 week with treatment)
■ Seborrheic dermatitis (also occurs on the trunk, but not exclusively)
■ Insect bites (rarely persistent and limited to the trunk)
■ Darier's disease.

Treatment
■ Grover's is self-limited, treatment is symptomatic.
■ Older patients will likely have more extensive eruptions of longer duration.
■ The extent and severity fluctuates, and some cases are persistent or recurrent (seasonal).

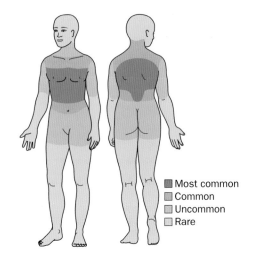

■ Most common
■ Common
■ Uncommon
■ Rare

- Strenuous exercise and exposure to excessive heat should be avoided.
- Advise minimal use of soap and liberal use of moisturizers.
- Colloidal oatmeal baths may relieve itching as will cool wet dressings and mentholated lotions (Sarna).
- Antihistamines are of limited value in controlling itching.
- Oral antibiotics and dapsone are not effective.
- A group I–V topical steroid may be used for initial control in most cases, and can then be used as needed for recurrences.
- Oral vitamin A 50,000 international units three times daily for 2 weeks, then reduced to 50,000 international units daily for a maximum of 12 weeks may be effective for extensive and severely pruritic cases.
- Isotretinoin 40 mg daily for 2–12 weeks then taper the dosage to 10 mg daily once the patient improves and continue for 12 weeks.
- Prednisone 20 mg twice daily controls extensive inflammation and itching, although relapse is common.

Pearls

- Because Grover's disease mimics many other diseases, consider skin biopsy to establish the diagnosis.

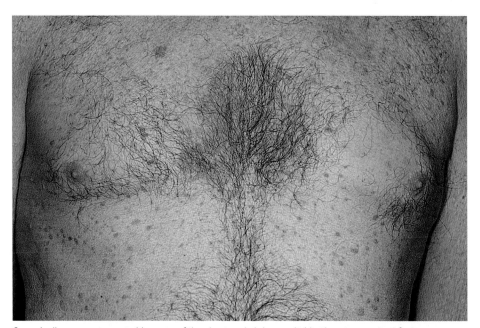

Grover's disease may cover wide areas of the chest and abdomen. Itching is not a constant feature.

Pityriasis Rosea

Description
- Common, self-limited, usually asymptomatic, clinically distinctive papulosquamous eruption.

History
- More than 75% of patients are between 10 and 35 years of age.
- Many patients report a mild prodrome or upper respiratory illness within a month of onset.
- The first lesion or herald patch appears, most often on the trunk.
- The lesion is an oval plaque of 1–2 cm in diameter, which develops a thin collarette of residual scale inside the border.
- 1–2 weeks later numerous similar but smaller lesions begin to appear and reach a maximum number within 2 weeks while the herald patch is still present.
- Lesions usually clear spontaneously in 4–12 weeks, without scarring, although postinflammatory pigmentary changes may take months to resolve in darker-skinned people.
- Seasonal cases in the spring and fall within the community suggest a viral etiology, though this has not been confirmed.
- Limited outbreaks have occurred in close quarters such as fraternity houses and military barracks.

Skin Findings
- Early lesions are broad-based papules that subsequently develop a thin collarette of scale as the center of the papule desquamates.
- Lesions are salmon colored on Caucasian skin and dark brown on African–American skin.
- Lesions are usually confined to the trunk and proximal extremities, often concentrated on the lower abdomen.
- The long axis of the oval lesions is oriented along skin lines reminiscent of drooping pine branches.
- When fully developed, most cases of pityriasis rosea are clinically distinct and may seem obvious.

- Atypical cases do occur and may be confused with other disorders.

Pediatric Considerations
- Children often have numerous lesions that can have varying morphologies: purpuric, vesicular and papular.
- Children can have lesions that predominate in the groin, elbows and knees (inverse pityriasis rosea).

Laboratory
- Skin biopsy is not usually necessary but is helpful in atypical cases.
- Potassium hydroxide examination may be useful in early cases (herald patch) to exclude a diagnosis of tinea.
- A serologic test for syphilis should be considered in the right clinical setting, especially if lesions are present on the palms and soles.

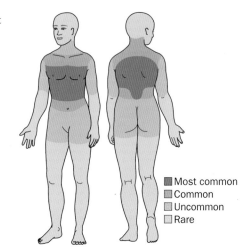

Most common
Common
Uncommon
Rare

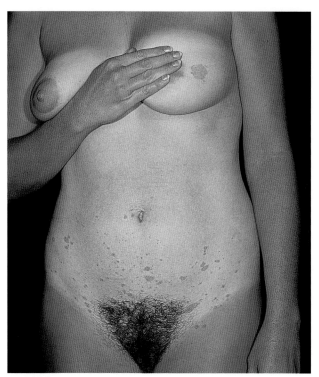

The first lesion is usually the largest. It is called the herald patch. It can be located anywhere but is typically found on the trunk. Here the herald patch is found on the left breast. Lesions that follow are smaller and usually confined to the trunk. Concentration of lesions in the lower abdominal and pubic area is highly characteristic of pityriasis rosea. Exposure to sunlight is an effective treatment. Here the lesions only appear on unexposed skin.

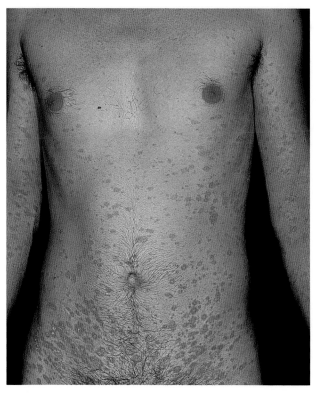

An extensive case in a typical distribution with lesions in the lower abdominal region. Here lesions are also found on the upper arms. It is very unusual to find lesions on the forearms or the lower legs. Most patients experience little or no itching.

Differential Diagnosis

- Tinea corporis (exclude by potassium hydroxide examination early in the course)
- Secondary syphilis (exclude by serology)
- Tinea versicolor (exclude by potassium hydroxide examination)
- Drug eruption (some medications are known to cause a pityriasis rosea-like eruption; consult an appropriate drug reference)
- Guttate psoriasis (often follows streptococcal infection; different lesion morphology and distribution)

Treatment

- Pityriasis rosea is self-limited and usually asymptomatic.
- Treatment is indicated for itching.
- Oral erythromycin stearate 250 mg four times daily (for adults) for 2 weeks effectively controls the eruption.
- Mentholated lotions (Sarna) or sprays (Eucerin AntiItch) are helpful.
- Group V topical steroids and oral antihistamines provide some relief.

- Prednisone (20 mg twice a day) is rarely needed and only in extensive cases with itching that is refractory to topical therapy.
- Ultraviolet B light, either from natural sunlight or administered in metered doses by a dermatologist, hastens resolution.

When to Refer

- Consider referral to a dermatologist when the lesion morphology is variable, when the lesions are more extensive than expected or the eruption is lasting longer than expected.
- 2% of cases are thought to be recurrent and should be referred for skin biopsy.

Pearls

- The herald patch is characteristic of pityriasis rosea, but is often misdiagnosed as tinea.
- Pityriasis may be indistinguishable from secondary syphilis.

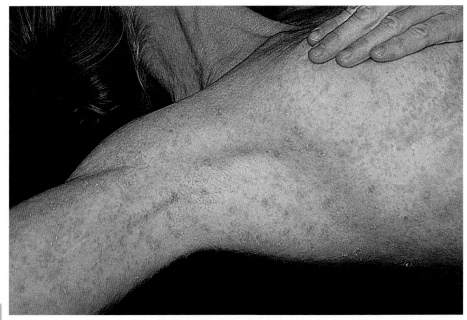

Highly active disease involving the neck, trunk, and extremities. The circular scale supports the diagnosis. Erythromycin 250 mg every day for 2 weeks was effective.

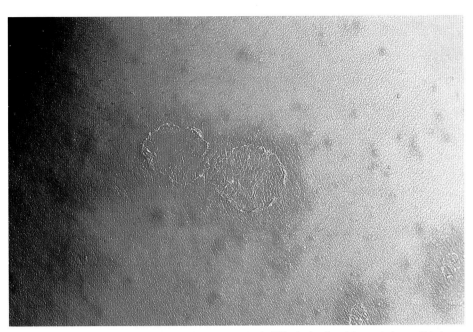

A ring of tissue-like scale (collarette scale) remains attached within the border of the oval plaque. This is almost pathognomonic of pityriasis rosea. The scale appears at the border with fungal infections.

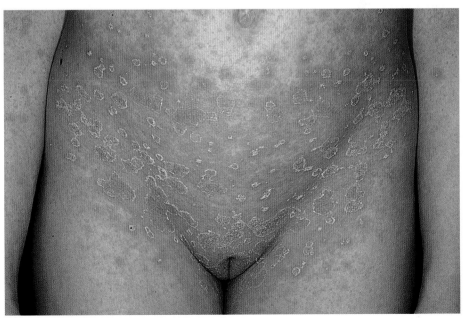

Lesions are typically concentrated in the lower abdomen and groin. Eruptions may be intense and widespread. The circular scale is a clue to the diagnosis.

Lichen Planus

Description
- An uncommon, inflammatory papulosquamous disorder of unknown etiology.
- Skin, nails, hair and mucous membranes may be affected.

History
- Rare in children aged under 5 years; more common in women.
- 10% of patients have a positive family history.
- Course is variable and unpredictable in all types.
- Itching is variable, most often intermittent, and insatiable.
- Can occur abruptly as generalized disease; may be secondary to a drug.
- Severe oral lichen planus may degenerate to squamous cell carcinoma (in 3% of cases).

Skin Findings
- The primary lesion is a 2–10 mm flat-topped papule with an irregular, angulated border (polygonal papules).
- New lesions are pink to white, but over time they become purple and sharply defined.
- Surface shows a lacy reticulated pattern of whitish lines (Wickham's striae).
- New lesions may develop in areas of injury (the Koebner phenomenon).
- There are several clinical forms.

Papular Lichen Planus
- The most common form.
- Papules are located on the flexor surfaces of the wrists and forearms, the ankles and the lumbar region.

Hypertrophic Lichen Planus
- Lesions that persist become thicker and dark red.
- Most often they are on the shins.
- Papules aggregate into different patterns.
- Vesicles or bullae may appear.
- Persistent brown staining develops after the lesions resolve.

Follicular Lichen Planus
- Follicle-based papules on the scalp.
- Permanent hair loss with marked scarring (scarring alopecia).

Mucosal Lichen Planus
- Most common form is the non-erosive with a white lacy pattern.
- The erosive form is painful with beefy desquamation.
- Oral lesions primarily involve the buccal mucosa and lateral edge of the tongue.
- This may extend to involve the mucosal lip, but rarely extends beyond the vermillion border.
- The penis and vulva may be involved, with intense itching and burning, marked mucosal fragility, and erythema.
- Secondary candidiasis occurs frequently, likely as a side effect of topical treatment.

Nail Involvement
- Changes may be present in the absence of skin findings.
- There are proximal to distal linear depressions in the nail plate.
- Inflammation of the matrix results in adhesion of the proximal nail fold to the scarred matrix to form a pterygium (scar).

Laboratory
- Skin biopsy shows an accumulation of mononuclear cells obscuring the dermoepidermal interface and a T cell-mediated cytotoxic reaction against basal layer keratinocytes.

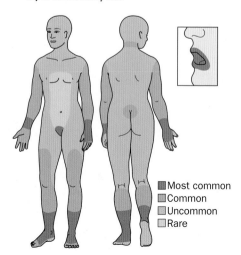

- Most common
- Common
- Uncommon
- Rare

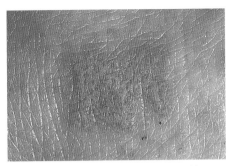

The primary lesion is a flat-topped papule with an irregular, angulated border (polygonal papule).

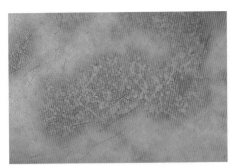

Close inspection of the surface shows a lacy reticular pattern of criss-crossed whitish lines (Wickham's striae) that can be accentuated with a drop of immersion oil.

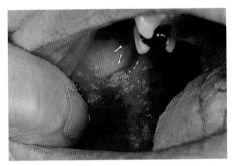

White plaques are located on the buccal mucosa. The classic presentation is a lacy net-like pattern.

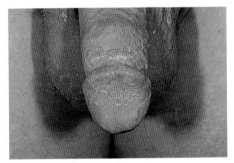

White lacy reticular pattern is present on the glans and shaft. Lesions are asymptomatic.

Lichen planus. Lesions are concentrated about the wrists and ankles. Itching varies in intensity and may not be present.

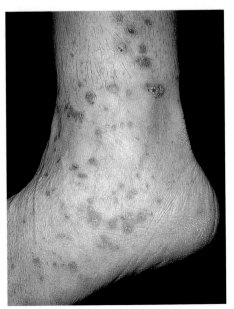

- Routine immunofluorescence biopsy of scalp skin helps rule out lupus.
- Antibodies to hepatitis C virus are detected in about 16% of patients with cutaneous lichen planus and about 30% of patients with mucosal involvement.

Differential Diagnosis

- Papular form may be confused with psoriasis and papular eczema though the epidermal changes are quite different
- Hypertrophic lichen planus is distinguished from psoriasis, lichen simplex chronicus, and stasis dermatitis with verrucous changes
- Scarring alopecia is discerned from discoid lupus by biopsy and immunofluorescence
- Mucosal non-erosive lesions may resemble leukoplakia or candidiasis and penile lesions can be difficult to distinguish from psoriasis papules
- Erosive lesions should be discerned from pemphigus vulgaris, paraneoplastic pemphigus and fixed drug eruption

Treatment

- Sedating antihistamines (hydroxyzine 10–25 mg every 4 hours) for pruritus.
- Group I or II topical steroids twice daily as initial topical treatment for localized disease.
- Intralesional triamcinolone acetonide (Kenalog 5–10 mg/ml) for hypertrophic lesions
- Prednisone for generalized skin or erosive mucosal involvement; a 4-week course starting at 1 mg/kg/day and gradually decrease of the dosage.
- Corticosteroids (fluocinonide, fluocinolone acetonide, triamcinolone acetonide) in an adhesive base (Orabase) for initial treatment for oral lesions, applied directly to the lesions.
- Inhaled corticosteroids (e.g. Azmacort) are alternatives to cream Orabase preparations. Simply spray onto lesions.
- Prednisolone tablets, the active form of prednisone; 5 mg tablet dissolved in the mouth. Swish and swallow.

- Retinoids (Acitretin) 1 mg/kg/day, cyclosporine (5–6 mg/kg/day) may be considered for severe recalcitrant forms of lichen planus.
- Tacrolimus (Protopic) 0.1% ointment twice daily has been used with some success for erosive oral lesions.
- Dapsone, azathioprine and hydroxychloroquine have been used for severe recalcitrant oral lesions.

When to Refer

- Scarring alopecia, erosive mucosal involvement, and refractory cases should be referred to a dermatologist for management.
- Gastroenterology referral should be considered for hepatitis C infection management.

Pearls

- There are five Ps of lichen planus:
  - Pruritic
  - Planar (flat-topped)
  - Polygonal
  - Purple
  - Papules
- White lacy patches of the oral mucosa are virtually diagnostic of oral lichen planus.

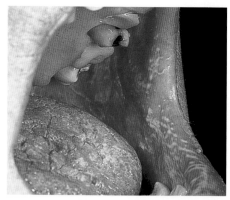

Mucous membrane lichen planus. A lacy white pattern is present on the buccal mucosa.

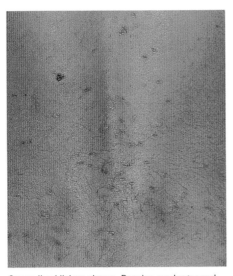

Generalized lichen planus. Papules are larger and are confluent in the lower back region.

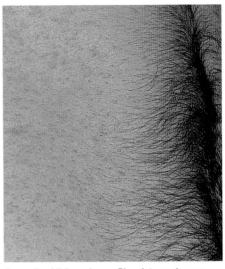

Generalized lichen planus. Pinpoint papules are numerous and widespread.

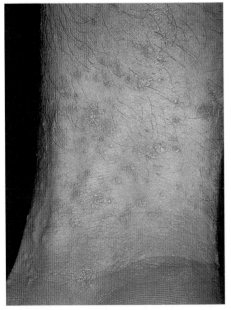

Localized lichen planus. Early lesions are present on the wrist, which is a common site for localized lichen planus.

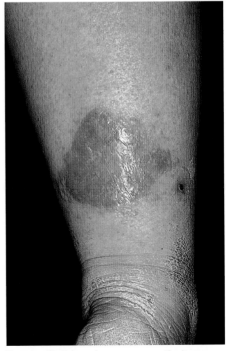

Hypertrophic lichen planus occurs on the lower legs. These plaques have a violaceous hue and are thick. Itching may be intense.

Lichen Sclerosus

Description

- An uncommon chronic inflammatory disease of unknown etiology which affects both skin and mucosal surfaces.

History

- The female to male ratio is 10 to 1.
- The disease has predilection for the anogenital skin.
- It is more common in women over 60 years of age, but can occur at any age.
- Affected women complain of chronic vulvar pruritus, dysuria or dyspareunia that interferes with sexual activity.
- Men have persistent balanitis which, if untreated, tends to progress to phimosis.
- Skin lesions are often asymptomatic.
- Squamous cell carcinoma develops in 3% of genital lesions.

Skin Findings

- The primary lesion is an ivory white, atrophic papule with a faint pink rim.
- On the skin, flat-topped, slightly raised papules coalesce into small oval plaques with a dull or glistening, smooth, white, atrophic, wrinkled surface.
- Focal hemorrhage may be seen among plaques.
- Keratotic follicular plugs appear on the surface (delling).
- On mucosal surfaces, papules are fragile, atrophic, white, and glistening with a wrinkled surface.
- Penile lesions favor the glans and coronal sulcus, but may extend to the shaft.
- Surface trauma leads to focal subepidermal hemorrhages and erosions.
- Atrophy leads to phimosis of the foreskin with pain on retraction of the foreskin or erection.
- Male genital lichen sclerosus is referred to as balanitis xerotica obliterans.
- The urethral meatus may become stenotic, and malignant degeneration may occur.
- Vulvar papules tend to coalesce, forming a white atrophic plaque with an hour-glass shape, which encircles the vagina and anus.

- Focal purpura is common, mucosal lesions may erode.
- Itching is the most frequent complaint which may be severe enough to interfere with sleep or daily activities.
- Scratching may lead to secondary infection and lichenification among areas of atrophy.
- Atrophy and scarring can lead to shrunken and fused tissues obliterating normal anatomic structures.

Pediatric Considerations

- Purpura of the vulva is an occasional manifestation of lichen sclerosus in prepubertal girls.
- This may be misdiagnosed as child abuse, thus lichen sclerosus should be carefully ruled out in such cases.
- Prepubertal cases usually resolve without sequelae, other than hyperpigmentation.

Laboratory Findings

- Biopsy is helpful in early cases and for areas suspicious for squamous cell carcinoma.
- Secondary candidiasis can occur as a consequence of treatment and a potassium hydroxide examination should be considered.

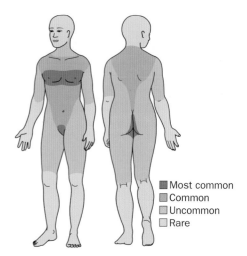

Most common
Common
Uncommon
Rare

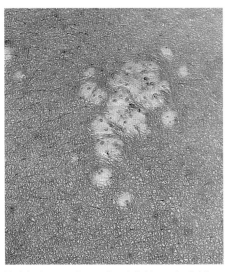

Early lesions are ivory-colored, flat-topped, slightly raised papules with follicular plugs.

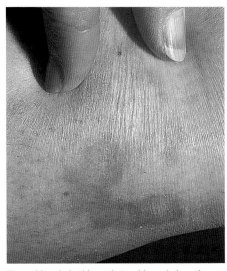

The epidermis is thin and atrophic and gives the appearance of wrinkled tissue paper when compressed.

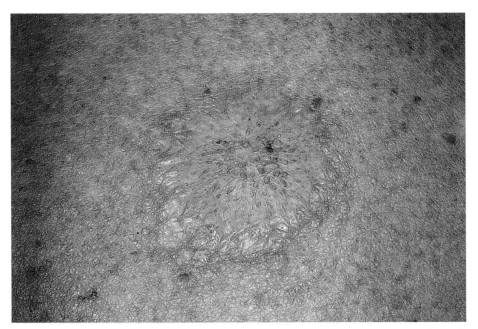

This is the classic presentation for a lesion that has been present for months. The plaque is white, firm and dense. Large follicular plugs are present in the center.

Differential Diagnosis

- Morphea and lichen sclerosis are similar on the skin (while both conditions may be present in some patients, the presence of mucosal lesions favors lichen sclerosus)
- Lichen planus and pemphigus vulgaris (especially for erosive mucosal lesions)
- Lichen simplex chronicus (vulvar involvement from scratching)
- Allergic contact dermatitis (typically fragrance allergy from personal hygiene products)
- Extramammary Paget's disease (should be considered for chronic anogenital itching with erosions)
- Steroid-induced atrophy (can be confused with lichen sclerosus)

Treatment

- Advise gentle cleansing of involved areas using gentle cleansers such as Cetaphil, wearing of ventilated cotton underwear, and liberal use of bland emollients and lubricants.
- Avoid panty liners, pre-mixed douches and sprays, and scented toilet paper.
- Topical steroid creams (group V twice daily for 2 weeks) is initial treatment for uncomplicated skin lesions and prepubertal mucosal lesions.
- Clobetasol propionate 0.05% (short intermittent courses) is effective for vaginal and penile disease in adults.
- Clobetasol propionate 0.05% (short intermittent courses) is effective for vaginal and penile disease in adults. Dermatologists are experienced in the use of this superpotent steroid.
- Intralesional triamcinolone acetonide (Kenalog, 2.5–5.0 mg/ml) are useful for unresponsive areas.
- Tacrolimus ointment (Protopic) 0.1% may be very effective for vaginal and penile disease. This non-steroidal antiinflammatory agent, unlike topical steroids, may be used on an "as needed" basis.
- Testosterone propionate 2% ointment has been used for years. Many experts now doubt its effectiveness.
- Acitretin (20–30 mg/day for 16 weeks) may be considered in severe lichen sclerosus atrophicus.
- Selected refractory medical cases may benefit from surgical reconstruction of scarred areas.

Pearls

- Chronic vulvar itching in the absence of infection should raise the suspicion of lichen sclerosus.
- Consider lichen sclerosus to be a pre-cancerous condition requiring regular follow-up and biopsy of areas suspicious for malignant change.

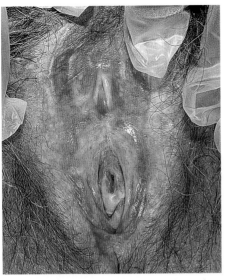

A white atrophic plaque encircles the vagina and rectum. The skin is fragile and easily erodes.

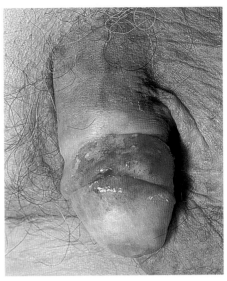

The glans is smooth, white and atrophic. Erosions are present on the prepuce.

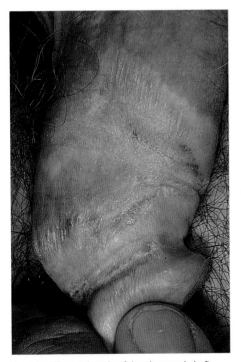

There is diffuse sclerosis of the glans and shaft. Several linear erosions are present.

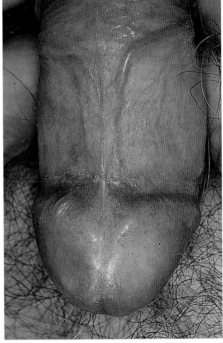

Sclerosis is limited to the glans. Note the ivory white color of the glans.

Pityriasis Lichenoides et Varioliformis Acuta

Description
- A rare inflammatory T cell-mediated disease of unknown etiology.
- There are two variants of pityriasis lichenoides et varioliformis—acute and chronic.
- The acute form, pityriasis lichenoides et varioliformis acuta, is also known as Mucha–Habermann disease.
- The chronic form is called pityriasis lichenoides chronica.
- The terms acute and chronic refer to the characteristics of the individual lesions and not to the course of the disease.

History
- Can occur at any age; most cases occur in the second and third decades.
- Pityriasis lichenoides et varioliformis acuta is usually a benign, self-limited papulosquamous disorder.
- Some evidence suggests that it is a hypersensitivity reaction to an infectious agent.

Skin Findings
- It occurs in crops of round 2–8 mm red-brown papules, singly or in clusters.
- Papules have a violaceous hue and adherent thin scale.
- Individual lesions can become vesicular and undergo hemorrhagic necrosis usually within 2–5 weeks, often leaving post-inflammatory hyperpigmentation.
- Lesions favor the trunk, thighs, and proximal extremities; face, scalp, palms, and soles are involved in approximately 10% of cases.
- Though the onset of lesions, their appearance and evolution is acute, the disease tends to be chronic with crops of lesions recurring over several months or years.
- Lesions are usually asymptomatic although mild itching may occur.
- High fever is a rare complication, but may be associated with an ulceronecrotic type of lesion.

- Complications include a self-limited arthritis and secondary infection of the skin lesions if excoriated.
- The chronic form also occurs primarily on the trunk, and consists of brown-red papules with fine, mica-like, adherent scale.
- In the chronic form lesions do not ulcerate or become necrotic and usually regress spontaneously within 3–6 weeks.

Laboratory
- Skin biopsy confirms the diagnosis.
- There is parakeratosis, regular acanthosis, and mild papillary dermal edema.
- There is superficial and deep perivascular lymphocytic infiltrate, along with exocytosis of normal appearing lymphocytes and extravasation of erythrocytes.
- Gene rearrangement studies have confirmed T cell clonality in some chronic cases though the significance of this finding is unclear.
- A relationship to cutaneous T cell lymphoma has been postulated, but not confirmed.

Differential Diagnosis
- Pityriasis rosea (also favors the trunk; lesion morphology is similar to chronic form)
- Lymphomatoid papulosis (lesions may undergo necrosis like those of the acute form)

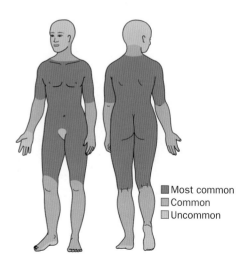

■ Most common
□ Common
□ Uncommon

- Insect bite reactions and scabies (may be confused with acute form)
- Varicella lesions: these occur in crops, with or without systemic symptoms

Treatment

- Prognosis for both forms is good.
- Acute exacerbation is common and the disease may wax and wane for months or years.
- Individual lesions may resolve, but new lesions continue to appear.
- Therapy is directed at itch relief, as the disease is self-limited.
- Oral erythromycin may produce a remission in some acute cases at a dose of 30–50 mg/kg daily over several weeks.
- Phototherapy with psoralen plus ultraviolet A and ultraviolet B,

tetracycline, gold, methotrexate, oral corticosteroids, and dapsone have all been used with some success in the acute form.
- The chronic form often responds to topical group I–III steroids applied twice daily.
- Ultraviolet B and narrow-band ultraviolet B are also effective for the chronic form.

Pearls

- Natural sunlight may help hasten resolution but tends to prolong post-inflammatory hyperpigmentation.
- An association between pityriasis lichenoides and cutaneous T cell lymphoma has been proposed, but it is controversial.

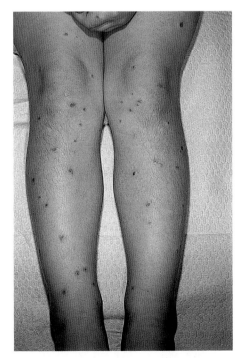

Crops of papules, colored red to brown, can become hemorrhagic, pustular, or necrotic. Acute exacerbations are common, and the disease may wax and wane for months or years.

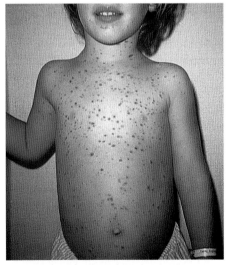

Lesions in children are vesicular or pustular and then undergo hemorrhagic necrosis. They appear on the trunk, thighs, and upper arms.

135

6 Bacterial Infections

Impetigo

Description
- Impetigo is a common, contagious, superficial skin infection produced by *Streptococcus pyogenes, Staphylococcus aureus*, or a combination of both bacteria.
- Bullous impetigo and nonbullous impetigo represent two clinical forms of the disease.
- *Staphylococcus aureus* is the primary pathogen.

History
- Impetigo may occur after a minor skin injury such as an insect bite, or within lesions of atopic or another dermatitis; it often develops on normal skin.
- Children in close physical contact with one another have a higher rate of infection.
- Responsible staphylococci may colonize the nose and serve as reservoir for skin infection.
- Warm, moist climates and poor hygiene predispose to this condition.

Skin Findings
- Lesions may be localized or widespread. Impetigo is common on the face.

Bullous Impetigo
- Thin-roofed bullae may turn from clear to cloudy. Bulla collapse, leading to an inner-tube-shaped rim with a central thin, flat, honey-colored crust.
- Lesions enlarge and often coalesce. There is minimal surrounding erythema. The thick crust accumulates in longer-lasting lesions.
- Lesions are found in all stages of evolution.

Non-Bullous Impetigo (Crusted)
- Vesicles or pustules rupture, exposing a red and moist base. A tinea-like scaling border forms as the round lesions enlarge.
- The firmly adherent crust is honey-yellow to white-brown in color; it accumulates as the lesion extends radially, and there is little surrounding erythema.
- Satellite lesions appear beyond the periphery.

Non-skin Findings
- Systemic symptoms are infrequent.
- Lesions are generally asymptomatic and painless.
- The incidence of acute nephritis is between 2% and 5%; in the presence of a nephritogenic strain of streptococci, the rate varies between 10% and 15%.
- Rheumatic fever has not been reported as a complication of impetigo.
- *Staphylococcus aureus* is a common infection with potential serious complications in people infected with human immunodeficiency virus.

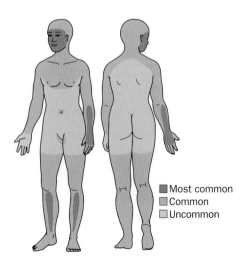

■ Most common
□ Common
□ Uncommon

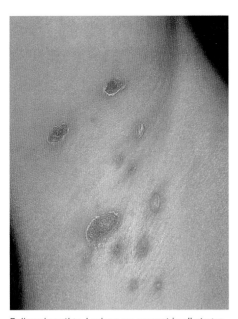

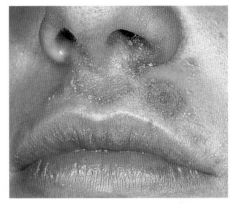

Bullous impetigo. Lesions are present in all stages of development. Bullae rupture, exposing a lesion with an eroded surface and peripheral scale.

A tinea-like scaling border forms as the round lesions enlarge.

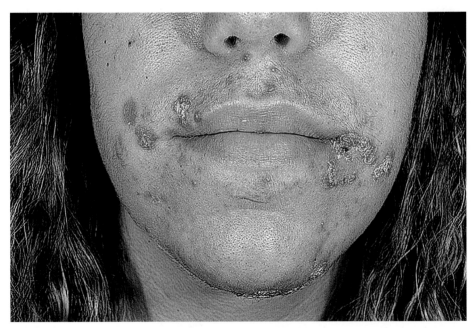

Impetigo occurs most often on the face. Here, lesions are found in all stages of development.

Recurrence following therapy is common.

Laboratory

- Cultures of lesions will reveal *Staphylococcus aureus* or group A *Streptococcus*. Sensitivity information is useful given the increasing incidence of antibiotic resistance and methicillin-resistant *Staphylococcus aureus*.

Differential Diagnosis

- Perioral dermatitis
- Allergic contact dermatitis
- Herpes simplex and herpes zoster
- Pemphigus foliaceus and pemphigus vulgaris
- Tinea infection

Course and Prognosis

- The disease is self-limiting, but if untreated it may spread and may last for weeks or months. Systemic complications are uncommon.
- Ecthyma (deeper, dermal infected lesions) may result from chronic, untreated impetigo infection, and is most common on the leg. There is an increased risk of pyoderma, folliculitis, cellulitis, lymphadenitis, and ecthyma in carriers of *Staphylococcus aureus* or group A *Streptococcus*.

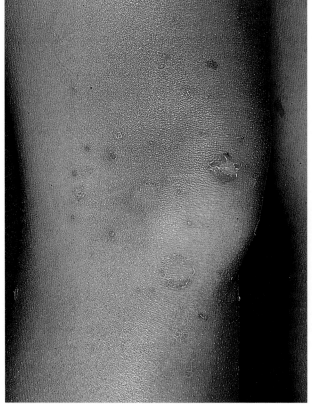

Pustules and round plaques with peripheral crust appeared spontaneously. They cleared with Mupirocin cream.

Treatment

- For limited, localized infections, Mupirocin 2% ointment or cream (Bactroban) is used three times a day for 10 days.
- Neomycin-bacitracin creams are also effective.
- For widespread infections, oral antibiotics are administered. An antibiotic such as dicloxacillin 250 mg, or cephalexin (Keflex) 250 mg, is prescribed four times a day for 5–10 days. Pediatric doses are cephalexin 40–50 mg/kg/day divided three times daily for 10 days, amoxicillin plus clavulanic acid 20 mg/kg/day divided three times daily for 10 days. Antibiotic-resistant staphylococci are a concern with oral erythromycin. For penicillin-allergic patients, azithromycin given over 5 days (500 mg on day 1 and 250 mg on days 2–5), or clarithromycin 250–500 mg twice daily for 10 days may be effective.
- For recurrent impetigo, the presence of *Staphylococcus aureus* is sought; the most common sites are the nares. Less commonly, it can be found in the perineum, axillae, and toe webs.
- Recurrent disease may be stopped with Mupirocin 2% ointment to nares twice a day for 5 days. This course is repeated monthly for several months to eradicate nasal carriers of *Staphylococcus aureus*.
- Fusidic acid cream has been used successfully for impetigo, though there are concerns related to development of bacterial resistance.

Discussion

- *Staphylococcus aureus* transiently colonizes the nares of 20–40% of healthy people, and the skin of atopic individuals.
- Bullous impetigo is primarily a staphylococcal disease.
- Non-bullous impetigo was once thought to be primarily a streptococcal disease, but staphylococci are isolated from most lesions of bullous and non-bullous impetigo.
- An epidermolytic toxin produced at the site of infection, most commonly by staphylococci of phage group II, causes intra-epidermal cleavage below or within the stratum granulosum, resulting in bulla formation in bullous impetigo.
- Guttate psoriasis is an uncommon sequelae of impetigo.

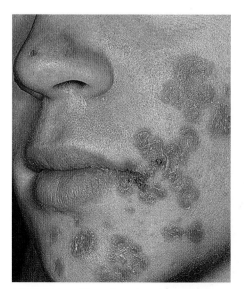

A thick, honey-yellow, adherent crust covers the entire eroded surface.

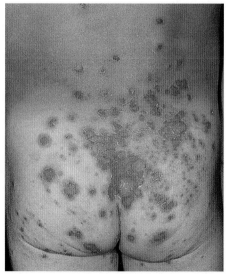

Widespread dissemination followed 3 weeks of treatment with a group IV topical steroid.

Pediatric Considerations

- Impetigo is the most common bacterial skin infection of children.
- For localized impetigo, topical therapy with Mupirocin (Bactroban) is generally well accepted by children.
- For widespread impetigo, systemic antistaphylococcal or antistreptococcal antibiotics (cephalexin 20–40 mg/kg/day divided three times daily) should be given orally for 7–10 days.
- Rarely, post-streptococcal glomerulonephritis may follow impetigo, typically 1–5 weeks after infection, and most commonly in children age 2–4 years.
- Group A streptococcal serotypes associated with nephritis can be determined and are most commonly M-T serotypes 2, 49, 55, 57 and 60.
- Serious secondary infections (e.g. osteomyelitis, septic arthritis, pneumonia) may follow seemingly trivial superficial infections in infants.
- For recurrent impetigo, antibacterial soaps used twice daily are useful adjuncts.
- Bacterial culture can be helpful to evaluate for carrier state (nares) and resistant organisms (methicillin-resistant *Staphylococcus aureus*).

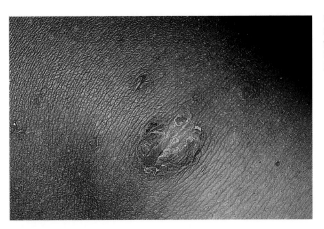

Excoriation of insect bites resulted in a secondary infection with impetigo. The infection was localized and responded to Mupirocin ointment.

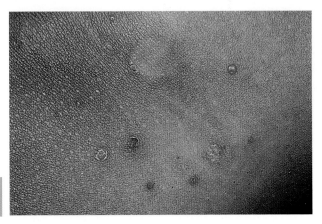

This patient had molluscum contagiosum. Lesions were excoriated and became impetiginized. Lesions cleared with Mupirocin ointment.

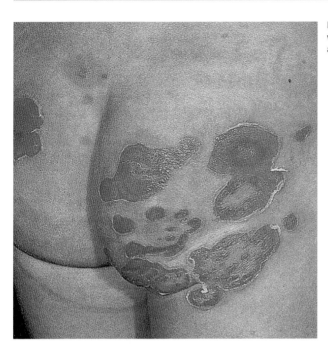

Bullous impetigo. Huge lesions with a glistening eroded base, and a collarette of moist scale.

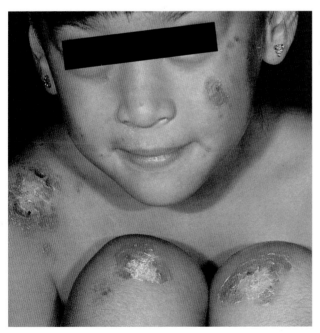

A bullous rim extended slowly for weeks. No topical or oral treatment had been attempted.

Cellulitis

Description
■ Cellulitis is an infection of the dermis and subcutaneous tissues characterized by fever, erythema, edema, and pain.

History
■ Localized pain and tenderness occur for a few days before presentation.
■ The most susceptible populations are people with diabetes, cirrhosis, renal failure, malnourishment, and human immunodeficiency virus. Patients who have cancer and are on chemotherapy or who abuse intravenous drugs and alcohol are also at increased risk.
■ Cellulitis typically occurs near surgical wounds and trauma sites (e.g. bites, burns, abrasions, lacerations, and ulcers).
■ It may develop in apparently normal skin or at sites of other dermatoses.
■ Recurrent episodes occur with local anatomic abnormalities that compromise the venous or lymphatic circulation (i.e. chronic stasis dermatitis).
■ The pinna and lower legs are particularly susceptible to recurrence.

Skin Findings
■ A pre-existing lesion such as an ulcer or erosion may act as a portal of entry for the infecting organism.
■ Athlete's foot may be a common predisposing condition for cellulitis of the lower extremities.
■ An expanding red, swollen, tender or painful plaque with an indefinite border may cover a small or wide area.
■ Palpation produces pain, but rarely crepitus.
■ Vesicles, blisters, hemorrhage, necrosis, or abscesses may occur.
■ Regional lymphadenopathy sometimes occurs; lymphangitis and adenitis are common with infection with *Streptococcus pyogenes*.
■ Repeated attacks on the legs can impair lymphatic drainage, leading to chronically swollen legs.
■ The end stage of repeated infection of the leg includes dermal fibrosis, lymphedema, and epidermal thickening. This is known as elephantiasis nostras.

Laboratory
■ Mild to moderate leukocytosis and a mildly elevated erythrocyte sedimentation rate may be present.
■ Cellulitis is most often caused by a group A streptococcus and *Staphylococcus aureus*. Many other bacteria can cause cellulitis. Less common causative organisms include *Erysipelothrix rhusiopathiae* (erysipeloid) in fish handlers, *Aeromonas hydrophilia* after swimming in fresh water, *Vibrio* species after swimming in salt water, *Pasteurella multocida* from an animal bite or scratch.
■ Culture of the lesion is a more predictable source of information than needle-aspirate cultures.

Differential Diagnosis
■ Stasis dermatitis
■ Thrombophlebitis
■ Deep venous thrombosis
■ Contact dermatitis
■ Erythema nodosum

Treatment
■ Pain can be relieved with cool Burrow's wet dressings.
■ Elevation of the affected limb assists with drainage and will hasten recovery. Rest with elevation of the affected limb is advised.

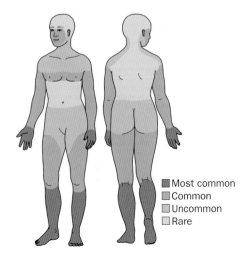

■ Most common
■ Common
■ Uncommon
□ Rare

- Empiric treatment with antibiotics aimed at staphylococcal and streptococcal organisms is appropriate, since it is difficult clinically to distinguish between streptococcal and staphylococcal infections.
- A penicillinase-resistant penicillin such as dicloxacillin 500 to 1000 mg orally every 6 hours
- Oral amoxicillin/clavulanate 875/125 mg twice daily or 500/125 mg three times daily (adult dose)
- A first generation cephalosporin such as cephalexin 250–500 mg four times daily.
- Azithromycin 500 mg initial dose, then 250 mg on days 2–5, or clarithromycin 500 mg every 12 hours.
- The mean time for healing after treatment is initiated is 12 days.
- Most cases improve when the patient is on simple oral antibiotic therapy. Non-responding cases require re-evaluation and consideration of intravenous antibiotics.
- Severe infections may require hospitalization and intravenous antibiotics. Intravenous empiric therapy with coverage for group A streptococci, and *Staphylococcus aureus* with cefazolin 1.0 g every 8 hours, or Nafcillin 2 g every 4–6 hours.
- Clostridial anaerobic cellulitis is most commonly caused by *Clostridia perfringens*, sometimes by other clostridia. Pain, soft tissue swelling and systemic toxicity are prominent features. Gas may be palpable or visible by x-ray. Treatment comprises of high-dose intravenous penicillin, in addition to prompt surgical exploration and debridement of devitalized tissue.
- Prolonged antimicrobial prophylaxis may be effective in preventing recurrent episodes. This may be continued for months or years using erythromycin (250 mg twice a day) or phenoxymethyl penicillin (250–500 mg twice a day).

Secondary bacterial cellulitis from pre-existing wounds, trauma, or skin lesions

- In eczema and lacerations infecting organisms are typically *Staphylococcus aureus* or group A streptococci.

- Infected decubitus ulcers are often malodorous and necrotic and are complicated by increasing tenderness and fever. Organisms most commonly present are mixed bowel flora (gram-negatives, streptococci, anaerobes).
- Infection of burns is most commonly due to *Pseudomonas aeruginosa*, other gram-negatives, *Staphylococcus aureus* and *Candida*.
- Post-surgical cellulitis may be due to Gram-negative organisms, and complicated by wound dehiscence and sepsis. Coverage for *Staphylococcus aureus*, group A streptococci, and gram-negative bacilli is recommended.

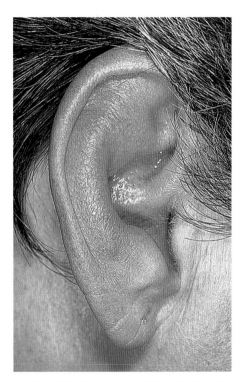

Cellulitis of the pinna may result from infection with *Pseudomonas* species or staphylococci and streptococci. The lymphatics may be permanently damaged during an attack, predisposing the patient to recurrent episodes of streptococcal erysipelas of the pinna. Recurrent attacks are brought on by manipulation, or even the slightest trauma.

143

- Gangrenous cellulitis involves extensive necrosis of subcutaneous tissue and overlying skin, and is a rapidly progressive form of cellulitis most commonly caused by group A streptococci. Such streptococcal gangrene most commonly occurs at the site of trauma. Painful erythema is followed by edema, bullae and necrosis, and may be complicated by rapid development of bacteremia and septic shock. Prompt management is critical.
- Treat infections from dog and cat bites with oral amoxicillin/clavulanic acid 875 mg/175 mg twice daily for 7–10 days or 500 mg/125 mg three times daily; an alternative is oral doxycycline 100 mg twice daily for 10 days. Cephalosporins are less effective.

Pearls

- Interdigital athlete's foot may be a predisposing condition for cellulitis of the lower extremity. Cultures from the interdigital spaces may yield the pathogenic bacteria.
- Cellulitis is characterized by erythema, edema and pain. Patients with cellulitis of the leg often have a pre-existing lesion, such as an ulcer or erosion, that acts as a portal of entry for the infecting organism.
- Empiric therapy of cellulitis must give good coverage for *Staphylococcus aureus*.
- Cellulitis of the pinna may result from infection with *Pseudomonas* species or with staphylococci and streptococci. The lymphatics may be permanently damaged during an attack, predisposing the patient to recurrent episodes of streptococcal erysipelas of the pinna. Recurrent attacks are brought on by manipulation, or even by the slightest trauma.

Pediatric Considerations

- Perianal cellulitis due to group A beta-hemolytic streptococci can be misdiagnosed as candidiasis. Children develop moist, edematous, pink skin around the anus and frequently complain of itch and pain with bowel movements.
- Cellulitis can complicate any cutaneous wound. Some children with varicella are at risk of acquiring invasive forms of group A beta-hemolytic streptococcus (necrotizing fasciitis)—return of fever, tachycardia and severe skin tenderness are signs that should prompt immediate evaluation for invasive group A streptococcus.
- Necrotizing fasciitis can occur after circumcision.

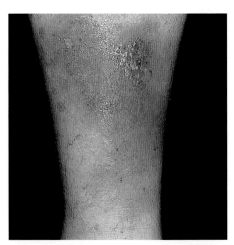

Cellulitis is characterized by erythema, edema, and pain. Patients with cellulitis of the leg often have a pre-existing lesion, such as an ulcer or erosion, that acts as a portal of entry for the infecting organism.

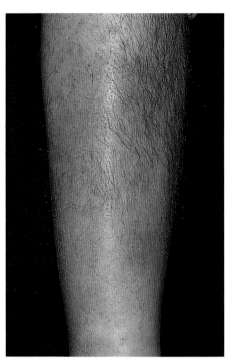

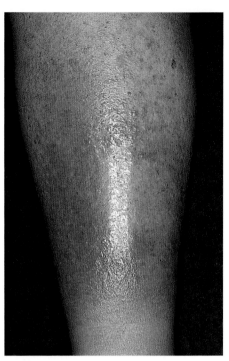

Cellulitis. An early case with diffuse erythema and minimal swelling. Pain was elicited with palpation.

Cellulitis. A more advanced case with edema and intense erythema. The lesion was painful. There was no regional lymphadenopathy.

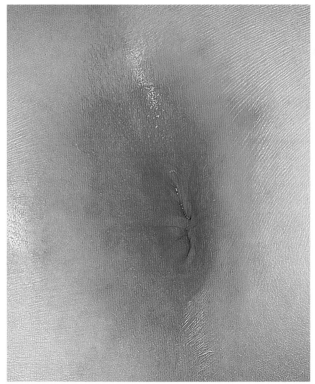

Perianal cellulitis. Cellulitis (group A beta-hemolytic streptococci) around the anal orifice is often misdiagnosed as candidiasis. It occurs more frequently in children. They are not systemically ill. Culture confirms the diagnosis. Systemic therapy is required.

Erysipelas

Description
- Erysipelas is an acute, inflammatory form of cellulitis that differs from other types of cellulitis in that lymphatic involvement ("streaking") is prominent.
- It is more superficial, involving the dermis and upper subcutaneous tissue, and the margins are more clearly demarcated from normal skin than those in classical cellulitis.
- The most common pathogen are group A streptococci.
- Infection may start at a break in the skin caused by a trauma, a surgical wound, an ulcer or bite, or superficial fungal infection. The site of entry is not always identified.

History
- Onset of the condition is sudden.
- Prodromal symptoms last for 4–48 hours and consist of malaise, myalgias, chills, high fever (38–40° C), and occasionally, anorexia and vomiting.
- Adenopathy and lymphangitis may also occur.

Skin Findings
- The most common site of involvement is the lower leg. The face, arm and upper thigh are other common sites. In the neonate, the periumbilical skin is a common site.
- One (or more) red, tender and firm spots rapidly increases in size, to form a tense and deeply erythematous, hot, sharply demarcated and uniformly elevated shiny patch with an irregular outline and raised border.
- The color becomes dark and deeply erythematous, and vesicles may appear at the advancing border and over the surface.
- Itching, burning, tenderness, and pain may be moderate or severe.
- Red, sometimes painful, streaks of lymphangitis may extend toward the regional lymph nodes.
- Repeated attacks can impair lymphatic drainage, which predisposes the patient to more infection and permanent swelling. This series of events takes place most commonly in the lower legs of patients with venous stasis and ulceration.

Non-skin Findings
- Predisposing diseases are lymphatic or venous circulatory problems, diabetes, renal failure, alcohol abuse, and immunosuppression.

Laboratory
- Streptococci cause 80% of cases; most often the culprits are group A streptococci, followed by group G and other non-group A streptococci. Group G streptococci may be common pathogens, especially in patients older than 50 years.
- *Streptococcus aureus, Pneumococcus, Klebsiella pneumoniae, Yersinia enterocolitica*, and *Haemophilus influenzae* are other causative agents.
- The diagnosis is based on the clinical findings; identification of the organism is difficult.
- Only a small percentage of cultures taken from the portal of entry and fluid from intact pustules or bullae are positive. The injection–aspiration method is unreliable.
- Blood cultures are sometimes positive if there is a high fever.
- The white blood cell count and erythrocyte sedimentation rate are frequently elevated.

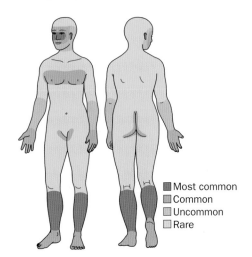

■ Most common
☐ Common
☐ Uncommon
☐ Rare

Course and Prognosis

■ Recurrences are common in people suffering from local impairment of circulation (e.g. post-mastectomy or with chronic venous stasis).

■ A relapse may occur in pharyngeal carriers of group A streptococci.

■ Post-streptococcal glomerulonephritis is a serious potential complication; streptococcal spread to distant sites is rare but has been reported. Cavernous sinus thrombosis is a serious and rare complication of erysipelas of the face.

Discussion

■ Erysipelas differs from cellulitis by exhibiting raised, clearly marginated borders and frequent lymphangitic streaking.

Treatment

■ In acute episodes, penicillin V orally 250–500 mg four times a day for 2 weeks is the drug of choice. Amoxicillin is also effective. Diagnosis of a streptococcal origin should be reconsidered if the response to penicillin is not rapid. Two alternatives for patients who cannot take penicillin are azithromycin (Zithromax) 500 mg on day 1 and 250 mg on day 2 to day 5, or clarithromycin (Biaxin) 250–500 mg every 12 hours for 7–14 days.

■ Bed rest and elevation of the affected limb is also indicated. Anticoagulant therapy should be considered in people taking bedrest who are at risk for venous thromboembolism.

■ Continuous antibiotic prophylaxis is indicated for patients with high recurrence rates. Daily administration of penicillin V orally 250–500 mg twice a day, or intramuscularly with benzathine penicillin 2.4 mUnits every 3 weeks for 1–2 years can be of help.

Pearls

■ Hospitalization for intravenous antibiotics, rest, and elevation should be considered if there are indications of severe advancing disease, comorbidity, or potential social barriers to appropriate and successful treatment.

■ Athlete's foot predisposes to erysipelas; it is the most common site for bacterial entry. Treatment of athlete's foot (tinea infection) is important to heal the otherwise compromised skin barrier.

■ A common complication of erysipelas is recurrence—due to lymphatic damage, subsequent swelling, and lymphedema—which predispose to repeated infection.

Pediatric Considerations

● Children do not often develop erysipelas.

● Erysipelas due to *Haemophilus influenzae* rarely occurs due to the introduction of the *Haemophilus* vaccine.

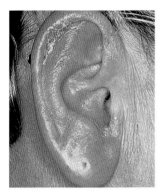

Recurrent episodes of infection have resulted in lymphatic obstruction and have caused permanent thickening of the skin.

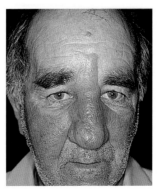

Erysipelas is an acute inflammatory form of cellulitis in which lymphatic involvement or "streaking" is prominent. Erysipelas is more superficial than cellulitis and has margins that are more clearly demarcated from normal skin.

147

Folliculitis

Description
- *Folliculitis* means an inflammation of the hair follicle, and there are several types.
- Common types include mechanical folliculitis from persistent trauma or tight clothing; another common type is bacterial folliculitis.
- Fungal folliculitis is less common but can result from untreated tinea corporis, or tinea infection in the beard or hair-bearing skin.
- Bacterial folliculitis includes follicular impetigo, a superficial form, and sycosis barbae, a deep form occurring in the beard area.

History
- Usually the eruption is abrupt.
- Bacterial folliculitis can spread by trauma, scratching, or shaving.
- The distribution is variable; often the scalp, arms, legs, axillae and trunk are involved.

Skin Findings
- Dome-shaped pustules with small erythematous halos arise in the follicle. These lesions are sometimes tender.
- In sycosis barbae, the inflammation is intense and deep; there is marked tenderness.

Laboratory
- Culture is not routinely necessary. *Staphylococcus aureus* is the most common infecting organism.
- Potassium hydroxide examination of the hair and surrounding scale is performed to exclude an infection by a dermatophyte.

Course and Prognosis
- Most folliculitis responds to antibiotics and hygienic measures. However, bacterial folliculitis may be recurrent if there is a source of bacteria (nasal vestibule in carriers of *Staphylococcus aureus*).

Discussion
- In a dermatophyte infection (Majocchi granuloma) hair follicle infection is caused by a dermatophyte fungus. There are inflammatory papules and pustules with surrounding scale and eczematous papules. The results of a potassium hydroxide examination of the hair and surrounding scale are positive.
- In eosinophilic folliculitis, pruritic, extensive follicular papules suddenly appear on the face, neck, and chest. Testing for the human immunodeficiency virus should be performed. The diagnosis of eosinophilic folliculitis is usually confirmed or suspected by lesional biopsy findings.
- In Gram-negative folliculitis, an acneiform eruption suddenly worsens and becomes pustular. Superficial Gram-negative bacterial overgrowth occurs in people on chronic antibiotics (often for treatment of acne).
- In hot tub folliculitis, erythematous papules and pustules appear, primarily on the trunk. *Pseudomonas* follicular infection is acquired from improperly sanitized hot tubs.
- Mechanical folliculitis results from chronic frictional exposure, such as occurs from tight pants.
- Occlusion folliculitis results from occlusion, for example from exposure to oil, greases or occlusive ointments.
- *Pityrosporum* folliculitis often appears on the back and chest. The results of potassium hydroxide testing are positive for short hyphae and round spores.
- In steroid folliculitis, multiple monomorphic small pustules and red

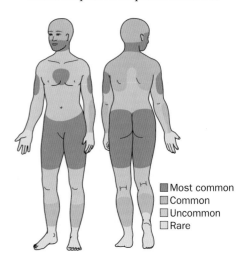

Most common
Common
Uncommon
Rare

papules appear within 2 weeks of using systemic corticosteroids; a neutrophilic inflammation of the hair follicles occurs.

Treatment

- Heat, friction, and occlusion should be minimized.
- Antibacterial soap and warm wet dressings are helpful. Razors should be changed frequently to avoid reinfection.
- Mupirocin (Bactroban) applied three times daily for 5 days is effective for limited, superficial involvement. Treat intranasally as well if culture confirms carriage of *Staphylococcus aureus*.
- Oral antistaphylococcal antibiotics (oxacillin, dicloxacillin, cefuroxime) are indicated for extensive or spreading disease, or for deep involvement of sycosis barbae.
- *Pityrosporum* folliculitis can be treated with topical or oral anti-yeast antibiotics such as clotrimazole lotion and econazole cream. Two tablets of 200 mg ketoconazole taken once and repeated after 1 week is also an effective regimen for widespread *Pityrosporum* folliculitis.
- Follicular dermatophyte infection (Majocchi granuloma) responds best to oral antifungal therapy. Griseofulvin or terbinafine (Lamisil) are good therapeutic choices.

Pearls

- Potassium hydroxide examination of the hair and any surrounding scaling should be performed to exclude a dermatophyte infection; failure to consider a dermatophyte infection can result in persistent and sometimes destructive follicular inflammation.
- Staphylococcal folliculitis is the most common form of infectious folliculitis. A group of pustules may appear, usually without fever or other systemic symptoms, on any body surface.
- Nasal carriage of *Staphylococcus aureus* is a common reason for recurrent bacterial folliculitis. Successful treatment must address the nasal carrier state.

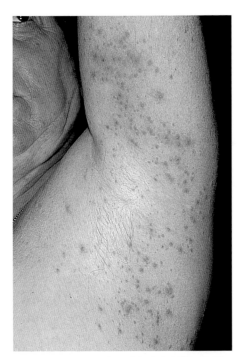

Folliculitis is inflammation of the hair follicle that is caused by infection, chemical irritation, or physical injury.

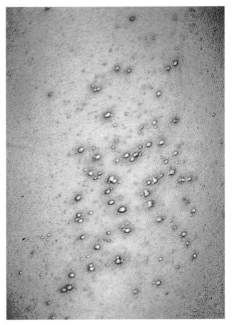

Staphylococcal folliculitis is the most common form of infectious folliculitis. A group of pustules may appear, usually without fever or other systemic symptoms, on any body surface. It may be a complication of occlusive topical steroid therapy, as in this case.

Pseudofolliculitis Barbae (Razor Bumps, Ingrown Hairs)

Description
- Pseudofolliculitis barbae is a papular and pustular, foreign body, inflammatory reaction that can affect any individual who has curly hair and who shaves closely on a regular basis.
- This condition is a particular problem in people of Hispanic or African-American background.
- It is often chronic, and can be disfiguring.

History
- Pseudofolliculitis barbae is a significant problem in predisposed individuals who are required to shave closely.
- It is found in 50-75% of African-American people and 3-5% of Caucasian people who shave.
- It is found in both men and women.
- The most severely affected site is the neck area.
- This is a chronic problem unless close shaving is avoided.

Skin Findings
- Pseudofolliculitis barbae affects people with curly hair or those with hair follicles oriented at an oblique angle to the skin surface.
- A sharp, shaved, tapered hair re-enters the skin as it grows from below the skin surface and induces a foreign body reaction, producing a microabscess.
- Perifollicular red papules or pustules appear in the affected skin, most commonly the beard area. The lesions can be both painful and/or pruritic.
- This condition occurs in any area where the hair is shaved (scalp, posterior neck, groin, legs).
- Scarring and hyperpigmentation may result from this chronic condition.
- Keloid formation is often a problem in affected skin, especially in African-American people.

Laboratory
- Typically the lesions are sterile inflammatory papules. The diagnosis is clinical, based on lesion location and appearance.
- Cultured lesions may reveal secondary staphylococcal infection as normal flora may be replaced by pathogenic organisms.

Differential Diagnosis
- Acne
- Folliculitis, bacterial or fungal (culture of a pustule may be helpful, and in resistant, severe or spreading conditions a perifollicular scraping or skin biopsy may reveal tinea infection)

Treatment
- The imbedded hair shaft must be dislodged. A needle is inserted under the hair loop, and the hair is firmly elevated.
- A Buff Puff or toothbrush can be used to gently massage in a circular fashion and thus dislodge any ingrown hair.
- Shaving should be discontinued until inflammation is under control.
- Topical azelaic acid cream (Finacea) will help reduce post-inflammatory hyperpigmentation while reducing bacterial colonization.
- Topical antibiotic preparations (clindamycin, benzoyl peroxide 5% or 10%, erythromycin) reduce bacterial colonization and may be beneficial in some patients.
- A short course of antistaphylococcal antibiotics may decrease inflammation and hasten the resolution.
- Intralesional triamcinolone acetonide 2.5 mg/ml is used for persistent papules. Atrophy may result temporarily.
- Once lesions resolve shaving may be resumed.
- Topical eflorinithine hydrochloride 13.9% cream (Vaniqa) inhibits ornithine decarboxylase—an enzyme important in

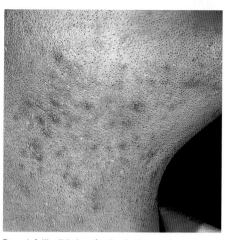

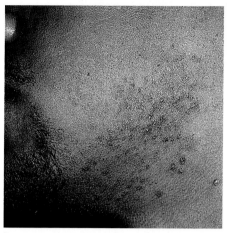

Pseudofolliculitis is a foreign body reaction to hair. The disease occurs only in men who have commenced shaving. It begins with the appearance of small follicular papules or pustules and rapidly becomes more diffuse as shaving continues.

The problem is more severe in the neck area, where hair follicles are more likely to be oriented at low angles to the skin surface, making re-penetration of the skin more likely.

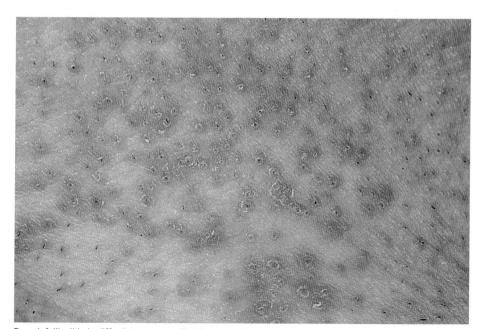

Pseudofolliculitis is difficult to manage. Hair is trapped just beneath the skin and initiates an inflammatory reaction. Shaving against the grain is a cause in predisposed people. This patient eventually had to stop shaving.

hair cell division—and retards hair growth. It is applied twice daily to affected skin. It is well tolerated in most, although a few users develop a mild irritant dermatitis.

- Depilatories (Nair, Neet) with barium sulfide or calcium thioglycolate are effective alternatives to shaving. They are applied to the skin for 3–10 minutes and then wiped off. These products are irritating and can be tolerated only once or twice each week.
- If all measures fail, shaving must be discontinued indefinitely.
- The only cure is permanent removal of the hair follicle. Laser-assisted hair removal may provide a safe, effective means of treating recalcitrant cases. Laser hair removal can be performed with the diode laser (800–810 nm), pulsed alexandrite (755 nm), neodynium-yttrium-aluminum garnet (Nd-YAG) (1064 nm) and pulsed noncoherent light source. Adverse effects include pigmentary alteration, including post-inflammatory hypopigmentation in people with dark skin, since melanin is the target of laser hair removal.

Shaving Instructions

- The goal is to avoid close shaves and the production of sharply angled hair tips.
- The patient should hydrate the beard before shaving. Shower before shaving and keep the beard hair in contact with warm water for at least 2 minutes.

- Dislodge any hair tips that are beginning to pierce the skin. A soft-bristled toothbrush in a circular motion or a needle cleaned with rubbing alcohol should be used. This is done before shaving and at bedtime.
- Use thick-lathering shaving gels (Aveeno Therapeutic Shave Gel, Edge Gel for Tough Beards).
- The Bump Fighter razor (http://www.asrco.com) cuts the hair slightly above the skin surface.
- Alternatively an electric razor can be used, but avoiding the "closest" shave setting.
- The patient should shave in the direction of hair growth. The skin should not be stretched.
- Multiple razor strokes should be avoided.
- A moisturizing lotion should be used after shaving. LactiCare-HC (1% or 2.5%) can be used intermittently to reduce inflammation.

Pearls

- Pseudofolliculitis is a foreign body reaction to hair. The problem is more severe in the neck area, where hair follicles are more likely to be oriented at low angles relative to the skin surface, making re-penetration of the skin more likely.
- The avoidance of close shaving is recommended.
- Presently, laser hair removal appears to offer the best long-term results in this otherwise chronic condition.

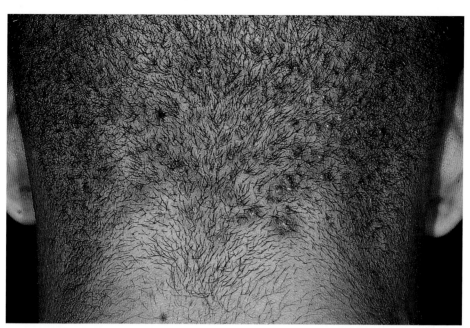

Acne keloidalis is an eruption that appears on the back of the neck. It is most often found in African-American men. The eruption is often mistaken for pseudofolliculitis but it is not caused by shaving.

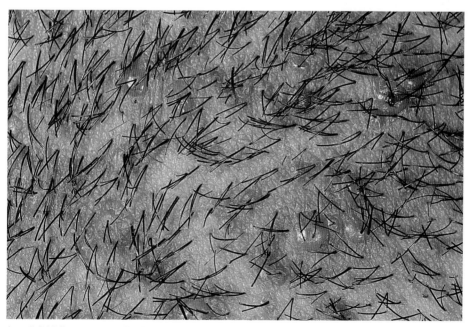

Acne keloidalis presents as hard papules with hair emerging from the center. This chronic progressive disease is managed with long-term suppression with antibiotics, topical and intralesional steroids.

Furuncles and Carbuncles

Description
- A furuncle (boil) is a walled-off, deep and painful, firm or fluctuant mass enclosing a collection of pus; often, it evolves from a superficial folliculitis.
- *Staphylococcus aureus* is the most commonly associated organism, but other organisms (*Escherichia coli, Pseudomonas aeruginosa, Streptococcus faecalis*) and anaerobes (*Peptostreptococcus, Peptococcus,* and *Lactobacillus* species) may cause lesions.
- Usually, a bacteriologic study of the abscess identifies the local flora.
- A carbuncle is an extremely painful, deep, interconnected aggregate of infected, abscessed follicles.

History
- Furuncles and carbuncles are uncommon in children.
- Occlusion and hyperhidrosis promote bacterial colonization.
- Most affected patients have normal immune systems, although certain conditions and immune defects may predispose the patient to furuncles and carbuncles (e.g. hyperimmunoglobulin E syndrome, chronic granulomatous disease, Wiskott–Aldrich syndrome, Chediak–Higashi syndrome, diabetes, leukemia, therapeutic immunosuppression, malnutrition, obesity).

Skin Findings
- Any hair-bearing site can be affected. Sites of high friction and sweating are most typically affected; these include the areas under the belt, the anterior thighs, the buttocks, the groin, the axillae, and the waist.
- With a furuncle, a deep dermal or subcutaneous, red, swollen and painful mass later points towards the surface and drains through multiple openings.
- With a carbuncle, deep, tender, firm subcutaneous erythematous papules enlarge to deep-seated nodules that can be stable or become fluctuant within several days.

- Favored sites for carbuncles are the back of the neck, the upper back, and the lateral thighs.

Non-skin Findings
- With a furuncle, the patient remains afebrile.
- With a carbuncle, malaise, chills and fever may precede or occur during the height of inflammation.

Laboratory
- Gram stain, culture and sensitivity are indicated and will help guide appropriate antibiotic therapy.

Differential Diagnosis
- Ruptured pilar or epidermal cyst
- Cystic acne
- Hidradenitis suppurativa
- Early lesion of pyoderma gangrenosum

Course and Prognosis
- The abscess either remains deep and is reabsorbed, or points toward the surface and ruptures.
- A ruptured lesion heals with a depressed, violaceous scar.
- Infection can spread to other sites.
- Recurrent furunculosis can be difficult to eradicate.

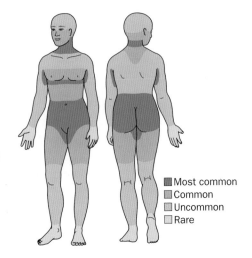

■ Most common
□ Common
□ Uncommon
□ Rare

Treatment
Furuncles and Carbuncles

- ▨ Warm, moist dressings are applied to the lesion 15–30 minutes several times a day. A culture and sensitivity is often appropriate for large or atypical lesions.
- ▨ Incision and drainage is the primary management for pointing, fluctuant lesions.
- ▨ Local anesthesia is required. Iodoform gauze is used for packing large abscesses; it is removed daily followed by cleansing of the wound, or it should be replaced when saturated.
- ▨ Periodic follow-up and re-evaluation is recommended to ensure wound improvement and treatment response.
- ▨ Systemic antibiotic therapy is indicated for most cases with an appropriate antistaphylococcal antibiotic, as shown below.
  - Dicloxacillin 250–500 mg four times daily for 10 days in adults.
  - Cephalexin 250–500 mg four times daily for 10 days in adults; 40–50 mg/kg/day divided three times daily in children.
  - Amoxicillin and clavulanate 875 mg twice daily for 10 days in adults; children aged more than 3 months and weighing less than 40 kg can be given 45 mg/kg/day divided twice or three times daily.
  - Clindamycin 150–300 mg four times daily for 10 days in adults; 15 mg/kg/day divided four times daily for 10 days in children.
  - Nafcillin or oxacillin 2 g intravenously every 6 hours is the drug of choice for moderate to severe infections with furunculosis and cellulitis with methicillin-sensitive *Staphylococcus aureus*. The incidence of methicillin-resistant *Staphylococcus aureus* (MRSA) is increasing, making culture and sensitivity data increasingly important.

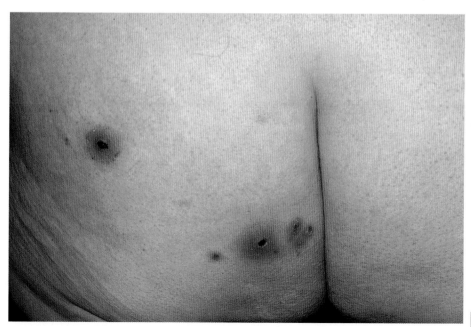

Boils (furuncles) are present on the buttock. They were all superficial and drained onto the surface. The surface of each lesion has crusted. All lesions were painful.

■ The patient should be advised of warning signs and symptoms of possible advancing or systemic infection—fever, malaise, spreading redness, increasing discomfort. Re-evaluation and hospitalization for intravenous antibiotic therapy should be considered.

Recurrent Furuncles and Carbuncles

■ To eradicate the carrier state of *Staphylococcus aureus*, Mupirocin cream (Bactroban) or ointment is applied to affected skin wounds and nares twice daily for 5 days or rifampin 600 mg for 10 days and either dicloxacillin 500 mg four times daily or trimethoprim–sulfamethoxasole one double-strength tablet twice daily for 10 days.

■ Methicillin-resistant carrier state can be treated with Mupirocin 2% on nares and wounds twice daily for 1–2 weeks, or one trimethoprim–sulfamethoxasole double-strength tablet twice daily orally for 10 days, and rifampin 600 mg every day for 10 days.

■ Maintenance regimens with Mupirocin may induce resistance in roughly 10% of patients.

■ Other measures include washing the entire body and fingernails each day for 1–3 weeks with Betadine and changing and washing the towels, washcloths, and bed sheets daily. The patient should change the wound dressings frequently, clean or replace shaving tools daily, and avoid nose picking.

■ Applicable predisposing factors must be addressed, including friction, tight clothing, exposure to industrial chemicals, obesity, poor hygiene, and diabetes.

Pearls

■ The primary management for a solitary furuncle is incision and drainage.

■ Secondary dissemination due to bacteremia can occur and is a greater risk in people who are immunocompromised, or those with alcoholism or diabetes. Seeding of artificial valves, grafts, long bones, kidneys or joints is a risk.

■ The nasal carriage of *Staphylococcus aureus*, or carriage of the bacterium in the folds or perineum, should be evaluated by culture in cases of chronic recurrent furunculosis.

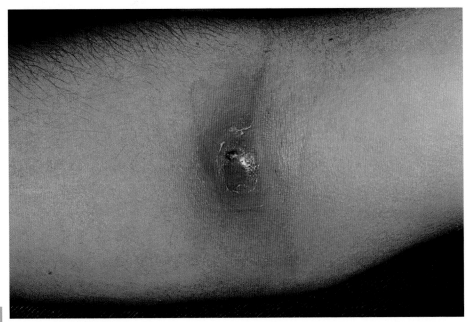

A furuncle has rapidly evolved in a plaque of atopic dermatitis. The center is swollen and soft and will soon rupture and exude purulent material.

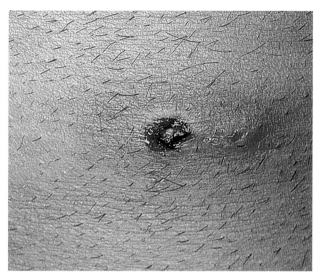

The abscess either remains deep and reabsorbs, or points and ruptures through the surface. This lesion ruptured and formed a crust. Oral antibiotics were not required and the lesion resolved without treatment.

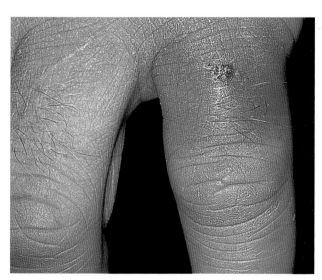

A single lesion on the finger. Surrounding erythema became more extensive and the patient was treated with cefadroxil 500 mg twice a day for 6 days.

Pseudomonas Folliculitis

Description
- *Pseudomonas* folliculitis is an acute skin infection that follows exposure to contaminated water.
- The urticarial red plaque with a central papule or pustule is highly distinctive.
- This is also called "hot tub folliculitis".

History
- The attack rate is significantly higher in children than in adults, possibly because children tend to spend more time in the water.
- *Pseudomonas* folliculitis occurs 8 hours to 5 days (or longer) after using a contaminated pool (whirlpool, hot tub, physiotherapy pool) or water slide, or a contaminated loofah sponge. The attack rate is variable; 7% to 100% of those exposed to *Pseudomonas* species develop the disease.
- The spread of infection from person to person is unlikely.
- Prolonged exposure to the water, excessive numbers of bathers, and inadequate pool care predispose to infection.
- Desquamated skin cells in the water provide a rich, organic nutrient source for bacteria.
- In most cases, the eruption clears in 7–10 days without any treatment, but recurrent crops of lesions may occur for as long as 3 months.

Skin Findings
- Plaques are 0.5–3 cm, and are red, pruritic, round and urticarial with a central papule or pustule.
- A few plaques to more than 50 occur primarily on the trunk.
- The rash may be a follicular, maculopapular, vesicular, or pustular, or a polymorphous eruption that includes all of these types of lesions.
- The rash is most severe in areas occluded by snug bathing suits.
- Occlusion and super-hydration of the stratum corneum favors colonization of the skin with *Pseudomonas aeruginosa*.
- Women who wear one-piece bathing suits are at an increased risk.
- The rash resolves, leaving round spots of red to brown, post-inflammatory hyperpigmentation.

Non-skin Findings
- Fever, malaise and fatigue may occur during the initial few days of the eruption, but this is uncommon.

Laboratory
- *Pseudomonas aeruginosa* serotypes 0:9 and 0:11 are most commonly isolated from skin lesions, but other serotypes have been reported.

Differential Diagnosis
- Staphylococcal folliculitis
- Hives
- Insect bites

Treatment
- The infection is self-limited; treatment is usually not required.
- A wet dressing of acetic acid 5% (white vinegar) is applied for 20 minutes twice or four times a day. Silver sulfadiazine cream (Silvadene) can help.
- Cases resistant to topical therapy can be treated orally with ciprofloxacin (Cipro) 500 mg or 750 mg twice each day for 5–10 days.

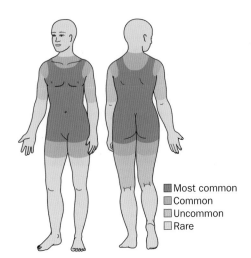

■ Most common
□ Common
□ Uncommon
□ Rare

Preventative Measures

- Continuous water filtration eliminates desquamated skin.
- Adequate chlorine levels should be maintained.

- The water in private hot tubs should be changed every 4–8 weeks.
- Public hot tubs should be drained daily.
- Showering after using the contaminated facility offers no protection.

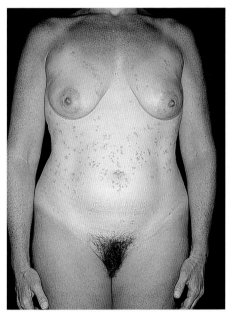

Occlusion and superhydration of the stratum corneum favors colonization of the skin with *Pseudomonas aeruginosa*. This may explain why the rash is most severe in areas occluded by a snug bathing suit. Women who wear one-piece bathing suits are at an increased risk.

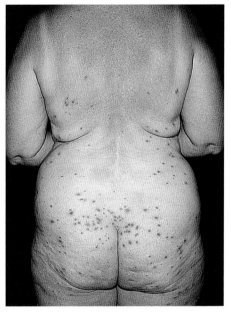

About 48 hours after the patient used a contaminated whirlpool, pruritic, round, urticarial plaques with a central papule or pustule appeared.

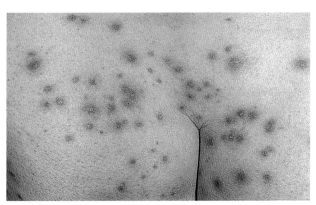

The rash may be a follicular, maculopapular, vesicular, pustular, or a polymorphous eruption that includes all of these types of lesions.

Otitis Externa

Description

■ Otitis externa is an inflammation of the external auditory canal, usually with secondary infection.

History

■ Otitis externa is found equally among males and females.

■ A mild self-limited form known as swimmer's ear is especially common in children, often in the summer.

■ No racial or genetic predisposition has been reported.

■ Symptoms range from itch and irritation to severe pain.

■ Mechanical cleansing of the external canal and medicaments used to relieve symptoms can mask or exacerbate the condition.

■ Cerumen is produced by modified apocrine glands of the external auditory canal. It forms a water-resistant barrier for the thin skin that lines the canal. It inhibits bacterial growth by maintaining a low pH environment. When this protective barrier is disrupted, bacterial overgrowth can occur.

■ The usual pathogen is *Pseudomonas*, but mixed infections with *Staphylococcus* and *Pseudomonas* species are common.

■ Swimmer's ear is typically caused by *Pseudomonas* species, Enterobacteriaceae, or *Proteus* species. Acute infection is usually due to *Staphylococcus aureus*.

■ Secondary infections with *Candida* species may also occur, but are uncommon.

Skin Findings

■ Dull pain is localized to the external auditory canal.

■ The external auditory canal is inflamed with erythema and edema.

■ Keratin and inflammatory cell debris accumulate within the canal. Most cases do not progress beyond this point.

■ With progression, the pinna becomes red, hot, and edematous.

■ Cellulitis involves the entire pinna and often extends to the preauricular skin. At this point, pain becomes sharp and constant.

■ Purulent drainage exudes from the external auditory canal.

Non-skin Findings

■ The regional lymph nodes are usually palpable and tender.

Laboratory

■ A skin biopsy is not recommended.

■ The external auditory canal should be cultured.

Course and Prognosis

■ The protective barrier of cerumen may be compromised by any number of mechanisms.

■ Mechanical disruption (i.e. vigorous cleansing of the canal), inflammatory conditions (e.g. psoriasis, seborrheic dermatitis), and contact dermatitis (irritant and allergic) may all lead to disruption of the barrier.

■ A rare and severe form of otitis, referred to as malignant external otitis, may develop in patients who have diabetes or who have had ear surgery. Cellulitis extends from the external auditory canal into the bone at the base of the skull. The ipsilateral facial nerve becomes involved.

■ Lymphatic drainage from the pinna may be altered by cellulitis. Such patients may be predisposed to future episodes of streptococcal erysipelas of the pinna.

Discussion

■ Early in the course, the differential diagnosis includes psoriasis, seborrheic dermatitis, and contact dermatitis. Any of these conditions can lead to compromise of the natural barrier and ultimately to otitis externa.

■ Herpes zoster infection involving the geniculate ganglion and Ramsay–Hunt syndrome can mimic early otitis externa with localized pain and inflammation. Careful examination reveals vesicles within the external auditory canal. Usually an ipsilateral Bell's palsy is present, or it develops soon after onset.

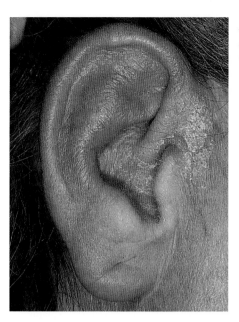

Otitis externa. Erythema begins in the ear canal. Traction on the ear produces pain. The canal usually contains moist debris. Eczema of the pinna, as occurs in this case, may be present.

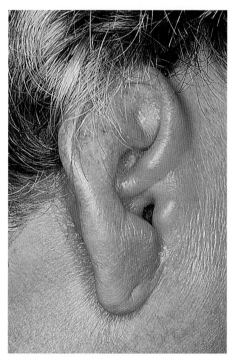

Pseudomonas cellulitis. The entire pinna and surrounding skin have become inflamed after an episode of external otitis.

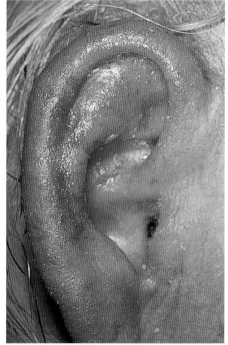

Malignant external otitis. Patients have a history of non-resolving otitis externa of many weeks' duration. Most patients are diabetic. *Pseudomonas* organisms invade underlying soft tissues. There is severe ear pain, a purulent exudate, and granulation tissue. Nuclear scanning studies and computerized tomography scans may reveal osteomyelitis of the skull base.

- When cellulitis involves the ear, the differential diagnosis includes relapsing polychondritis, a recurrent phenomenon presumably of autoimmune origin. Purulent discharge is not seen in this condition.

Treatment

- Treatment involves re-establishing the natural protective barrier.
- Cellular debris is flushed from the external canal with gentle irrigation.
- An acetic acid solution (VoSol otic solution or VoSol HC otic solution) helps lower the pH and inhibits bacterial and fungal growth.
- Ofloxacin otic solution 0.3% (Floxin otic solution twice daily) or ciprofloxacin and hydrocortisone (Cipro HC otic) are instilled twice a day. For acute disease, oral dicloxacillin 500 mg four times daily.
- Topical steroids, or wet dressings using an astringent such as Domeboro, or Bluboro wet dressings applied for half an hour three times daily, and oral antibiotics such as ciprofloxacin (Cipro) are of value when cellulitis involves the pinna.
- Avoidance of the more common contact allergens (such as topicals bacitracin, neomycin, and hydrocortisone) and review of other topical product contents for possible contact allergens can minimize the chance of a contact allergy complicating this problem.

- Vigorous scratching, rubbing, or mechanical debridement of the external auditory canal can remove protective wax defenses and should be strongly discouraged.
- Malignant external otitis requires hospitalization, the administration of intravenous antibiotics, and debridement—as well as consideration of a computerized scan or magnetic resonance imaging scan to evaluate possible osteomyelitis.
- An otolaryngology consultation is recommended.

Pearls

- Chronic otitis externa is often secondary to an underlying skin condition, such as seborrhea, psoriasis, or contact allergy. Seborrhea should be controlled with an antidandruff shampoo, such as selenium 2.5% or ketoconazole shampoo, and a medium-potency steroid solution, such as fluocinolone acetonide solution 0.01% twice daily. Consider patch testing for contact allergy that aggravates this problem.
- In malignant otitis externa there is typically a history of non-resolving otitis externa of many weeks' duration. Most patients are diabetic. *Pseudomonas* organisms invade underlying soft tissues. There is severe ear pain, purulent exudate, and granulation tissue.

7 Sexually Transmitted Infections

Sexually Transmitted Diseases

Treatment Guidelines 2002

(Summary of treatment of most common sexually transmitted diseases. Consult www.cdc.gov for complete details and latest guidelines.)

Genital Herpes Simplex Virus (HSV) Infections

First Clinical Episode of Genital Herpes
Acyclovir 400 mg orally three times a day for 7–10 days
    OR
Acyclovir 200 mg orally five times a day for 7–10 days,
    OR
Famciclovir 250 mg orally three times a day for 7–10 days,
    OR
Valacyclovir 1 g orally twice a day for 7–10 days.

NOTE: Treatment may be extended if healing is incomplete after 10 days of therapy.

Recurrent Episodes of HSV Disease
Acyclovir 400 mg orally three times a day for 5 days,
    OR
Acyclovir 200 mg orally five times a day for 5 days,
    OR
Acyclovir 800 mg orally twice a day for 5 days,
    OR
Famciclovir 125 mg orally twice a day for 5 days,
    OR
Valacyclovir 500mg orally twice a day for 3–5 days,
    OR
Valacyclovir 1 g orally once a day for 5 days.

Suppressive Therapy for Recurrent Genital Herpes
Acyclovir 400 mg orally twice a day
    OR
Famciclovir 250 mg orally twice a day,
    OR
Valacyclovir 500 mg orally once a day,
    OR
Valacyclovir 1 g orally once a day.

Valacyclovir 500 mg once a day might be less effective than other valacyclovir or acyclovir dosing regimens in patients who have very frequent recurrences (i.e. >10 episodes per year).

Syphilis

Primary and Secondary Syphilis (Recommended Regimen for Adults)
Benzathine penicillin G 2.4 million units IM in a single dose.

Latent Syphilis (Recommended Regimen for Adults)

Early latent syphilis
Benzathine penicillin G 2.4 million units intramuscularly in a single dose.

Late latent syphilis or latent syphilis of unknown duration
Benzathine penicillin G 7.2 million units total, administered as three doses of 2.4 million units intramuscularly each at 1 week intervals.

Chancroid

Azithromycin 1 g orally in a single dose,
   OR
Ceftriaxone 250 mg intramuscularly in a single dose,
   OR
Ciprofloxacin 500 mg orally twice a day for 3 days,
   OR
Erythromycin base 500 mg orally three times a day for 7 days.

Management of Patients who have Nongonococcal Urethritis

Azithromycin 1 g orally in a single dose
   OR
Doxycycline 100 mg orally twice a day for 7 days.

Alternative regimens

Erythromycin base 500 mg orally four times a day for 7 days,
   OR
Erythromycin ethylsuccinate 800 mg orally four times a day for 7 days,
   OR
Ofloxacin 300 mg twice a day for 7 days,
   OR
Levofloxacin 500 mg once daily for 7 days.

Recurrent and Persistent Urethritis

Recommended Regimens

Metronidazole 2 g orally in a single dose
   PLUS
Erythromycin base 500 mg orally four times a day for 7 days
   OR
Erythromycin ethylsuccinate 800 mg orally four times a day for 7 days.

Uncomplicated Gonococcal Infections of the Cervix, Urethra, and Rectum

Recommended regimens

Cefixime 400 mg orally in a single dose,
   OR
Ceftriaxone 125 mg intramuscularly in a single dose,
   OR
Ciprofloxacin 500 mg orally in a single dose,*
   OR
Ofloxacin 400 mg orally in a single dose,*
   OR
Levofloxacin 250 mg orally in a single dose,*
   PLUS (IF CHLAMYDIAL INFECTION IS NOT RULED OUT)
Azithromycin 1 g orally in a single dose
   OR
Doxycycline 100 mg orally twice a day for 7 days.

*Quinolones should not be used for infections acquired in Asia or the Pacific, including Hawaii. In addition, use of quinolones is probably inadvisable for treating infections acquired in California and in other areas with increased prevalence of quinolone resistance.

Syphilis

Description
- Syphilis is a sexually transmitted infectious disease caused by the spirochete *Treponema pallidum*.
- It can affect virtually every organ in the body and mimic various other diseases.
- Untreated, syphilis passes through three stages: primary infectious, secondary, and latent, or progression to a rare tertiary stage.
- Syphilis is also called lues.

History
- Syphilis is of great historical importance. It was named after an afflicted sheep herder named Syphilus in 1530.
- It is believed the disease was introduced to Europe by Columbus after returning from the West Indies, and its spread within Europe was blamed on the frequent wars within the region at that time. Incidence declined after World War II because of penicillin treatment.
- The Tuskegee study is a dark part of syphilis history. In 1932, penicillin therapy for black men who were infected with syphilis was withheld in order to study the short-term and long-term effects of the disease.
- Syphilis has become more common with the introduction of the acquired immune deficiency syndrome (AIDS) and is more common in homosexual men, bisexual men, and prostitutes.

Primary Syphilis
- A cutaneous ulcer (chancre) is acquired by direct contact with an infectious lesion.
- The chancre appears 10–90 days (average 21 days) after exposure. It develops at the site of initial contact.
- Chancres are usually solitary, but multiple lesions can occur.
- Untreated primary chancres resolve in 75% of cases, but the spirochete remains within the host.

Secondary Syphilis
- Secondary syphilis results from hematogenous and lymphatic spread of the spirochete.
- The secondary stage begins approximately 6 weeks after the chancre appears and it lasts for 2–10 weeks.
- An influenza-like syndrome occurs with mucocutaneous lesions, hepatosplenomegaly, and generalized adenopathy.
- The distribution and morphologic characteristics of individual lesions vary.
- Syphilis in this stage is easily confused with numerous other cutaneous and systemic diseases, and therefore it has been termed the "great imitator".

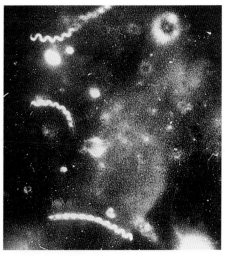

Treponema pallidum is the organism responsible for syphilis, seen here photographed through a dark-field microscope.

Latent Syphilis

- The results of serologic tests are positive (not false positive) without evidence of active disease.
- The early latent period begins 1 year or less from the onset of primary disease; late latent syphilis may last more than 4 years.
- About 25% of untreated cases in the secondary stage relapse during the first year; a small percentage relapse in the second year.

Tertiary Syphilis

- Tertiary syphilis is characterized by a small number of organisms eliciting a large or brisk cellular immune response.
- Systemic disease develops in about 25% of untreated or inadequately treated cases.
- Cardiovascular and central nervous system involvement, with systemic granulomas or gummas may occur.

Congenital Syphilis

- *Treponema pallidum* can be transmitted from an infected mother to her fetus.

- In untreated cases, 25% of neonates are stillborn, 25% die shortly after birth, 10% have no symptoms, and 40% will have late symptomatic congenital syphilis.
- In early congenital syphilis, rash, hepatosplenomegaly, bone and joint changes occur before age 2 years.
- In late congenital syphilis, bone and joint changes, neural deafness and interstitial keratitis occur after age 5 years.
- Therapy before the 16th week of gestation usually prevents infection of the fetus.
- A fetus is at greatest risk when the mother has syphilis for less than 2 years.

Skin Findings

Primary Syphilis

- The chancre begins as a papule, undergoes ischemic necrosis, and erodes.
- A painless (sometimes tender), hard and indurated chancre of 0.3–2.0 cm forms.
- The borders are raised, smooth, and sharply defined.
- These lesions may be asymptomatic and undetected on the cervix of women, allowing transmission to the unsuspecting.

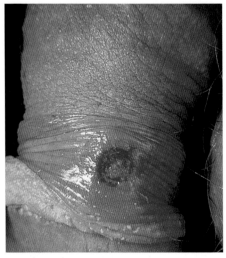

Primary syphilis. The lesion begins as a papule that undergoes ischemic necrosis and erodes, forming a 0.3–2.0 cm, painless to tender, hard, indurated ulcer. The base is clean, with a scant yellow serous discharge.

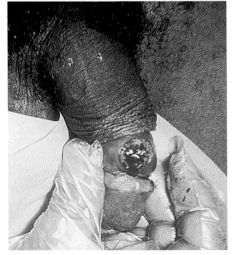

Primary syphilis. The borders of the ulcer are raised, smooth, and sharply defined.

- Painless, hard, discrete, non-suppurative regional lymphadenopathy develops in 1-2 weeks.
- The chancre heals with scarring, typically in 3-6 weeks.

Secondary Syphilis

- This stage of syphilis is characterized by systemic, cutaneous and mucosal signs and symptoms.
- Fever, malaise, pharyngitis, adenopathy and weight loss and meningeal signs (headache) are common.
- The most common sign is a non-pruritic generalized, pink, scaly papular eruption (80%).
- The lesions develop slowly, appear in a variety of shapes, including round, ellipsoid, and annular and persist for weeks or months.
- Symmetric hyperpigmented oval papules with a collarette of scale appear on the palms or the soles in most patients.
- Irregular alopecia of the beard, scalp, and eyelashes occurs which is sometimes referred to as "moth-eaten alopecia."
- Whitish, moist, anal condyloma lata lesions are highly infectious wart-like papules that are characteristic of syphilis.
- Classic split papules appear at the angle or commissures of the mouth.
- All secondary lesions are infectious with direct contact or palpation.
- Without treatment, lesions of this stage relapse in about 20% of patients within a year.

Latent Syphilis

- Very few if any clinical signs of syphilis in this stage.

Tertiary Syphilis

- Gummas or granulomatous lesions develop subcutaneously, expand and ulcerate in the skin.
- These lesions also occur in the liver, bones and other organs.

Laboratory

- Direct detection of treponemes is diagnostic.
- Detection of the treponeme from skin lesions can be achieved under dark-field microscopy, which shows corkscrew rotation motility of the small, spiral syphilis spirochete.
- There are two serologic screening tests: the rapid plasma reagin test and the Venereal Disease Research Laboratory, or VDRL, test.
- These screening tests are reactive by day 7 of the chancre and are easy to perform.
- Latent syphilis can be diagnosed by a reactive screening test.
- Positive results from the screening tests should be confirmed with a fluorescent treponemal antibody absorption test.
- One-third of latent syphilis-infected people have a negative or non-reactive result in the rapid plasma reagin test. They show no signs of disease and only have a positive result on the microhemagglutination-*Treponema pallidum* antibody test. Another third have a positive rapid plasma reagin test and microhemagglutination-*Treponema pallidum* test, and the remaining third have clinical symptoms of tertiary disease.
- Tertiary syphilis is diagnosed by elevated cerebrospinal fluid pressure, protein concentration and specific antitreponemal antibodies.
- False-positive results are possible with all serologic tests.

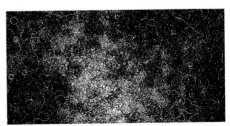

Secondary syphilis. Temporary and irregular ("moth eaten") alopecia of the beard, scalp, or eyelashes may occur.

167

Differential Diagnosis

Primary Syphilis

- Herpes simplex
- Chancroid
- Behçet syndrome
- Fixed drug eruption
- Traumatic ulcers

Secondary Syphilis

- Pityriasis rosea
- Guttate psoriasis
- Lichen planus
- Tinea versicolor
- Exanthematous drug eruption
- Viral eruptions

Treatment

- In early disease (primary, secondary, latent less than 1 year) the drug of choice is benzathine penicillin G 2.4 million units intramuscularly, given once.

- In late disease (lasting more than 1 year) the drug of choice is benzathine penicillin G 2.4 million units intramuscularly once a week for 3 weeks consecutively.
- People who are allergic to penicillin can be given doxycycline 100 mg twice a day for 2 weeks, or tetracycline, 500 mg four times a day for 2 weeks.
- Successful therapy is indicated by a falling rapid plasma reagin titer.
- Rapid plasma reagin testing should be repeated 3, 6, and 12 months after treatment is complete.
- Treatment is repeated when there is a sustained fourfold increase in the rapid plasma reagin titer.
- Therapy is repeated when a high titer does not show a fourfold decrease within 1 year.
- In most patients infected with the human immunodeficiency virus, syphilis responds to standard treatment regimens.

Pediatric Considerations

- Congenital syphilis (early and late) is acquired from an untreated or inadequately treated pregnant woman.
- Early adequate treatment of the mother can prevent severe birth defects.
- Early congenital syphilis appears in the perinatal period (up to 2 years of age) but typically manifests itself in the first 3 months of life.
- Children develop the following main symptoms:
  - Skin: scaling of palms and soles (51%), papulosquamous eruption (44%), eroded intertriginous papules (17%), periorificial rhagades (14%)
  - Bone: osteochondritis periostosis (80%)
  - Pain with handling (38%)
  - Nasal congestion (snuffles) (18%)
  - Hepatosplenomegaly (48%)
- Late congenital syphilis begins at age 2 with the following manifestations:
  - Frontal bossing (81%)
  - Underdeveloped maxillae (83%)
  - High-arched palate (76%)
  - Saddle nose (73%)
  - Dome-shaped molars with multiple poorly formed molars (65%) and notched incisors, or Hutchinson's teeth (63%)
  - Proximal clavicular thickening (39%)
  - Interstitial keratitis (9%)
  - Sabot shins (4%)
  - Deafness (3%)
- All patients with syphilis should be tested for human immunodeficiency virus.

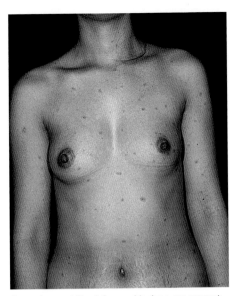

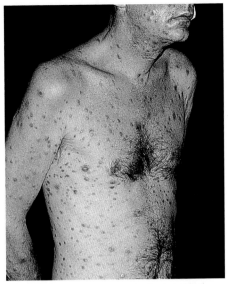

Secondary syphilis. A few oval lesions are present on the trunk. The initial diagnosis was pityriasis rosea.

The lesions of secondary syphilis have marked tendency to polymorphism, with various types of lesions presenting simultaneously. They have a coppery tint and assume a variety of shapes. Eruptions may be limited and discrete, or profuse and generalized.

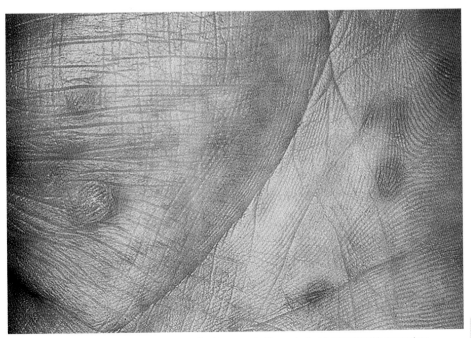

Secondary syphilis. Lesions on the palms and soles occur in the majority of patients with secondary syphilis. A coppery color resembling that of clean-cut ham is characteristic of secondary syphilis.

Chancroid

Description

- Chancroid is a rare sexually transmitted disease caused by *Haemophilus ducreyi*.
- It is characterized by painful genital ulceration and inguinal lymphadenopathy.

History

- The male to female ratio is 10 to 1.
- It is more common in heterosexual men, who obtain it from asymptomatic carriers, usually prostitutes.
- It is common in certain developing countries but is rare in the United States.
- Co-infection with human immunodeficiency virus can occur.

Skin Findings

- A painful red papule first appears at the site of inoculation, followed by a pustule, which may rupture, forming an ulcer with a bright red base.
- The ulcer of chancroid is deep, bleeds easily and may spread laterally. It is covered by a yellow to gray fibrinous exudate.
- These ulcers are highly infectious and may become multiple via autoinoculation. This can occur on the thighs, buttocks and anal area.

Non-skin Findings

- Patients may feel ill, with fever, anorexia and malaise.
- Unilateral or bilateral inguinal lymphadenopathy develops in 50% about 1 week after infection.
- Lymph nodes may suppurate and ulcerate or resolve spontaneously.
- Women may carry the organism, but display no clinically detectable lesions and have no symptoms.
- Untreated cases either resolve spontaneously or become chronic and require a long time to heal.

Laboratory

- *Haemophilus ducreyi* cannot be cultured on routine media.
- Newly formulated transport media can maintain the viability of the organism.
- A cotton swab is used to obtain a specimen at the base of the ulcer, which is then rolled over a glass slide. Gram-negative clumped organisms, resembling a "school of fish" can be seen and is diagnostic.
- There is a high rate of coinfection with human immunodeficiency virus among patients with chancroid, so a test for this virus is reasonable in these patients. Syphilis serologies should be considered.

Differential Diagnosis

- Herpes simplex
- Syphilis
- Lymphogranuloma venereum
- Granuloma inguinale
- Traumatic ulceration

Treatment

- Azithromycin 1 g orally in a single dose.
- Ceftriaxone 250 mg intramuscularly in a single dose.
- Ciprofloxacin 500 g orally twice daily for 3 days.
- Erythromycin 500 mg orally four times daily for 7 days.

Pearls

- Herpes simplex is the most common form of genital ulceration in North America.
- The combination of painful genital ulceration and ulcerative or suppurative inguinal adenopathy is highly suggestive of a diagnosis of chancroid in high-risk geographic areas.
- Chancroid infection is strongly associated with co-infection with human immunodeficiency virus.
- Treatment of chancroid should not be delayed for culture results if the disease is suspected. Prolonged genital ulceration from the disease may increase the risk and susceptibility for transmission of human immunodeficiency virus.

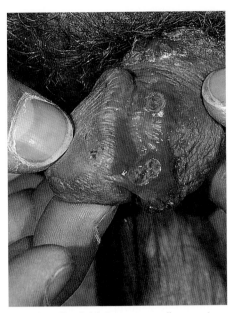

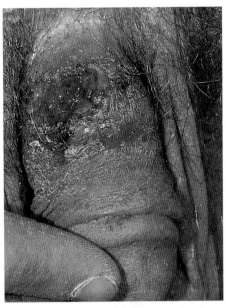

Several small, painful ulcers are usually present. The base is purulent, in contrast to the chancre of syphilis, which is not painful.

The ulcers have coalesced during a 4-week period without treatment.

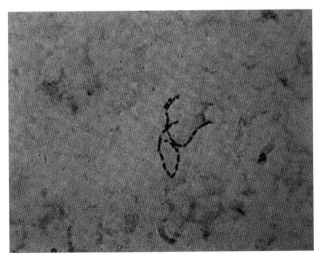

Wright's stain of purulent material of the base of the ulcer shows a chain of coccobacilli in a "school of fish" pattern.

Genital Warts (Condyloma Acuminata or Venereal Warts)

Description
- Genital warts are due to infection of genital or anal skin by the human papilloma virus.
- Warts in these locations can be difficult to eradicate and can lead to carcinoma.

History
- Warts spread rapidly over moist areas and may therefore be symmetric on opposing surfaces of the labia or rectum.
- Common warts can be the source of genital warts, although they are usually caused by different types of virus.
- Genital warts frequently recur after treatment.
- Latent virus exists beyond the treatment areas in clinically normal skin.
- Half of patients who have multiple and widespread infection with genital human papilloma virus and who practice orogenital sex have oral condylomata. The lesions are asymptomatic. Magnification may be necessary to detect oral lesions.

- The course is highly variable. Spontaneous resolution may occur but warts may persist for long periods.

Skin Findings
- Genital wart lesions may vary from person to person.
- Lesions tend to be pale pink to white, and rough barely raised papules.
- Some lesions may have projections on a broad base.
- The surface may be smooth, velvety and moist, and it lacks the hyperkeratosis of warts found elsewhere.
- The lesions may coalesce in the rectal or perineal area to form a large, cauliflower-like mass.
- Warts may extend into the vaginal tract, urethra and rectum, in which case a speculum or sigmoidoscope is required for visualization and treatment.

Differential Diagnosis
- Pearly penile papules are dome-shaped or hair-like projections that appear on the corona of the penis and sometimes on the shaft, just proximal to the corona, and they occur in up to 10% of male patients (these small angiofibromas are normal

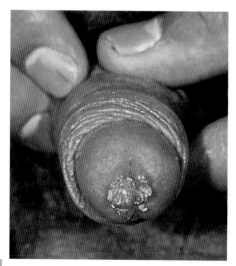

Wart at the urethral meatus.

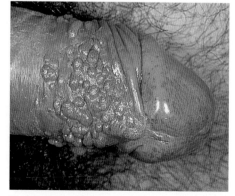

Warts spread rapidly over moist areas, such as under the foreskin and on the vulva, and tend to be more numerous than on skin in other areas.

variants but are sometimes mistaken for warts)

- Molluscum contagiosum (a dome-shaped, firm, white papule that usually has a central depression)

Treatment

- Warts that are flat and inconspicuous, especially on the penile shaft and urethral meatus can be difficult to visualize without magnification.
- Treatment can be difficult, and multiple visits and treatments are often necessary for success.
- Liquid nitrogen cryotherapy can be performed. The wart is frozen until a rim of 1 mm appears around it. Repeat treatment is performed in 2–3 weeks. The treatment is painful, and blisters may form.
- Electrocautery and curettage involves a light touch with monopolar electrocautery; this is effective for treating a few isolated lesions, but scarring is possible.
- Podofilox (Condylox gel) is applied to the external genital warts twice a day for 3 days consecutively, followed by 4 days without treatment. This cycle is repeated at weekly intervals for a maximum of 4 weeks. Local adverse effects of the drug, such as pain, burning, inflammation and erosion have occurred in more than 50% of patients.
- Imiquimod cream 5% is an immune response modifier. It is applied every other night at bedtime, left on the wart for 8–12 hours, and removed by washing with mild soap and water. This regimen is repeated until the warts have resolved which usually takes 2–3 months. Treatment may have to be temporarily interrupted if irritation occurs.
- The use of condoms may reduce transmission to partners who are likely to be uninfected (such as new partners).

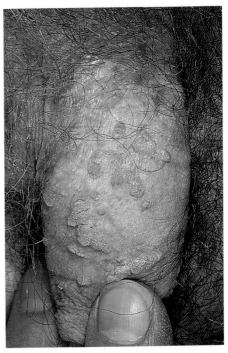

Multiple discrete warts on the shaft of the penis.

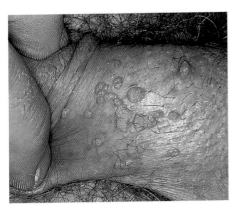

These warts are similar in appearance to common warts.

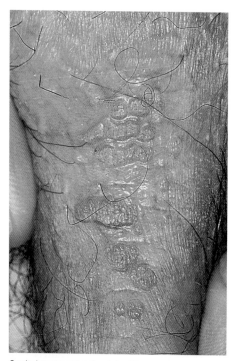

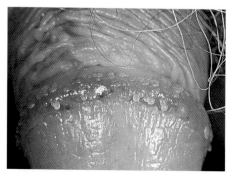

Pearly penile papules. An anatomic variant of normal, most commonly found on the corona of the penis. They are sometimes mistaken for warts. No treatment is required.

Genital warts are pale pink with numerous, discrete, narrow to wide projections on a broad base.

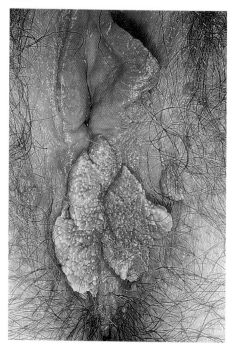

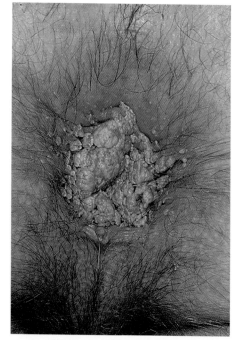

A large cauliflower-like wart projects from the vagina.

Warts in the anal area may be numerous and very large. Infection to this extent is painful. Podophyllin or imiquimod (Aldara) would be reasonable initial therapy. Consider excision if topical therapy fails.

- Over 90% of cervical carcinomas are related to human papilloma virus infection.
- For this reason women who have no visible external warts, but have a sexual partner with genital warts, should have a complete gynecologic exam and a Papanicolaou (Pap) smear.

Pearls

- Individual variations in cell-mediated immunity may explain differences in severity and duration.
- Warts occur more frequently, last longer, and appear in greater numbers in people with acquired immunodeficiency syndrome and cancers, and in those who are taking immunosuppressive medications, such as transplant patients.

Pediatric Considerations

- The rates of perinatal transmission from mother to child are not known and are likely to be lower than previously thought.
- Genital warts that are seen in children under 3 years of age can be perinatally acquired from the mother.
- If genital or anal warts are seen in older children (less than 4 years) for the first time, the child should be referred to a sexual abuse team to investigate further sexually transmitted infections and the possibility of sexual abuse.
- The presence of genital warts does not "prove" sexual abuse, and human papilloma virus typing is generally not helpful.

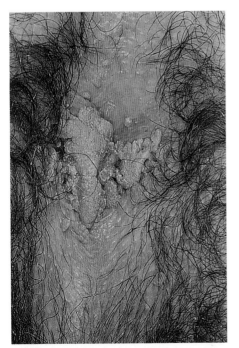

Anal warts are often numerous and very large. The patient responded to the application of 20% podophyllin in benzoin that was applied in the physician's office.

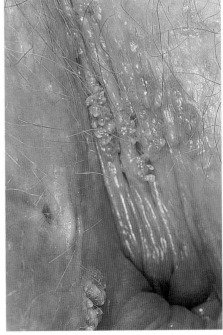

Many small warts may be found in the anal area. Topical therapy or electrocautery should be effective.

Genital Herpes Simplex

Description

- Genital herpes simplex is a common sexually transmitted disease caused by the herpes simplex virus (HSV-2).
- The primary infection is followed by recurrent outbreaks of grouped vesicles on an inflamed red base.
- Many cases are transmitted by people who are unaware that they have the infection or are asymptomatic when transmission occurs.

History

Primary Infection

- After a total of 2–20 days after exposure, influenza-like systemic signs begin (e.g. fever, headache, malaise, myalgia); the complaints peak 3–4 days after viral vesicles develop.
- Tender lymphadenopathy occurs in the second and third weeks.

Recurrent Infection

- Influenza-like symptoms are less intense or most often are absent.
- The prodrome is described as a burning or itching in the infected area.
- A chronic relapsing course is common.

Skin Findings

- Symptoms of a primary infection are more severe (greater number of lesions) and more extensive than recurrent infection.
- The lesions in recurrent infection occur in the same region and sequence but on a diminished scale.
- The condition presents with a red swollen plaque followed by grouped vesicles that evolve into pustules.
- Umbilication (a central depression) is a characteristic feature of herpetic vesicles.
- The pustules rupture or break, may crust, and then form shallow, painful erosions.
- Large confluent erosions and ulcers can occur.
- The lesions heal in 2–4 weeks; recurrent lesions heal in 1–2 weeks.
- Hypopigmentation, hyperpigmentation, and sometimes scars may be left behind.
- Primary infection is often the most extensive and severe in women; lesions are seen on the labia majora and minora, perineum, and inner thighs. Infections may also occur on the labia and buttocks.
- Regional lymphadenopathy (painful) occurs with primary infection.

Laboratory

- The most definite method is viral culture.
- Lesions must be sampled in the vesicular or early ulcerative stage.
- A rapid test is the Tzanck smear. The best results are obtained from intact vesicles, and multinucleated giant cells are the characteristic finding.
- A Papanicolaou (Pap) smear is useful for detecting herpes simplex virus in women without symptoms.
- An intact vesicle can be biopsied.
- Type-specific antibody titres can be ordered (for herpes simplex virus types 1 or 2).
- A rapid direct fluorescent antibody examination is available.

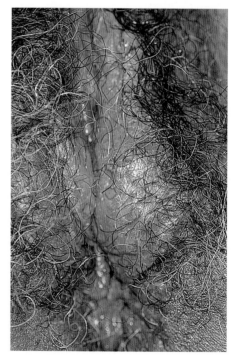

Primary herpes simplex. Numerous lesions form on moist surfaces.

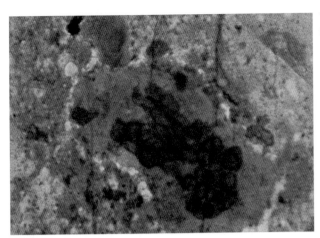

Tzanck smear. Multinucleated giant cell.

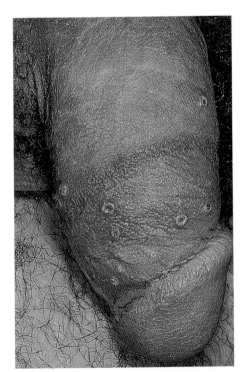

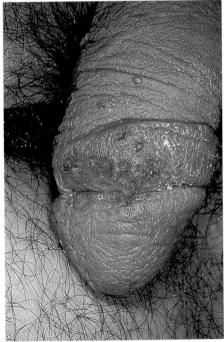

Primary herpes simplex. Lesions spread over a wide area.

Primary herpes simplex. Vesicles became confluent and then eroded.

Differential Diagnosis
- Syphilis
- Chancroid

Treatment
Counseling
- There is currently no permanent cure for herpes simplex.
- The natural history of the disease, the potential for recurrent episodes, asymptomatic viral shedding, and sexual transmission should be explained.
- The patient should be instructed to use condoms during all sexual exposures with new or unaffected sex partners. Condoms are not 100% effective in protecting males. Vaginal secretions may infect males on the thighs and pubic areas.

Systemic Therapy
- Systemic antiviral drugs partially control the symptoms and signs of herpes eruptions.

- These drugs neither eradicate latent virus nor affect the risk, frequency, or severity of recurrences after the drug is discontinued.

Primary Infection
- Treatment should be initiated within 72 hours of the onset of signs and symptoms.
- Valacyclovir (Valtrex) 1 g every 12 hours for 10 days can be prescribed.
- Famciclovir (Famvir) 250 mg can be administered every 8 hours for 10 days.
- Acyclovir (Zovirax) 200 mg every 4 hours five times a day, 400 mg every 8 hours, or 800 mg orally every 12 hours for 10 days, can be administered.
- Cool, wet water dressings may suppress inflammation.

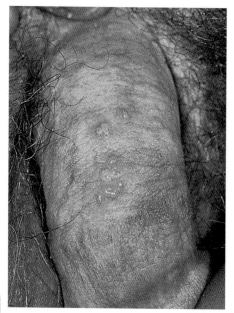

Recurrent herpes simplex. Vesicles on a red base.

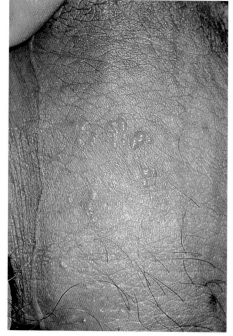

Recurrent herpes simplex. A group of vesicles on a red base.

- Severe primary infections can be treated intravenously with acyclovir 5 mg/kg every 8 hours for 7 days. This regimen should be considered in immunocompromised patients.

Recurrent Infection
- Treatment with one of the following regimens is initiated within 24–48 hours of the onset of signs and symptoms.
  - Valacyclovir (Valtrex) 500 mg every 12 hours for 5 days
  - Famciclovir (Famvir) 125 mg every 12 hours for 5 days
  - Acyclovir (Zovirax) 400 mg every 8 hours for 5 days
- Patients should be provided with a prescription for the medication so that treatment can be started at the first sign of prodrome or genital lesion.

Long-Term Suppressive Therapy
- Valacyclovir (Valtrex) 1 g daily or 500 mg daily can be prescribed for fewer than nine recurrences a year.

- Famciclovir (Famvir) 250 mg twice daily.
- Acyclovir (Zovirax) 400 mg twice daily.
- Treatment is continued for at least 6–12 months.
- If treatment is successful, a trial without medication may be considered.
- Daily suppressive therapy reduces the frequency of genital herpes recurrences by at least 75% among patients who have frequent recurrences (six or more occurrences per year).
- Suppressive treatment reduces but does not eliminate asymptomatic viral shedding.

Reducing the Risk of Transmission
- Valacyclovir (Valtrex) 500 mg taken once daily by immunocompetent persons with recurrent genital herpes simplex virus type 2 infection significantly reduces the rates of viral transmission of genital herpes to a susceptible partner.

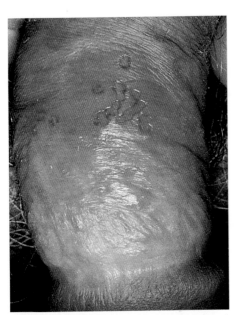

Recurrent herpes simplex under the foreskin. A group of discrete erosions is present. Crusts do not form on this moist surface.

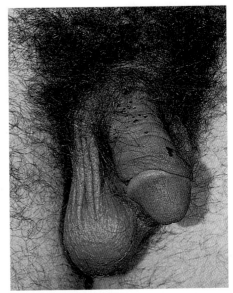

Recurrent herpes simplex with scattered small crusts and lack of vesicles.

Pubic Lice (*pediculosis pubis*)

Description
- Pubic lice are the most contagious sexually transmitted disease.
- The chance of acquiring pubic lice from an infested partner is more than 90%.
- Direct contact is the primary source of transmission.
- Additional information can be obtained from the National Pediculosis Association (http://www.head-lice.org).

History
- Fomite transmission occurs from sheets and clothing.
- The majority of patients complain of pruritus.
- Many patients are aware that something is crawling on the groin but are not familiar with the disease and have never seen lice.
- Up to 30% of patients infested with pubic lice have at least one other sexually transmitted disease.
- Eggs (nits) are cemented to the hair shaft 1 cm from the skin surface.
- Nits hatch in 8–10 days.

Skin Findings
- Nits are firmly cemented to hair shafts.
- Lice may be difficult to see with close inspection or magnification.
- The pubic hair is the most common site of louse infestation, but lice frequently spread to the hair around the anus.
- On hairy people, lice may spread to the upper thighs, abdominal area, axillae, chest, and beard.
- Occasionally, gray to blue macules (maculae ceruleae) that vary in size from 1 cm to 2 cm are seen in the groin and at sites distant from the infestation. Their cause is not known, but they may represent altered blood pigment.
- Most infected patients have very little if any inflammatory changes, but those who delay seeking help may develop widespread inflammation and infection of the groin with regional adenopathy.

Standard Treatments
- An over-the-counter permethrin rinse 1% (Nix cream rinse) is often the drug of first choice. It is applied and washed off after 10 minutes.
- Over-the-counter synergized pyrethrin shampoos (RID, A-200, R&C) are also used.
- Permethrin 5% (Elimite cream) is prescribed when over-the-counter treatment fails. It is left on the hair overnight.
- Lindane (Kwell) shampoo is left on for 5 minutes and then washed out; treatment is repeated in 1 week. It is used if over-the-counter treatments fail. Lindane-resistant lice have emerged.
- Malathion lotion (Ovide) is highly effective. It is applied to dry hair and shampooed out after 8–12 hours.
- All agents attack the louse nervous system, but nits are not affected.
- Treatment should be repeated in 1 week to kill nits that have not hatched.
- Oral medication with ivermectin 200 μg/kg/day is given in a single oral dose that is repeated in 10 days. The average adult dose is 12 mg. It attacks invertebrate nerve and muscle cells in the louse and causes paralysis and death. It has selective activity against parasites but no systemic effects on mammals.

Nit Removal
- It is important to remove all nits.
- Shaving the pubic and abdominal hair may be helpful.
- Fomite control is essential.

Pediatric Considerations
- Infested adults may spread pubic lice or crab lice to the eyelashes of prepubertal children.
- Sexual abuse is a possible cause of crab lice infestation in prepubertal children.

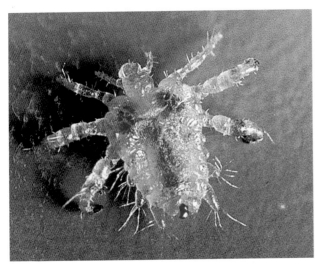

Phthirus pubis (pubic louse, or crab louse). The crab louse is the smallest louse, with a short oval body and prominent claws resembling those of sea crabs.

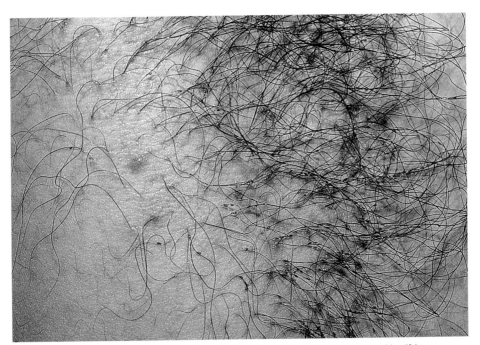

Pediculosis pubis. Lice become rust-colored from the ingestion of blood; their color is an identifying characteristic. Lice feces can be seen on the skin as small, rust-colored flecks.

Molluscum Contagiosum

Description

■ Molluscum contagiosum is a poxvirus infection of the skin characterized by discrete umbilicated papules.

History

■ Molluscum contagiosum is very common in children.
■ It is spread by direct contact or by autoinoculation.
■ Lesions tend to be more numerous and spread rapidly in patients with atopic dermatitis.
■ Lesions may become large, numerous and disfiguring in patients with the human immunodeficiency virus. It is often a marker of late-stage disease.
■ Genital molluscum contagiosum in adults can be acquired by sexual transmission.

Skin Findings

■ Discrete 2–5 mm lesions appear, which are slightly umbilicated, flesh-colored, and dome-shaped.
■ The pubic and genital areas are most commonly involved in adults.
■ The lesions are frequently grouped and cover a wide area.
■ Inflammation, erythema and scaling at the periphery of a single or several lesions may occur. This may be the result of inflammation from scratching, or it may be a hypersensitivity reaction.
■ Trauma may decrease the characteristic appearance of some lesions.
■ Papules are often camouflaged by pubic hair. Most patients have just a few lesions that can be easily overlooked.
■ The focus of examination is the pubic hair, genitals, anal area, thighs, and trunk. Lesions may appear anywhere except the palms and soles.

Differential Diagnosis

■ Warts and flat warts
■ Milia

Treatment

■ Genital lesions should be treated to prevent spread through sexual contact.
■ New lesions too small to be detected at the first examination may appear after treatment and require attention at a subsequent visit.
■ Small papules can be quickly removed with a curette with or without local anesthesia. Bleeding is controlled with gauze pressure or Monsel's solution. Curettage is useful when there are a few lesions because it provides the quickest, most reliable treatment, but may be too painful for small children. A small scar may form; therefore this technique should be avoided in cosmetically important areas.
■ Lidocaine/prilocaine (EMLA) cream applied 30–60 minutes before treatment helps prevent the pain of curettage for children.

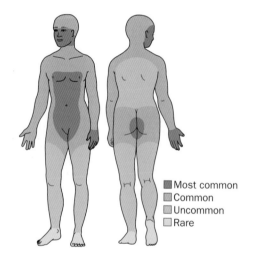

■ Most common
□ Common
□ Uncommon
□ Rare

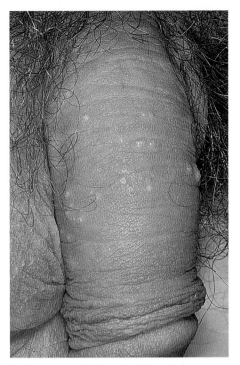

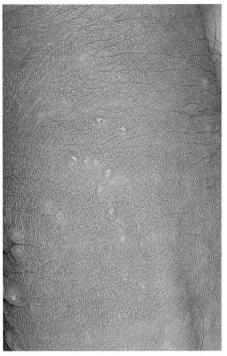

Lesions are usually discrete, white, and dome shaped. They lack the many small projections found on the surface of warts.

Close observation of individual lesions is necessary to confirm the diagnosis. Lesions are often misdiagnosed as warts.

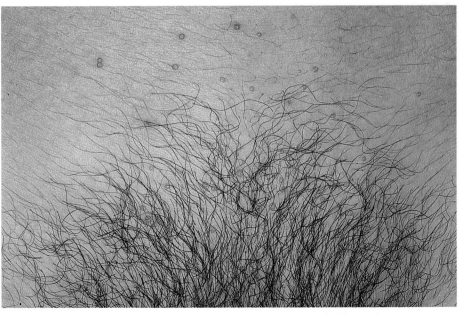

Molluscum are difficult to see through pubic hair. These lesions were removed with a number one curette.

- Cryosurgery with liquid nitrogen is effective for patients who do not object to the pain. The papule is sprayed or touched lightly with a nitrogen-bathed cotton swab until the advancing, white, frozen border has progressed down the side of the papule to form a 1 mm halo on the normal skin surrounding the lesion. This should take approximately 5 seconds. A conservative approach is necessary because excessive freezing produces hypopigmentation or hyperpigmentation.
- A small drop of cantharidin 0.7% (Cantharone) is applied with the stick end of a cotton swab over the surface of the lesion, and contamination of normal skin is avoided. This should be washed off 4–6 hours later. Lesions blister and may resolve without scarring. New lesions occasionally appear at the site of the blister created by cantharidin. Hypopigmentation or hyperpigmentation may occur.
- Imiquimod (Aldara) 5% cream can be effective when applied three times weekly at night for 2–3 months. This is especially effective for treating facial molluscum in children where scarring procedures are contraindicated.
- In atopic dermatitis patients with molluscum, the dermatitis must also be treated at the same time, because the altered skin barrier will promote autoinoculation.

Pediatric Considerations

- Genital molluscum contagiosum is common in children and this finding alone does not warrant further evaluation for sexual abuse.
- One should look for other evidence of molluscum in other regions and in other siblings, especially if they bathe together.
- Children with molluscum contagiosum should not bathe with their siblings.
- Cantharone should not be used on the face.

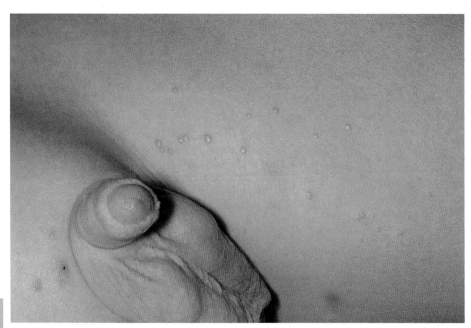

Molluscum are commonly found in the genital area in young children.

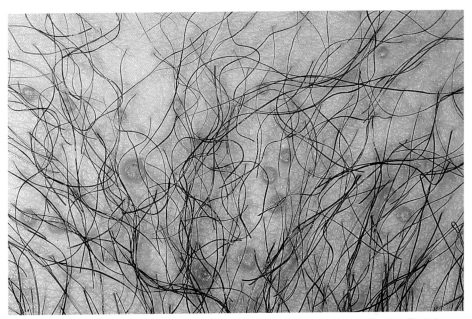

Molluscum are commonly found in the pubic area in adults. Exam this area with magnification. The hair obscures the view and many lesions can be hidden from view.

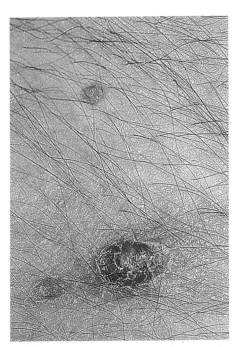

A single lesion became inflamed and disappeared 10 days later.

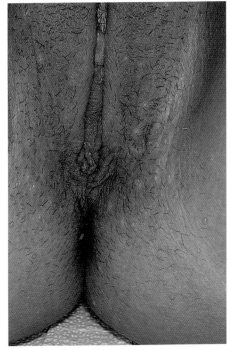

Molluscum spread rapidly over warm, moist intertriginous areas on the upper thigh near the vulva.

8 Viral Infections

Warts (Verruca Vulgaris)

Description

- Warts are benign epidermal proliferations caused by human papilloma virus (human papilloma virus) infection, a double-stranded DNA virus, which infects skin and mucous membranes.
- There are over 150 different types of human papilloma virus. New subtypes are defined by DNA hybridization. Some subtypes are associated with a particular typical location and characteristic clinical and pathologic presentation.
- Transmission is by simple contact, often at sites with small skin breaks, abrasions, or other trauma. The virus must contact basal epithelial cells for infection to occur.
- Local spread is often by autoinoculation.

History

- The estimated incidence of infection is 10% in children and young adults.
- The peak incidence is age 12–16 years.
- The incubation period is variable: 1–6 months for common warts.

Skin Findings

- Flesh-colored papules evolve into dome-shaped, gray to brown, hyperkeratotic, discreet and rough papules, often with black dots on the surface.
- The black dots are thrombosed capillaries.
- Warts are usually few in number but may be numerous.
- Common sites are the hands, periungual skin, elbows, knees, and plantar surfaces.
- Filiform warts are growths with finger-like, flesh-colored projections on a narrow or broad base; they often occur on the face.

Laboratory

- Human papilloma virus subtyping is not routine, readily available, or necessary for common warts. Subtype associations are:
  - Common warts with human papilloma virus 2, 4, 7
  - Plantar warts with human papilloma virus 1, 4
  - Genital warts with human papilloma virus: 1, 2, 6, 10, 11, 16, 18, 31, 32, 33, 34
- Genital human papilloma virus subtypes 16, 18, and 31 are high-risk subtypes and account for approximately 75% of invasive genital cancers.
- A non-resolving wart on the hand, periungual unit, or the foot, should be biopsied to rule out squamous cell carcinoma, which can mimic a wart, particularly in the region of the nail unit.

Course and Prognosis

- The course is highly variable; spontaneous resolution with time and the development of a cell-mediated immune response is the rule.
- In children approximately two thirds of all warts spontaneously regress within 2 years.

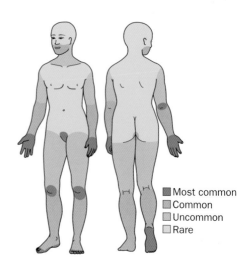

- Most common
- Common
- Uncommon
- Rare

- Warts in the immunocompromised patient can be widespread, intractable, and chronic.

Treatment

- Multiple treatments are available for warts. No single treatment is consistently highly effective. Painful treatment should be avoided, especially in children. Since warts will resolve spontaneously with no treatment, this may be comfortably recommended; however, many patients seek treatment due to the unsightly appearance, fear of spread or enlargement, or discomfort from pressure.
- Duct tape can be cut to wart size and applied. It should be left in place for 6 days, then removed, and skin washed and gently debrided. Reapply and continue this cycle for 1 month if necessary.
- Over-the-counter topical salicylic acid preparations (15–40%) are applied once a day; they are safe and effective. The preparations may be occluded with tape to increase penetration. The duration of treatment is often lengthy (8–12 weeks). Soreness and irritation are minor side effects. Cure rate with salicylic acid preparations is 75% compared with 48% with placebo. Some options are Mediplast (40% salicylic acid), DuoFilm solution (17% salicylic acid) or patch (40% salicylic acid) and Occlusal HP solution (17% salicylic acid).
- Multiple visits and treatments are often necessary for success when treating with ablative therapy. With liquid nitrogen cryotherapy, the 15-second freeze time is repeated once. A follow-up visit for retreatment occurs in 2–3 weeks. Cure rate in the range of 52% is reported. Side

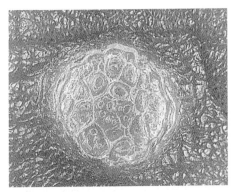

Warts form cylindric projections. The projections become fused in common warts on thicker skin and form a highly organized mosaic pattern on the surface.

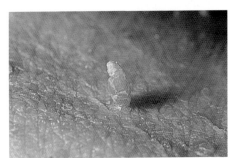

This digitate wart has a single projection that resembles a finger.

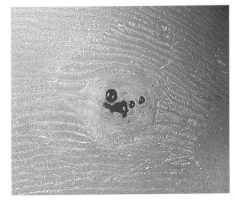

Warts remain confined to the epidermis and interrupt normal skin lines. The wart is gone when normal skin lines reappear.

Thrombosed black vessels become trapped in the projections and are seen as black dots on the surface. They bleed when pared with a blade.

effects are pain and a blister after treatment. Caution treating warts around the nail unit is advised. Older children may tolerate gentle cryotherapy; consider this for longstanding warts, or if other child-friendly treatments have failed.

■ Imiquimod 5% cream (Aldara) is an immune response modifier with limited use in common warts; efficacy is limited by poor penetration in non-mucosal skin. Treat with liquid nitrogen, then apply a 17% salicylic acid preparation at night, and imiquimod in the morning with occlusion. Continue for 6–9 weeks. Efficacy is 50–100% anecdotally.

■ The limitations of electrocautery and curettage are pain, secondary infection, and scarring.

■ Intralesional bleomycin has been used in the treatment of refractory warts; efficacy is limited. Contact immunotherapy of warts using dinitrochlorobenzene, squaric acid and *Candida* antigen has been employed by some dermatologists.

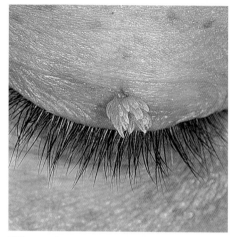

The hands are the most commonly involved area. Warts become confluent and obscure large areas of normal skin. Biting or picking the skin around the nails can spread the warts.

Filiform and digitate warts consist of a few or several finger-like flesh-colored projections emanating from a narrow or broad base. They are most commonly observed about the mouth, the beard, eyes, and nose.

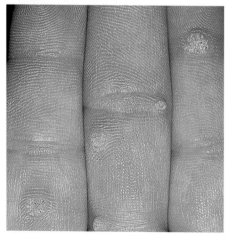

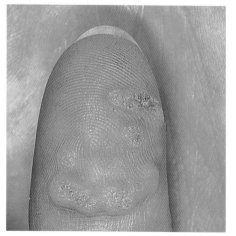

Warts on the palms have a similar appearance to those on the soles. The skin is thick, and the warts are more difficult to treat with liquid nitrogen and salicylic acid.

These warts have become confluent. Freezing a wide area of the fingertip is very painful. Localized areas should be treated in two or three treatment sessions

- The limitations of laser surgery are pain and potential scarring. Pulsed dye laser has been used but shows no significant advantage over conventional treatment.
- Filiform warts are the easiest to treat. Local anesthesia can be used and the lesion removed with a snip or a curette. Light electrocautery and cryotherapy are other alternatives.

Pediatric Considerations

- Warts are common in children. Treatment—if offered—should be child friendly; painful therapy should be avoided.

Pearls

- Individual variations in cell-mediated immunity may explain differences in wart severity and duration.
- Warts remain confined to the epidermis and interrupt normal skin lines. The wart is gone when normal skin lines reappear.
- Biting, shaving, or picking the wart-infected skin can spread warts. Inform your patients and discourage them from these habits.
- Warts occur more frequently, last longer, and appear in greater numbers in patients with acquired immunodeficiency syndrome and lymphoma and in patients on immunosuppressive medications.

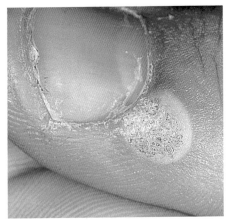

Warts are frozen until the "freeze front" extends for about 1–2 mm beyond the growth. Using two freeze–thaw cycles during one treatment session may increase the cure rate.

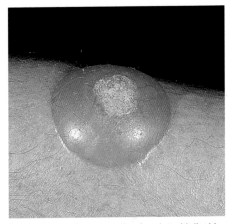

Warts blister a day or two after freezing with liquid nitrogen. The size of the blister varies depending on the location and the individual. Blisters are often filled with blood and are painful. These may be punctured and drained with a #11 surgical blade.

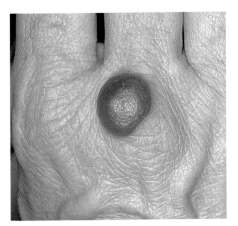

Large blisters commonly form on the backs of the hands after treatment with liquid nitrogen.

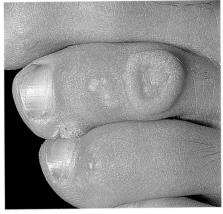

The wart virus spread to the edge of the blister and formed a wart larger than the lesion that was originally treated. This is one possible side effect of cryosurgery.

Flat Warts

Description
- Flat warts are benign cutaneous hyperproliferations due to infection with human papilloma virus. Common subtypes are types 3 and 10.

History
- Flat warts are common in children and young adults.
- Flat warts spread in a local region often through mildly traumatized skin, such as within an area of shaving.

Skin Findings
- These pink, light brown or light yellow papules are slightly elevated and flat-topped. They vary in size from 0.1–0.3 cm. They may be few or numerous and often occur grouped or in a line as a result of spread from scratching.
- Typical sites are the forehead, the back of the hands, the chin, neck, and legs.
- Flat warts are typically asymptomatic.

Course and Prognosis
- The duration may be lengthy; flat warts may be very resistant to treatment. They are generally located in cosmetically important areas where aggressive, scarring treatment procedures must be avoided.
- Immunocompromised patients often have a protracted course.

Treatment
- If sparse numbers of lesions, a salicylic acid preparation may be applied daily directly to each lesion. This treatment is limited by irritation.
- Imiquimod 5% cream (Aldara) applied to affected skin at night. Decrease frequency of application if excessive irritation. Treatment may be required for weeks.
- Tretinoin cream 0.025%, 0.05%, or 0.1% is applied at bedtime over the entire involved area. The frequency of application is adjusted to produce fine scaling and mild erythema. Treatment may be required for weeks or months.
- Liquid nitrogen or a very light touch with an electrocautery needle may be

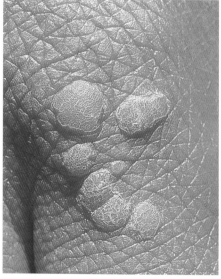

Warts are often grouped and are easily spread by scratching. The surface projections in these warts are very small and require magnification to be seen.

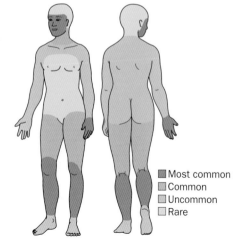

- ■ Most common
- ☐ Common
- ☐ Uncommon
- ☐ Rare

performed for quick results. Flat warts may not respond to cryotherapy, even after many treatment sessions.

■ Applied once or twice a day for 3–5 weeks, 5-fluorouracil cream 5% (Efudix) may produce dramatic clearing of flat warts. Persistent hyperpigmentation may follow the use of 5-fluorouracil and is minimized by applying it to individual lesions with a cotton-tipped applicator.

Pearls

■ Inform patients that flat warts are easily spread within areas of shaving. Shaving over affected skin should be discouraged.

■ Unlike common warts, the face is a common location for flat warts.

■ Imiquimod appears promising in the treatment of flat warts; its use may be limited by high cost and erythema and skin discomfort. Use is off-label.

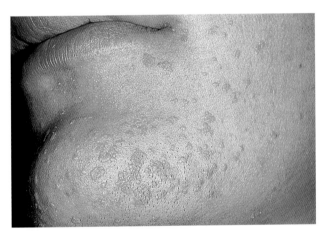

Flat warts are pink, light brown, or light yellow, and are slightly elevated, flat-topped papules that vary in size from 0.1 cm to 0.3 cm. There may be only a few, but generally there are many.

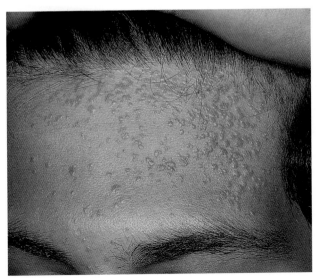

The face is a commonly involved site. Flat warts are difficult to treat. Many different treatment modalities may be tried before a response is obtained.

Plantar Warts

Description

- Plantar warts are caused by human papilloma virus infection on the plantar foot.
- Infection frequently occurs at points of maximal pressure, such as over the heads of the metatarsal bones, the heels or the toes.
- A cluster of many warts is referred to as a "mosaic wart".

Skin Findings

- The round, single or multiple, coalescing, flesh-colored, rough keratotic papules often look depressed.
- Punctate black dots within the wart, often seen on paring, are capillary loops.
- The papules may be tender with pressure.
- Some plantar warts are depressed, resembling numerous small pits.

Laboratory

- Biopsy may be indicated in warts that are rapidly growing, ulcerated, atypical, or resistant to treatment; squamous cell carcinoma or melanoma may mimic a wart.
- Human papilloma virus types 1, 2, and 4 are typically associated with plantar warts.

Course and Prognosis

- Treatment is often difficult; plantar warts can be very refractory and recurrent. Often, multiple treatment sessions are required.
- Hyperhidrosis is associated with a more widespread distribution of warts that are often refractory to treatment.

Treatment

- Plantar warts do not require therapy as long as they are painless. Spontaneous resolution with time is the rule.
- There are multiple treatment options, indicating no single best option.
- Keratolytic therapy with salicylic acid (DuoPlant, Occlusal) is a conservative initial treatment. There is no scarring. The wart is pared, the affected part is soaked in warm water, and the salicylic acid preparation is applied to the wart surface. Limitations include irritation and soreness. Treatment may require 6–8 weeks.
- Plasters with salicylic acid 40% (Mediplast) are useful in treating plantar warts. They are left on for 24–48 hours and replaced. Treatment may require 6–8 weeks.
- Imiquimod 5% cream (Aldara) may help hasten resolution; one method is to use cryotherapy first, then apply Imiquimod every night under duct tape occlusion for 6–12 weeks.
- Blunt dissection is a fast, effective surgical treatment (90% cure rate) and

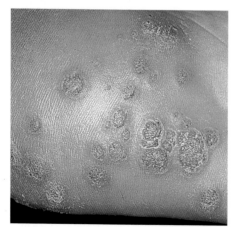

Plantar warts frequently occur at points of maximal pressure, such as over the heads of the metatarsal bones or on the heels. A cluster of many warts that appear to fuse is referred to as a mosaic wart.

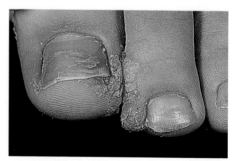

"Kissing lesions." Warts on one toe have spread to the adjacent toe. Apposition of the two surfaces would enhance the effect of salicylic acid liquid.

usually produces no scarring. It is superior to both electrodesiccation/curettage and excision because normal tissue is not disturbed. Many podiatrists are experienced at this procedure.

■ In cryosurgery with liquid nitrogen, the nitrogen is applied for 15–30 seconds, twice to a wart. The resultant painful blister can interfere with mobility. Repeated light applications of liquid nitrogen are optimal. Treatment is painful.

■ Carbon dioxide and pulsed-dye laser treatment is also available but is expensive, and probably no more effective than other treatments.

■ Electrodesiccation/curettage is sometimes used; it is infrequently chosen due to pain from the anesthesia, postoperative pain, and a risk of scarring.

■ Bleomycin 0.5 units/ml is injected into the wart to achieve blanching. The size of the wart determines the injection quantity. Responsive warts show hemorrhagic eschars that heal without scarring. Treatment is very painful; necrosis or severe vasospasm may occur. Pregnancy is a contraindication. This is an aggressive treatment option which is reserved for those experienced in its use.

Pediatric Considerations

● Choose a painless treatment option (duct tape occlusion, or salicylic acid) or no treatment for plantar warts in children; in time the warts will resolve spontaneously.

● Aggressive treatment is not appropriate; it can result in marked pain, difficulty walking, scarring, and fear of future medical care providers.

Pearls

■ A clavus (corn) can be mistaken for warts.

■ A wart lacks surface skin lines and has centrally located black dots that bleed with paring. Corns have a hard, painful, translucent central core.

■ Gentle paring of a wart to remove debris or using a pumice stone to whittle away debris improves penetration of topical therapies.

■ Caution your patient not to pick at the warty skin, and to clean any paring tool so not to spread wart virus from the debrided skin to other areas.

■ Persistence in treating plantar warts can pay off; the slow process of salicylic acid debridement can take as long as 12 weeks to resolve a wart.

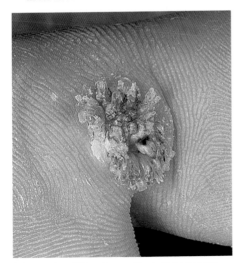

This wart has little callus on the surface and will bleed if pared with a blade.

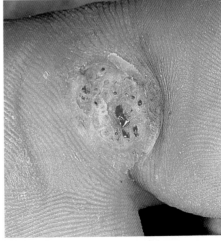

Care should be used when removing the callus. Some warts have a thick surface callus, but others are fragile and bleed easily when pared.

Molluscum Contagiosum

Description

- Molluscum contagiosum is a localized, self-limited viral infection of the skin; it is spread on the skin by autoinoculation and is transmitted to others by skin-to-skin contact.
- The cause of infection is a DNA virus of the pox virus family.

History

- Molluscum contagiosum may occur at any age.
- It peaks in ages between 3 and 9 years and again between 16 and 24.
- Lesions tend to occur in different areas of the body within different age groups.
- Most lesions are asymptomatic, although tenderness and itching can occur and are usually associated with mild local inflammation.
- The risk of transmission appears to be lower than that of herpes virus and papilloma virus.

Skin Findings

- Molluscum contagiosum begins as a 1-2 mm shiny, white to flesh-colored, dome-shaped firm papule.
- There is a small central whitish umbilication that is best seen with magnification or when the epidermis is lightly frozen with ethyl chloride or liquid nitrogen.
- Over some weeks, the lesion maintains its discrete dome shape with central punctum, attaining a maximum size of 2-5 mm.
- With time the papule becomes softer and more pink in color, and the central umbilication becomes more obvious.
- Untreated lesions usually persist for 6-9 months before slowly involuting, not usually leaving any mark, but rarely a minute pitted scar remains.
- Inflammation surrounding a lesion of molluscum contagiosum implies a host immune response and predicts resolution.
- Excoriations as well as crusting from secondary impetiginization may be present.

- The body area involved varies with age.
- Children tend to have lesions on the upper trunk, extremities, and especially on the face.
- Larger lesions occur in immunocompromised hosts.

Laboratory

- Skin biopsy is rarely needed to establish the diagnosis in an immunocompetent host.
- Biopsy confirms the presence of large intracytoplasmic viral inclusions known as "molluscum bodies" within infected keratinocytes.
- Curettage of a lesion expresses a white, rubbery core of infected keratinocytes suitable for potassium hydroxide examination.
- Infected keratinocytes are strikingly round and separate easily from one another.
- Normal keratinocytes are flat and cohesive, forming a sheet of adherent cells.
- Lesions occurring in an immunocompromised host such as those infected with human immunodeficiency virus should be biopsied to confirm the diagnosis. Other infections that also occur in such patients may mimic molluscum contagiosum.

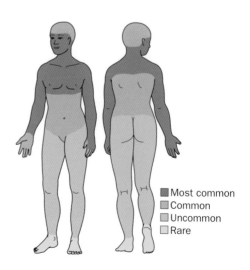

■ Most common
☐ Common
☐ Uncommon
☐ Rare

Course and Prognosis

- Individual lesions often resolve spontaneously within 6–9 months but may persist for up to 24 months.
- Individuals with atopic dermatitis are prone to developing numerous lesions within eczematous areas through inoculation of inflamed skin. Such lesions are notoriously difficult to clear until the eczema is brought under control.

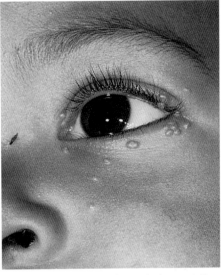

Inoculation around the eye is a typical presentation for children.

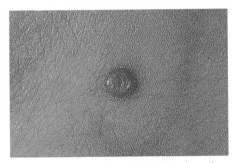

Molluscum are dome-shaped flesh-colored papules. Most lesions have a central umbilication. The central depression can be accentuated and more easily identified during treatment with nitrogen.

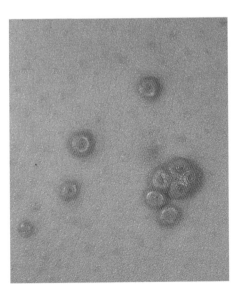

Molluscum contagiosum is characterized by discrete 2–5 mm, slightly umbilicated, flesh-colored, dome-shaped papules. It spreads by autoinoculation, by scratching, or by touching a lesion.

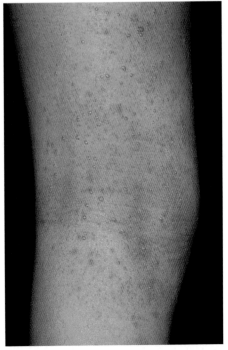

Lesions spread to inflamed skin, such as areas of atopic dermatitis. Most lesions are self-limiting and clear spontaneously in 6–9 months. However, they may last much longer.

- Molluscum contagiosum is similarly difficult to treat in immunocompromised hosts such as in the setting of the human immunodeficiency virus. Lesions are often more numerous and widespread, and individual lesions can become quite large and persistent.

Differential Diagnosis

- Differential diagnosis of molluscum lesions in immunocompetent hosts includes:
  - Flat warts
  - Genital warts
  - Herpes simplex infection
- Warts lack the central umbilication and may occur on the palms and soles.
- Herpes lesions are vesicles and are only transiently umbilicated, and they are usually tender and have a more rapid onset and shorter clinical course.
- In human immunodeficiency virus disease, other opportunistic fungal infections, including cryptococcosis and histoplasmosis, may produce lesions resembling those of molluscum contagiosum.

Treatment

- Skin-to-skin contact should be avoided to minimize transmission of the virus.
- Because lesions resolve spontaneously in healthy individuals and because there is some risk of scarring with treatment, the decision to treat must be made on an individual basis.
- In children, lesions should be kept covered by clothing if possible. Picking is discouraged.
- Genital lesions in sexually active adults should be treated.
- Sexual partners of affected individuals should be checked for lesions.
- The use of condoms should be encouraged because lesions may be too small to detect during the initial examination of the skin surrounding the genitalia.
- Depending on the location of lesions, the patient should be advised not to shave lesional areas because it can also lead to autoinoculation.
- Curettage to remove the infectious central core of the lesions is fairly painless and clears the lesions immediately.
- Anesthesia may not be required but is recommended, especially in children.
- Curettage is particularly useful for genital lesions.
- There is some risk of scarring, and caution should be used, especially on the face.
- Cryosurgery with liquid nitrogen is effective and in trained hands, rarely produces scarring. Treatment can be painful, especially for genital lesions.
- Cantharidin 0.7% solution is painless, effective, and well tolerated, especially by children. A wooden stick applicator is used to cautiously place a drop on each lesion, in order to avoid normal skin. The treated lesion develops a small blister within 24 hours, which then resolves along with the lesion; scarring rarely occurs. A mild temporary burning pain may occur.
- Imiquimod 5% cream (Aldara), a topical immune response modifier, can be applied to the lesions daily (or less frequently depending on degree of irritation). Duration of treatment is up to 12 weeks.
- Topical tretinoin cream (0.025%, 0.05%) applied daily to individual lesions may hasten resolution. A month or more of continuous treatment is usually required. Significant local irritation from the tretinoin may develop.
- Hypoallergenic surgical adhesive tape may be used. The tape is applied to each lesion. The tape is changed each day after showering. Treatment is continued until the lesion has ruptured, which may require several weeks.
- Cimetidine may enhance lymphocyte proliferation and immune response. Its use is controversial. A dose of 40 mg/kg/day appears to be of variable efficacy.

Pediatric Consideration

- Autoinoculation around the eyes is particularly common, especially in children. These lesions are best left to resolve spontaneously.
- Lesions will resolve spontaneously as cell-mediated immunity develops so treatment is not absolutely necessary.
- If treatment is desired, the best options for treating molluscum in children include cautiously applied cantharidin, imiquimod, or low strength tretinoin.
- Eutectic mixture of prilocaine and lidocaine (EMLA) or 4% lidocaine (LMX) should be applied 60–90 minutes before ablative procedures such as liquid nitrogen or curettage.
- The dose of EMLA cream should be limited (especially in neonates and infants) because of the small risk of methemoglobinemia.
- Molluscum contagiosum is primarily a sexually transmitted disease in young adults.
- Lesions tend to occur on the lower abdomen, pubic area (including the genitalia), and thighs.

Pearls

- A drop of mineral oil on lesions and use of a magnifier or dermatoscope will often allow confirmation of the diagnosis by accentuating the lesion's central core.
- Treatment should be individualized; lesions are self-limited.
- Significant scarring may result from overtreatment.
- It is common to see erythema and scaling at the periphery of a single or several lesions. This may be the result of inflammation from scratching or may be a hypersensitivity reaction. Inflamed molluscum often spontaneously clear coincident to the inflammation.

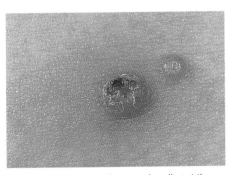

It is common to see erythema and scaling at the periphery of a single lesion or several lesions. This may be the result of inflammation from scratching, or may be a hypersensitivity reaction. Inflamed molluscum may clear spontaneously. This inflammation is often misinterpreted as infection.

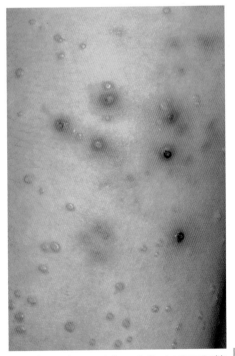

Several warts became inflamed after treatment with imiquimod cream. Note small scars from resolved lesions.

Herpes Simplex (Cold Sores, Fever Blisters)

Description

- Herpes simplex virus is a double stranded DNA virus with two different virus types (types 1 and 2) that can be distinguished in the laboratory.
- Type 1 is generally associated with vesicular ulcerative oral infections and type 2 with genital infections.
- Type 1 genital infections and type 2 oral infections are becoming more common, possibly as a result of increased incidence of oral–genital sexual contact.
- Herpes simplex virus infections have two phases: the primary infection, after which the virus becomes established in a nerve ganglion, and the secondary phase, characterized by recurrent disease at the same site.

Primary Infection

- The majority of primary infections are asymptomatic and can be detected only by an elevated immunoglobulin G antibody titer.
- The virus may be spread by respiratory droplets, direct contact with an active lesion, or contact with virus-containing fluid, such as saliva or cervical secretions in people with no evidence of active disease.
- Symptoms occur from 3–7 or more days after contact.
- Tenderness, pain, mild paresthesias, or burning occurs before the onset of lesions at the site of inoculation.
- Gingivostomatitis and pharyngitis are the most frequent manifestations of the first episode of type-1 infection.
- Localized pain, tender lymphadenopathy, headache, generalized aching, and fever are characteristic prodromal symptoms.
- Women with symptomatic primary genital infection may experience vulvovaginitis, vaginal and cervical erosions with pain, edema and dysuria.
- Men or women may also experience proctitis, anorectal pain, discharge, constipation, or tenesmus.
- Grouped vesicles on an erythematous base appear and subsequently erode.

- The vesicles in primary herpes simplex are more numerous and scattered than in the recurrent infection.
- Lesions on the mucus membrane accumulate exudate, whereas lesions on the skin form a crust.
- Lesions last for 2–6 weeks and heal without scarring.
- During this primary infection, the virus enters the nerve endings in the skin directly below the lesions and ascends through peripheral nerves to the dorsal root ganglia, where it remains in a latent stage.

Recurrent Infection

- The recurrence rate is the same as for patients who had a symptomatic or asymptomatic primary infection.
- Local skin trauma (e.g. ultraviolet light exposure, chapping, abrasion) or systemic changes (e.g. menses, fatigue, fever) reactivate the virus, which then travels down the peripheral nerves to the site of initial infection and causes the characteristic focal, recurrent infection.
- Recurrent infection is not inevitable. In many individuals, there is a rise in the antibody titer, but no clinical evidence or recurrence.
- The prodromal symptoms, lasting 2–24 hours, can resemble those of the primary infection. Tenderness, pain, mild paresthesias, or burning occurs before the onset of lesions in the focal area of the primary infection.
- Within 12 hours a group of lesions evolves rapidly from an erythematous base to form papules and then vesicles.
- The dome-shaped, tense vesicles rapidly umbilicate.
- In 2–4 days the vesicles rupture, forming aphthae-like erosions in the mouth and vaginal area or erosions covered by crusts on the lips and skin.
- Crusts are shed in approximately 8 days to reveal a pink, re-epithelialized surface.
- In contrast to the primary infection, systemic symptoms and lymphadenopathy are rare unless there is secondary infection.

- Many people experience a decrease in the frequency of recurrences with time, though some experience an increase.

Laboratory

- In culture testing, the base of the vesicle is swabbed with the special viral culture kits provided by the laboratory. Results can be available in 24 hours. Culture will identify the virus and its type (1 or 2).
- In Tzanck smears, the base of the vesicle is swabbed with a cotton swab and smeared onto a glass slide. The sample can be stained directly or the slide submitted to the laboratory. The characteristic multinucleated giant cells help confirm the diagnosis.
- Rapid direct fluorescent antibody testing of material swabbed from a lesional base is also available in some centers.
- Serology can be performed for virus types 1 and 2.

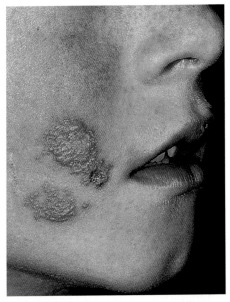

Primary herpes simplex infection. Primary infections in children typically begin in or about the oral cavity. Blisters are numerous.

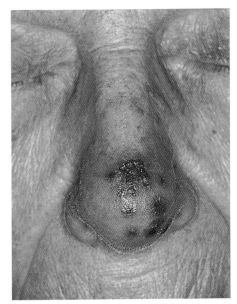

Recurrent herpes. The diagnosis of herpes can be made at any stage in the evolution of lesions.

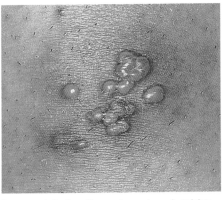

Recurrent infection. Tense, dome-shaped vesicles.

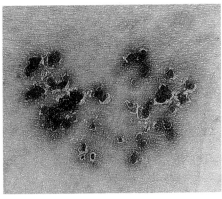

Recurrent infection. A group of crusts.

Differential Diagnosis
- Hand, foot and mouth disease
- Aphthous stomatitis
- Erythema multiforme
- Impetigo
- Herpes zoster

Course and Prognosis
- About 80–90% of people with symptomatic first episode of type 2 genital infection will experience a recurrent infection within the following year, compared to 50–60% of patients with type 1 infection.
- An average of four recurrences a year occur in patients with type 2 infection, compared with one per year in type 1 genital infection.
- Other complications of herpes simplex virus infection include ocular keratitis, encephalitis, meningitis, hepatitis, and pneumonitis.

Discussion
- HSV is the most common cause of genital ulcerations in the industrialized world. At least one in five Americans has herpes simplex type 2 infection.
- Most transmission of the virus occurs during periods of unrecognized, asymptomatic shedding of the virus.
- Infections can occur anywhere on the skin. Infection in one area does not protect the patient from subsequent infection at a different site.
- Herpes labialis (infection of the lips) is the most common presentation.
- Herpetic whitlow (herpes simplex of the fingertips) can resemble a group of warts or a bacterial infection. It is most often reported in pediatric patients with gingivostomatitis and in women with genital herpes.
- Herpes gladiatorum (cutaneous herpes in athletes involved in contact sports) is transmitted by direct skin-to-skin contact. This is a recognized health risk for wrestlers.
- Herpes simplex of the buttock area is more common in women.
- Herpes simplex of the lumbosacral region or trunk may be very difficult to differentiate from herpes zoster; the diagnosis becomes apparent only at the time of recurrence.
- Eczema herpeticum (Kaposi's varicelliform eruption) is the association of two common conditions: atopic dermatitis and herpes simplex virus infection. The disease is most common in areas of active or recently healed atopic dermatitis, particularly the face, but normal skin can be involved. In most cases, the disease is a primary herpes simplex infection. Herpes infections may spread within areas of other widespread dermatoses (Darier's disease); such spread may be camouflaged, heralded by an increase in lesional pain and worsening of disease with new erosions or crusted

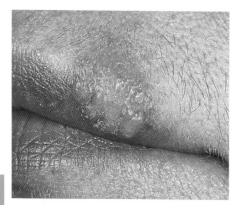
Recurrent herpes. Vesicles are confluent.

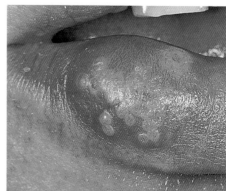
Recurrent herpes. Umbilicated vesicles.

areas. The spread is more common on corticosteroid-treated skin and in the setting of immunocompromise.

■ Herpes simplex genital lesions are a risk factor for transmission of human immunodeficiency virus.

■ Attempts to develop a preventive vaccine are ongoing; thus far primary vaccination has been unsuccessful.

Treatment

■ The patient should be advised of measures to prevent spread of the virus to others: contact with open lesions should be avoided; glasses, razors should not be shared, condoms should be used; kissing while a lesion is open or has a moist crust may spread the disease.

■ Infections resolve without treatment. The need for treatment of first-episode infections, recurrent infections, and suppressive therapy is based on each patient's needs.

■ Long-term suppressive therapy can greatly improve the quality of life for people with frequent and painful recurrences.

■ Subsequent recurrence rate off medication is not influenced by any topical or oral medication.

Topical Agents

■ These can be used for relief of pain. When applied frequently, tetracaine cream 1.8% (Cepacol Viractin Cream; which can be obtained over the counter) reduces the healing time of recurrent herpes labialis lesions by about 2 days.

■ Abreva (docosanol) is a non-prescription topical cold-sore medication approved by the Food and Drug Administration. It shortens healing time to about the same extent as penciclovir cream.

■ When applied several times each day, penciclovir cream (Denavir) reduces the duration of herpes labialis by about half a day. It is very expensive.

■ Topical acyclovir is not approved for use on cold sores in the immunocompetent host because of its lack of efficacy. Use of topical antivirals may potentiate resistance to antiviral therapy, and since efficacy is lacking, such use should be discouraged.

■ The lips should be protected from sun exposure with opaque creams such as zinc oxide or with sun-blocking agents incorporated into a lip balm.

■ A wet dressing with cool water decreases erythema and debrides crusts to promote healing.

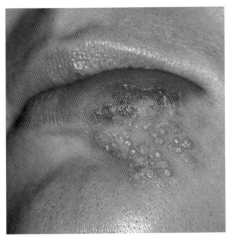

Recurrent herpes. A large group of vesicles followed sun exposure.

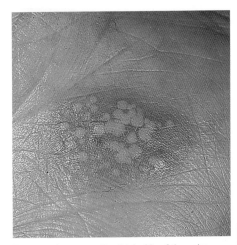

Recurrent herpes on the thick skin of the palm.

Oral Antiviral Agents

- Therapy is initiated at the first sign or symptom.
- Therapy is most effective when administered within 48 hours of the onset of signs and symptoms.
- The frequency and severity of episodes of untreated herpes may change over time. After 1 year of suppressive therapy, the frequency and severity of the infection should be reevaluated to assess the need for continued therapy.
- Valacyclovir (Valtrex)
  - For initial episodes, 1 g is given twice a day for 10 days.
  - For recurrent episodes, 500 mg is administered twice a day for 3 days.
  - Recurrent oral–labial infection may be treated with 1 g, two tablets twice a day for just 1 day.
  - Suppressive therapy requires the administration of 1 g per day. In patients with a history of no more than nine recurrences a year, an alternative dose is 500 mg per day.
- Famciclovir (Famvir)
  - For recurrent episodes, 125 mg twice a day is given for 5 days.
  - For suppressive therapy, 250 mg is administered twice a day for up to 1 year.
- Acyclovir (Zovirax)
  - For initial episodes, 200 mg is given every 4 hours five times a day for 10 days.
  - For suppressive therapy, 400 mg is administered twice a day for up to 12 months. Then the case is re-evaluated. Alternative regimens have included doses ranging from 200 mg three times a day to 200 mg five times a day.
  - For recurrent episodes, 400 mg is administered every 8 hours three times a day for 5 days.
- L-Lysine is ineffective
- Long-term use of acyclovir topically or orally in people infected with human immunodeficiency virus-infected is a risk factor for the development of acyclovir resistance. Diagnosis of acyclovir-resistant viral lesions should be considered when lesions are longer in duration of healing.

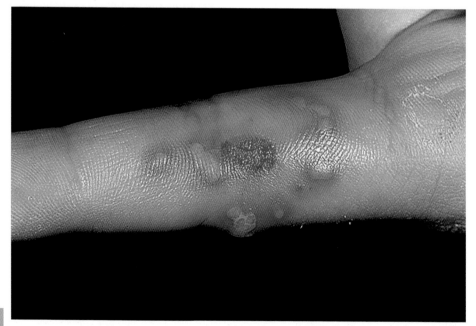

Recurrent herpes on the finger. Herpes can infect any skin surface. A diagnosis of poison ivy was made but the patient reported that this eruption had occurred several times in the past.

Pediatric Considerations

- Infants with suspected herpes simplex infection should be treated with antiviral therapy and treated early to prevent disseminated infection.
- Infants who acquire the virus in utero have a poor prognosis with high morbidity (mental retardation, seizures, deafness) and high mortality rates.
- Infants who acquire the virus perinatally have a much better prognosis with more than 90% developing normally.
- The part of the infant's body which presents in delivery is most likely to come into contact with maternal virus-containing secretions and is more apt to show the first signs of infection.
- Cutaneous signs often lag behind other signs such as poor feeding and irritability.

Pearls

- Viral shedding occurs intermittently and in most cases without symptoms. It is the major cause of the ongoing epidemic.
- Umbilicated vesicles (dome-shaped with a slight central depression) are the hallmark of herpes virus infections.
- Most infections are acquired from people who shed the virus but have no symptoms.
- Most primary infections are asymptomatic.
- Recurrent infection with herpes simplex is the most common cause of recurrent erythema multiforme.
- Time spent on the emotional impact and practical aspects preventing spread of the disease is time well spent.
- Time spent trying to pinpoint the source of an infection is usually fruitless and unproductive since most primary infections are asymptomatic.

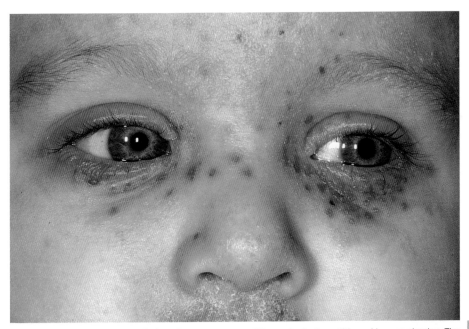

Eczema herpeticum is the association of two common conditions, atopic dermatitis and herpes simplex. The virus infects areas where atopic dermatitis is commonly found. The infection can spread rapidly over wide areas.

Varicella (Chicken Pox)

Description

- Varicella, a highly contagious infection, is caused by the varicella zoster virus and most commonly results in lifetime immunity.

History

- Transmission is via airborne droplets or vesicular fluid.
- Patients are contagious from 2 days before the onset of the rash until all lesions have crusted.
- The incubation period is approximately 14–16 days.
- In children, prodromal symptoms are absent or consist of low-grade fever, headache, and malaise; fever, malaise, and a generalized vesicular rash develop and last 4–7 days. Photophobia may be present.
- Adolescents, adults, and immunocompromised persons have more severe disease and are at risk for complications.
- Moderate to intense pruritus is present during the vesicular stage.
- Temperature varies from 38–40° C but returns to normal when the vesicles disappear.

Skin Findings

- There is a simultaneous presence of lesions (vesicles, pustules and crusts) in all stages.
- The rash begins on the trunk and spreads to the face and extremities. The extent of involvement varies considerably.
- A lesion starts as a 2–4-mm red papule, and then a thin-walled, clear vesicle appears on the surface. The vesicle becomes umbilicated (a central dell occurs) and cloudy, breaking after 8–12 hours to form a crust as the red base disappears. The formation of new lesions ceases by the fourth day.
- Crusts fall off in about 7 days and usually heal without scarring.
- Secondary infection or excoriation extends the process into the dermis.

- Vesicles often form in the oral cavity and vagina and rupture quickly to form multiple, aphthae-like ulcers.

Non-skin Findings

- Pneumonia is the most common serious complication in normal adults.
- Hepatitis is the most common complication in immunosuppressed patients.

Laboratory

- Culture or a Tzanck smear is performed for questionable cases.
- A direct immunofluorescence test of scrapings obtained from the vesicle base is a rapid and sensitive test, but not widely available.

Complications

- Bacterial superinfection with *Streptococcus pyogenes* or *Staphylococcus aureus*, pneumonia, dehydration, encephalitis, and hepatitis are possible complications. The most common neurologic complication is ataxia secondary to cerebellar inflammation. Roughly 15% of healthy adults develop pulmonary involvement.

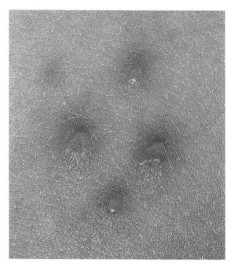

The lesion starts as a 2–4-mm red papule, which develops an irregular outline (rose petal) as a thin-walled clear vesicle appears on the surface (dew drop).

- Since the association between Reye syndrome and aspirin use was identified, the occurrence of Reye syndrome has become more rare.
- Suspected ocular involvement should be evaluated by an ophthalmologist.
- Thrombocytopenia, transient thrombocytopenic purpura, and Henoch-Schönlein purpura are rare complications.
- Maternal infection with varicella zoster virus during the first 20 weeks of gestation poses a risk of fetal congenital varicella syndrome.

Differential Diagnosis
- Disseminated varicella zoster
- Disseminated herpes simplex
- Eczema herpeticum
- Henoch-Schönlein purpura
- Smallpox
- Folliculitis
- Impetigo

Treatment
- Symptomatic treatment consists of bland antipruritic lotions (e.g. Sarna). Antihistamines (hydroxyzine) may help control excoriation.
- Other antiviral medication includes acyclovir 10 mg/kg intravenously every 8 hours for 7 days. Other antivirals, such as valacyclovir 1 g t.i.d. for 7 days and famciclovir 500 mg t.i.d. for 7 days, may have a role in treatment of varicella, though they are presently approved in the United States for treatment of varicella zoster infection.

American Academy of Pediatrics Recommendations for Acyclovir Therapy of Varicella Zoster Infections	
Indications	**Recommended Therapy**
· Non-pregnant, healthy adolescents ≥ 13 years of age who have varicella	Consider acyclovir: should be initiated within 24 hours of onset of rash
· Children > 12 months of age who have chronic cutaneous or pulmonary disorder or are on long-term term salicylate therapy	Dosage: 20 mg/kg (800 mg maximum) orally four times a day for 5 days
· Children receiving short, intermittent, or aerosolized courses of corticosteroids	
· Children infected from household contact	
· Healthy children and adults with complications of varicella	Intravenous acyclovir
· Immunocompromised children (including secondary to high-dose corticosteroids) with primary varicella	Dosage: 10 mg/kg intravenously every 8 hours for 7 days
· Immunocompromised children with recurrent zoster	
· Pregnant patients with complications of varicella	
· Healthy children with varicella	Routinely, no therapy
· Pregnant patients with uncomplicated varicella	
· Healthy children exposed to varicella	

Treatment of Adolescents and Adults

▪ Early therapy with oral acyclovir decreases the time to cutaneous healing of adult varicella, decreases the duration of fever, and reduces the severity of symptoms but does not alter viral shedding. The initiation of therapy after the first day of illness is of no value in uncomplicated cases of adult varicella.

▪ There is a high morbidity rate even in normal patients with clinically evident varicella pneumonia; intravenous acyclovir 10 mg/kg intravenously every 8 hours for 7 days may help.

Immunocompromised Patients

▪ Immunosuppressed patients treated with acyclovir have decreased morbidity from visceral dissemination; there is a modest effect on cutaneous disease. The recommended schedule is acyclovir 10 mg/kg intravenously every 8 hours for 7-10 days.

▪ The use of varicella zoster immune globulin is recommended for post-exposure prophylaxis. It may be administered within 96 hours after exposure.

Recommendations for the Use of Varicella Zoster Immunoglobulin for Post-Exposure Prophylaxis	
Persons < 13 Years of Age	**Persons > 13 Years of Age**
Used for passive immunization of susceptible, immunocompromised children after substantial exposure to varicella or herpes zoster, including: 1. Children with primary and acquired immuno-deficiency disorders 2. Children with neoplastic diseases who are receiving immunosuppressive treatment 3. Neonates whose mothers have signs and symptoms of varicella within 5 days before and 2 days after delivery 4. Premature infants who have substantial postnatal exposure and who should be evaluated on an individual basis	A healthy, unvaccinated adolescent or adult who has had substantial exposure and is determined as being susceptible Varicella zoster immunoglobulin should be considered for susceptible pregnant women who have been exposed, in order to prevent complications of varicella in the mother, rather than to protect the fetus Note: If varicella is prevented through the use of varicella zoster immunoglobulin, vaccination should be offered later

Immunization: Varicella Vaccine Recommendations (Varivax)

Persons < 13 Years of Age	Persons > 13 Years of Age
A single, 0.5 ml subcutaneous dose is recommended for all healthy children aged 1–12 years old with no history of varicella Children with a reliable history are considered immune Those with an uncertain history are immunized Serologic testing is not warranted because the vaccine is well tolerated in seropositive persons	Two 0.5 ml doses of varicella vaccine given 4–8 weeks apart are recommended for healthy adolescents and adults with no history of the disease Those with a reliable history of previous infection are considered immune Those who do not have such histories are considered susceptible and can be tested to determine immune status or can be vaccinated without testing

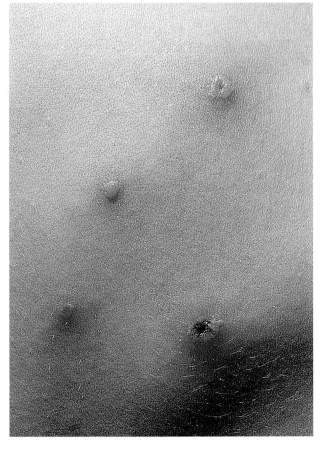

Vesicles become umbilicated and cloudy and break in 8–12 hours to form a crust as the red base disappears.

Pediatric Considerations

- The varicella vaccine is highly efficacious, with a 96% seroconversion rate in healthy children; the efficacy is 71–91%.
- Children who have been immunized with the live attenuated vaccine may develop a mild afebrile illness—varicella-like syndrome—consisting of erythematous macules and papules, and few vesicles roughly 15 days after exposure. The lesions are much less numerous.

Pearls

- In varicella (chicken pox), lesions of different stages (vesicles, crusts, and pustules) are present at the same time in any given body area. This is in contrast to the rash of variola (smallpox) where lesions are all in the same stage during the eruption course. Small pox lesions are the same size and extend into deep dermis.
- In chicken pox, lesions are centripetal (more heavily distributed on the trunk); however, in small pox lesions are centrifugal (more lesions on the face and extremities than the trunk).
- Varicella is highly contagious; patients hospitalized for complications or therapy require strict isolation procedures.
- Acyclovir-resistant varicella may occur in people infected with human immunodeficiency virus on chronic topical or oral therapy; such should be considered in severe atypical or disseminated disease.

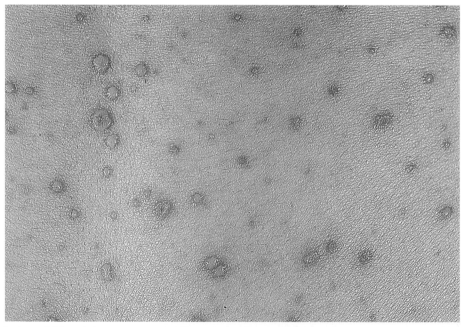

Lesions of different stages are present at the same time in any given body area.

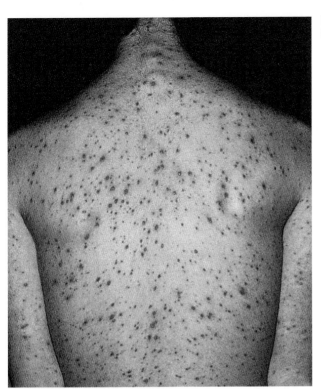

Numerous lesions on the trunk (centripetal distribution).

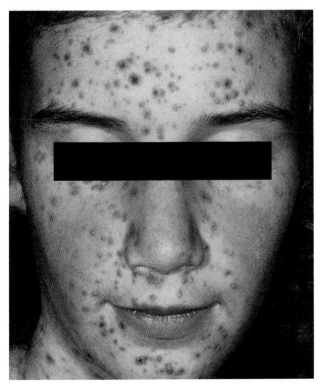

Lesions present in all stages of development.

Herpes Zoster (Shingles)

Description

- Herpes zoster is a cutaneous viral infection generally involving the skin of a single or adjacent dermatomes.
- Herpes zoster results from the reactivation of varicella virus that entered the cutaneous nerves during an earlier episode of chicken pox.
- Shingles is another name for herpes zoster.

History

- This condition occurs during the lifetime of 10–20% of all people.
- People of all ages may be afflicted; the incidence increases with age.
- Patients with zoster are not more likely to have an unknown underlying malignancy.
- Zoster may be the earliest clinical sign of the development of the acquired immunodeficiency syndrome in high-risk individuals.
- Age, immunosuppressive drugs, lymphoma, fatigue, emotional upsets, and radiation therapy have been implicated in reactivating the virus.
- The elderly are at greater risk for developing segmental pain, which can continue for months after the skin lesions have healed.
- Patients with Hodgkin's lymphoma are uniquely susceptible to herpes zoster.
- The pain may simulate pleurisy, myocardial infarction, abdominal disease, or migraine headache and may present a difficult diagnostic problem until the characteristic eruption provides the answer.
- The constitutional symptoms of headache, photophobia and malaise may precede the eruption by several days. Fever is uncommon. Regional lymphadenopathy may be present.
- An attack of herpes zoster does not confer lasting immunity, and it is not abnormal to have two or three episodes in a lifetime.

Skin Findings

- Pre-eruptive tenderness or hyperesthesia throughout the dermatome is a useful predictive sign.
- Pain, itching, or burning, generally localized to the dermatome, may precede the eruption by 4 or 5 days.
- Although generally limited to the skin of a single dermatome, the eruption may involve one or two adjacent dermatomes. Non-contiguous multidermatomal lesions are most often associated with immunosuppressed individuals.
- Occasionally, a few vesicles appear across the midline.
- Approximately 50% of patients with uncomplicated zoster have a viremia, with the appearance of 20 or 30 vesicles scattered over the skin surface outside the affected dermatome.
- The thoracic region is affected in two-thirds of cases.
- The eruption begins with red swollen plaques of various sizes and spreads to involve part or all of a dermatome.
- The vesicles arise in clusters from the erythematous base and become cloudy with purulent fluid by the third or fourth day.
- The vesicles vary in size, in contrast to the cluster of uniformly sized vesicles noted in herpes simplex.
- Vesicles either umbilicate or rupture before forming crusts, which fall off in 2 or 3 weeks.
- Elderly or debilitated patients may have a prolonged and difficult course. For them, the eruption is typically more extensive and inflammatory, occasionally resulting in hemorrhagic blisters, skin necrosis, secondary bacterial infection, or extensive scarring.
- Complications of herpes zoster in immune competent individuals can include peripheral nerve palsies, encephalitis, myelitis, and a contralateral hemiparesis syndrome. Disseminated disease may result in death.
- Acute retinal necrosis, heralded by visual changes within weeks or months of an episode of zoster, is a complication more often associated with patients seropositive for human immunodeficiency virus.

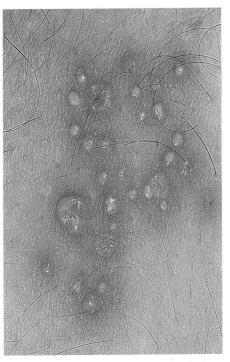

The vesicles vary in size, in contrast to the cluster of uniformly sized vesicles noted in herpes simplex.

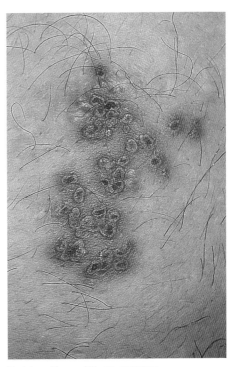

Vesicles either umbilicate or rupture.

A crust forms. It falls off in 2–3 weeks.

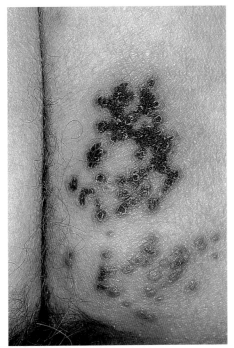

Ophthalmic Zoster
- Involvement of any branch of the ophthalmic nerve is called herpes zoster ophthalmicus.
- With ophthalmic zoster, the rash extends from eye level to the vertex of the skull but does not cross the midline.
- Vesicles on the side or tip of the nose (Hutchinson's sign) are associated with the most serious ocular complications.
- Of patients who are not treated with antiviral therapy 50% will develop ocular complications (keratopathy, episcleritis, iritis). Oral antiviral therapy results in decreased frequency of late ocular complications.
- Patients with ophthalmic zoster should be referred to an ophthalmologist.

Post-Herpetic Neuralgia
- Pain is the major cause of morbidity in zoster; post-herpetic neuralgia is pain that persists more than 30 days after the rash.
- The incidence and duration of pain increase with age.
- Pain can persist in a dermatome for months or years after lesions have disappeared.
- The pain is often severe, intractable, and exhausting. The patient protects areas of hyperesthesia to avoid the slightest pressure, which activates another wave of pain.
- The majority of patients under 30 years of age experience no pain. By age 40, the risk of prolonged pain lasting longer than 1 month increases to 33%. By age 70, the risk increases to 74%.
- The degree of pain is related neither to the extent of involvement nor to the number of vesicles or degree of inflammation or fibrosis in peripheral nerves.

Laboratory
- Culture is specific, but the virus is labile and not easily isolated.
- Complement fixation tests can be used for retrospective diagnosis.
- Direct immunofluorescence of cellular material from skin lesions can be performed.
- In a Tzanck smear, the base of a vesicle is scraped with a cotton swab, and the material is smeared onto a glass slide. It is submitted to the laboratory or stained directly to see multinucleated giant cells.

Treatment
Suppression of Inflammation, Pain, and Infection
- Topical therapy is tried. Cool tap water can be used in a wet dressing. The wet dressings are applied for 20 minutes several times a day; they macerate the vesicles, remove serum and crust, and discourage bacterial growth.
- With oral steroids, there is a decrease of acute pain and a quicker rash resolution but no effect on post-herpetic neuralgia. There is no difference in pain at 6 months when acyclovir and prednisone are used together, compared with acyclovir alone or prednisone alone. There are no significant differences between steroid-treated and non-steroid-treated patients in the time to a first or a complete cessation of pain. The incidence of adverse effects is higher in patients treated with corticosteroids.
- Sympathetic blocks (stellate ganglion or epidural) with bupivacaine 0.25% may terminate the pain of acute herpes zoster and prevent or relieve post-herpetic neuralgia.

Attenuation of the Acute Phase
- Oral antiviral drugs decrease acute pain, inflammation, vesicle formation, and viral shedding.
- The duration and severity of post-herpetic neuralgia may be reduced by treating acute herpes zoster with valacyclovir or famciclovir.
- Treatment is most effective when started within the first 48 hours of infection.
- It is reasonable to use antiviral therapy in the patient seeking medical treatment more than 48 hours after the vesicles appear if the lesions are not completely crusted.
- The recommended oral dosage for adults is a 7–10-day course of acyclovir (Zovirax) 800 mg five times a day; valacyclovir (Valtrex) 1000 mg three times

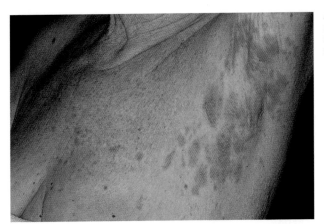

A large group of vesicles involving several dermatomes. It is not unusual for shingles to involve more than one dermatome.

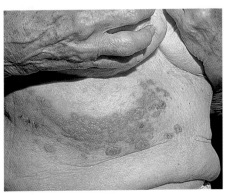

The eruption begins with red swollen plaques of various sizes and spreads to involve part or all of a dermatome. Elderly or debilitated patients may have a prolonged and difficult course. For them, the eruption is typically more extensive and inflammatory.

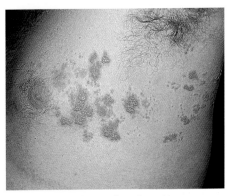

Vesicles arise in clusters from the red base. Lesions often involve more than one dermatome.

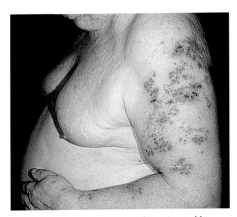

Herpes zoster may involve any dermatome. Many patients think that "shingles" involves only the trunk.

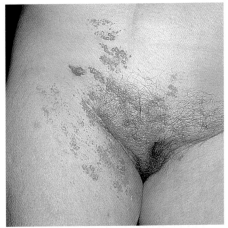

Sacral zoster. A neurogenic bladder with urinary hesitancy or urinary retention can be associated with zoster of the sacral dermatome S2, S3, or S4. Migration of virus to the adjacent autonomic nerves is responsible for these symptoms.

a day; or famciclovir (Famvir) 500 mg three times a day. Valacyclovir and Famciclovir are equal in ability to increase healing and pain resolution; their simpler dosing regimen and pharmacokinetic profile makes them preferable to acyclovir. All three drugs are safe and well tolerated. Dosage adjustments are necessary for patients with renal insufficiency.

■ The drugs are given empirically to patients who are older than 50 years of age, are immunocompromised, or have trigeminal zoster.

■ Topical antivirals play no role in the management of herpes zoster.

Post-Herpetic Neuralgia

Prevention

■ Famciclovir and valacyclovir may decrease the duration of post-herpetic neuralgia.

■ Oral steroids used to prevent post-herpetic neuralgia have not been proven to be effective.

■ Some authors recommend starting amitriptyline at low doses (10–25 mg) and gradually increasing this to doses of 50–75 mg over 2–3 weeks in all patients older than 60 years of age as soon as shingles is diagnosed. A 50% decrease in the incidence of post-herpetic neuralgia has been reported.

Treatment

■ There is no reliable treatment for post-herpetic neuralgia. Consultation with a pain management specialist can be helpful.

■ Oral analgesics (e.g. acetaminophen, oxycodone) are first-line therapy.

■ The topical lidocaine patch is the first drug approved for post-herpetic neuralgia by the United States Food and Drug Administration.

■ Tricyclic antidepressants, such as amitriptyline 75 mg/day, nortriptyline 25–75 mg/day, and desipramine, and the anticonvulsant gabapentin, relieve pain in some patients.

■ Some clinicians advocate a short course of steroids (e.g. prednisone, 40–60 mg/day for 3–5 days or longer).

■ Narcotics and analgesics are effective in many patients.

■ Topical capsaicin cream (Zostrix, Zostrix HP) acts by enhancing the release or inhibiting the re-accumulation of substance P from cell bodies and nerve terminals. Patients experience some pain relief but may not be able to tolerate the burning. Applying EMLA or topical lignocaine (lidocaine) before capsaicin use may make the treatment more tolerable. Capsaicin should not be applied to unhealed skin lesions.

Pediatric Considerations

● More than 20,000 healthy children in the United States will develop herpes zoster each year.

● Children with a history of chicken pox developing before age 1 are at an increased risk for herpes zoster.

● Children with zoster do not have a higher incidence of underlying immune compromise; laboratory studies in healthy children with zoster are not routinely necessary.

● Otherwise healthy children with zoster do not require a serologic test for human immunodeficiency virus.

Pearls

■ Sacral zoster can occur. A neurogenic bladder with urinary hesitancy or urinary retention can be associated with zoster of the sacral dermatome S2, S3, or S4. Migration of virus to the adjacent autonomic nerves is responsible for these symptoms.

■ Varicella zoster of the geniculate ganglion is called Ramsay–Hunt syndrome. There is involvement of the sensory and motor portions of the VIIth cranial nerve. There may be unilateral loss of taste on the anterior two-thirds of the tongue, and vesicles on the tympanic membrane, external auditory meatus, concha, and pinna.

- Herpes zoster in people infected with human immunodeficiency virus is associated with frequent recurrences, and atypical lesions. Treatment should be continued until all lesions have completely resolved.

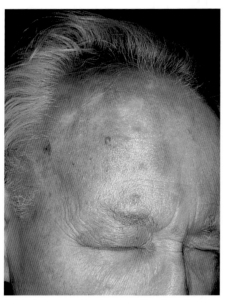

Ophthalmic zoster. Involvement of any branch of the ophthalmic nerve is called herpes zoster ophthalmicus. The rash extends from eye level to the vertex of the skull but does not cross the midline. This is the initial vesicular stage.

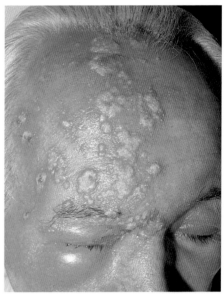

Ophthalmic zoster. Vesicles on the side or tip of the nose (Hutchinson's sign) that occur during an episode of zoster are associated with the most serious ocular complications, including conjunctival, corneal, scleral, and other ocular diseases, although this is not invariable.

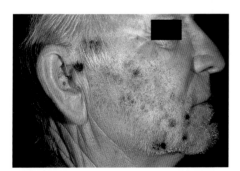

Varicella zoster of the geniculate ganglion is called Ramsay–Hunt syndrome. There is involvement of the sensory and motor portions of the VIIth cranial nerve. There may be unilateral loss of taste on the anterior two thirds of the tongue and vesicles on the tympanic membrane, external auditory meatus, concha, and pinna.

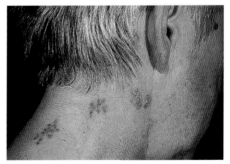

A classic presentation of grouped vesicles and crusts involving a cervical dermatome.

Hand, Foot, and Mouth Disease

Description

■ Hand, foot and mouth disease is a highly contagious viral infection that causes aphthae-like oral erosions and a vesicular eruption on the hands and feet.

■ The classic benign, self-limited form of this disease is associated with coxsackie A16 virus.

■ Enterovirus 71 is a picornavirus genetically related to coxsackie A16. It can cause oral ulcers and similar skin exanthem, but epidemic outbreaks have associated potentially serious neurologic and cardiopulmonary complications, particularly in children under 4 years.

History

■ The incubation period is 4–6 days.

■ Coxsackie A16 related hand, foot, and mouth disease usually presents with acute stomatitis and a mild fever.

■ There may be mild symptoms of sore throat and malaise or abdominal pain for 1 or 2 days.

■ About 20% patients develop submandibular lymphadenopathy, cervical lymphadenopathy, or both.

■ Epidemics usually occur in the summer and autumn but may appear at any time.

■ Children younger than 5 years of age are most commonly affected, but the rate of infection among close household contacts is high.

■ Epidemics of disease associated with enterovirus 71-related disease have occurred in Bulgaria, Hungary, Malaysia, Taiwan, and Australia. Genotypes responsible for this disease in the Far East have arisen since 1997.

■ Enterovirus 71 outbreaks commonly include fever, oral ulcers and/or extremity rash, vomiting and cough.

Skin Findings

■ The number of oral aphthae-like erosions (3–6 mm) varies from a few to ten or more. They are irregularly distributed anywhere in the oral cavity. They are more painful in younger children. Each erosion lasts 3–5 days.

■ Cutaneous lesions in coxsackie-induced hand, foot and mouth disease occur in two-thirds of patients and appear less than 24 hours after the oral lesions.

■ They begin as 3–7-mm red macules that rapidly become pale, white oval vesicles with red areolae. The vesicles have a unique rhomboidal shape of "square blisters." There may be a few inconspicuous lesions, or there may be dozens.

■ The vesicles occur on the palms, soles, dorsal aspects of the fingers and toes, and occasionally on the face, buttocks, and legs.

■ They heal in approximately 7 days, usually without crusting or scarring.

Course

■ Hand, foot, and mouth disease caused by coxsackie A16 is usually mild and self-limited. It resolves without treatment in about 10 days.

■ Oral ulcerations are painful in infants and interfere with feeding.

■ Recent emergence of epidemics of hand, foot and mouth disease caused by enterovirus 71 are associated with varied neurological syndromes including aseptic meningitis, Guillain–Barré syndrome, polio-like paralysis, acute transverse myelitis, acute cerebellar ataxia,

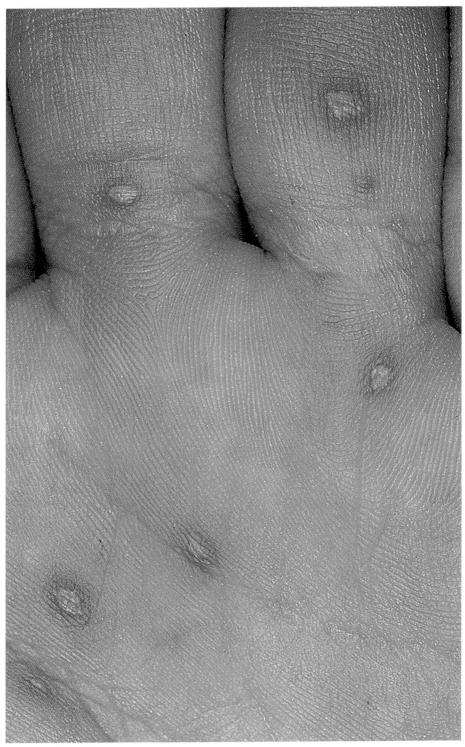

Cloudy vesicles with red halos are highly characteristic of this disease.

intracranial hypertension, and febrile convulsions. The prodrome is 1–7 days prior to the neurologic disease and has associated fever, coryza, malaise, headache, and diarrhea. Two-thirds of those affected may have a rash; often truncal, herpangina-type lesions may occur in the mouth.

Laboratory

- The diagnosis is usually made clinically.
- Laboratory studies are usually unnecessary for the benign presentation of the disease.
- Virus can be cultured from the vesicles, throat, and stool. Viral isolates can be detected by neutralization assay.
- Convalescent sera show elevated titers of specific complement-fixing viral antibodies. Serum for serology can be examined for enterovirus 71-specific antibody by means of a serum neutralization assay, and may be detected in the sera of as many as 50% of acute, and 70% of convalescent patients.
- Both varicella and herpes simplex have multinucleated, giant cells in smears taken from the moist skin exposed when a vesicle is removed and the base scraped (Tzanck smear). Giant cells are not present in the lesions of hand, foot, and mouth disease.

Differential Diagnosis

- Herpangina (lesions limited to the posterior oral cavity, tonsils, and soft palate; disease is associated with a higher temperature)
- Aphthous stomatitis (patients are afebrile and tend to have recurrences)

Pediatric Considerations

- Herpetic gingivostomatitis is the most common cause of stomatitis in children younger than 5 years of age. Gingival involvement is severe and associated with lymphadenopathy and a high fever. The oral erosions of hand, foot, and mouth disease are usually small and uniform.
- Enterovirus 71 infection should be considered in the young child with neurologic manifestations (as described above) and diffuse rash, sometimes petechial, or manifestations of herpangina.

Treatment

- Children may be isolated during the most contagious period, usually for 3–7 days. Some may be carriers up to 3 months after the infection. Symptomatic relief is important in infants to prevent dehydration. Fever and pain are controlled with acetaminophen. Cool fluids are best tolerated; acidic foods are avoided.
- Acyclovir suspension 200–300 mg five times a day for 5 days is anecdotally reported to provide rapid relief of signs and symptoms in children age 9 months to 5 years.
- Effective antiviral therapy for enterovirus 71-induced diseased is not presently available. Intravenous immunoglobulin has been of little benefit. Vaccine development is needed for this disease.

Pearls

- Cloudy vesicles with red halos on the palms and soles are highly characteristic.
- Increasing epidemics of enterovirus 71 disease in the Asia–Pacific region have been associated with severe neurologic and cardiopulmonary disease.
- Enterovirus 71 infection should be considered in the young child with fever, neurologic sequelae, and oral ulcers and/or extremity rash.

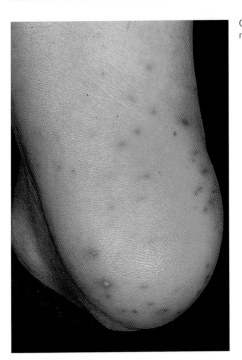

Cloudy vesicles with red halos in hand, foot, and mouth disease.

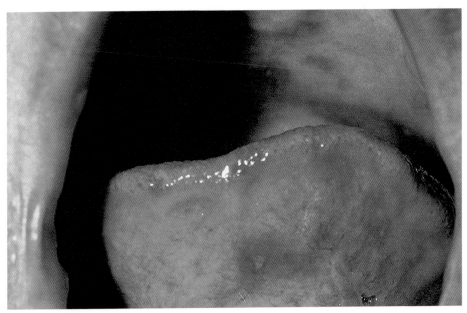

Pale white oval vesicles with red areolae in hand, foot, and mouth disease.

9 Fungal Infections

Candidiasis (Moniliasis)

Description
- *Candida albicans* and a few other *Candida* species are capable of producing skin and mucous membrane infections.
- The organism lives among the normal flora of the mouth, vaginal tract, and lower gastrointestinal tract.
- It reproduces through the budding of oval yeast forms, forming elongated pseudohyphae.
- Factors that predispose to infection include infancy, pregnancy, oral contraceptive use, systemic antibiotic therapy, diabetes, skin maceration, topical and systemic steroid therapy, and decreased cell-mediated immunity.

Skin Findings
- The yeast infects only the outer layers of the epithelium of mucous membrane and skin (the stratum corneum).
- The primary lesion is a pustule, the contents of which dissect horizontally under the stratum corneum and peel it away.
- Clinically, this process results in a red, denuded, glistening surface with a long, cigarette paper-like, scaling and advancing border.
- Yeast grows best in a warm, moist environment; thus infection is usually confined to the mucous membranes and intertriginous areas.

Laboratory
- In potassium wet mount preparation and culture, the pseudohyphae and hyphae may be difficult to distinguish from dermatophytes in potassium hydroxide preparations.
- Culture results must be interpreted carefully because the yeast is part of the normal flora in many areas.
- Nickerson's media is used to isolate and identify *Candida* species.

Candidal Balanitis

Description
- A localized, acute infection of the foreskin and glans penis caused by *Candida* organisms.

History
- Occurs more frequently in uncircumcised men than in circumcised men.
- Diabetics are at greater risk.
- Intercourse with an infected woman is probably a risk factor, though infections occur and persist without sexual exposure.
- Yeast invades the superficial epidermis, producing pustules and exudate.

Skin Findings
- Pinpoint red papules evolving into umbilicated pustules on the glans and coronal sulcus with pasty macerated debris under the foreskin.
- Pustules rupture under the foreskin and leave 1–2 mm, white doughnut-shaped erosions.
- Ulceration and fissures may follow.
- Edema and pain can be intense enough to limit retraction of the foreskin.

Laboratory
- Potassium hydroxide examination reveals numerous yeast forms (pseudohyphae and blastospores).
- Bacterial culture may reveal coexistent bacterial infection.

Differential Diagnosis
- Herpes simplex (forms umbilicated pustules that erode)

- Molluscum contagiosum (forms umbilicated papules that persist)
- Inverse psoriasis may be masked by a superimposed *Candida* infection
- Irritant contact dermatitis (due to detergents and allergic contact dermatitis due to medicaments)

Course and Prognosis
- Persistent and recurrent if not treated, especially in people with diabetes.
- Sexual contact is best avoided until the infection resolves.

Treatment
- Topical therapy usually suffices
- Miconazole, clotrimazole, ketoconazole, oxiconazole, or econazole cream twice daily for 10 days.
- Relief is almost immediate, but treatment should be continued for 10 days.

- Preparations containing topical steroids (Lotrisone: clotrimazole and betamethasone diproprionate) give temporary relief by suppressing inflammation, but the eruption rebounds and worsens, sometimes even before the cortisone cream is discontinued. These preparations are *not* recommended.
- Resistant cases may respond to systemic therapy with itraconazole 200 mg every day for 3–7 days or fluconazole 150 mg every day for 1–3 days.

Pearls
- Umbilicated pustules occur with herpes simplex and acute *Candida* infection. They may be clinically indistinguishable.
- Satellite pustules or bright pink papules are highly suggestive of candidiasis.

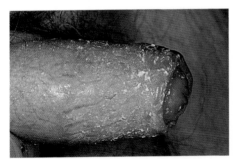

The uncircumcised penis provides the warm moist environment ideally suited for yeast infection. Here, the inflammation is intense, causing fissuring. The white exudate is highly characteristic.

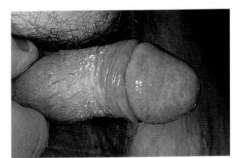

Candida balanitis. Tender pinpoint red papules and pustules appear on the glans and are macerated by the overlying foreskin to form erosion.

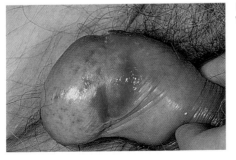

Infection and inflammation are more intense on this warm and moist intertriginous surface.

221

Candidiasis (Diaper Dermatitis)

Description
- Diaper dermatitis is a term that encompasses a number of skin conditions, causing red scaly rashes on the diaper area.

History
- Diapers occlude the skin, leading to skin maceration and predisposing to skin infection and inflammation.
- Frequent diaper changes decrease the incidence of diaper dermatitis.
- Highly absorbent disposable diapers effectively draw moisture away from the skin.
- Elevations in skin pH occur when urine is mixed with stools (especially diarrhea), predisposing to breakdown of the epidermal barrier.

Skin Findings
Clinical Patterns
Irritant Contact Diaper Dermatitis
- This is the most common form.
- Red, scaly, eroded, painful plaques occur on the convex surfaces.
- The creases are spared.

Candidal Diaper Dermatitis
- *Candida* can be a primary cause of diaper dermatitis, occurring as bright red (beefy red) plaques in the inguinal and gluteal folds.
- *Candida* infection can occur in the setting of seborrheic dermatitis or psoriasis.
- Satellite pustules are the hallmark of *Candida* dermatitis.
- Pustules rupture to form a superficial collarette of scale.
- Chronic, poorly treated *Candida* diaper dermatitis can form granulomatous nodules.
- *Candida* dermatitis can rarely result in a psoriasis-like eruption at distant sites such as the cheeks and torso.

Seborrheic Dermatitis and Psoriasis
- Seborrheic dermatitis affects the scalp and intertriginous areas, including the diaper area.
- Red, scaly plaques occur on the scrotum, penis, labia majora, pubis and inguinal and gluteal folds.
- Psoriasis can be isolated to the diaper area and appear identical to seborrheic dermatitis.

Erosions
- Erosions can be a manifestation of herpes, bullous impetigo or fungal infection.
- Infants who stool frequently often develop erosive perianal eruptions.

Discussion
- There are several causes of inflammation in the diaper area.
- Diaper candidiasis is an acute infection of the superficial layers of the skin.

Laboratory
- Potassium hydroxide examination will confirm the presence of pseudohyphae and spores if present.
- Culture results are often mixed with bacterial superinfection as well as *Candida* species.

Differential Diagnosis
- Streptococcal anal cellulitis and staphylococcal impetigo (best discerned by culture)
- Rare causes of diaper dermatitis include cystic fibrosis, histiocytosis, and nutritional deficiency (especially zinc deficiency)

Treatment
- Therapy should be directed at minimizing wetness in the diaper area.
- Frequent diaper changes and brief diaper-free time periods should be encouraged.
- Barrier ointments such as petrolatum, Aquaphor ointment or zinc oxide are useful for prophylaxis.
- Avoid overzealous cleaning with irritating baby wipes.
- Initially apply 1% hydrocortisone cream twice daily until inflammation is controlled.
- Avoid Lotrisone in the diaper area—the steroid component is too potent.
- Elidel (pimecrolimus) 1% cream and

Protopic (tacrolimus) 0.03% ointment are steroid-free anti-inflammatory alternatives.

■ Candida infection is treated with miconazole, clotrimazole, ketoconazole, oxiconazole, or Spectazole cream applied twice daily for a week or two.

■ Do not apply at the same time as the anti-inflammatory therapy; consider alternating applications with successive diaper changes.

■ Localized bacterial infection can be treated with Mupirocin cream (Bactroban).

■ Extensive infection requires oral antibiotic therapy.

■ Consider recommending Pampers Rash Guard diapers (Procter & Gamble).

■ These diapers reduce the severity and frequency of diaper rash by delivering petrolatum to the diaper area.

■ Petrolatum transferred to the baby's skin provide a moisture barrier, and breathable fabric between the stripes absorbs the moisture.

Pearls

■ Think of psoriasis when diaper dermatitis fails to respond to antifungal topical medication.

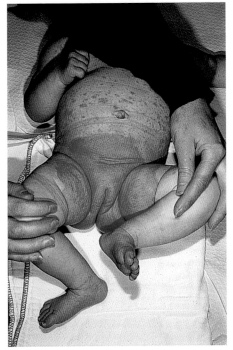

Intense erythema under the entire diaper area. Disease may progress to this extent if topical steroids are the only treatment. Psoriasis would be in the differential diagnosis for this patient.

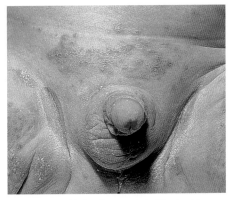

Diaper dermatitis is often treated with steroid combination creams. The cortisone component may alter the clinical presentation and prolong the disease.

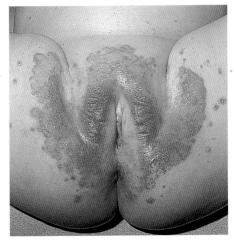

An artificial intertriginous area is created under a wet diaper, predisposing the area to a yeast infection with the characteristic red base and satellite pustules.

Candidiasis of Large Skinfolds (Candidal Intertrigo)

Description
- Yeast thrive in intertriginous areas where skin touches skin.
- Large skinfolds retain heat and moisture, providing the environment suited for yeast infection.

History
- Predisposed individuals include older women with pendulous breasts, obese men and women with overhanging skinfolds below the abdomen, in the groin and rectal areas, and in the axillae.
- Predisposing factors are hot, humid weather; tight or abrasive underclothing; diabetes; poor hygiene. Inflammatory diseases occurring in the skinfolds, such as psoriasis, and the use of topical steroids favor yeast growth within fold areas.

Skin Findings
- Pustules form but become macerated under apposing skin surfaces and develop into red papules with a fringe of moist scale at the border.
- Intact pustules may be found outside the apposing skin surfaces.
- Red, moist, glistening plaques extend to or just beyond the limits of the apposing skinfolds.
- The advancing border is long, sharply defined, and has an ocean wave-shaped fringe of macerated scale.
- Satellite papules dot the normal skin just beyond the plaques.
- There is a tendency for painful fissuring in the skin creases.

Laboratory
- Potassium hydroxide examination is performed by collecting material from the pustule or advancing border with a cotton swab or gently scraping the surface with the blade of a #15 surgical scalpel.
- Material is placed on a glass slide, a drop of 10% potassium hydroxide solution is applied, then a cover slip.

- Gentle pressure disperses the material for easier viewing.
- Gentle heat may be applied but is not usually necessary.
- Pseudohyphae and spores are often numerous.
- Culture material is obtained by sterile cotton swab of pustules or moist areas of the plaque.
- Yeast survive in the commonly available transportable bacterial culture tube kits.
- Bacterial superinfection may be identified by culture.

Course and Prognosis
- *Candida intertrigo* may persist or recur after treatment.

Differential Diagnosis
- Inverse psoriasis (may have superimposed candidal infection, especially if treated with topical steroids)
- Seborrheic dermatitis (usually involves the scalp and central face as well as fold areas)
- Intertrigo from other causes (likely if the potassium hydroxide examination is negative)
- Erythrasma caused by *Corynebacterium* (coral red fluorescence under Wood's light)
- Eczema (particularly if treated with topical steroids) may be masked by an overlying *Candida* infection

Treatment
- Wet dressings with either tap water or with Burrow's (aluminum acetate solution) applied for 20–30 minutes several times each day will help to dry the involved areas.
- Application of wet dressings should be continued until the pustules clear.
- Antifungal creams (miconazole, clotrimazole, ketoconazole, oxiconazole, econazole) applied in a thin layer twice a day until the rash clears.
- Fluconazole 100 mg daily for 7 days is used for resistant cases.
- An absorbent powder, not necessarily medicated, such as Zeasorb, may be applied after the inflammation is gone.

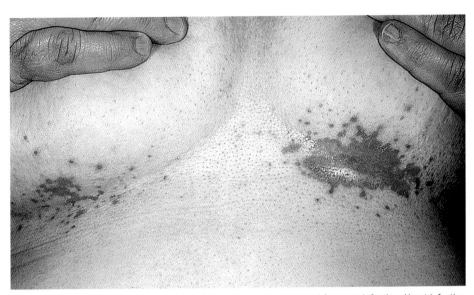

Skinfolds contain heat and moisture, providing an environment well suited for yeast infection. Yeast infection is made more likely with hot, humid weather, with tight or abrasive underclothing, with poor hygiene, or with inflammatory diseases occurring in the skinfolds, such as psoriasis.

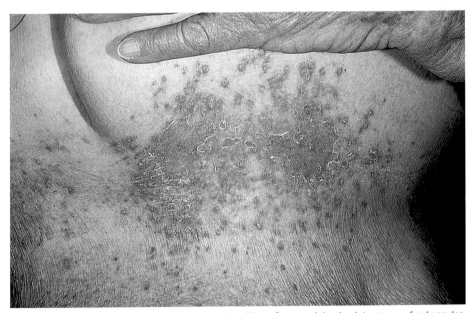

Pustules form, but become macerated under apposing skin surfaces and develop into groups of red papules with a fringe of moist scale at the border. Intact pustules may be found outside the apposing skin surfaces.

■ The powder absorbs a small amount of moisture and acts as a dry lubricant, allowing skin surfaces to slide freely, thus preventing moisture accumulation in a potentially stagnant area.

Pearls

■ Obese diabetic patients are susceptible to recurrent *Candida* infections.

■ There is a potential interaction between oral hypoglycemic agents and fluconazole which requires careful monitoring of blood sugars with concomitant use.

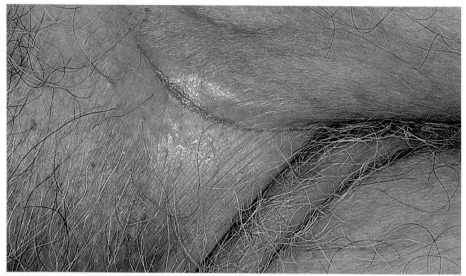

A shallow to deep fissure is commonly found in groin intertrigo. Intermittent use of a group VII topical steroid is effective. Powder may absorb moisture. A cool wet dressing dries the area and encourages healing.

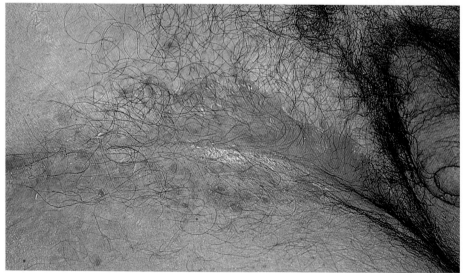

Intertrigo in the groin is common especially in obese individuals. The warm, moist apposing surfaces become red and sore. Yeast infection with papules and pustules may follow. Fungal infections usually do not cause inflammation on symmetrical apposing surfaces.

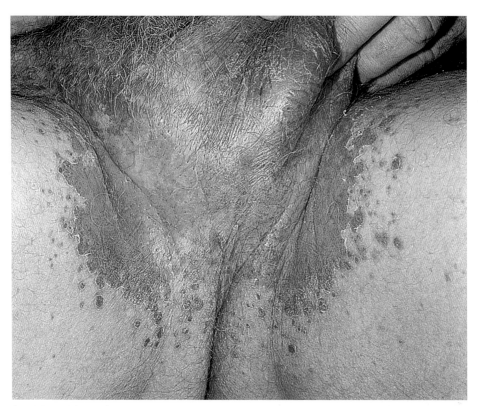

Candidiasis. A fringe of moist scale is present at the border. A red, moist, glistening plaque extends to the limits of the opposing thigh and scrotum. Compare this to tinea of the groin (see p. 249).

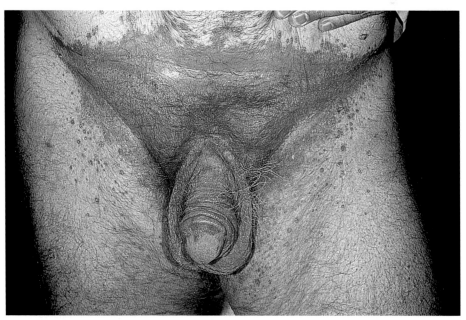

Candidiasis. Papules and pustules are found outside the opposing skin surfaces. A red plaque extends to the border of all apposing skinfolds.

Tinea Versicolor

Description
- A common infection caused by the lipophilic yeast *Pityrosporum orbiculare* (*Malassezia furfur*).
- The organism is part of the normal skin flora.
- It is possibly contagious and people with oily skin may be more susceptible.
- Excess heat and humidity predispose to infection.

History
- More common during the years of higher sebaceous activity (adolescence and young adulthood).
- Very common especially in tropical and semi-tropical regions.
- Varies in activity for years, diminishes or disappears with advancing age.
- May itch, but is usually asymptomatic.
- Appearance is often the patient's major concern.

Skin Findings
- Numerous small, circular, white, scaling papules on the upper trunk is the common presentation.
- May involve the upper arms, neck, and abdomen.
- Facial involvement more common in the skin of children and black people.
- Powdery scale that may not be obvious on inspection can easily be shown by scraping lightly with the blade of a #15 surgical scalpel.
- Lesions are hypopigmented in tanned skin, and pink or fawn colored in untanned skin.
- Color is uniform in each person but may vary between people.
- Lesions may be inconspicuous in fair-complexioned people during the winter months.
- Wood's light examination shows hypopigmented areas of infection.

Non-skin Findings
- Adrenalectomy, Cushing's disease, pregnancy, malnutrition, burns, corticosteroid therapy, immunosuppression, and oral contraceptives may lower the patient's resistance, allowing this normally non-pathogenic resident yeast to proliferate in the upper layers of the stratum corneum.

Laboratory
- Potassium hydroxide examination of the scale shows numerous hyphae that tend to break into short, rod-shaped fragments intermixed with round spores in grape-like clusters, giving the so-called "spaghetti and meatballs" pattern.

Differential Diagnosis
- Vitiligo macules (depigmented and do not scale)
- Post-inflammatory hypopigmentation following nummular eczema or pityriasis rosea (does not fluoresce or scale)
- Pityriasis rosea, nummular eczema and guttate psoriasis (papules are similar in size and pink in color; potassium hydroxide examination is negative)

Course and Prognosis
- A variety of topical and oral agents eliminate the organism, but relief is usually temporary and recurrences are common (40–60%).
- Dyspigmentation persists for several weeks after the yeast is eliminated.

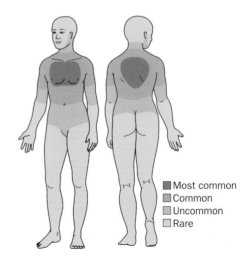

■ Most common
□ Common
□ Uncommon
□ Rare

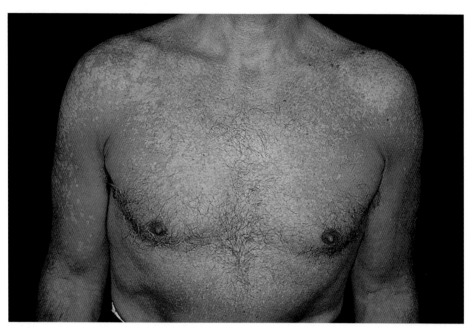

An extensive eruption in a dark-skinned person. Lesion are lighter than normal skin. They become accentuated when uninfected skin tans. Demonstration of the fine scale helps differentiate this from vitiligo.

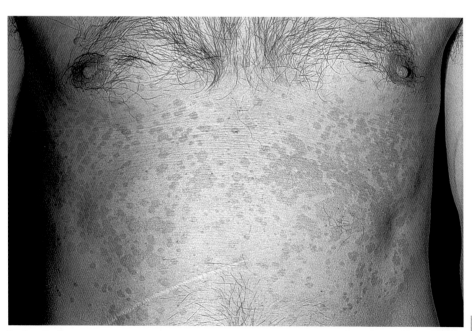

Lesions begin as multiple small circular macules in various colors (white, pink, brown) that enlarge radially. The lesions may be inconspicuous in fair-complexioned individuals during the winter.

- Sun exposure helps to blend in the dyspigmented areas after treatment.

Treatment

- Topical treatment is indicated for limited disease.
- Selenium sulfide lotion 2.5% is applied to the entire skin surface from the lower posterior scalp area down to the thighs and washed off in 10 minutes. This can be repeated every day for 7 consecutive days.
- Ketoconazole 2% shampoo is applied to dampened skin, lathered and left on for 5 minutes, and then rinsed. This has a clinical response rate of about 70% when used as a single application or daily for 3 days.
- Zinc pyrithione soap (ZNP bar) is applied in the shower, lathered and left on for 5 minutes, then rinsed off. This is a low-cost, convenient treatment.
- Miconazole, clotrimazole, econazole, ketoconazole applied to the entire affected area at bedtime for 2–4 weeks is effective, odorless and non-greasy, but expensive.
- Oral treatment is used in patients with extensive disease and those who do not respond to topical treatment or have frequent recurrences.
- Cure rates may be greater than 90%.

- Sweating may improve transfer of ketoconazole and fluconazole to the skin surface and the patient should not bathe for at least 12 hours after treatment. Refraining from bathing allows the medication to accumulate in the skin.
- Itraconazole 200 mg twice daily on one day, or 200 mg every day for 5 days, taken with food to enhance absorption.
- Ketoconazole 400 mg in a single dose or 200 mg every day for 5 days, taken at breakfast with a fruit juice.
- Fluconazole 150 mg (two capsules per week for 4 weeks) or (two capsules as an initial dose to be repeated after 2 weeks).
- Oral Lamisil is not effective in this condition.
- Patients without obvious involvement who have a history of multiple recurrences might consider repeating a treatment program just before the summer months.

Pearls

- The diagnosis of tinea versicolor is often made in any patient presenting with white spots on the trunk.
- A potassium hydroxide examination can quickly establish the correct diagnosis.

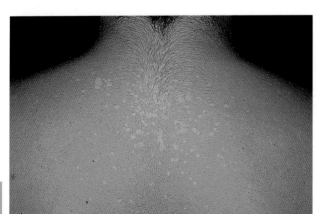

Tinea versicolor varies in extent. Some patients have a few lesions that may resemble vitiligo, pityriasis alba or ringworm (tinea corporis). This patient had no involvement of the chest and was not aware of the infection.

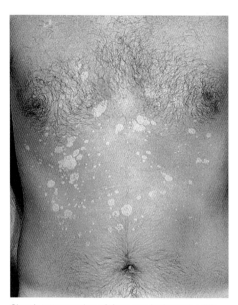

Classic presentation of tinea versicolor with white, oval or circular patches on tan skin.

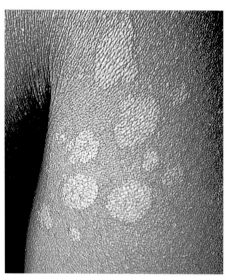

Lesions may be hyperpigmented or hypopigmented in African–American people. The color is uniform in each individual. The lesions may be inconspicuous in fair-complexioned people during the winter.

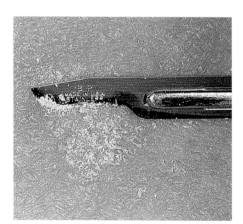

A powdery scale that may not be obvious on inspection can easily be demonstrated by scraping lightly with a #15 surgical blade.

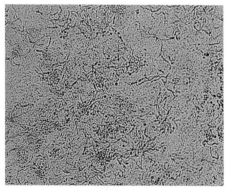

Tinea versicolor. A potassium hydroxide wet mount. A low-power view showing numerous, short, broad hyphae and clusters of budding cells, which have been described as having the appearance of "spaghetti and meatballs."

Pityrosporum (Malassezia) Folliculitis

Description
■ An infection of the hair follicle caused by the yeast *Pityrosporum orbiculare*, also known as *Malassezia furfur*, the same organism that causes tinea versicolor.
■ A discrete, sometimes itchy, papulopustular eruption, which is localized mainly to the upper portion of the trunk and shoulders.

History
■ Occurs in young and middle-aged adults.
■ Occurs in a male to female ratio of 1 to 3.
■ Follicular occlusion may be a primary event, with yeast overgrowth as a secondary occurrence.
■ Diabetes mellitus and administration of broad-spectrum antibiotics or corticosteroids are predisposing factors.
■ Can occur as a localized eruption on the forehead, appearing as treatment-resistant acne.

Skin Findings
■ Asymptomatic or slightly itchy dome-shaped follicular papules and pustules, 2–4 mm in diameter.
■ Occurs on the upper back, chest, and upper arms.
■ More common in the tropics, where it presents with follicular papules, pustules, nodules, and cysts.
■ It has been suggested that "pomade acne" on the forehead represents *Pityrosporum* folliculitis rather than true acne.

Laboratory
■ Potassium hydroxide examination confirms abundant round spores and, less commonly, short hyphae.
■ Skin biopsy is rarely needed, but it demonstrates abundant spores and occasionally hyphae in a dilated follicle. Methenamine silver is used to stain the hyphae.
■ Fungal culture is possible with special media but is rarely performed.

Differential Diagnosis
■ Acne (especially treatment-resistant acne and pustular acne limited to the forehead)
■ Lack of comedones differentiates *Pityrosporum* folliculitis from acne
■ Bacterial folliculitis including *Staphylococcus* and *Pseudomonas* species

Course and Prognosis
■ Discontinuing oral antibacterial antibiotics increases the rate of success with topical and oral anti-yeast agents.
■ Facial involvement is more persistent, is more likely to recur, and requires persistent suppression with topical anti-yeast medications.

Discussion
■ Patients may have associated tinea versicolor, seborrheic dermatitis or acne.
■ Their active sebaceous glands presumably provide the lipid-rich environment required by the yeast.
■ Occlusion and greasy skin may be important predisposing factors.

Treatment
■ Selenium sulfide shampoo (Selsun) is applied and showered off 30 minutes later; this is repeated each day for 3 days to clear and then once each week for maintenance.

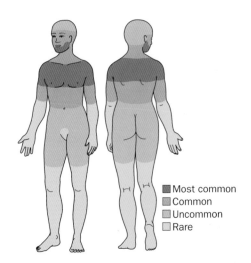

■ Most common
■ Common
□ Uncommon
□ Rare

- Zinc pyrithione soap (ZNP bar) in the shower is also effective.
- Topical antifungal agents, such as e.g. Loprox (ciclopirox) gel or cream, or Spectazole (econazole) cream, applied at bedtime each night for 1 week and then once a week for several weeks or months.
- A combination of oral and topical therapy is the most effective treatment. Combined ketoconazole shampoo and systemic ketoconazole (200 mg daily for 4 weeks) is reported to be 100% effective.
- Oral therapy with itraconazole (Sporanox) 200 mg for 5 days is also effective.

- Response to treatment is shown by relief of the itching in the first week of treatment, but the papules remain for up to 3–4 weeks.
- Recurrence is seen in most cases if topical treatment is not maintained intermittently.

Pearls

- Patients who appear to have acne may instead have *Pityrosporum* folliculitis.
- *Pityrosporum folliculitis* should be considered in young and middle-aged adults with itching and follicular lesions located on the trunk.

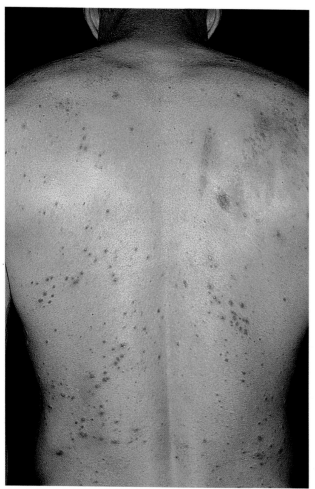

Pityrosporum folliculitis. This infection is seen in young people and presents with papulopustules similar to those found in acne except that there are no comedones or cysts. Lesions occur on the back, chest, upper arms and face. A KOH examination shows aggregates of spores.

Tinea of the Nails (Onychomycosis)

Description

- Tinea of the nails is a fungal infection of the nail plate of the finger or toe caused by many different species of fungus.
- Once established, it tends to become chronic and asymptomatic.

History

- Prevalence increases with age.
- It affects 15-20% of the population aged 40-60 years.
- Life-long infection, with no spontaneous remission.
- Trauma, especially from tight-fitting shoes, predisposes to infection.
- A large mass composed of thick nail plate and underlying debris may cause discomfort with footwear.

Skin Findings

- There are four distinct clinical patterns of infection.
- These patterns are not exclusive and may occur simultaneously in the same or in adjacent nail plates.
- Nail infection may occur simultaneously with hand or foot tinea or may occur as an isolated phenomenon.

Distal Subungual Onychomycosis

- This is the most common pattern.
- Fungi invade the distal area of the nail bed.
- The distal plate turns yellow or white as an accumulation of hyperkeratotic debris causes the nail to rise and separate from the underlying bed.

White Superficial Onychomycosis

- Caused by surface invasion of the nail plate, most often by *Trichophyton mentagrophytes*.
- The nail surface is soft, dry and powdery, and can easily be scraped away.
- The nail plate is not thickened and remains adherent to the nail bed.

Proximal Subungual Onychomycosis

- Microorganisms enter the posterior cuticle are of the nail fold and invade the nail plate from below.
- The surface of the nail plate remains intact.
- Hyperkeratotic debris causes the nail to separate.
- *Trichophyton rubrum* is the most common cause.
- This is the most common pattern seen in patients with human immunodeficiency virus infection.

Candida Onychomycosis

- Nail plate infection caused by *Candida albicans* is seen almost exclusively in chronic mucocutaneous candidiasis—a rare disease.
- It generally involves all of the fingernails.
- The nail plate thickens and turns yellow to brown.

Diagnosis

- Examine all nails and the skin to rule out other diseases that mimic onychomycosis.
- The diagnosis of fungal nail infection should be established with a potassium hydroxide examination.
- The diagnosis should be confirmed with either fungal culture (preferable) or nail plate clippings submitted for histology stained with either Grocott's methenamine silver or periodic acid–Schiff reaction.

Laboratory

- Potassium hydroxide examination of subungual debris and nail plate will confirm presence of hyphae.
- Fungal culture will confirm the species of fungus and establish the presence of dermatophytes (organisms susceptible to itraconazole, terbinafine, and fluconazole).
- There are no clear guidelines for laboratory monitoring of patients being treated with terbinafine, itraconazole or fluconazole.
- A prudent approach would be to order a complete blood count and liver function

tests before treatment and 6 weeks into treatment.

Differential Diagnosis

- Psoriasis (most commonly; the two diseases may coexist)
- Psoriatic nail disease (may present as an isolated phenomenon without other cutaneous signs)
- Pitting of the nail plate surface (distinctive sign of psoriasis, not fungal infection)
- Leukonychia (trauma-induced white spots or bands that appear proximally and migrate distally with growth)
- Eczema, or habitual picking of the proximal nail fold induces the nail plate to be wavy and ridged
- Thick nails (50% are not infected with fungus)
- Onycholysis (very common in women with long fingernails, caused by separation of the nail plate from the nail bed)

Course and Prognosis

- Indications for treatment include pain with thick nails, functional limitations, secondary bacterial infection, diabetes, and cosmesis.

- Oral therapy has the highest success rate with nail infections.
- Systemic therapy is 50% effective to more than 80% effective with a relapse rate of approximately 15–20% in 1 year.

Discussion

- Dermatophytes *Trichophyton rubrum* and *Trichophyton mentagrophytes* are responsible for most infections of fingernails and toenails.
- *Aspergillus, Cephalosporium, Fusarium* and *Scopulariopsis* are considered to be contaminants or non-pathogens, but are also capable of infecting the nail plate.
- Multiple pathogens may be present in a single nail.

Treatment

- Topical antifungal treatments are less effective than systemic agents. Antifungal solutions and lacquers (Penlac) are more effective than creams.

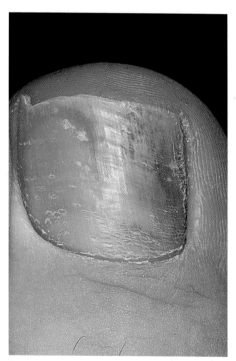

Distal subungual onychomycosis. Yellow to brown color extends down one side of the nail.

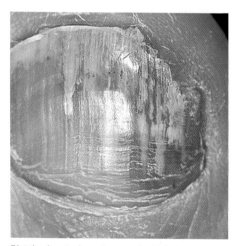

Distal subungual onychomycosis. Various patterns are produced as the fungi grow proximally. Yellow longitudinal channels are highly characteristic of tinea.

- Topical therapy is best reserved for single nail involvement and for patients who are reluctant to treat systemically.
- Prolonged use of a topical antifungal agent, after clinical response of onychomycosis to an oral agent, may prevent nail re-infection.
- Lamisil 250 mg daily on fingernails for 6 weeks, toenails for 12 weeks. Lamisil may provide the highest cure rates and longest remission. It is not effective for some *Candida* species.
- Sporanox 200 mg every day on fingernails for 6 weeks, toenails for 12 weeks, or pulse-dosing 200 mg twice daily for 1 week on and 3 weeks off (fingernails two or three pulses; toenails three or four pulses).
- Fluconazole 300 mg once a week for 6–9 months or until the nail is normal.
- Griseofulvin may be effective at very high doses used for many months but the above drugs are clearly superior.

- Know the potential interactions between oral antifungal agents and medications the patient may be taking.
- Patient follow-up visit at 6 weeks and at the end of oral therapy.
- Nail debridement should be performed at each office visit.
- A nail clipper with "pliers" handles may be used to remove substantial amounts of hard, thick debris.
- Insert the pointed tip of the instrument as far down as is comfortably possible between the diseased nail and the nail bed.
- Removing infected nail plate provides higher cure rates and longer remissions.

Pearls
- Nails in most cases will not appear clear at 12 weeks and the patient needs to know that the drug remains in the nail plate for months and will continue to kill fungus.

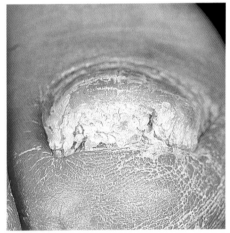

Distal subungual onychomycosis. A large mass composed of thick nail plate and underlying debris may cause discomfort with footwear.

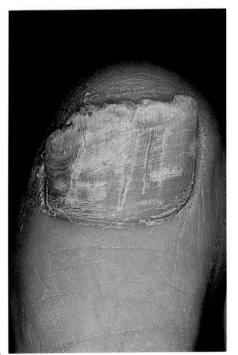

Distal subungual onychomycosis. Infection involves the entire distal plate. Hyphae have invaded the full thickness of the nail and have caused it to crumble.

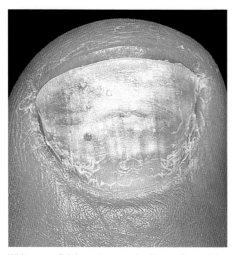

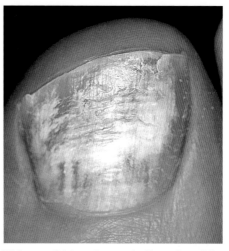

White superficial onychomycosis. The surface of the nail is soft, dry, and powdery and can easily be scraped away. The nail plate is not thickened and remains adherent to the nail bed.

White superficial onychomycosis. The surface of the nail plate has been invaded and is crumbling away.

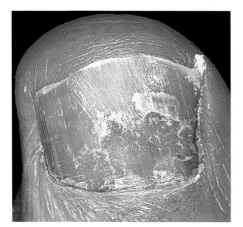

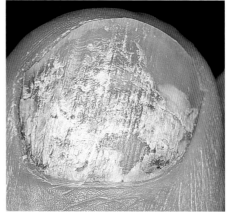

Proximal subungual onychomycosis. Microorganisms enter the cuticle area of the posterior nail fold, migrate to the underlying matrix, and finally invade the nail plate from below.

Proximal subungual onychomycosis. Hyperkeratotic debris accumulates and causes the nail to separate. This is the most common pattern seen in patients with HIV.

Angular Cheilitis (Perlèche)

Description
- Angular cheilitis is a chronic recurring inflammation at the angles of the mouth.
- Saliva macerates and irritates this small intertriginous area leading to eczema, fissuring and secondary bacterial and yeast infections.

History
- More common in the elderly.
- Occurs frequently in patients treated with Accutane.
- May be longstanding; recurrences are common.
- Irritation, pain and itching.
- The presence of saliva at the angles of the mouth is the most important factor.
- Deep perioral rhytides predispose to recurrences.
- Saliva collects at the angles as a result of mouth breathing while sleeping, often as a consequence of nasal congestion.
- Malocclusion of poorly fitting dentures and compulsive lip licking also predispose to recurrence.
- Aggressive use of dental floss may cause mechanical trauma to mouth angles.

Young Patients
- Lip licking, biting the corners of the mouth, or thumb sucking causes perlèche.
- Continued irritation may lead to eczematous inflammation.

Older Patients
- A moist, intertriginous space forms in skinfolds at the angles of the mouth as a result of advancing age and sagging facial contours.
- Sagging also occurs with weight loss, or abnormal vertical shortening of the lower one-third of the face from loss of teeth and resultant resorption of the alveolar bone.
- Capillary action draws saliva from the mouth into the fold, creating maceration, chapping, fissures, erythema, exudation, and secondary infection with *Candida* organisms and/or staphylococci.

Skin Findings
- Papules and pustules surrounding a fissure.
- Edema, erythema with scaling develop with persistent inflammation, may progress onto erosion and then ulceration.

Laboratory
- Culture usually shows mixed bacterial infection and yeast.

Differential Diagnosis
- Allergic contact dermatitis (especially to flavorings in lip balms, toothpastes and mouthwash; more often circumoral in distribution; excluded by patch testing)

Course and Prognosis
- The inflammation starts as a sore fissure in the depth of the skinfold.
- Erythema, moist scale, and crust form at the sides of the fold.
- Patients lick and moisten the area in an attempt to prevent further cracking.
- This attempt at relief aggravates the problem and may lead to eczematous inflammation, staphylococcal infection, or hypertrophy of the skinfold.

Treatment
- Applying anti-yeast creams twice daily (e.g. clotrimazole, miconazole) followed in a few hours by a group V–VI steroid cream or lotion—such as Locoid (hydrocortisone butyrate) cream 0.1% or DesOwen (desonide) lotion 0.05%, or Elidel 1% cream—until the area is dry and free of inflammation.
- Discontinue topical therapies when inflammation has resolved.
- Thereafter, a thick, protective lip balm (Chapstick) or ointment (Aquaphor or plain petrolatum or zinc oxide ointment) is applied prophylactically at bedtime.
- Secondary bacterial infection requires topical antibiotics e.g. Bactroban or systemic antibiotics active against staphylococci.
- Injectable fillers or surgically placed (Gore-Tex) soft-tissue fillers and laser ablation may reduce deep perioral folds which predispose the patient to relapse.

Pearls

■ Avoid mixing topical therapies for convenience of application as this dilutes the concentrations of active ingredients and reduces their effectiveness.

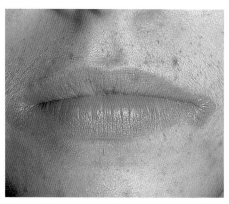

Patients lick and moisten the area in an attempt to prevent cracking. This only aggravates the problem and may lead to eczematous inflammation, staphylococcal infection, or hypertrophy of the skinfold.

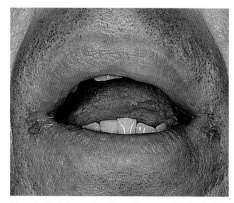

Chronically inflamed surfaces become infected with a mixed flora of yeast and bacteria. Crust and exudate form, and the site becomes painful.

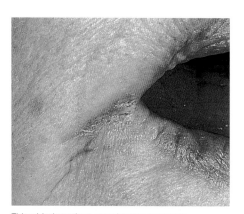

This elderly patient experiences recurrent inflammation from saliva flowing into the deep skinfold at the angle of the mouth.

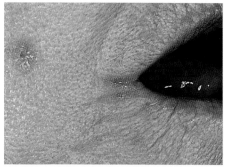

Fissures have formed in the valleys of the skin creases at the mouth angle. These tiny intertriginous surfaces become macerated and inflamed when constantly exposed to saliva.

Cutaneous Fungal Infections

Description
- Dermatophyte fungi are the main cause.
- Tinea is the clinical term for dermatophyte infection.
- Dermatophytes have the ability to infect and survive only on dead keratin; that is, the top layer of the skin (stratum corneum), the hair, and the nails.
- They cannot survive in the mouth or vagina where the keratin layer does not form.
- They are responsible for the vast majority of fungal infections of the skin, nail, and hair.
- Genetic susceptibility may predispose a patient to infection.

Classifications
Biologic
- There are three genera: *Microsporum*, *Trichophyton*, and *Epidermophyton*.
- There are several species of *Microsporum* and *Trichophyton* and one species of *Epidermophyton*.

Origin
- Anthropophilic dermatophytes grow only on human skin, hair, or nails.
- Zoophilic varieties originate from animals, but may infect humans.
- Geophilic dermatophytes live in soil but may infect humans.

Type of Inflammation
- Zoophilic and geophilic dermatophytes elicit a brisk inflammatory response.
- Anthropophilic fungi elicit a mild response.

Type of Hair Invasion
- Some species are able to infect the hair shaft.
- Endothrix pattern fungal hyphae inside the hair shaft.
- Ectothrix pattern fungal hyphae inside and on the surface of the hair shaft.
- Spores of fungi are either large or small.
- The type of hair invasion is further classified into large-spored or small-spored ectothrix, and large-spored endothrix.

Body Region
- Dermatophytes produce a variety of disease patterns that vary with the location.
- It is important to know the general patterns of inflammation in different body regions. These are:
- Tinea of the foot (tinea pedis)
- Tinea of the groin (tinea cruris)
- Tinea of the body (tinea corporis)
- Tinea of the face (tinea faciei)
- Tinea of the hand (tinea manuum)
- Tinea of the scalp (tinea capitis)
- Tinea of the beard (tinea barbae)
- Tinea of the nails (onychomycosis)

Diagnosis
- The greatest number of hyphae are located in the active border.
- This is the best area to get a sample for a potassium hydroxide examination.
- The active border is scaly and red, and slightly elevated.
- Vesicles appear at the active border when inflammation is intense.

Potassium Hydroxide Wet Mount Preparation
- The most important test for diagnosis is direct visualization under the microscope of the branching hyphae in keratinized material.
- Hold a #15 surgical blade perpendicular to the skin surface and smoothly but firmly draw the blade with several short strokes against the scale.
- If an active border is present, the blade is drawn along the border at right angles to the fringe of the scale.
- The scale is placed on a microscope slide, gently separated, and a coverslip is applied.
- Potassium hydroxide (10% or 20% solution) is applied with a toothpick or eye-dropper to the edge of the coverslip and allowed to run under by capillary action.
- The preparation is gently heated under a low flame and then pressed to facilitate separation of the epithelial cells and fungal hyphae.
- Lowering the condenser of the microscope and dimming the light enhances contrast, thus making hyphae easier to identify.

- Nail plate keratin can be softened by leaving the fragments along with several drops of potassium hydroxide in a watch glass covered with a Petri dish for 24 hours.
- A Nail Micronizer can be used to pulverize nails for microscopy and culture.

- Hair specimens require no special preparation and can be examined immediately.

Microscopy
- Scan the entire area under the coverslip at low power (10 ×).

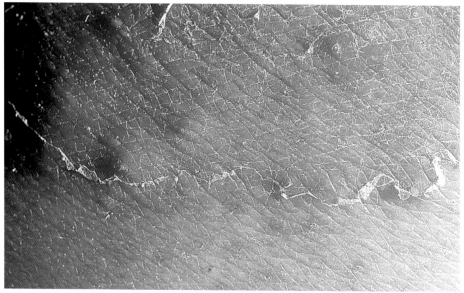

A very characteristic pattern of inflammation is the active border of infection. The highest numbers of hyphae are located in the active border, and this is the best area to get a sample for a potassium hydroxide examination. This pattern is present in all locations except the palms and soles.

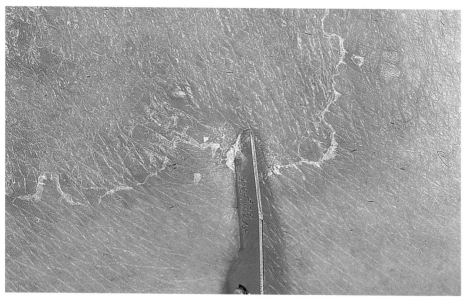

Scale is obtained by holding a #15 surgical blade perpendicular to the skin surface, and smoothly but firmly drawing the blade with several short strokes against the scale.

- The presence of hyphae is confirmed by examination with the 40 × objective.
- Slight back-and-forth rotation of the focusing knob aids visualization of the entire segment of the hyphae.
- Dermatophytes appear as translucent, branching, rod-shaped filaments (hyphae) of uniform width, with lines of separation (septa) spanning the width and appearing at irregular intervals.
- The uniform width and branching distinguish hyphae from hair and other debris.
- A mosaic artifact produced by lipid droplets appearing in a single-file line between cells, especially from specimens taken from the palms and soles may cause confusion.
- Artifact disappears when the cells are separated further by additional heating and pressure.
- Longitudinal, rod-shaped potassium hydroxide crystals that simulate hyphae may appear if the wet mount is heated excessively or too rapidly.
- A drop of Parker's blue ink added to the wet mount will clearly stain hyphae, rendering them visible under low power.

Culture

- It is usually not necessary to know the species of dermatophyte infecting skin in most cases because the same oral and topical agents are active against all of them.
- Fungal culture is necessary for hair and nail fungal infections.
- The sampling technique involves taking a sterile cotton swab moistened with sterile water or on an agar plate and rubbing vigorously over the active part of the lesion, which is then wiped over the surface of the agar.

Culture Media

- Dermatophytes are aerobic and grow on the surface of media.
- Cultures usually become positive in 1–2 weeks.
- Three types of culture media are used for tinea, Mycosel agar, Sabouraud's dextrose agar, and dermatophyte test medium.

Mycosel Agar

- Mycosel agar is Sabouraud's medium that contains cycloheximide and chloramphenicol to prevent the growth of bacteria and saprophytic fungi.
- Mycosel agar is best for evaluation of hair tinea because only dermatophytes cause hair tinea.

Sabouraud's Dextrose Agar

- Sabouraud's agar does not contain antibiotics, and allows the growth of most fungi, including non-dermatophytes.
- It is useful for nail infections because the detection of non-dermatophytes is desirable in nail infections.

Dermatophyte Test Medium

- This culture can be performed in the physician's office as the medium is supplied in vials. This produces fast but slightly less accurate results.
- The yellow medium turns pink in the presence of dermatophytes in 6–7 days, but remains yellow in the presence of non-pathogenic fungi.
- Must be discarded after 2 weeks because saprophytes can induce a similar color change from this time on.
- Species identification is possible but is more accurately determined with Mycosel agar and Sabouraud's dextrose agar.

Culture Media for Yeast

- Initial isolation can occur on Sabouraud's agar.
- Nickerson's media is for isolation and identification of *Candida* species.

Wood's Light Examination

- Hair, but not the skin of the scalp, fluoresces with a blue to green color if infected with *Microsporum canis* or *Microsporum audouinii*.
- No other dermatophytes that infect hair produce fluorescence.
- Fungal infections of the skin do not fluoresce, although tinea versicolor, caused by *Pityrosporum* yeast, produces a pale white to yellow fluorescence.
- Erythrasma, a non-inflammatory, pale brown, scaly eruption of the toe webs,

groin, and axillae caused by the bacteria *Corynebacterium minutissimum* show a brilliant coral red fluorescence with the Wood's light.

■ Wood's light examination should be performed in a dark room with a high-intensity instrument.

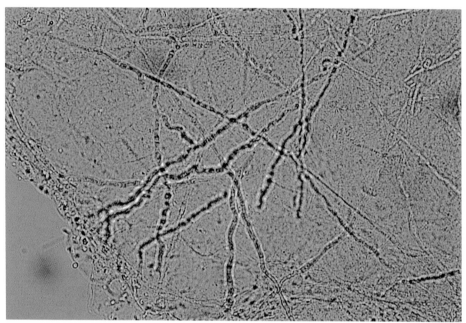

Dermatophytes appear as translucent, branching, rod-shaped filaments (hyphae) of uniform width, with lines of separation (septa) spanning the width and appearing at irregular intervals.

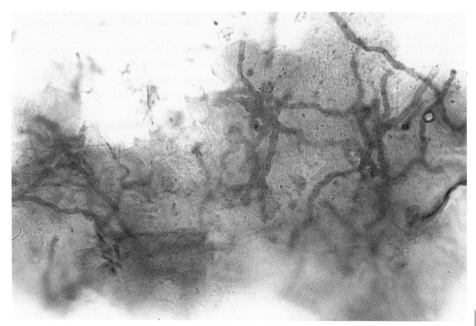

Hyphae may be difficult to find in a potassium hydroxide wet mount. Parker's blue ink and other stains easily stain the hyphae, rendering them visible under low power.

Tinea of the Foot (Tinea Pedis)

Description
- The feet are the most common area infected by dermatophytes.
- There are many different clinical presentations.
- Tinea pedis is also referred to as "athlete's foot."

History
- Common in young and middle-aged adults.
- Uncommon in prepubertal children.
- More common in adult men than in women.
- Probably inevitable in immunologically predisposed individuals regardless of elaborate precautions taken to avoid the infecting organism

Predisposing factors
- Shoes promote warmth and sweating, which encourage fungal growth.
- Locker-room floors contain fungal elements.
- Communal baths may create an ideal condition for repeated exposure to infected material.

Skin Findings
- Tinea of the feet may present with the classic "ringworm" pattern, but most infections are found in the toe webs or on the soles.
- There are three classic clinical presentations: interdigital tinea pedis (toe web infection), chronic scaly infection of the plantar surface, and acute vesicular tinea pedis.

Interdigital Tinea Pedis (Toe Web Infection)
- The web between the fourth and fifth toes is most commonly involved, but all webs may be infected.
- Tight-fitting shoes compress the toes, creating a warm, moist environment.
- The webs become dry, scaly, and fissured or white, macerated, and soggy.
- Itching is most intense when the shoes and socks are removed.
- Overgrowth of bacterial population determines the severity of infection.
- Extension out of the web space onto the plantar surface or the dorsum of the foot is common and occurs with the typical, chronic, ringworm type of scaly, advancing border or with an acute, vesicular eruption.

Chronic Scaly Infection of the Plantar Surface
- Plantar hyperkeratotic or moccasin-type tinea pedis is a chronic form of tinea that is resistant to treatment.
- The entire sole is usually infected and covered with a fine, silvery white scale.
- The skin is pink and tender, and/or pruritic.
- The hands may be similarly infected.
- It is rare to see both palms and soles infected simultaneously; rather, the pattern is infection of two feet and one hand or of two hands and one foot.
- *Trichophyton rubrum* is the usual pathogen.

Acute Vesicular Tinea Pedis
- A highly inflammatory infection may originate from a more chronic web infection.
- Vesicles evolve rapidly on the sole or on the dorsal foot.
- Vesicles may fuse into bullae or remain intact as collections of fluid under the thick scale of the sole.
- Secondary bacterial infection occurs.
- Toenail or fingernail fungal infection (onychomycosis) may accompany tinea pedis.
- "Id reaction": a second wave of vesicles may follow in the same areas or at distant sites such as the arms, chest, and along the sides of the fingers.
- These itchy sterile vesicles represent an allergic response to the fungus and are termed a dermatophytid or id reaction.
- Occasionally, the id reaction is the only clinical manifestation of a fungus infection.
- Examination of these patients may show an asymptomatic fissure or area of maceration in the toe webs.

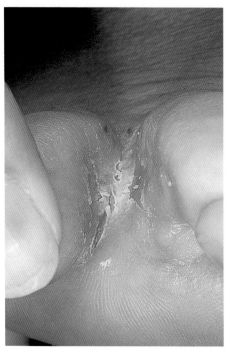

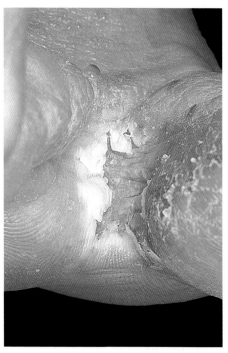

Interdigital tinea pedis (toe web infection). Tight-fitting shoes compress the toes, creating a warm and moist environment in the toe webs; this environment is suited to fungal growth.

Interdigital tinea pedis (toe web infection). The web can become dry, scaly, and fissured or white, macerated, and soggy.

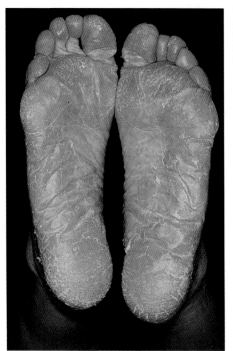

Tinea of the soles often presents with a dry, scaling surface. The entire sole of one or both feet may be involved. It is sometimes difficult to demonstrate hyphae in a potassium hydroxide preparation. The infection is difficult to treat with topical medication.

Laboratory

■ Potassium hydroxide examination to confirm the presence of fungal elements.

■ Interpretation of potassium hydroxide examination is difficult in the macerated skin of the toe webs and in severely inflamed skin.

■ Fungal culture difficult to diagnosis cases.

Differential Diagnosis

■ Localized psoriasis and eczema may be confused with tinea pedis.

■ Tinea should be considered in the differential diagnosis of children with foot dermatitis.

Course and Prognosis

■ Once established, the individual becomes a carrier and is more susceptible to recurrences.

■ Atopic individuals are particularly prone to chronic or recurrent *Trichophyton rubrum* infections.

Treatment

■ Topical medications include butenafine (Mentax, Lotrimin Ultra), terbinafine (Lamisil), sertaconazole (Ertaczo). They are applied twice daily for 2-4 weeks.

■ These agents produce higher cure rates and lower relapse rate than the antifungal-corticosteroid combination (Lotrisone).

■ Econazole nitrate (Spectazole) has activity against several bacterial species associated with severely macerated interdigital interspaces.

■ Acute vesicular tinea pedis responds to Burrow's wet dressings applied for 30 minutes several times each day in combination with topical antifungal creams applied twice daily

■ An oral antifungal agent may be started and topical antifungal agents applied twice daily for acute or extensive infection.

■ Oral therapy with Lamisil 250 mg every day for 2 weeks, or Sporanox Pulse Pack 200 mg twice daily for 1 week, or Diflucan 150 mg once a week for 2 weeks.

■ Secondary bacterial infection is treated with oral antibiotics and culture is recommended.

■ A vesicular "id reaction" sometimes occurs at distant sites during an inflammatory foot infection

■ Cool wet dressings, group V topical steroids and, occasionally, a short course of prednisone are required for control of such id reactions.

■ Recurrence is prevented by wearing wider shoes and expanding the web space with a small strand of lamb's wool (Dr Scholl's Lamb's Wool) or a cotton ball.

■ Powders, not necessarily medicated, absorb moisture (Zeasorb).

■ Powders should be applied to the feet rather than to the shoes.

■ Wet socks should be changed

Pearls

■ The id reaction sometimes seen with successful oral or topical treatment may be confused with a drug rash if an oral antifungal agent is used.

■ In fact, the allergic reaction is to the fungus and treatment to eradicate the infection should be continued.

■ If in doubt, use topical antifungal creams.

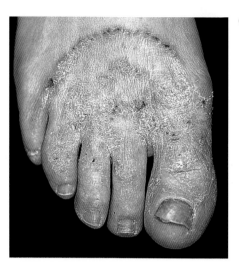

Classic ringworm pattern of fungal infection.

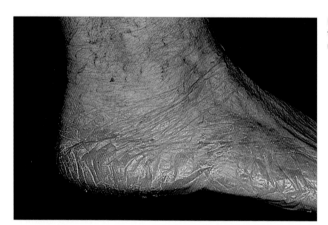

Erythema and scale extend onto the sides of the foot. This pattern resembles eczema.

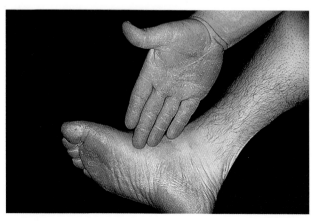

The classic presentation of hand and foot eczema. The typical pattern is to see infection of two hands and one foot or two feet and one hand. Both palms and soles show involvement of the entire surface and resemble dry skin.

247

Tinea of the Groin (Tinea Cruris, Jock Itch)

Description
- A dermatophyte infection of the crural fold is known as tinea cruris or "jock itch".

History
- It occurs almost exclusively in postpubertal males.
- It occurs in the summer after sweating or in the winter after wearing layers of clothing.
- Many patients are unaware of the infection.
- Itching becomes worse as moisture accumulates.

Skin Findings
- Often bilateral, begins in the crural fold.
- Half moon-shaped patch forms as a well-defined scaling, and sometimes a vesicular border advances out of the crural fold onto the thigh.
- It is rare for dermatophyte infections to extend onto the scrotum.
- Skin within the border turns red-brown, is less scaly, and may develop red papules.
- Acute inflammation may appear after wearing occlusive clothing.
- The infection occasionally migrates to the buttocks and gluteal cleft.

Laboratory
- Specimens for potassium hydroxide examination should be taken from the advancing scaling border.
- Culture can be taken if the wet mount is negative.

Differential Diagnosis
- Intertrigo (this is symmetric, involving both the inner thigh and scrotum)
- Inverse psoriasis (may be masked by tinea; tends to be asymptomatic)
- Erythrasma (a *Corynebacterium* infection of the crural folds; lacks a scaling border, but fluoresces red under a Wood's light)

Course and Prognosis
- The infection may improve or resolve if the moist environment is eliminated.

Treatment
- Antifungal creams with activity against *Candida* and dermatophytes (such as Spectazole, Oxistat, Micatin, Lotrimin) applied twice daily for 10–14 days are effective.
- Moist lesions may be treated with a cool wet water or a Burrow's dressing for 20–30 minutes two to six times daily until skin has been dried.
- Resistant infections respond to itraconazole 200 mg every day for 1–2 weeks, or terbinafine 250 mg every day for 2 weeks, or fluconazole 150 mg once a week for 2–4 weeks.
- A pure antifungal cream should be used once symptoms are controlled.
- Prolonged use of a steroid/antifungal cream may not cure the infection and cause striae in this intertriginous area.
- Absorbent powders—not necessarily medicated (Zeasorb)—help to control moisture and prevent re-infection.

Pearls
- Steroid creams are frequently prescribed for inflammatory disease of the groin and can modify the typical clinical presentation of dermatophyte infection (tinea incognito).

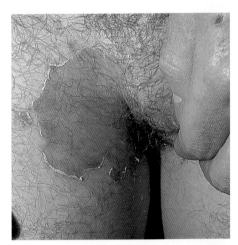

A half-moon-shaped plaque forms as a well-defined scaling, and sometimes a vesicular border advances out of the crural fold onto the thigh. The skin within the border turns red-brown, is less scaly, and may develop red papules.

- Prolonged use of combination steroid/antifungal preparations should be avoided as striae will develop.
- Patients have difficulty discerning between early striae and tinea and may unknowingly continue to worsen striae irreversibly with continued steroid use.

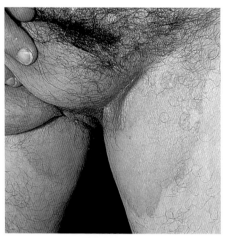

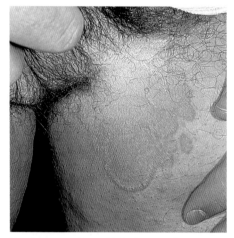

The entire surface of this lesion is dry and scaling. Involvement of the scrotum is unusual, unlike candidal reactions in which it is common.

The ringworm pattern of infection may also appear in the groin.

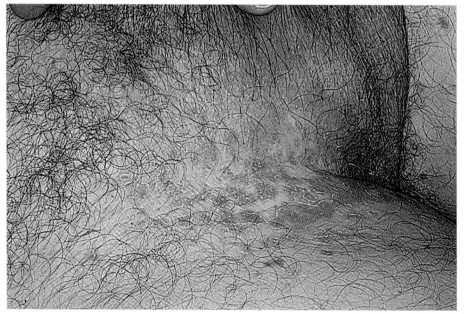

The ringworm pattern of infection with multiple round superficial plaques with scaling borders. Lesions are present on the thighs and scrotum.

Tinea of the Body (Tinea Corporis) and Face (Tinea Faciei)

Description
■ Dermatophyte infection of the body, trunk, and limbs is called tinea corporis.

History
■ More common in warm climates.
■ Epidemics can occur among wrestlers.

Skin Findings
■ Lesions varying in size, degree of inflammation, and depth of involvement.
■ There are two general clinical patterns: round annular lesions (classic ringworm) and deep inflammatory lesions.

Round Annular Lesions (Classic Ringworm)
● Lesions begin as flat, scaly papules which slowly develop a raised border that extends at variable rates in all directions.
● Advancing, scaly border may have red raised papules or vesicles.
● The central area becomes brown or hypopigmented and less scaly as the active border progresses outward.
● Red papules may occur in the central area.
● Several annular lesions may enlarge to cover large areas of the body surface.
● Larger lesions tend to be mildly itchy or asymptomatic.
● They may reach a certain size and remain for years with no tendency to resolve.

Deep Inflammatory Lesions
● Zoophilic fungi from animals such as *Trichophyton verrucosum* from cattle may produce a very inflammatory skin infection.
● The round, intensely inflamed lesion has a uniformly elevated, red, boggy, pustular surface.
● The pustules are follicular and represent deep penetration of the fungus into the hair follicle.
● Secondary bacterial infection can occur, usually with *Staphylococcus*.

● The process ends with brown hyperpigmentation and scarring.
● Majocchi's granuloma is a deep fungal infection of the hair follicle, typically occurring on the lower legs, more often in women; shaving and superficial trauma are felt to play a role.

Laboratory
■ Potassium hydroxide examinations usually show abundant hyphae.
■ Bacterial and fungal culture of deep inflammatory lesions helps confirm the diagnosis and genus and species of the fungus.

Differential Diagnosis
■ Nummular eczema and psoriasis are best ruled out by a positive potassium hydroxide examination; neither has an advancing border.
■ Pityriasis rosea has a collarette of scale which does not reach the edge of the red border as it does in tinea.

Course and Prognosis
■ With treatment, the scaling resolves before the erythema fades.
■ Post-inflammatory dyspigmentation blends away over several months.
■ Re-infection is common, especially among wrestlers and other athletes where direct

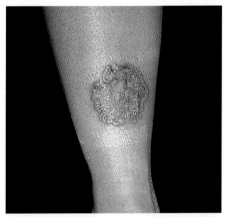

Inflammatory lesions. In classic ringworm, lesions begin as flat scaly spots that develop a raised border which extends out at variable rates in all directions. The advancing scaly border may have red raised papules or vesicles.

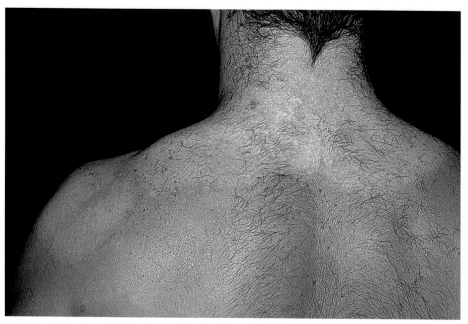

Round annular lesions. Larger lesions tend to be mildly itchy or asymptomatic. They may reach a certain size and remain for years with no tendency to resolve.

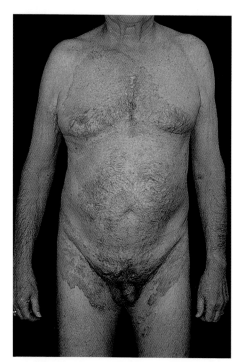

Tinea may be asymptomatic or itchy. Infection can be subtle and present for years. Very large areas may be infected.

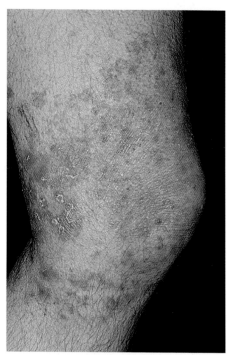

Tinea incognito. A diagnosis of psoriasis was incorrectly made months ago. Repeated treatment with the group I topical steroid clobetasol caused this widespread infection.

251

skin contact occurs, where it may lead to disqualification from competition.

Treatment

- Superficial lesions respond to antifungal creams (clotrimazole, miconazole, econazole, butenafine or terbinafine) applied twice each day for a minimum of two weeks.
- Continue treatment for at least 1 week after resolution of the infection.
- Extensive lesions or those with red papules require oral therapy.
- Griseofulvin (ultramicrosize) 333 mg every day or 250 mg every day or twice daily are all acceptable options for an adult; 5–7 mg/kg/day for 2–6 weeks or Sporanox 200 mg every day for 2 weeks, or Lamisil 250 mg every day for 2 weeks or Diflucan 150 mg once a week for 3–4 weeks are all acceptable options for a child.
- Secondary bacterial infection is treated with oral antibiotics.
- A short course of prednisone may be considered for highly inflamed lesions to minimize scarring.

Pearls

- It may be necessary to treat wrestlers throughout the season to prevent re-infection in an epidemic of tinea corporis.

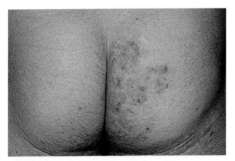

Plaques covering a wide area appear to be eczema. The papules and pustules represent invasion of infection deep into the hair follicles. Topical antifungal medications may not penetrate deep enough to be effective.

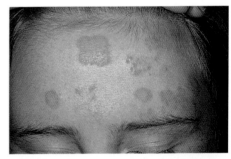

Tinea can occur on the face and look like eczema, psoriasis or seborrheic dermatitis. Application of topical steroids will result in a widespread bizarre pattern of infection.

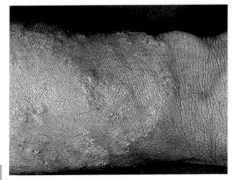

Round annular lesions. The border and central area are papular and vesicular.

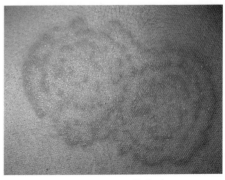

The classic ringworm pattern of infection.

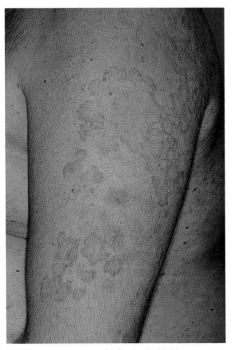

The ringworm pattern of infection is highly characteristic.

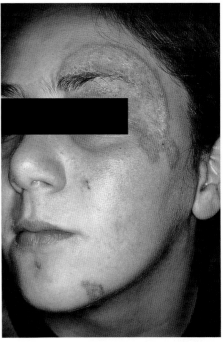

Ringworm of the face is not common. It is often misdiagnosed as eczema or seborrheic dermatitis. Look for the sharp scaling border.

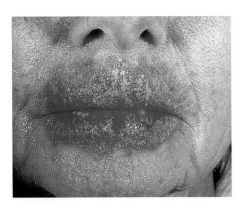

Tinea incognito. Fungal infections treated with topical steroids often lose some of their characteristic features. Diffuse erythema, diffuse scale, scattered pustules or papules, and brown hyperpigmentation may all result.

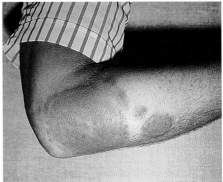

This large plaque was diagnosed as psoriasis. However, it lacks the silvery surface scale seen in psoriatic plaques. The scaling border is the diagnostic feature.

Tinea of the Hand (Tinea Manuum)

History
- Tinea manuum is a fungal infection of the hand.
- Children are rarely affected.
- May be insidious and progresses slowly over a period of weeks, months or years.
- Itching is moderate, minimal or absent.

Skin Findings
- Tinea involving the dorsal hand has all of the features of classic ringworm lesions of the body.
- A raised, red, scaly advancing border is typical.
- Papules or vesicles may be present at the border or in the central area.
- Tinea involving the palm has the same appearance as the dry, diffuse, keratotic form of tinea on the soles.
- Frequently seen in association with tinea pedis.
- The usual pattern of infection is involvement of one hand and two feet or of two hands and one foot.
- Hyperkeratotic tinea of the palms may be asymptomatic and the patient may be unaware of the infection, attributing the dry, thick, scaly surface to hard physical labor.
- The diagnosis is subtle and easily missed.
- Fingernail fungal infection (onychomycosis) may accompany tinea manuum.

Laboratory
- Diagnosis is established by performing a microscopic examination of skin scrapings with a potassium hydroxide wet mount.
- Fungal cultures are required if the diagnosis cannot be confirmed by the wet mount.

Differential Diagnosis
- Tinea of the hands may look like eczema or psoriasis, especially if the border is not distinct.
- If there is any doubt, obtain skin scrapings and prepare a potassium hydroxide wet mount.

Course and Prognosis
- Annular lesions on the back of the hand respond to treatment sooner than the palms and tend not to recur.
- Hyperkeratotic scaling palms respond more slowly to treatment and may recur.
- The thickened palms may be severely dry and develop cracks and fissures.

Treatment
- Topical antifungal creams ketoconazole 2% cream (Nizoral), clotrimazole 1% cream or lotion (Lotrimin, Mycelex), econazole 1% cream or lotion (Spectazole), miconazole 2% cream (Monistat), terbinafine (Lamisil), butenafine hydrochloride (Mentax Cream 1%, Lotrimin Ultra) may be effective, but oral medication is more reliable.
- Adults are treated with ultramicrosized griseofulvin 250 mg or 330 mg every day, or twice daily for 3-6 weeks.
- Alternate therapies include Sporanox 200 or 400 mg daily for 1-2 weeks or Lamisil 250 mg every day for 2 weeks or 4 weeks

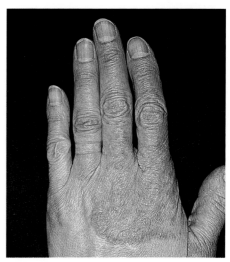

Tinea of the dorsal aspect of the hand (tinea manuum) has all of the features of tinea corporis. The nails are also frequently infected.

or Diflucan 150 mg once weekly for 2 or 4 weeks.
- Treatment of nail infections requires a longer course of treatment.

Pearls

- Reevaluate patients with palm infections in 6 months as there is a significant recurrence rate.

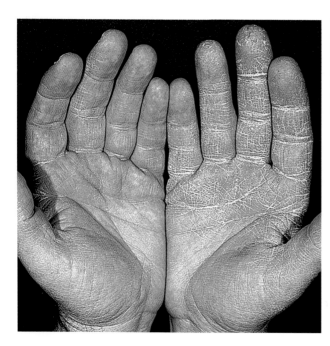

Tinea of the palms has the same appearance as the dry, diffuse, keratotic form of tinea on the soles. It may be asymptomatic, and the patient may be unaware of the infection, attributing the dry, thick, scaly surface to hard physical labor.

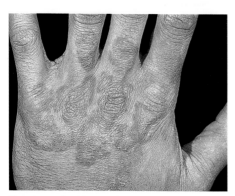

Tinea incognito. Fungal infections treated with topical steroids often lose some of their characteristic features. Multiple rings have appeared.

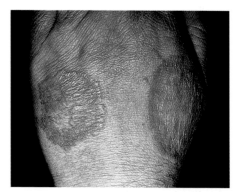

Ringworm pattern of infection. Lesions had been present for months. They responded to topical antifungal creams.

Tinea Incognito

Description

■ Tinea incognito is a localized cutaneous fungal infection, the appearance of which has been altered by application of topical corticosteroids.

History

■ Cortisone creams applied to cutaneous fungal infections decrease inflammation, alter the usual clinical presentation, and produce unusual atypical eruptions.
■ This altered clinical picture is called tinea incognito.
■ The intensity of itching is variable.

Skin Findings

■ The groin, face, and dorsal aspect of the hand are most commonly involved.
■ Tinea infections of the hands are often misdiagnosed as hand eczema and treated with topical steroids.
■ Appearance changes depending on the stage of the treatment cycle.
■ Treatment with topical steroids.
  ● Topical steroids decrease inflammation and give the false impression that the rash is improving early in the course.
  ● The fungus flourishes secondary to cortisone-induced local immunosuppression.
■ Treatment is stopped.
  ● The rash returns when treatment is stopped, but it has changed in appearance.
  ● Scaling at the margins may be absent.
  ● Diffuse erythema, diffuse scale, scattered pustules or papules, and brown hyperpigmentation may all result.
  ● A well-defined border may not be present and a once-localized process may have expanded greatly.
■ The cycle continues.
  ● Memory of the good initial response prompts re-use of the steroid cream and the repetitive cycle continues.
  ● The dermatophyte infection extends creating a clinical pattern which may simulate another dermatologic condition becoming entirely unrecognizable as a dermatophyte infection.

Laboratory

■ Potassium hydroxide examination reveals numerous hyphae, especially a few days after discontinuing use of the steroid cream when scaling reappears.
■ Fungal culture is usually not necessary because the potassium hydroxide examination preparation is almost always positive.

Differential Diagnosis

■ Eczema
■ Folliculitis
■ Rosacea
■ Pityriasis rosea
■ Psoriasis

Treatment

■ It is important to discontinue the topical steroid.
■ Superficial lesions respond to antifungal creams (e.g. clotrimazole, miconazole, econazole, oxiconazole, terbinafine) applied twice each day.

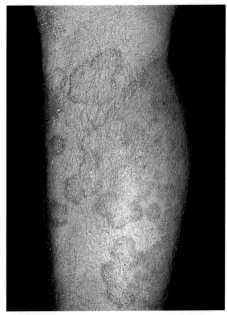

Tinea incognito. Fungal infections treated with topical steroids can lose some of their characteristic features. Here, a once localized process has expanded greatly.

- Continue treatment for at least 1 week after resolution of the infection.
- Extensive lesions, those with red papules or pustules, require oral therapy with one of several possible agents:
  - Lamisil 250 mg every day for 2 weeks
  - Sporanox 200 mg every day for 2 weeks
  - Diflucan 100 mg every day for 2 weeks
  - Griseofulvin (ultramicrosize) 333 mg four times daily or twice daily or 250 mg every day or twice daily for an adult; 5-7 mg/kg/day for 2-6 weeks for a child

- Secondary bacterial infection is treated with oral antibiotics.
- Cool-water wet dressings suppress inflammation and control itching.

Pearls

- If tinea is in your differential diagnosis for a rash, you should perform a potassium hydroxide examination.
- If the rash you are treating with topical steroids is not clearing as expected, perform a potassium hydroxide examination.

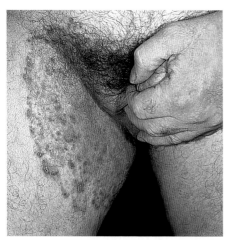

Tinea incognito. Topical steroid creams modify the typical clinical presentation of tinea. Red papules sometimes appear at the edges and center of the lesions. This modified form may not be immediately recognized as tinea.

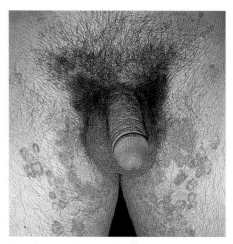

Tinea incognito. The eruption may be much more extensive, and the advancing scaly border may not be present.

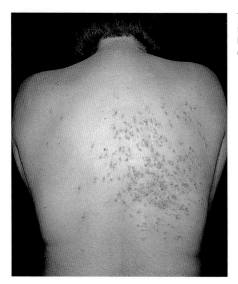

Tinea incognito. Diffuse erythema, diffuse scaling, scattered pustules or papules, and brown hyperpigmentation may all result. All of the characteristic features of tinea have been lost.

Tinea of the Scalp (Tinea Capitis)

Description
■ Tinea of the scalp is caused by the invasion of the stratum corneum and the hair shaft with fungal hyphae.

History
■ More than 90% of tinea capitis in the United States is caused by *Trichophyton tonsurans*.
■ Tinea capitis occurs most frequently in children.
■ It is seen in crowded inner cities, especially in Black or Hispanic people.
■ It is acquired by close contact with an infected person, often in the same household.
■ Spores are shed in the air, and remain viable for long periods on combs, brushes, blankets, and telephones.
■ Zoophilic *Microsporum canis* infection is acquired from infected household pets (particularly cats).

Skin Findings
■ *Trichophyton tonsurans* has four different clinical infection patterns.

Seborrheic Dermatitis Type
■ This is the most common type.
■ It resembles seborrheic dermatitis.
■ There is diffuse or patchy, fine, white, adherent scale on the scalp.
■ Adenopathy is often present.
■ Potassium hydroxide examination is often negative; culture is necessary to make diagnosis.

Inflammatory Tinea Capitis (Kerion)
■ One or more inflamed boggy, tender areas of alopecia with pustules.
■ Scarring alopecia may occur.
■ Fever, occipital adenopathy, and leukocytosis may occur.
■ Potassium hydroxide wet mounts and fungal cultures are often negative.
■ Treatment may have to be initiated based on clinical appearance.

"Black Dot" Pattern
■ This is uncommon.
■ Large areas of alopecia are present without inflammation.
■ There is a mild to moderate amount of scalp scale.
■ Occipital adenopathy may be present.
■ Arthrospores weaken the hair and cause it to break off at the scalp surface, resulting in a "black dot" appearance.

Pustular Type
■ There are pustules or scabbed areas without scaling or significant hair loss.
■ Cultures and potassium hydroxide wet mounts may be negative.

Laboratory
■ The brush culture method involves gently rubbing a previously sterilized toothbrush in a circular motion over areas where scale is present or over the margins of patches of alopecia. The brush fibers are then pressed into the culture media and the brush is discarded.
■ Cotton culturette is an effective method to culture in children.

Differential Diagnosis
■ Tinea amiantacea, a form of seborrheic dermatitis that occurs in children, is frequently misdiagnosed as tinea capitis. This is a localized non-inflammatory 2–8-cm patch of large brown polygon-shaped scales that adheres to the scalp and mats the hair.
■ Scalp psoriasis and other forms of seborrheic dermatitis may be confused with tinea capitis and neither excludes the possibility of tinea capitis.

Course and Prognosis
■ Close living quarters increase the risk of infecting household contacts.
■ Successful intervention requires that all household members be evaluated and treated accordingly.
■ Risk of reinfection is minimized by scrupulous cleaning of all possibly contaminated objects.
■ Combs, towels and bedding should be cleaned regularly and not shared.

Treatment

- Management requires both oral and topical approach.
- Griseofulvin is usually the drug of first choice, but many children cannot tolerate the high doses, and others do not respond.
- Griseofulvin 20–25 mg/kg/day of the microsize liquid formulation, or 15–20 mg/kg/day of the ultramicrosized capsule, administered once as a single dose or divided into two doses daily and taken for a minimum of 6–8 weeks.
- Griseofulvin is absorbed more efficiently with a fatty meal; children can be given the medicine with ice cream or whole milk.

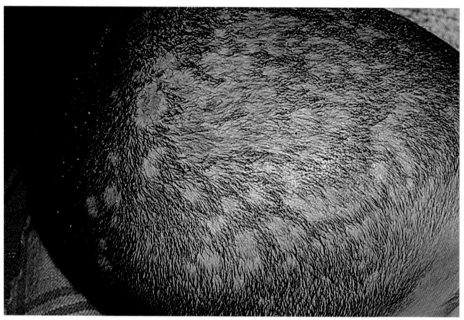

Tinea of the scalp with many round areas of scale and alopecia. Wood's light examination showed green hairs. *Microsporum canis* from a pet cat grew in the culture.

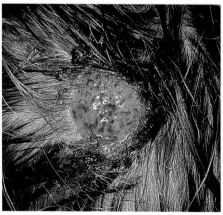

Inflammatory tinea capitis (kerion). There is an inflamed, boggy, tender area of alopecia with pustules. Occipital adenopathy was present.

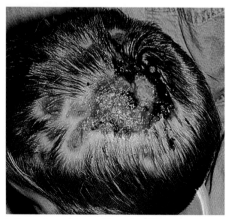

Inflammatory tinea capitis caused by *trichophyton tonsurans*. Permanent hair loss occurred after this destructive infection.

- Treat 2 weeks beyond the time that cultures and potassium hydroxide preparations become negative, generally after 6–12 weeks.
- Terbinafine 3–6 mg/kg/day for 4–8 weeks may be the most cost-effective treatment.
- There is no liquid formulation.
- Itraconazole 25–100 mg/day (2.5–5 mg/kg/day) taken with food for 4–8 weeks.
- Sprinkle the contents of a capsule into food for children who cannot swallow capsules.
- Fluconazole 6–8 mg/kg/d for 4–8 weeks.
- Fluconazole is available in a pediatric liquid formulation.
- A single dose of 150 mg once weekly for 4 weeks may also be effective for older children.
- Suppressing the inflammation of a kerion may be accomplished with topical, oral, or intralesional steroids.
- Prednisone 1–2 mg/kg/day may hasten resolution and reduces or prevents scarring.
- Topical treatment with shampoos reduces the risk of shedding of spores and is believed to be protective of other household contacts.
- Shampoo with selenium sulfide 1% (Selsun Blue; Head & Shoulders Intensive Care) or ketoconazole (Nizoral) every other day for the first 2 weeks, then twice weekly throughout the rest of the course of oral therapy.
- Shampoo should be applied, left on for 5 minutes, and then rinsed off.
- Other family members should also use the shampoo two to three times a week.

Daily Dosage of Terbinafine	
Body Weight	**Daily dose**
Less than 20 kg (44 lb)	62.5 mg (one quarter of a tablet)
20–40 kg (44–88 lb)	125 mg (one half of a tablet)
More than 40 kg (88 lb)	250 mg (one whole tablet)

Dosage of Itraconazole	
Body Weight	**Dosage**
10–18 kg (22–40 lb)	100 mg every other day
18–27 kg (40–60 lb)	100 mg daily
27–41 kg (60–90 lb)	100 mg daily or 100 mg and 200 mg on alternate days
41–50 kg (90–110 lb)	100 mg and 200 mg on alternate days
More than 50 kg (110 lb)	200 mg daily

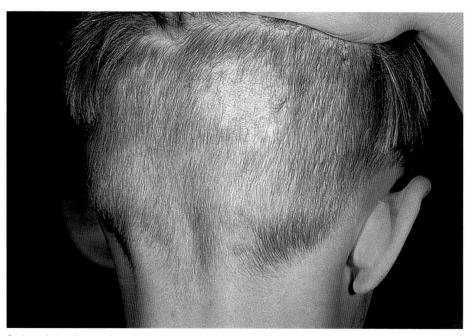

Scale and pustules may be seen. A once chronic infection can become inflammatory.

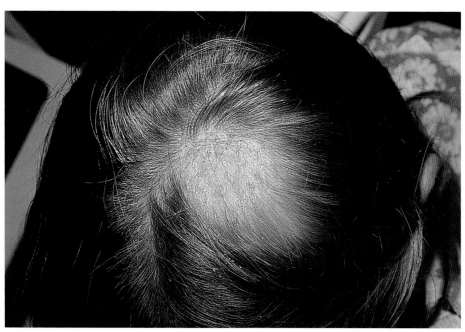

Non-inflammatory lesions tend to be chronic and last for months. Hairs break off at or below the scalp surface, resulting in a "black dot" appearance of the scalp surface.

Tinea of the Beard (Tinea Barbae)

Description
- Tinea barbae is an uncommon, often misdiagnosed dermatophyte infection of the skin and hair in the beard area.

History
- Tinea is a slowly evolving disease in contrast to bacterial infections.
- Infection of the skin causes some itching while infection of the follicle causes pain and swelling.
- Outside of rural farming areas, it is most common among wrestlers.

Skin Findings
- There are two clinical patterns, the ringworm pattern and the follicular pattern.

Ringworm Pattern
- Superficial infection resembles the annular plaques of tinea corporis with a sharply defined scaling border.
- The hair follicles within the plaque are also usually infected, with adherent crusting, or may appear to be broken off.
- *Trichophyton rubrum* and *Trichophyton violaceum* are the most common causes although *Trichophyton rubrum* does not actually infect the hairs.

Follicular Pattern
- Deep follicular infection resembles bacterial folliculitis.
- Pustules and draining nodules may lead to kerion formation and permanent scarring.
- *Trichophyton mentagrophytes* and *Trichophyton verrucosum* are the most common organisms.

Non-skin Findings
- Regional lymphadenopathy occurs when there is secondary bacterial infection.

Laboratory
- Potassium hydroxide examination of skin and plucked hairs.

- Hairs are loosened and easily removed from follicles infected with fungi; it is more difficult to extract hairs from follicles infected with bacteria.
- Fungal cultures are required if the diagnosis is suspected but cannot be confirmed by potassium hydroxide examination.
- A skin biopsy is occasionally required to establish the diagnosis.

Differential Diagnosis
- Bacterial folliculitis (especially staphylococcal) tends to spread quickly and involve the entire beard area
- Furunculosis (a deeper infection can resemble a kerion)
- Actinomycosis (an uncommon deep bacterial infection, usually mandibular from a dental source; can mimic a kerion)

Course and Prognosis
- Dermatophyte (tinea) infections are slow to evolve and are usually limited to one area of the beard.
- The infection begins insidiously with a small group of follicular pustules.
- The process becomes confluent in time with the development of a boggy, erythematous, tumor-like abscess covered with dense, superficial crust similar to fungal kerions seen in tinea capitis.
- Scarring may occur in advanced cases.

Treatment
- Topical antifungal agents are not reliably effective because they do not penetrate deep enough into the hair follicle.
- Adult men are treated with Lamisil (terbinafine) 250 mg every day for 2–4 weeks, or Sporanox (itraconazole) 200 mg every day for 2–4 weeks, or Diflucan (fluconazole) 150 mg once a week for 3–4 weeks, or ultramicrosized griseofulvin 250 mg or 330 mg every day or twice daily for 4 weeks.

Pearls
- A positive culture for staphylococcus does not rule out tinea, in which purulent lesions may be infected secondarily with bacteria.

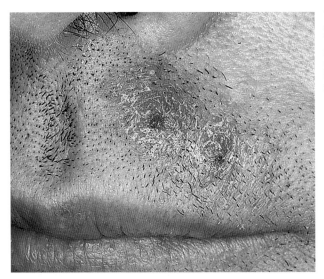

Tinea begins insidiously with a small group of follicular pustules. The process becomes confluent and resembles bacterial infection or seborrheic dermatitis. Potassium hydroxide examination proves the diagnosis.

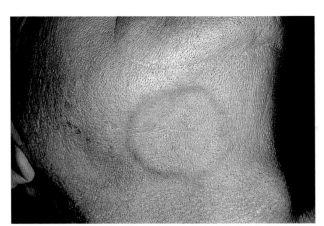

Superficial infection. This pattern resembles the annular lesions of tinea corporis. The hair is usually infected.

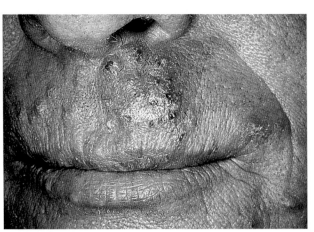

Deep follicular infection. This pattern clinically resembles bacterial folliculitis except that it is slower to evolve and is usually restricted to one area of the beard. Look carefully for the well-defined sharp advancing border.

10 Exanthems and Drug Reactions

Non-Specific Viral Rash

Description
- An exanthem is a rash that occurs as a sign of a systemic disease. A viral exanthem is a rash that arises due to a viral infection.
- Most viruses produce similar rashes, leading to the term "non-specific viral rash."

History
- Non-specific viral rashes are the most common viral exanthems and are challenging to diagnose.
- Historical elements such as season, exposure history, and local and regional epidemiology are extremely important in the evaluation of a patient with a suspected viral exanthem.
- Most non-specific viral exanthems in the winter are due to respiratory viruses; in the summer and fall they are due to the enteroviruses.
- Examples of viruses capable of causing non-specific viral exanthems include non-polio enteroviruses (enterovirus, coxsackievirus, echovirus), Epstein–Barr virus, human herpes virus-6, human herpes virus-7, parvovirus B-19, and respiratory viruses (rhinovirus, adenovirus, parainfluenza virus, respiratory syncytial virus, influenza virus).

Skin Findings
- Non-polio enterovirus can produce generalized erythematous macules and papules.
- Sometimes, these viruses produce petechial rashes that can mimic meningococcemia.
- Epstein–Barr virus causes pharyngitis, morbilliform (5–15%), vesicular, urticarial, and petechial rashes. Periorbital edema occurs in 35% of patients with this virus. Erythematous to copper-colored macules and papules occur 1–2 days after treatment with amoxicillin in 90–100% of patients. This rash is not associated with amoxicillin allergy.
- All respiratory viruses can cause diffuse pink macules and papules that coalesce to plaques. Many patients with adenovirus infection develop keratoconjunctivitis that is highly contagious.
- Papular acrodermatitis of childhood (Gianotti–Crosti syndrome) is a viral exanthem characterized by monomorphic, discrete papules and vesicles coalescing on the face, extremities, and buttocks.
- Unilateral laterothoracic exanthem (asymmetric periflexural exanthem) is a rash occurring on the lateral thorax, near the axilla. Sometimes this viral exanthem will spread to the other hemi-thorax and the extremities.
- Papular-purpuric gloves and socks syndrome is an acute self-limiting rash characterized by petechial erythema on the palms and soles. Patients with this may have fevers and flu-like symptoms. The vast majority of cases are caused by parvovirus B19.

Non-skin Findings
- Non-skin findings vary according to the specific virus. Most non-specific viruses are associated with fever and constitutional symptoms.
- Non-polio enteroviruses cause fever, abdominal pain and vomiting. There can be multi-organ involvement, involving the central nervous system, and the pulmonary and cardiac systems. These viruses can mimic serious bacterial illness.
- Epstein–Barr virus can produce fever, sore throat, lymphadenopathy, abdominal pain, myalgias, and hepatosplenomegaly.

Laboratory and Biopsy
- The laboratory evaluation should be focused and directed by the history and physical examination.

- Skin biopsy findings are not specific, but can be helpful to distinguish between staphylococcal scalded skin syndrome and drug hypersensitivity reaction.

Differential Diagnosis

- Drug hypersensitivity reaction
- Kawasaki disease
- Staphylococcal scalded skin syndrome
- Toxin-mediated erythema (toxic shock syndrome, staphylococcal toxic shock syndrome)

Course and Prognosis

- Most non-specific viral exanthems are self-limiting and resolve in 1–2 weeks.

- The rash of Gianotti–Crosti syndrome can last up to 8 weeks.

Pediatric Considerations

- Viral exanthems are extremely common in childhood and can be difficult to distinguish from morbilliform drug reactions.
- Measles vaccination exanthem occurs in 5% of those receiving the vaccine.
- Kawasaki disease should be considered in small infants with exanthems and prolonged fever.

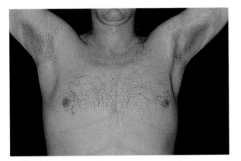

Viral exanthems and drug rashes may have the same appearance. They are symmetrical and widespread.

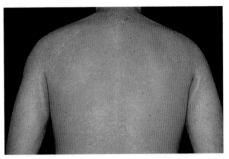

Viral exanthems may have different presentations. This symmetrical maculopapular eruption appeared suddenly with other viral symptoms. Oral medications had not been used.

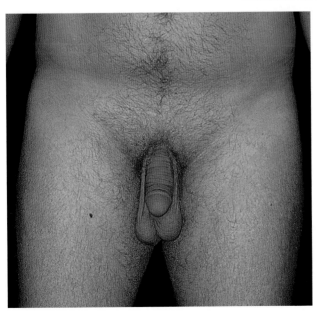

This symmetrical eruption of sudden onset produces only mild itching. It resolved in 2 weeks without any treatment.

Roseola Infantum

Description
- Roseola infantum is a viral exanthem characterized by high fever followed by the abrupt appearance of a diffuse rash as the fever resolves.

History
- Roseola infantum occurs in infants from the ages of 6 months to 3 years, with a peak incidence at 6 months.
- It is caused by human herpes virus 6 and human herpes virus 7.
- Most cases occur during early spring, although Roseola infantum can occur anytime during the year.
- The incubation period is 12 days (range 5–15 days).
- Infants appear well, except for a high fever (38.3–41.1° C).

Skin Findings
- Within 2 days of defervescence, small pink almond-shaped macules occur on the neck, the trunk, the proximal extremities and face.
- The rash is not itchy and fades within several days or a week.
- Eyelid edema is seen in 30% of children.
- The vast majority of patients have pink papules on the uvula and soft palate.

Non-skin Findings
- Irritability can occur in up to 14% of patients.
- Posterior cervical, occipital, and posterior auricular adenopathy are common.
- Open fontanelles are sometimes bulging.
- Complications include febrile seizures, aseptic meningitis, hemiplegia, and encephalitis or encephalopathy.

Laboratory and Biopsy
- Leukocytosis develops at the onset of fever.
- Leukopenia with a granulocytopenia and relative lymphocytosis appears as the temperature increases and persists until the eruption fades.
- Serologic testing is available, but typically is not helpful.
- Skin biopsy findings are not specific.

Differential Diagnosis
- Other viral exanthems (such as parainfluenza virus, parvovirus B19, rubella, enterovirus)
- Drug eruptions

Course and Prognosis
- Prodromal symptoms include a sudden onset of high fever of 39.4–41.1° C.
- Most children appear to be inappropriately well, given the high fever.
- Roseola is a major cause of visits to the emergency department, of febrile seizures, and of hospitalizations.

Treatment
- Acetaminophen and ibuprofen are effective antipyretics.
- Immunocompromised hosts or children with a severe illness may require antiviral treatment.

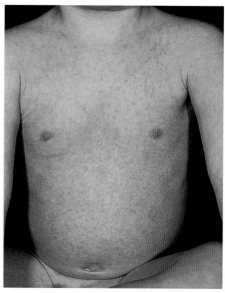

Numerous pale pink, almond-shaped macules.

Pearls

- Infections by herpes virus types 6 and 7 should be suspected in infants with febrile convulsions—even those without the exanthem.

- People with acquired immunodeficiency syndrome can have disseminated multisystem involvement, and transplant patients can have re-activation of latent virus.

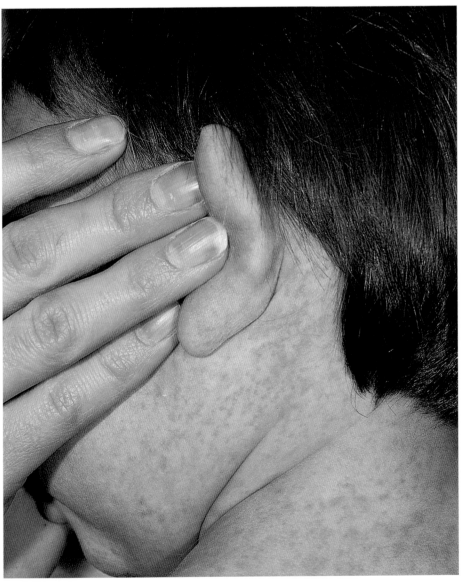

Pale pink macules may first appear on the neck.

Erythema Infectiosum (Fifth Disease)

Description
■ Erythema infectiosum, also known as "fifth disease" or "slapped cheek syndrome," is a common viral exanthem that causes bright red cheeks and lacy erythema of the arms.

History
■ Erythema infectiosum occurs in the winter and spring and is associated with community outbreaks.
■ It is caused by parvovirus B19 and is transmitted via respiratory secretions, blood, or vertically from mother to fetus.
■ Peak attack rates occur in children aged 5–14 years.
■ During outbreaks, 60% of susceptible school children and 30% of susceptible adults acquire the infection. Asymptomatic infection is common.
■ The incubation period is 4–14 days.
■ Prodromal symptoms are usually mild or absent. Pruritus, low-grade fever, malaise, and sore throat precede the eruption in approximately 10% of cases. Lymphadenopathy is absent. Older persons may complain of joint pain.

Skin Findings
■ There is facial erythema—the slapped-cheek appearance. Red papules on the cheeks rapidly coalesce in hours, forming red, slightly edematous, warm, erysipelas-like plaques that are symmetric on both cheeks and spare the nasolabial fold and the circumoral region (circumoral pallor). The slapped-cheek appearance fades in 4 days.
■ Approximately 2 days after the slapped-cheek rash, lacy erythema in a "fish net" pattern begins on the proximal extremities and extends to the trunk and buttocks, fading in 6–14 days.
■ For the next 2–3 weeks the eruption fades and reappears in previously affected sites. Factors such as sunlight, hot water, physical and emotional exertion exacerbate the rash.

■ The rash fades without scaling or pigmentation and the palms and soles are spared.

Non-skin Findings
Adults
■ Women may develop itching and arthritis. The itching varies from mild to intense and is localized or generalized.
■ Women tend to develop a moderate to severe, symmetric migratory polyarthritis (especially the small joints of the hands and knees), similar to rheumatoid arthritis. The duration of the arthritis is variable, lasting from 2 weeks to 4 years.
■ Generally, men do not develop arthritis.
■ The arthritis is preceded by a non-specific macular eruption, unlike the typical lacy rash.
■ Flu-like symptoms and joint pains coincide with immunoglobulin G antibody production (18–24 days after exposure), suggesting that immune complexes play an important role in extracutaneous disease.

Children
■ Unlike adult women, who commonly experience arthritis and arthralgias, only 8–10% of children develop joint symptoms.
■ In children, large joints are affected more often than the small joints. The knees are the most commonly affected joints (82%) followed by ankles, wrists, elbows, neck, hands and feet, hips, shoulders, and sternoclavicular joints.

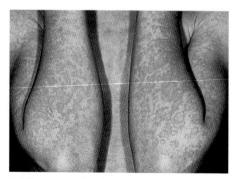

Net-like pattern of erythema.

- The duration of joint symptoms is usually less than 4 months, but some have persistent arthritis for extended periods (2-13 months), fulfilling criteria for juvenile rheumatoid arthritis.

Pregnancy

- Approximately 60% of pregnant women are immune to parvovirus B19.
- When infection occurs during pregnancy, only 30-44% report signs (arthralgias and rash) of acute infection.
- The overall risk of fetal loss is 8-10% and is greatest when infection occurs before 20 weeks' gestation, since most fetal losses occur between 20 and 28 weeks' gestation.
- An affected fetus can develop anemia, high output cardiac failure, pleural effusions, polyhydramnios, and non-immune hydrops fetalis.
- Overall, the vast majority of parvovirus B19 infected mothers deliver healthy term infants.

Laboratory and Biopsy

- Detection of serum immunoglobulin M antibodies to parvovirus B19 using enzyme immunoassay is the most sensitive indicator of acute parvovirus B19 infection in immunocompetent hosts. These antibodies persist for up to 6 months.
- Polymerase chain reaction is the most sensitive method to detect parvovirus B19 and is the preferred method in immunocompromised hosts. These studies can be used to test fetal and maternal blood, and amniotic fluid.
- Exposed pregnant women should have serologic or other diagnostic testing.
- Serial fetal ultrasounds should be performed on all pregnant women infected with parvovirus B19.

Differential Diagnosis

- Scarlet fever
- Enterovirus infection
- Rubella
- Rheumatoid arthritis (when there are joints symptoms)

Course and Prognosis

- Patients are not considered infectious after the rash develops.
- Most infections are self-limited without adverse sequelae.

Treatment

- Non-steroidal anti-inflammatory drugs can control joint symptoms for most patients.
- Patients should be assured that this unusual eruption will fade and does not require treatment.
- If a fetus is affected, intrauterine evaluation and treatment are available at tertiary care centers.

Pediatric Considerations

- Children can return to day-care and school when the rash appears.

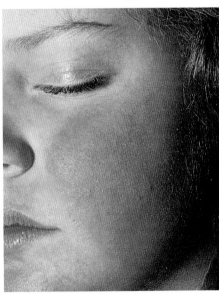

Facial erythema "slapped cheek." The red plaque covers the cheek and spares the nasolabial fold and the circumoral region.

269

Kawasaki Disease

Description

- Kawasaki disease, also known as mucocutaneous lymph node syndrome, is an acute multisystem vasculitis of unknown origin that occurs in infants and young children.
- The major causes of short-term and long-term morbidity are the cardiovascular manifestations.
- This condition occurs in both endemic and epidemic forms worldwide, but is most common in Japan.
- Ages range from 7 weeks to 12 years (mean 2.6 years); adult cases are rarely reported.
- Recurrences are rare.

Kawasaki Syndrome Centers for Disease Control and Prevention Diagnostic Criteria

- This diagnosis of the disease is based on having five of the following six clinical signs:
  - Fever of unknown origin for more than 5 days (95%)
  - Bilateral conjunctiva injection (87–90%)
  - Changes of the lips and oral cavity (85–95%)
  - Cervical lymphadenopathy (60–70%)
  - Polymorphous exanthem with vesicles or crusts (85–90%)
  - Changes of the peripheral extremities (90–95%)
- If other diseases have been excluded and the patient has a coronary artery aneurysm, Kawasaki disease can be diagnosed with less than five of the six clinical signs.
- Infants less than 6 months of age can have only prolonged fever and coronary artery aneurysms ("atypical Kawasaki disease"), making Kawasaki disease an important diagnostic consideration in all small infants with a fever of unknown origin.

Skin Findings

Conjunctival Injection

- Conjunctival injection occurs within 4 days of disease onset and subsides in 1 week.

- Uveitis occurs in 70% of cases.
- There is no purulent discharge or ulceration.

Changes in the Oral Mucous Membranes

- The lips and oral pharynx become red 3–5 days after the onset of the disease.
- The lips become dry, fissured, cracked, and crusted.
- Hypertrophic tongue papillae result in the "strawberry tongue" (80%) which is similar to that seen in scarlet fever.

Changes in the Extremities

- Around 2–5 days after the onset of illness, the palms and soles become red, and the hands and feet become edematous (non-pitting). The tenderness can be severe enough to limit walking and use of the hands. The edema lasts for approximately 1 week.
- Desquamation of the hands and feet occurs 10–14 days after the onset of fever. The skin peels off in sheets, beginning around the fingernails and fingertips and progressing down to the palms and soles.
- Beau's lines may appear in the nails weeks later.

Rash

- A rash appears soon after the onset of fever.
- The rash is described as polymorphous because macules, papules, urticarial-like lesions, and erythema multiforme-like lesions have been described. Urticarial eruptions and diffuse, deep red, maculopapular eruptions are the most common.
- Dermatitis in the diaper area is common and occurs in the first week. Red macules and papules become confluent. Desquamation occurs within 5–7 days.
- In children with inflammation of the diaper area, the skin peels at the margins of the rash and on the labia and scrotum.
- Perineal desquamation occurs 2–6 days before desquamation of the fingertips and toes.

Non-skin Findings

Fever

- Fever without chills or sweats lasts 5-30 days (mean 8.5 days).
- The fever begins abruptly and spikes from 38.3-40° C and does not respond to antibiotics or antipyretics.

Cervical Lymphadenopathy

- Firm, non-tender, non-suppurative lymphadenopathy is often limited to a single cervical lymph node.

Cardiac Involvement

- Kawasaki disease is the major cause of acquired heart disease in children in the United States. Clinical cardiac involvement occurs in 16.3% of patients.
- Early in the course of Kawasaki disease, more than 50% of patients develop myocarditis with tachycardia and gallop rhythms. These arrhythmias sometimes result in sudden death.
- In the subacute phase, aneurysm formation in medium-sized arteries, particularly the coronary arteries, is found in about a quarter of patients. These lesions may persist, scar with stenosis, or resolve angiographically. Aneurysms and thrombi form between 12 and 25 days after the onset and may result in congestive heart failure, pericardial effusions, arrhythmias, and death from myocardial ischemia or aneurysmal rupture.
- The abnormalities peak in the third week and often resolve thereafter.
- The prevalence of cardiac sequelae is high in male patients, in infants younger than 1 year of age, and children older than 5 years of age.
- Boys younger than age 1 year who have prolonged fever, elevated platelet counts, and high erythrocyte sedimentation rates are at greatest risk for coronary involvement.

Laboratory

- No diagnostic test exists.
- The acute phase is characterized leukocytosis (20,000–30,000 cells/mm^3) with a left shift (80%), thrombocytosis, and anemia.
- The erythrocyte sedimentation rate (90%), C reactive protein levels, and serum alpha l-antitrypsin levels are elevated with the onset of fever and persist for up to 10 weeks.
- The platelet count begins to rise on day 10 of the illness, peaks at 600,000 cells/ml to 1.6 million cells/ml, and returns to normal by day 30.

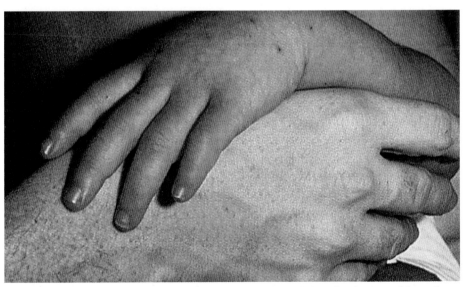

The hands become red and swollen. The hands began to peel about 14 days after the onset of the erythema and swelling. Courtesy of Nancy B Esterly, MD.

Course and Prognosis

- The worst prognosis occurs in children with so-called giant aneurysms, that is those with a maximum diameter of > 8 mm.
- Almost 10% of children do not improve clinically with treatment.

Treatment

- Intravenous immune globulin is given as a single infusion at a dose of 2 g/kg and aspirin (30–50 mg/kg) within the first 10 days from onset. The aspirin dose is decreased to 3-5 mg/kg as a single daily dose after the fever subsides.
- Approximately 10% of children are resistant to intravenous immune globulin. For these patients, methylprednisolone should be considered as an alternative to intravenous immune globulin.

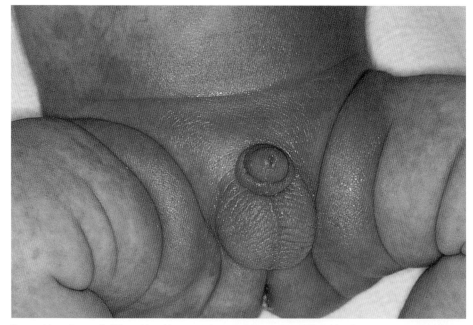

Kawasaki syndrome. A diffuse, blanching, macular exanthem can appear and is often concentrated in the perianal area. This occurs 3 to 4 days after the onset of the illness. The rash becomes confluent and desquamates in 5 to 7 days. Peeling begins to occur at the margin of the rash. Desquamation of the fingertips and toes occurs 2 to 6 days later.

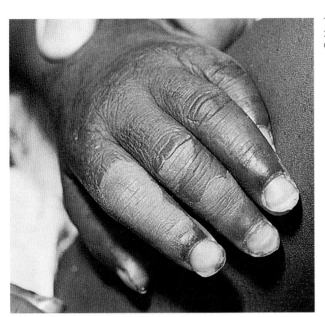

The hands peel approximately 2 weeks after the onset of fever. Courtesy of Nancy B Esterly, MD.

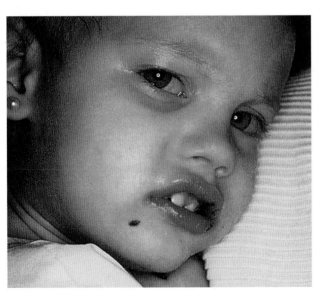

Non-purulent conjunctival injection and "cherry-red" lips with fissuring and crusting are early signs of the disease. Courtesy of Anne W Lucky, MD.

Cutaneous Drug Reactions

Description
- Cutaneous drug reactions are common complications of drug therapy, and they can occur in many forms and can mimic many dermatoses.

History
- Cutaneous drug reactions are seen in 2–3% of hospitalized patients, most of whom are on multiple medications.
- Fever may occur, and hours later a diffuse maculopapular rash, hives, generalized pruritus, or a combination of these develops.
- There is no correlation between the development of an adverse reaction and the patient's age, diagnosis, or survival.
- Drugs may be taken for weeks or years without ill effect, but once sensitization occurs a reaction may occur within minutes to 24–48 hours.
- Chemically related drugs may cross-react in a patient sensitized to one agent.
- Two groups of mechanisms are mostly involved: immunologic (with all four types of hypersensitivity reactions described) and non-immunologic (more common).

Morbilliform Eruptions
- The most frequent of all cutaneous drug reactions, maculopapular eruptions are often indistinguishable from viral exanthems.
- The onset occurs 7–10 days after starting the drug but may not occur until after the drug is stopped. The rash lasts 1–2 weeks and fades, in some cases even if the drug is continued.
- Maculopapular eruption, red macules, and papules become confluent in a symmetric, generalized distribution that often spares the face. Itching is common. The mucous membranes, palms, and soles may be involved.
- Symptoms are treated with antihistamines and cooling lotions (e.g. Sarna lotion).

Urticarial Drug Reactions
- Aspirin, penicillin, and blood products are the most frequent causes of urticarial drug eruptions, but almost any drug can cause hives.
- Anaphylactic immunoglobulin E-dependent reactions occur within minutes (immediate reactions) to hours (accelerated reactions) of drug administration.
- In circulating immune complex disease (serum sickness), urticaria occurs 4–21 days after drug ingestion; hives typically fade in less than 24 hours, only to recur in another area. Once the drug is stopped, this problem resolves over several weeks.
- Non-immunologic histamine reactions can occur in minutes; the allergenic drug or agent (e.g. morphine, codeine, polymyxin B, lobster, strawberries) may exert a direct action on the mast cell.
- Symptoms are treated with antihistamines and cooling lotions (e.g. Sarna lotion); topical steroids do not help.
- Hospitalization, observation, intubation, and epinephrine (adrenaline) all may be needed for severe reactions.

Internal–External Reactions
- The patient first develops a contact dermatitis with a topical agent and subsequently develops either a focal flare or a generalized eruption when exposed orally to the same or chemically related medication.

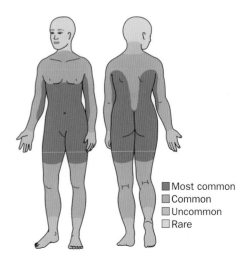

■ Most common
▨ Common
▢ Uncommon
▢ Rare

Box 10.1 Drug Reactions and the Drugs That Cause Them

Maculopapular (exanthematous) eruptions
Ampicillin
Barbiturates
Diflunisal (Dolobid)
Gentamicin
Gold salts
Isoniazid
Meclofenamate (Meclomen)
Phenothiazines
Phenylbutazone
Phenytoin (5% of children; dose dependent)
Quinidine
Sulfonamides
Thiazides
Thiouracil
Trimethoprim–sulfamethoxazole (in patients with acquired immunodeficiency syndrome)

Anaphylactic reactions
Aspirin
Penicillin
Radiographic dye
Sera (animal derived)

Serum sickness
Aspirin
Penicillin
Streptomycin
Sulfonamides
Thiouracils

Acneiform (pustular) eruptions
Bromides
Hormones
    Adrenocorticotropic hormone
    Androgens
    Corticosteroids
    Oral contraceptives
Iodides
Isoniazid
Lithium
Phenobarbital (aggravates acne)
Phenytoin

Alopecia
Allopurinol
Anticoagulants
Antithyroid drugs
Chemotherapeutic agents
    Alkylating agents
    Antimetabolites
    Cytotoxic agents
Colchicine
Hypocholesteremic drugs
Indomethacin

Levodopa
Oral contraceptives
Propranolol
Quinacrine
Retinoids
Thallium
Vitamin A

Erythema nodosum
Iodides
Oral contraceptives
Sulfonamides

Exfoliative erythroderma
Allopurinol
Arsenicals
Barbiturates
Captopril
Cefoxitin
Chloroquine
Cimetidine
Gold salts
Hydantoins
Isoniazid
Lithium
Mercurial diuretics
Para-aminosalicylic acid
Phenylbutazone
Sulfonamides
Sulfonylureas

Fixed drug eruptions
Aspirin
Barbiturates
Methaqualone
Phenazones
Phenolphthalein
Phynylbutazone
Sulfonamides
Tetracyclines
Trimethoprim–sulfamethoxazole
(Many others reported)

Lichen planus-like eruptions
Antimalarials
Arsenicals
Beta-blockers
Captopril
Furosemide
Gold salts
Methyldopa
Penicillamine
Quinidine
Sulfonylureas
Thiazides

Box 10.1 Drug Reactions and the Drugs That Cause Them (*continued*)

Erythema multiforme-like eruptions
Allopurinol
Barbiturates
Carbamazepine
Hydantoins
Minoxidil
Nitrofurantoin
Non-steroidal anti-inflammatory agents
Penicillin
Phenolphthalein
Phenothiazines
Rifampin
Sulfonamides
Sulfonylureas
Sulindac

Lupus-like eruptions

Common
Hydralazine
Procainamide

Probable
Acebutolol
Carbamazepine
Ethosuximide
Lithium carbonate
Penicillamine
Phenytoin
Propylthiouracil
Sulfasalazine

Uncommon
Chlorpromazine
Hydrochlorothiazide
Isoniazid
Methyldopa
Quinidine

Photosensitivity
Amiodarone
Carbamazepine
Chlorpropamide
Furosemide
Griseofulvin
Lomefloxacin
Methotrexate (sunburn reactivation)
Nalidixic acid
Naproxen
Phenothiazines
Piroxicam (Feldene)
Psoralens
Quinine
Sulfonamides
Tetracyclines
    Demeclocycline

Doxycycline (less frequently with
    tetracycline and minocycline)
Thiazides
Tolbutamide

Skin pigmentation disorders
Adrenocorticotropic hormone (brown as in
    Addison's disease)
Amiodarone (slate-gray)
Anticancer drugs
    Bleomycin (30%; brown, patchy, linear)
    Busulphan (diffuse as in Addison's
    disease)
    Cyclophosphamide (nails)
    Doxorubicin (nails)
Antimalarials (blue-gray or yellow)
Arsenic (diffuse, brown, macular)
Chlorpromazine (slate-gray in sun-exposed
areas)
Clofazimine (red)
Heavy metals
    Silver
    Gold
    Bismuth
    Mercury
Methysergide maleate (red)
Minocycline (patchy or diffuse blue-black)
Oral contraceptives (chloasma-brown)
Psoralens
Rifampin (very high dose; red man
syndrome)

Pityriasis rosea-like eruptions
Arsenicals
Barbiturates
Bismuth compounds
Captopril
Clonidine
Gold compounds
Methoxypromazine
Metronidazole
Pyribenzamine

Toxic epidermal necrolysis
Allopurinol
Phenylbutazone
Phenytoin
Sulfonamides
Sulindac

Small-vessel cutaneous vasculitis
Allopurinol
Diphenylhydantoin
Hydralazine
Penicillin

Box 10.1 Drug Reactions and the Drugs That Cause Them (*continued*)

Piroxicam (Feldene) (Henoch–Schönlein purpura)
Propylthiouracil
Quinidine
Sulfonamides
Thiazides

Vesicles and blisters
Barbiturates (pressure areas; comatose patients)
Bromides
Captopril (pemphigus-like)
Cephalosporins (pemphigus-like)
Clonidine (cicatricial pemphigoid-like)
Furosemide (phototoxic)
Iodides
Nalidixic acid (phototoxic)
Naproxen (like porphyria cutanea tarda)
Penicillamine (pemphigus foliaceus-like)
Phenazones

Piroxicam (Feldene)
Sulfonamides

Ocular pemphigoid
Demecarium bromide
Echothiophate iodide
Epinephrine
Idoxuridine
Pilocarpine
Timolol

Chemotherapy-induced acral erythema
Cyclophosphamide
Cytosine arabinoside
Doxorubicin
Fluorouracil
Hydroxyurea
Mercaptopurine
Methotrexate
Mitotane

- Continued use of the medication can intensify the reaction and lead to generalization of the eruption.
- Eczematous internal–external reaction usually presents as areas of redness, particularly in the axillae or groin.
- Topical or oral steroids control these eruptions

Erythema Multiforme and Toxic Epidermal Necrolysis Reactions

- The lesions of erythema multiforme look like targets. Bullae develop in severe forms of the disease.
- These reactions may be limited to the skin or mucous membranes, but can be generalized.
- Severe forms are often caused by medications. Mycoplasmal pneumonia, herpes simplex infections, and medications cause less severe forms.
- Toxic epidermal necrolysis can be severe and fatal. The cause of death is loss of large areas of skin, resulting in fluid loss and sepsis.
- Severe reactions are best managed in burns units or intensive care units.
- The use of oral steroids is controversial.

Exfoliative Erythroderma

- There are generalized redness and desquamation.
- The reaction is potentially life threatening.

Fixed Drug Eruptions

- Single or multiple, round, sharply demarcated, dusky red plaques appear soon after drug exposure and reappear in exactly the same site each time the drug is taken.
- The lesions are generally preceded or accompanied by itching and burning, which may be the only manifestations of reactivation in an old patch.
- The area often blisters and then erodes; desquamation or crusting (after bullous lesions) follows, and brown pigmentation forms with healing.
- Lesions can occur on any part of the skin or mucous membrane, but the glans penis is the most common site. Tetracycline and co-trimoxazole frequently cause fixed lesions or fixed drug eruptions on the glans penis.
- The length of time from re-exposure to a drug and the onset of symptoms is 30 minutes to 8 hours.

277

- After each exacerbation, some patients experience a refractory period (weeks to several months) during which time the offending drug does not activate the lesions.
- A careful history is important because patients often do not relate their complaints to the use of a drug.
- "Provoking" or challenging the appearance of the lesion with the suspected drug confirms the diagnosis, prevents recurrences, and allays the anxiety of the patient regarding a venereal origin of disease.

Drug-Induced Hyperpigmentation
- Drug-induced hyperpigmentation is caused by many different drugs, including antiarrhythmics (amiodarone), antimalarials, antibiotics (minocycline), antivirals (zidovudine), antiseizure agents (hydantoin), chemotherapy agents, heavy metals, hormones, and antipsychotics (chlorpromazine). The discoloration often fades with time (months to years).
- Amiodarone causes a dusky red coloration that with time becomes blue-gray or ashen. This is usually in photodistributed areas.
- Minocycline (Minocin) causes a blue-gray or slate-gray discoloration, often in acne lesions, but also on the gingiva and perhaps on teeth.
- Zidovudine causes brown longitudinal pigmentation on the nails and a similar brown color on the lips and oral mucosa.
- Antimalarial agents typically cause a brown discoloration on the shins or elsewhere.
- Hydantoin may cause melasma-like brown pigmentation on the face.
- Bleomycin causes a dramatic reaction, causing a flagellate, streaking hyperpigmentation on the trunk and extremities.
- Melasma, a typical brown pigmentation on the cheeks and central face, is associated with oral contraceptive use. The use of a broad-spectrum ultraviolet B and ultraviolet A sunscreen is advisable in many of these cases.

Lichenoid Drug Reactions
- The clinical and histologic patterns mimic those of lichen planus.
- The latent period between the beginning of administration of a drug and the eruption is 3 weeks to 3 years.
- There are multiple flat-topped, itchy violaceous papules; oral lesions may be present.
- Lesions heal with brown pigmentation.
- Gold and antimalarial agents are most often associated with drug-induced lichen planus.
- The lesions are chronic and persist for weeks or months after the offending drug is stopped.

Photosensitivity Drug Eruptions
- Both systemic and topical medications can induce photosensitivity.
- There are two main types: phototoxicity and photoallergy.
- Phototoxic reactions are related to drug concentration and can occur in anyone. They can occur on first administration and subside when the drug is stopped. The eruption is confined to sun-exposed areas. There is erythema within 24 hours of light exposure.
- Photoallergic reactions are less common and are not related to concentration. There is a delay of 48 hours after exposure before the eruption appears. The eruption can spread to non-sun-exposed regions.

Onycholysis
- Onycholysis is separation of the nail plate from the nail bed.
- It may occur from drug photosensitivity and has occurred after the administration of tetracyclines, psoralens, and fluoroquinolones.

Small-Vessel Necrotizing Vasculitis (Palpable Purpura)
- Small-vessel necrotizing vasculitis may be precipitated by drugs.
- Lesions are most often concentrated on the lower legs.
- Vessels of the kidneys, joints, and brain may be involved.

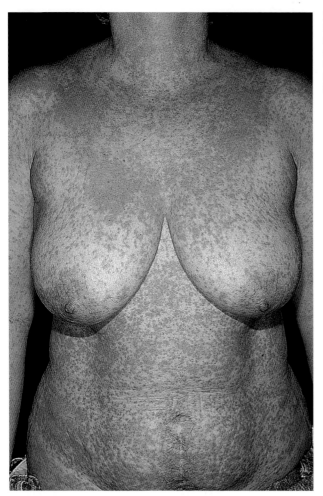

Maculopapular eruption. Maculopapular drug eruptions are often indistinguishable from viral exanthems. They are the classic ampicillin rashes, but several other drugs also cause this pattern.

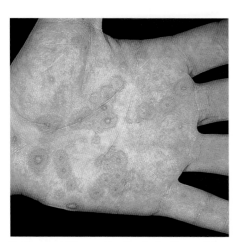

Erythema multiforme. The classic ring-like eruption on the palms.

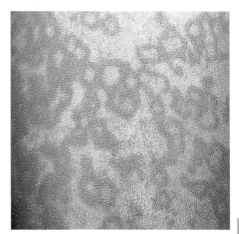

Urticarial eruption. Drugs are a common cause of hives.

279

Chemotherapy-Induced Acral Erythema

- Tingling on the palms and soles is followed in a few days by painful, symmetric, well-defined swelling and erythema.
- The hands are more severely affected than the feet.
- Areas of pallor develop, blister, desquamate, and re-epithelialize.
- Chemotherapy-induced acral erythema occurs most commonly after the administration of cytosine arabinoside, fluorouracil, and doxorubicin.
- The reaction is dose-dependent, and a direct toxic effect of the drug is likely.
- The time of onset is 24 hours to 10 months, and the severity varies.
- Cytosine arabinoside has a predilection to progress to blisters.
- Treatment is supportive and includes elevation and cold wet dressings.
- Systemic steroids have been used with variable success.
- Cooling the hands and feet during treatment to decrease blood flow may attenuate the reaction.
- Modification of the dosage schedule may also help.

Reactions to Gold

- There are many different forms of gold rashes. The most common is a non-specific, eczematous, papular, itchy eruption.
- Some 25% of gold rashes resemble lichen planus, but the distribution is atypical.
- A pityriasis rosea-like eruption occurs also.
- The rate of resolution correlates with the extent of the rash and not with the specific morphologic form. The median duration to resolution is 10 weeks. There is no increased risk of developing the rash when gold therapy is resumed.
- Group V topical steroids provide symptomatic relief for gold dermatitis.
- Systemic steroids may be required for severe reactions.

Acute Generalized Exanthematous Pustulosis

- Acute generalized exanthematous pustulosis is characterized by multiple tiny superficial pustules over most of the body.

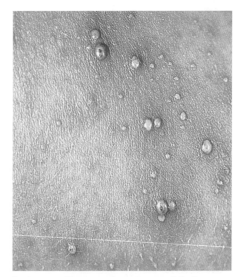

Acute generalized exanthematous pustulosis. Numerous pustules appeared 5 days after penicillin was started. The medication was stopped, and the pustules cleared spontaneously in 2 weeks.

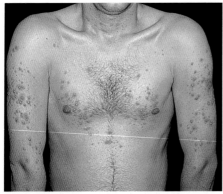

Acute generalized exanthematous pustulosis. Antibiotics, especially beta-lactams and macrolides, are the main culprits.

- The most common drugs are the antibacterial agents (mostly penicillin).
- There is a short interval between drug ingestion and the eruption (mean 5 days), and resolution occurs in less than 15 days.

- Fever, leukocytosis, and an ill-appearing patient are common.
- Desquamation occurs with no scarring.
- Simple lubrication of the skin along with removal of offending drug is all that is needed.

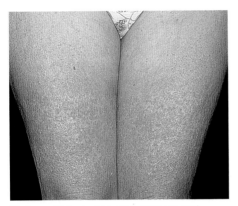

Photosensitivity drug eruption. Erythema and papules occurred on exposed areas in this patient who had been taking a thiazide antihypertensive medication.

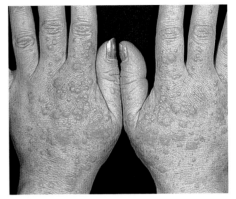

Photosensitivity drug eruption. Red papules in a symmetric photodistribution in a patient taking amiodarone.

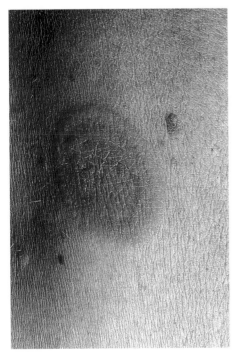

Fixed drug eruption. Single or multiple, round, sharply demarcated, dusky-red plaques appear soon after drug exposure and reappear in exactly the same site each time the drug is taken.

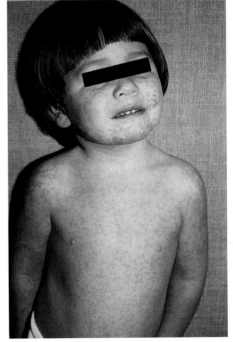

Classic viral, generalized, symmetrical, maculopapular eruption also involving the face, palms and soles. There was little itching.

Toxic Shock Syndrome

Description

■ Toxic shock syndrome is an acute toxin-mediated multisystem disease resulting in high fever, diffuse erythroderma, mucous membrane hyperemia, and profound hypotension (see Box 10.2).

History

■ In the past, the majority of patients with toxic shock syndrome were women of reproductive age who are vaginally infected or colonized with a toxin-producing strain of *Staphylococcus aureus* (phage group 1; TSST-1, enterotoxin B, A, C$_1$). Symptoms occur within 4 days of menses and the risk is higher with use of high-absorbency tampons.

■ Toxin-producing strains of *Streptococcus pyogenes* (M protein types 1, 3, 12, 28; toxins SPE-A or SPE-B) can produce toxic shock syndrome (streptococcal toxic shock syndrome). In this syndrome, the infectious focus is often the skin or soft tissue and many patients are bacteremic.

■ Non-menstrual-related toxic shock syndrome accounts for 20–30% of toxic shock syndrome cases. On average, symptoms occur 7 days after the precipitating event. Patients with bacterial tracheitis (especially after an infection with influenza B virus) and burns appear to be at higher risk for non-menstrual-related toxic shock syndrome.

■ Toxic shock syndrome has been described in association with surgical and non-surgical wound infections, with abortion, childbirth, and use of nasal packing, and contraceptive sponges.

■ In all forms of toxic shock syndrome, susceptible hosts appear to have low levels to absent levels of toxin-specific antibodies and local factors that favor toxin production.

Skin Findings

■ In toxic shock syndrome, a scarlatiniform rash develops on the torso and spreads to the extremities within 1–3 days of disease onset. Early in the course of the disease, there may be edema of the hands and feet (50%), petechiae (27%), conjunctival injection (85%), oropharyngeal hyperemia (90%), and genital hyperemia (100%). One or two weeks after disease onset, many patients develop a generalized itchy morbilliform eruption involving the palms and soles, but the face is spared. Desquamation of the palms, soles, fingertips, and toes occurs 10–21 days after the onset.

■ In streptococcal toxic shock syndrome, 80% of patients have cutaneous signs of soft tissue infection and 70% have deep soft tissue infections, such as necrotizing fasciitis, that require immediate surgical debridement.

Non-skin Findings

■ In toxic shock syndrome, patients acutely develop high fever, abdominal pain, vomiting, headache, and myalgias, leading to profound hypotension and multiorgan failure (Box 10.1).

■ In toxic shock syndrome children develop respiratory distress more commonly than adults.

Laboratory and Biopsy

■ Hematological and serum chemistry abnormalities reflect multi-organ damage (Box 10.1).

■ Skin microscopic findings are not specific for toxic shock syndrome. A skin biopsy should be done to distinguish toxic shock syndrome from toxic epidermal necrolysis and drug hypersensitivity reaction.

Diffential Diagnosis

■ Drug eruptions
■ Kawasaki syndrome
■ Infantile polyarteritis nodosa
■ Scarlet fever
■ Staphylococcal scalded skin syndrome
■ Toxic epidermal necrolysis
■ Viral exanthema

Course and Prognosis

■ With prompt antibiotic and supportive therapy, the mortality is low: overall 3.7%; in men 12.2%; and in women 2.6%.

Treatment

- The goal of therapy in toxic shock syndrome is to minimize organ damage though supportive management of shock, and medical and surgical treatment of infection.
- In toxic shock syndrome, beta-lactamase-resistant antimicrobial antibiotics (oxacillin, nafcillin, cefoxitin, vancomycin, clindamycin) are administered intravenously. In 3–5 days most patients are able to tolerate oral antibiotics, which are continued for a total of 10–14 days.
- Intravenous immune globulin has been helpful in some patients because of neutralizing antibodies

---

Box 10.2 Toxic Shock Syndrome Case Definition

Major criteria (all four must be met)
Fever: temperature > 38.9° C (102° F)
Rash: diffuse or palmar erythroderma progressing to subsequent peripheral desquamation (hands and feet)
Mucous membrane: non-purulent conjunctival hyperemia, or oropharyngeal hyperemia, or vaginal hyperemia or discharge
Hypotension: systolic blood pressure less than 90 mmHg for an adult (over 16 years of age) or less than 5th percentile for age for a child; or orthostatic hypotension as shown by a drop in diastolic blood pressure greater than 15 mmHg from recumbent to sitting; or history of orthostatic dizziness

Multisystem involvement (three or more must be present)
Gastrointestinal: history of vomiting or diarrhea at onset of illness
Muscular: creatinine phosphokinase > 2 × upper limit of normal for laboratory values 4–20 days after onset
Central nervous system: disorientation or alteration in consciousness without focal signs at a time when patient is not in shock or hyperpyrexic
Renal: blood urea nitrogen or serum creatinine clearance levels > 2 × upper limit of normal; and abnormal findings on urinalysis (> 5 white blood cells per high-power field; > 1 red blood cell per high-power field; protein > 1 +); or oliguria defined as urine output < 1 ml/kg/hour for 24 hours.
Hepatic: total serum bilirubin level of > 1.5 × upper limit of normal; or serum glutamate pyruvate transaminase levels of > 2 × upper limit of normal
Hematologic: thrombocytopenia (platelets less than 100,000/mm^3)
Cardiopulmonary: adult respiratory distress syndrome; or pulmonary edema; or new onset second-degree or third-degree heart block; or electrocardiogram criteria for myocarditis decreased voltage and ST–T wave changes; or heart failure shown by new onset of gallop rhythm, or by increase in size of cardiac silhouette from one chest roentgenogram to another during the course of the illness, or diagnosed by cardiologist
Metabolic: serum calcium level less than 7.0 mg/dl with serum phosphate level less than 2.5 mg/dl, and total serum protein level less than 5.0 mg/dl

Evidence for absence of other causes
When obtained: negative blood, throat, urine, or cerebrospinal fluid cultures
When obtained: absence of serologic evidence of leptospirosis, rickettsial disease, or rubeola
Evidence for absence of Kawasaki syndrome: no unilateral lymphadenopathy or fever lasting more than 10 days

---

Adapted from Chesney RW, Chesney PJ, Davis JP, Segar WE (1981) Clinical manifestations of toxic shock syndrome. *J Amer Med Assoc* 246(7):741–8.

11 Hypersensitivity Syndromes and Vasculitis

Erythema Multiforme

Description
■ Erythema multiforme is a relatively common, acute—often recurrent— inflammatory disease characterized by target-shaped skin lesions.

History
■ Commonly erythema multiforme is associated with herpes simplex, *Mycoplasma pneumoniae*, and upper respiratory tract infections.
■ Rarely, erythema multiforme is associated with contact allergens, drugs, connective tissue diseases, physical agents, x-ray therapy, pregnancy, and internal malignancies.
■ The cause of erythema multiforme is unknown in at least half of the patients.
■ A minority of patients with re-activation of herpes simplex develop recurrent erythema multiforme.
■ Erythema multiforme is thought to be produced by a cytotoxic immune response directed against keratinocytes expressing foreign viral or drug antigens.

Skin Findings
■ As its name suggests, erythema multiforme shows numerous lesion morphologies: target lesions, erythematous macules and papules, urticarial-like lesions, vesicles and bullae.
■ Patients should only be diagnosed clinically with erythema multiforme if target lesions are seen.
■ Target lesions begin as dusky red, round macules and papules that may burn and itch.
■ These early lesions appear suddenly in a symmetric pattern on the palms, soles, backs of the hands and feet and the extensor aspect of the forearms and legs. The diagnosis of erythema multiforme

may not be suspected until the nonspecific early lesions evolve into target lesions during a period of 24–48 hours.
■ The classic "iris" or target lesion results from centrifugal spread of the red maculopapule to a circumference of 1–3 cm. The center of the iris can appear dark red, purpuric or vesicular and is due to acute epidermal injury. This central area is surrounded by a pale area of edematous skin, which is in turn surrounded by a sharp discrete ring of erythema.
■ Lesions appear in crops, resolving in 1–2 weeks without scarring.
■ Post-inflammatory pigment changes are common (hypopigmentation and/or hyperpigmentation).
■ Bullae and erosions may be present in the oral cavity.
■ The urticarial plaques seen in erythema multiforme are distinguished from hives in that they are fixed and do not resolve in 24 hours.
■ Erythema multiforme lesions may occur in areas of trauma (Koebner phenomenon).

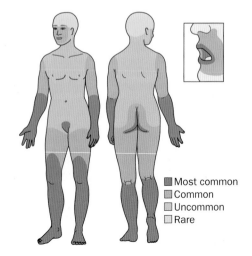

■ Most common
□ Common
□ Uncommon
□ Rare

Non-skin Findings

■ Erythema multiforme may be preceded by cough, malaise and fever and be associated with pneumonia.

Laboratory and Biopsy

■ Laboratory testing is not necessary. Vesicles or erosions suggestive of herpes simplex confirmed by viral culture or direct immunofluorescence.

■ Skin biopsy shows an interface reaction with necrotic keratinocytes and can be helpful when the diagnosis is uncertain.

Course and Prognosis

■ Usually erythema multiforme resolves within 1 month.

■ Patients who develop erythema multiforme associated with reactivated herpes simplex may require suppressive therapy to prevent recurrences.

Treatment

■ Most patients with erythema multiforme do not require treatment.

■ Ruptured blisters and eroded skin can be treated with local measures, such as topical antibiotics (bacitracin, Bactroban).

■ Widespread erythema multiforme responds rapidly to 1–3 weeks of systemic corticosteroids. Prednisone 40–80 mg/day should be administered until lesions resolve, and then tapered as appropriate.

■ Recurrent herpes associated erythema multiforme can be prevented by administering oral acyclovir (200 mg two or three times a day or 400 mg twice a day), valacyclovir (Valtrex), 500 mg/day, or famciclovir (Famvir) 125 mg twice daily as continuous suppressive therapy.

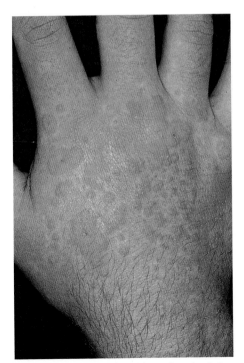

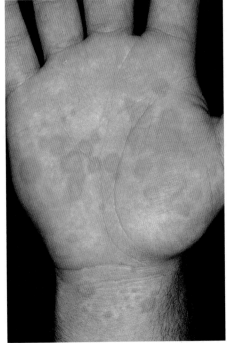

A dusky red macule or urticarial papule expands to about 2 cm over 24–48 hours. A papule, vesicle, or bulla develops in the center, then flattens and may clear. The periphery becomes cyanotic to form the classic target lesion.

The palms, back of the hands and extensor forearms are a common place to find the initial target lesions. They can resemble urticaria and drug eruptions. Symptoms of burning or itching are usually mild.

Stevens–Johnson Syndrome

Description
- Stevens-Johnson syndrome is a severe blistering mucocutaneous syndrome involving at least two mucous membranes.

History
- Stevens-Johnson syndrome occurs in all ages, but is more common in children and young adults.
- The syndrome is similar to erythema multiforme and is thought to be due to cytotoxic immune responses directed against keratinocytes expressing foreign infectious and drug antigens.
- *Mycoplasma pneumoniae* has been associated with Stevens-Johnson syndrome.
- Phenytoin, phenobarbital, carbamazepine, sulfonamides, and aminopenicillins are frequently implicated drugs.
- Medications started within 1 month of disease onset are more likely to cause Stevens-Johnson syndrome.
- Patients with human immunodeficiency virus infection, with systemic lupus erythematosus and malignancies treated with radiation are at increased risk for developing Stevens-Johnson syndrome.

Skin Findings
- Erythematous papules, dusky appearing vesicles, purpura, and target lesions erupt acutely.
- Patients frequently complain of skin tenderness and burning.
- Oral, genital, and perianal mucosa develop bullae and erosions.
- Thick hemorrhagic crusts can cover the lips.
- Patients develop conjunctivitis and are at risk for corneal ulceration and uveitis.
- Stevens-Johnson syndrome skin lesions are more centrally distributed on the face and trunk.
- Crops of lesions erupt for 10-14 days and slowly subside for the next 3-4 weeks.

Non-Skin Findings
- During the early phase, 10-30% of patients develop a high fever with marked constitutional symptoms.
- Pulmonary (pneumonitis (23%), bronchitis (6%), bronchiolitis obliterans), gastrointestinal (dysphagia, abdominal pain, diarrhea), central nervous (coma and seizures), and renal (renal failure) systems can be affected.
- With widespread skin breakdown, patients develop increased fluid and nutritional requirements and are at risk for sepsis.

Laboratory and Biopsy
- Skin biopsy shows full-thickness epidermal necrosis with a relatively normal dermis.

Differential Diagnosis
- Anticonvulsant hypersensitivity syndrome
- Paraneoplastic pemphigus
- Pemphigus vulgaris
- Herpetic gingivostomatitis
- Staphylococcal scalded skin syndrome

Course and Prognosis
- Uncomplicated Stevens-Johnson syndrome resolves in a month.
- In the case of limited disease and adequate supportive care, the mortality rate is less than 1%.
- Recurrence is not common unless there is re-exposure to a causative drug.

Treatment

- Treatment regimens focus on identifying and treating sources of infection, withdrawing suspected offending drugs, maintaining fluid and nutritional requirements, providing meticulous local wound care, and halting the progression of Stevens–Johnson syndrome.
- Lips can be soothed with frequent mouth rinses and applications of petroleum jelly (Vaseline) or Aquaphor. Viscous Xylocaine or Benadryl elixir can also be helpful.
- The eyes should be treated frequently with topical erythromycin ointment to prevent ocular adhesions. An ophthalmologist should be consulted.
- Eroded skin should be treated in the same manner as a burn by cleansing gently, removing necrotic tissue, and applying bland emollients.
- The role of systemic corticosteroids remains controversial.
- Narcotics may be necessary to control pain.
- Intravenous immunoglobulin G (IVIG) has been proposed and shown to be beneficial.

Pediatric Consideration

- Children have a slightly better prognosis than adults.

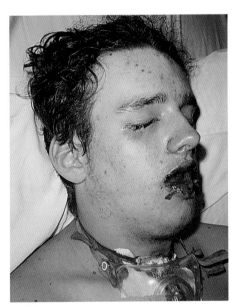

Severe bullous form. Bullae are present on the conjunctiva and in the mouth.

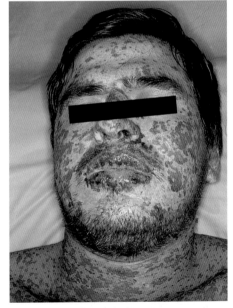

Skin lesions are flat atypical targets, or purpuric maculae, that are widespread or distributed on the trunk. Lesions in this extensive case have become eroded and infected.

Toxic Epidermal Necrolysis

Description
■ Toxic epidermal necrolysis is a rare life-threatening mucocutaneous disease characterized by widespread blistering and sloughing of the skin and mucous membranes.

History
■ Most patients with toxic epidermal necrolysis (80–90%) have taken a drug 1–3 weeks before the disease onset. The most frequently associated drugs are sulfonamides, antimalarials, anticonvulsants, non-steroidal anti-inflammatory drugs, and allopurinol.
■ Patients with human immunodeficiency virus infection and certain autoimmune conditions such as systemic lupus erythematosis appear to be at greater risk for drug-induced toxic epidermal necrolysis.
■ Toxic epidermal necrolysis can be precipitated by a recent immunization (diphtheria–pertussis–tetanus, measles, poliomyelitis, influenza), viral infection (cytomegalovirus, Epstein–Barr virus, herpes simplex, varicella zoster, hepatitis A), mycoplasmal infection, streptococcal infection, syphilis, histoplasmosis, coccidioidomycosis, and tuberculosis.
■ Acute graft-versus-host disease can be associated with toxic epidermal necrolysis.
■ The cause of toxic epidermal necrolysis is unknown. The marked skin sloughing seen may be due to an increase in keratinocyte programmed cell death (apoptosis), mediated by the cell-surface death receptor (Fas) and its ligand (FasL). Anti-Fas antibodies in intravenous immunoglobulin G (IVIG) are thought to block the Fas receptor and halt the progression of the disease.

Skin Findings
■ Most patients develop diffusely red "sunburn-like" tender skin with scattered target lesions and bullae. Bullae quickly coalesce, resulting in widespread skin sloughing.

■ Full-thickness epidermal necrosis and detachment (necrolysis) leave a tender glistening raw surface.
■ Gentle lateral pressure easily produces epidermal detachment.
■ Mucous membranes develop exquisitely painful erosions.

Non-skin Findings
■ Non-skin findings are identical in toxic epidermal necrolysis and Stevens–Johnson syndrome (see section 11.2 Stevens–Johnson Syndrome).

Laboratory and Biopsy
■ A skin biopsy can be helpful to distinguish between toxic epidermal necrolysis and staphylococcal scalded skin syndrome. Sloughed skin can be "jelly-rolled" onto a round wooden applicator and sent for frozen section. This quick and simple test will show a superficial epidermal split in staphylococcal scalded skin syndrome and a full-thickness necrotic epidermis in toxic epidermal necrolysis.
■ A skin biopsy sent for direct immunofluorescence can distinguish between toxic epidermal necrolysis and autoimmune blistering conditions such as paraneoplastic pemphigus.

Differential Diagnosis
■ Staphylococcal scalded skin syndrome
■ Graft-versus-host disease
■ Staphylococcal toxic shock syndrome
■ Kawasaki syndrome
■ Acute-onset paraneoplastic pemphigus

Course and prognosis
■ Like Stevens–Johnson syndrome, toxic epidermal necrolysis is preceded by fever, malaise, cough, and abdominal pain.
■ Predictors of poor outcome include old age, widespread blistering, neutropenia, impaired renal function and multiple medications.
■ Overall, the mortality rate for toxic epidermal necrolysis is 30–50%.
■ The mortality rate for acute graft-versus-host-disease-associated toxic epidermal necrolysis is nearly 100%.

Treatment

- Like Stevens-Johnson syndrome, treatment regimens focus on controlling pain, identifying and treating sources of infection, withdrawing suspected offending medications, maintaining fluid and nutritional requirements, providing meticulous local wound care, and halting the progression of toxic epidermal necrolysis. If possible, severely affected patients should be managed in a burn unit.
- Intravenous immunoglobulin G (IVIG) 1 gm/kg for 3 or 5 days improves survival if it is administered early in the course of toxic epidermal necrolysis.

- Systemic corticosteroids have been used for years to treat toxic epidermal necrolysis, but it is not known whether they worsen or improve outcomes. They may halt its progression, but increase the risk for infection. If used, systemic corticosteroids should be administered for a brief period and with prophylactic antibiotics.

Pediatric Considerations
- Treatment principles are the same in children as they are in adults.
- Overall, children have a lower mortality rate than adults.

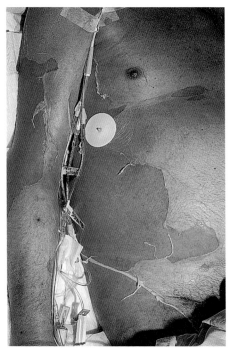

Shedding of full-thickness epidermis in toxic epidermal necrolysis.

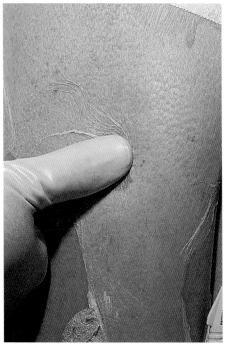

Wrinkling with slight pressure in toxic epidermal necrolysis (Nikolsky's sign).

Erythema Nodosum

Description
■ Erythema nodosum is a panniculitis characterized by tender pink nodules on the extensor surface of the lower legs.

History
■ In adults, erythema nodosum is five or six times more common in women, and the peak age of onset is in ages 20-30 years. In children, boys and girls are affected equally.
■ Erythema nodosum is thought to be due to a hypersensitivity reaction to a variety of antigenic stimuli.
■ Many bacteria, viruses, fungi, parasites, drugs, malignancies, and connective tissue diseases have been associated with erythema nodosum (see Box 11.1). In the United States, streptococcal infections and sarcoidosis are commonly associated with erythema nodosum.
■ Half of cases are idiopathic.

Skin Findings
■ Erythema nodosum is characterized by pink to dusky red firm nodules with indistinct edges, occurring symmetrically on the pretibial surfaces. Erythema nodosum can occur on the head, neck, torso, arms and thighs.
■ Erythema nodosum fades over a period of 1-2 weeks, similar to a bruise, and does not leave residual scars.
■ Ankle edema and leg pain are common.

Non-skin Findings
■ Erythema nodosum may be associated with fever, malaise, diarrhea, headache, conjunctivitis and cough.

Laboratory and Biopsy
■ Laboratory evaluation should be guided by history and physical examination. Initial tests should include a throat culture or rapid test for streptococcus, a complete blood count and a chest radiograph.
■ A deep skin biopsy to include fat can be helpful in patients with atypical lesions.

■ Chest x-ray may show bilateral hilar adenopathy. This finding can be present in erythema nodosum due to sarcoidosis as well as other diseases.

Differential Diagnosis
■ Cellulitis
■ Infected insect bites
■ Minor trauma
■ Other forms of panniculitis
■ Henoch–Schönlein purpura
■ Superficial and deep thrombophlebitis
■ Vasculitis

Course and Prognosis
■ New crops of lesions usually develop for 3-6 weeks, although, rarely erythema nodosum can persist for months to years.

Treatment
■ Associated diseases and infections should be identified and treated. Precipitating medications should be discontinued.
■ Usually symptoms can be relieved with rest, compressive bandages, and non-steroidal anti-inflammatory drugs (indomethacin, Naprosyn).
■ Supersaturated potassium iodide and systemic corticosteroids have been helpful for chronic recurrent erythema nodosum.

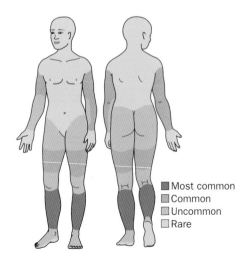

■ Most common
□ Common
▨ Uncommon
□ Rare

Box 11.1 Erythema Nodosum: Associated Conditions and Medications

Infections

Bacterial infections
Streptococcal
Tuberculosis
Yersinia
Mycoplasma
Psittacosis
Brucellosis
Campylobacter
Shigella
Salmonella
Leprosy
Leptospirosis
Tularemia

Viral infections
Epstein–Barr virus
Hepatitis B
Orf
Herpes simplex virus
Bartonella

Fungal infections
Coccidiomycosis
Blastomycosis
Histoplasmosis
Sporotrichosis
Dermatophytosis

Parasitic infections
Ascariasis
Amebiasis
Giardiasis

Drugs
Sulfonamides
Oral contraceptives
Bromides
Iodides
Minocycline
Gold
Penicillin
Salicylates

Malignancies
Lymphoma
Leukemia
Renal cell carcinoma
Post-radiation therapy

Inflammatory conditions
Sarcoidosis
Ulcerative colitis
Crohn's disease
Behçet's disease
Sweet's syndrome

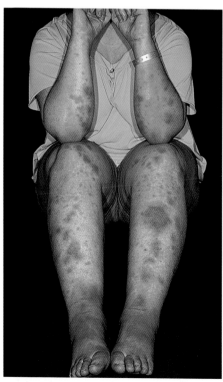

Red node-like swelling in the characteristic distribution.

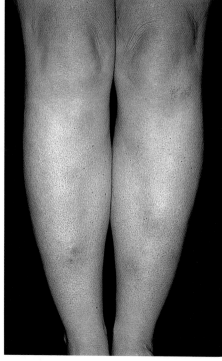

Lesions begin as red node-like swellings over the shins; as a rule, both legs are affected. The border is poorly defined, with size varying from 2 cm to 6 cm.

Cutaneous Small Vessel Vasculitis (Hypersensitivity Vasculitis)

Description

- Cutaneous small vessel vasculitis describes a group of disorders characterized by inflammation of small blood vessels in the skin, primarily post capillary venules. The principle skin lesion is palpable purpura.

History

- Cutaneous small vessel vasculitis is precipitated by many infectious agents, drugs, chemicals and food allergens (see Box 11.2) and is associated with many chronic connective tissue diseases and malignancies (see Box 11.3).
- In 60% of patients, no precipitating agent or coexistent disease is identified.
- Cutaneous small vessel vasculitis is caused by deposition of immunoglobulin G or immunoglobulin M immune complexes in small post-capillary venules.

Skin Findings

- Early lesions show minimal blood vessel damage and are seen as asymptomatic purpuric macules.
- With time and more vessel damage, lesions coalesce and become edematous and palpable, ranging in size from less than a millimeter to several centimeters. Purpuric papules, nodules, pustules, vesicles, bullae, and ulcerations can occur.
- Lesions may occur on any dependent area or an area under local pressure (e.g. the back and arms of supine patients). They are uncommon on the face, palms and soles.
- Lesions can be itchy, painful and occur in crops.
- Frequently, patients develop ankle and lower leg edema.

Non-skin Findings

- Commonly, arthralgias, myalgias, fever, and malaise accompany each crop of lesions.
- Immune complexes deposit in the kidneys, gastrointestinal tract, lungs, heart, nervous system, joints, and eyes, causing multiorgan damage.

Laboratory and Biopsy

- Laboratory testing should be directed by history and physical exam findings. Baseline laboratory testing should examine other organ systems for the presence of vasculitis and coexistent disease. Initial screening should include: a chest radiograph, a complete blood count, liver enzymes, total protein, blood urea nitrogen, creatinine, electrolytes, serum calcium, uric acid, erythrocyte sedimentation rate, antinuclear antibody and urinalysis.
- The erythrocyte sedimentation rate is always elevated during active vasculitis.
- A skin biopsy will show leukocytoclastic vasculitis.

Differential Diagnosis

- Thrombocytopenic purpura
- Drug eruptions
- Disseminated intravascular coagulation
- Purpura fulminans
- Septic vasculitis
- Septic emboli
- Bacteremia

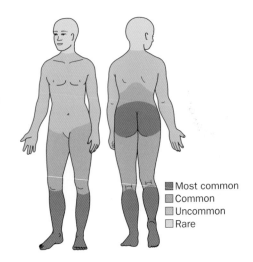

- Most common
- Common
- Uncommon
- Rare

Box 11.2 Precipitating Agents for Cutaneous Small Vessel Vasculitis

Infections

Bacteria
Beta-hemolytic *Streptococcus* group A
Staphylococcus aureus

Viruses
Hepatitis A, B, and C viruses
Herpes simplex virus
Influenza virus

Fungi
Candida albicans

Protozoa
Plasmodium malaria

Helminths
Schistosoma haematobium
Schistosoma mansoni
Onchocerca volvulus

Drugs
Insulin
Penicillin

Hydantoins
Streptomycin
Aminosalicylic acid
Sulfonamides
Thiazides
Phenothiazines
Vitamins
Phenylbutazone
Quinine
Streptokinase
Tamoxifen
Anti-influenza vaccines
Oral contraceptives
Serum

Chemicals
Insecticides
Petrolatum products

Foodstuff allergens
Milk proteins
Gluten

Adapted from Lotti T, Ghersetich I, Comacchi C, Jorizzo JL (1998) Cutaneous small-vessel vasculitis. *J Am Acad Dermatol* 39:667–87.

Box 11.3 Conditions Associated with Cutaneous Small Vessel Vasculitis

Chronic diseases
Systemic lupus erythematosis
Sjögren syndrome
Rheumatoid arthritis
Behçet's disease

Hyperglobulinemic states
Cryoglobulinemia
Bowel bypass syndrome
Ulcerative colitis
Cystic fibrosis
Primary biliary cirrhosis
Human immunodeficiency virus seropositivity and acquired immunodeficiency syndrome

Malignant neoplasms
Lymphoproliferative disorders
Hodgkin's disease
Mycosis fungoides
Lymphosarcoma
Adult T cell leukemia
Multiple myeloma

Solid tumors
Lung cancer
Colon carcinoma
Renal cancer
Prostate cancer
Head and neck cancer
Breast cancer

Adapted from Lotti T, Ghersetich I, Cornacchi C, Jorizzo JL (1998) Cutaneous small-vessel vasculitis. *J Am Acad Dermatol* 39:667–87.

Course and Prognosis

- Cutaneous small vessel vasculitis usually subsides within 1 month. However, some patients develop chronic, intermittent crops of lesions for years.

Treatment

- Removal of precipitating agents and appropriate treatment of coexistent disease usually results in resolution of cutaneous small vessel vasculitis.
- Local measures using topical steroids and antibiotics help some patients.
- Antihistamines and nonsteroidal anti-inflammatory drugs are useful to control fever, myalgias and arthralgias.
- Systemic corticosteroids (prednisone 60–80 mg/day) are helpful for managing systemic manifestations and skin ulceration. Rebound can be prevented with a slow taper over 3–6 weeks.
- Immunosuppressive agents (cyclophosphamide, methotrexate, azathioprine and cyclosporine) have been used when systemic corticosteroids fail.

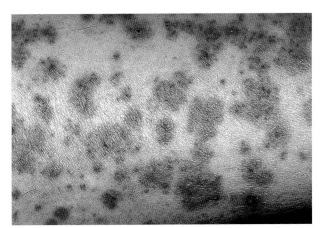

Purpura is the first sign of hypersensitivity vasculitis. Lesions vary in size from pinpoint to several centimeters. They then become papular, nodular, vesicular, bullous, pustular, or ulcerated as superficial infarctions occur. This gives the lesions substance which can be palpated, thus the term palpable purpura.

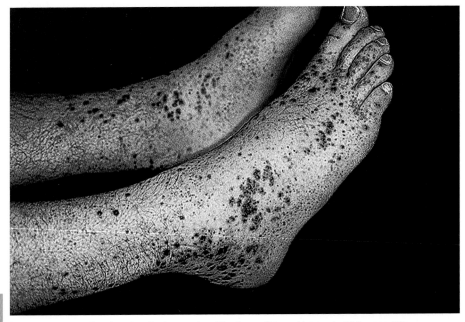

Purpura are most often found on the lower extremities in small vessel hypersensitivity vasculitis.

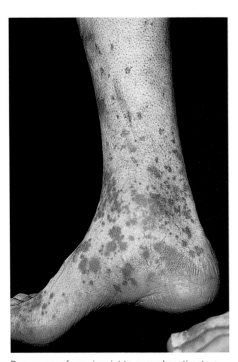

Purpura vary from pinpoint to several centimeters. This is an early case with little swelling.

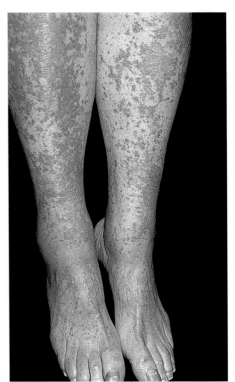

A few to numerous discrete, purpuric lesions are most commonly seen on the lower extremities, but may occur on any dependent area, including the back if the patient is bedridden, or the arms.

Lesions are most often found on the legs and about the ankles. They appear in crops and are all in the same stage. Edema usually occurs soon after the appearance of the palpable purpura. Lesions are mildly pruritic or painful. They resolve in 3 or 4 weeks and leave hyperpigmentation and atrophic scars.

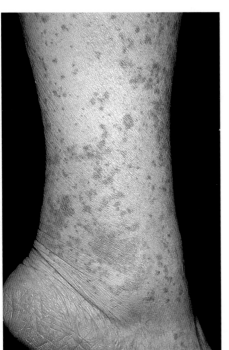

Henoch–Schönlein Purpura

Description

- Henoch-Schönlein purpura is a leukocytoclastic small vessel vasculitis due to deposition of immunoglobulin A immune complexes in postcapillary venules. It occurs primarily in children.
- Henoch-Schönlein purpura is characterized by palpable purpura, joint pain, abdominal pain, and glomerulonephritis.

History

- Henoch-Schönlein purpura and Kawasaki disease are the two most common forms of childhood vasculitis. Some 90% of all Henoch-Schönlein purpura occurs in children less than 10 years of age. Boys between 4-8 years of age are at highest risk.
- The peak incidence is during the winter months. Henoch-Schönlein purpura commonly follows an acute respiratory illness by 1-2 weeks, suggesting that infection is an important initiating factor.

Skin Findings

- Skin lesions begin as symmetric pink to red macules that quickly evolve into purpuric papules.
- They are pinhead sized to 2 cm and characteristically occur on the buttocks and lower extremities.
- Like other forms of cutaneous small vessel vasculitis, Henoch-Schönlein purpura lesions occur in crops and fade within 2 weeks.
- Edema of the hands and feet can be prominent.
- Children less than 3 years of age can develop striking edema around the eyes, scalp, and ears.

Non-skin Findings

- Up to 2 weeks before the onset of purpura, 40% of children develop low-grade fever, headache, arthralgias, and abdominal pain.
- Arthralgias (80%), abdominal pain (70%), renal changes (45%) are the most commonly affected extracutaneous organs.
- Rarely, patients develop other system disorders, of the central nervous system (seizures and neurological deficits) pulmonary (pulmonary hemorrhage), cardiac (myocarditis), hepatomegaly, parotitis, adrenal necrosis, and hydrops of the gallbladder.
- Less than 5% of children are at risk for massive gastrointestinal bleeding and ilio-ileal intussusception (especially older children).
- Boys can develop scrotal edema. Scrotal pain can occur prior to the purpura, making it difficult to distinguish from testicular torsion.

Laboratory and Biopsy

- Diagnosis is based on the typical clinical features.
- In atypical cases, a skin biopsy will show leukocytoclastic vasculitis. A skin biopsy should be sent for direct immunofluorescence, looking for immunoglobulin A immune complex deposition.
- Helpful initial laboratory tests include complete blood count, coagulation studies, blood urea nitrogen, creatinine, liver enzymes, bilirubin, amylase, lipase, and urinalysis.

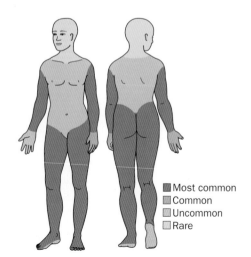

Most common
Common
Uncommon
Rare

- Patients with severe abdominal pain should be evaluated for intussusception with an abdominal ultrasound. Further diagnostic evaluation should be done in consultation with a specialist in gastroenterology and/or surgery.
- Patients with high blood pressure or laboratory signs of nephritis should be seen in consultation with a nephrologist.

Differential Diagnosis

- Bacterial sepsis
- Hemolytic uremic syndrome
- Post-streptococcal glomerulonephritis
- Rocky Mountain spotted fever or other rickettsial disease
- Other forms of cutaneous small vessel vasculitis

Course and Prognosis

- Most children have self-limited disease, lasting less than 1 month.
- Long-term prognosis may be determined by the degree of renal involvement.

Treatment

- Non-steroidal anti-inflammatory drugs can be helpful to manage arthralgias.
- Systemic corticosteroids and immunosuppressive agents may be indicated in patients with severe renal and gastrointestinal complications.
- Care must be given when they are used for gastrointestinal symptoms, since they can mask symptoms of intussusception and intestinal perforation.

Pediatric Considerations

- Quick referrals should be made to the appropriate specialists in children with severe abdominal pain and evidence of nephritis.
- Children should be followed closely for renal involvement, checking blood pressure and urinalysis for 3 months after the purpura resolves.

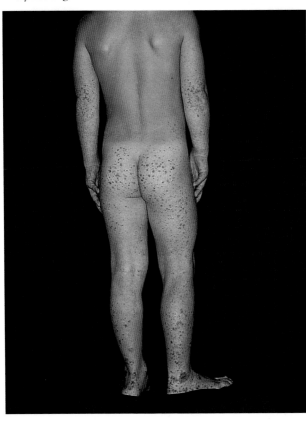

Henoch-Schönlein purpura is a systemic vasculitis characterized by palpable purpura, colicky abdominal pain, gastrointestinal hemorrhage, arthralgias, and renal involvement. Palpable purpura are most often seen on the lower extremities and buttocks but they may appear on the upper body.

Schamberg's Disease (Schamberg's Purpura)

Description

■ Schamberg's disease, a form of progressive pigmented purpura, is a lymphocytic capillaritis characterized by petechiae and brown purpuric patches, occurring most commonly on the lower extremities.

History

■ Schamberg's disease slowly evolves on the distal lower extremities and progresses proximally.

■ In adults, men are more commonly affected. In children, girls are more commonly affected.

■ Schamberg's disease is a lymphocytic capillaritis, suggesting a cell-mediated hypersensitivity.

Skin Findings

■ Patients develop multiple distinct orange-brown, pinhead-sized "cayenne pepper" macules with numerous petechiae. Lesions occur symmetrically on the lower extremities and sometimes on the upper body.

■ New petechiae are bright red, becoming violaceous with age and leaving brown dots of hemosiderin pigmentation.

■ Schamberg's disease can be asymmetric, especially when seen in adolescence.

■ There may be a slight amount of erythema, scale and itching.

Non-skin Findings

■ Schamberg's disease is an isolated skin disorder.

Laboratory and Biopsy

■ Laboratory testing is not necessary.

■ A skin biopsy can be done to exclude leukocytoclastic vasculitis.

■ Skin microscopy shows a perivascular mononuclear cell infiltrate with extravasated red blood cells.

Differential Diagnosis

■ Cutaneous T cell lymphoma
■ Nummular eczema
■ Scurvy
■ Senile purpura
■ Contact dermatitis
■ Drug-induced purpura
■ Stasis dermatitis
■ Facticial dermatitis

Course and Prognosis

■ Schamberg's disease is a chronic condition without internal disease. The vast majority of patients improve with time.

Treatment

■ Pigmentation can be covered with cosmetic creams such as DermaBlend.

■ There are no consistently effective therapies, although the following have been administered:
  ● Group V topical steroids
  ● Pentoxifylline (Trental) 300 mg per day for 8 weeks
  ● Rutoside (oral bioflavonoid) 50 mg twice daily and ascorbic acid 500 mg twice daily for 4 weeks

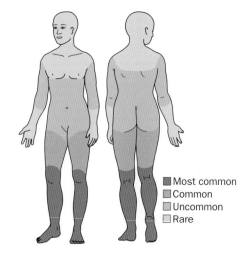

■ Most common
□ Common
□ Uncommon
□ Rare

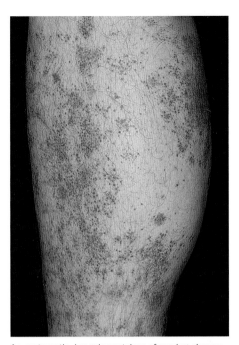

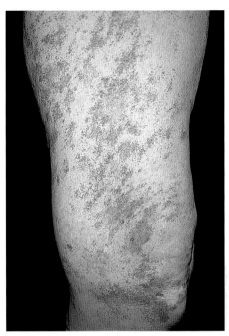

Asymptomatic, irregular patches of varying shapes and sizes occur most often on the lower extremities. The most characteristic feature is the orange-brown, pin-sized "cayenne pepper" spots.

The lesions begin as asymptomatic, localized areas of cutaneous hemorrhage that acquire substance and become palpable as blood leaks out of damaged vessels.

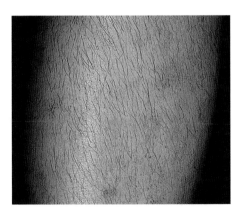

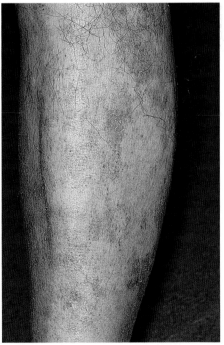

These changes are more subtle and resemble the hyperpigmentation seen with stasis dermatitis.

The distribution is haphazard. The "cayenne pepper" spots are not as prominent as is seen in the above figures.

Sweet's Syndrome

Description

■ Sweet's syndrome is an acute inflammatory eruption characterized by multiple pink to red tender plaques, associated with fever, malaise, and leukocytosis.

History

■ Sweet's syndrome occurs in adults of all ages (mean age 56 years) but is uncommon in children.

■ The disease onset is preceded by an upper respiratory infection in many patients.

■ Sweet's syndrome is paraneoplastic (hematologic malignancy, solid tumors) in 15–20% of patients and may precede the malignancy by up to 6 years.

■ Paraneoplastic Sweet's syndrome can affect mucous membranes, tends to be recurrent, and occurs more commonly in males.

■ Other associated conditions include streptococcal infection, inflammatory bowel disease, autoimmune disorders (Hashimoto's thyroiditis, Sjögren syndrome), myelodysplastic syndrome and acute myelomonocytic leukemia.

■ Sweet's syndrome has been associated with pregnancy.

Skin Findings

■ Sweet's syndrome lesions erupt acutely and can be painful. They are plum-colored and "juicy" (pseudovesicular) in appearance.

■ They can occur on any skin surface, but tend to occur on the head, neck, legs, arms, dorsal hands, and fingers.

Non-skin Findings

■ Systemic symptoms include fever higher than 38° C (50%), malaise, arthralgias or arthritis (62%), eye involvement (conjunctivitis, episcleritis, iridocyclitis) (33%), and oral aphthae (13%).

■ Rarely, neutrophilic infiltrates occur within the upper respiratory tract, lungs, liver, kidneys, and brain.

Laboratory and Biopsy

■ Common laboratory abnormalities include white blood cell count of > 8000 cells/ml with more than 70% polymorphonuclocytes, increased erythrocyte sedimentation rate, and elevated alkaline phosphatase (40%).

■ Skin biopsy shows an abundance of neutrophils in the dermis with marked subepidermal edema without vasculitis.

Differential Diagnosis

■ Erythema multiforme
■ Erythema nodosum
■ Adverse drug reaction
■ Urticaria

Course and Prognosis

■ Sweet's syndrome can be self-limiting in some patients.

■ Sweet's syndrome responds quickly to systemic corticosteroids. Typically, laboratory values correct within 72 hours and skin lesions clear within 3–9 days.

■ A minority of patients (15%) develop relapses for several years.

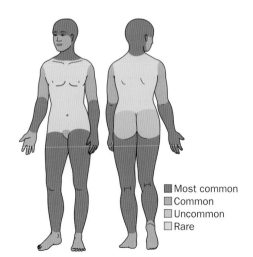

■ Most common
□ Common
□ Uncommon
□ Rare

Treatment

- Systemic corticosteroids (prednisone 0.5–1.5 mg/kg/day) produce rapid improvement and can be tapered over 2–6 weeks.
- Minocycline 100 mg twice a day, or doxycycline 100 mg twice a day, may be effective.
- Oral potassium iodide 15 mg/kg/day inhibits neutrophil chemotaxis and equals systemic corticosteroids in effectiveness.
- Other therapies include colchicine, dapsone, clofazimine, non-steroidal anti-inflammatory agents, and cyclosporine.

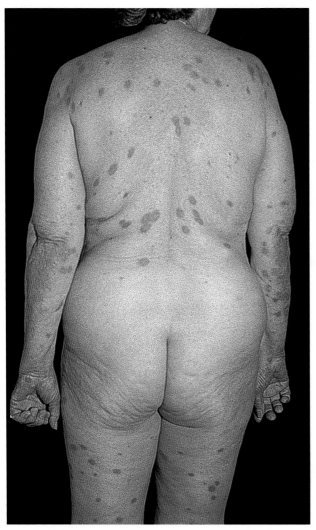

Acute, tender, erythematous plaques, nodes, pseudovesicles and, occasionally, blisters with an annular or arciform pattern occur on the extremities. The trunk is sometimes involved in extensive cases.

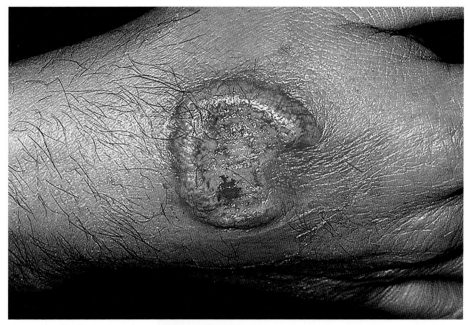

Skin lesions are tender erythematous papules and plaques that also can be pseudovesicular or pustular. Pustules occur on or adjacent to the lesions. Lesions tend to be multiple, but isolated lesions are seen. Plaques usually measure a few centimeters, but larger lesions up to 20 cm in diameter occur.

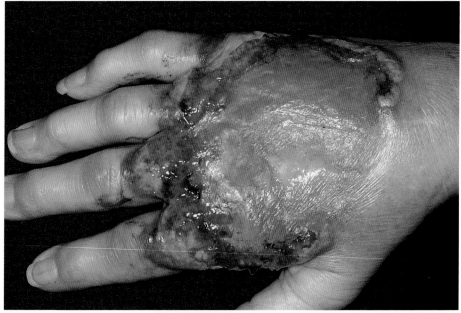

Atypical Sweet's syndrome (also known as neutrophilic dermatosis of the dorsal hands) is a recently described disorder. Severely painful, purulent blue to purple nodules and plaques frequently accompanied by ulceration occur on the dorsal hands. Oral corticosteroids are effective, antibiotics are not.

Panniculitis

Description
■ Panniculitis refers to a group of disorders that cause inflammation of the subcutaneous fat.

History
■ Typically panniculitis occurs in association with an underlying systemic disorder or in association with a cutaneous disease. Rarely, panniculitis occurs as a primary idiopathic process.

Skin Findings
■ Panniculitis manifests as discrete pink to deep red, tender nodules and firm plaques.
■ Some forms of panniculitis cause extensive skin necrosis and breakdown (calciphylaxis).

Non-skin Findings
■ Non-skin findings vary with the type of panniculitis.

Laboratory and Biopsy
■ Laboratory evaluation should be guided by the history and physical examination.
■ In most patients, a skin biopsy is an essential part of the diagnostic evaluation for panniculitis. An early lesion should be biopsied deep enough to include full-thickness skin and abundant fat. A deep excisional biopsy provides an adequate specimen.

Differential Diagnosis
Selected forms of panniculitis include:
■ Erythema nodosum
■ Alpha 1-antitrypsin deficiency panniculitis
■ Cold-induced panniculitis
■ Neonatal subcutaneous fat necrosis
■ Pancreatic panniculitis
■ Lupus panniculitis
■ Sarcoidosis
■ Calcifying panniculitis of renal failure (calciphylaxis)
■ Fungal and bacterial panniculitis
■ Polyarteritis nodosa
■ Lipodermatosclerosis
■ Leukemia and lymphoma

Course and Prognosis
■ The course and prognosis depends upon the type of panniculitis.

Treatment
■ Panniculitis associated with an underlying systemic condition improves with treatment of the condition. Other forms of panniculitis (erythema nodosum and cold-induced panniculitis) are self-limiting and do not require anything more than symptomatic treatment (see section 11.4 Erythema Nodosum).

12 Infestations and Bites

Scabies

Description
- Scabies is an intensely pruritic contagious infestation.
- It is caused by the mite *Sarcoptes scabiei* var. *hominis*.
- Historically, scabies is the most likely cause of "the seven-year itch."

History
- Patients with scabies complain of unremitting itching and cannot stop scratching, even while being examined.
- It is uncommon for scabies to present in just one member of a family. Usually, other members, especially bed partners, will also be symptomatic.
- Nodular lesions take the longest to heal.
- Crusted scabies (thousands of mites) may be the source of epidemic scabies or seen in institutionalized patients.
- Persistent itching after adequate treatment is due to a prolonged allergic response.

Skin Findings
- A burrow is the classic lesion of scabies; it is a linear, curved, or S-shaped slightly elevated vesicle or papule up to 1-2 mm wide.
- Burrows are most likely to be found in the finger webs, wrists, sides of the hands and feet, the penis, buttocks and scrotum, and the palms and soles of infants.
- Scabies may also present with scattered inflamed pustules, vesicles, papules and even larger nodules.
- Individual lesions may be excoriated.
- Scabies rash appears 2-6 weeks after exposure.
- Typical locations are the wrists, web space of the hands, sides of hands and feet, the genital area, warm intertriginous regions, and the abdomen.
- In infants, the scalp, palms, and soles are affected more often.
- Eczema and impetigo may appear as secondary lesions.
- A unique, advanced clinical variant is crusted (Norwegian) scabies. Patients— usually those with dementia, Down syndrome, and immunosuppression— experience thick crusting and eczematous dermatitis, especially on the hands and feet. These lesions contain numerous mites.

Laboratory
- Mites, eggs, or feces can be identified in a scabies preparation.
- Potassium hydroxide and heat will make mites easier to identify but will destroy mite feces.
- Mineral oil is applied to a burrow, vesicle, or papule to preserve the mite feces. The burrow is scraped with a #15 blade, rubbed on a glass slide, and a coverslip placed on top.

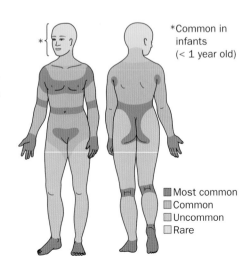

*Common in infants (< 1 year old)

■ Most common
□ Common
□ Uncommon
□ Rare

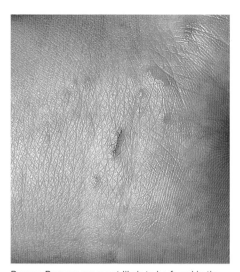

Burrow. Burrows are most likely to be found in the finger webs, wrists, sides of the hands and feet, the penis, buttocks, scrotum, and the palms and soles of infants.

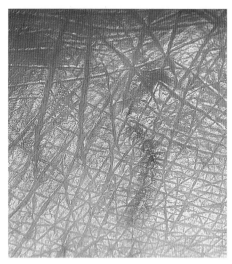

Burrow. The linear, curved or S-shaped burrows are approximately as wide as #2 suture material and are 2–15 mm long. A drop of ink can accentuate them.

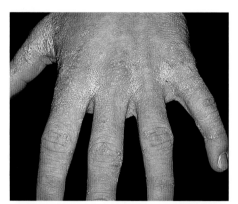

Vesicles and papules. Vesicles are isolated, pinpoint, and filled with serous rather than purulent fluid. The fact that they remain discrete is a key point in differentiating scabies from other vesicular diseases such as poison ivy.

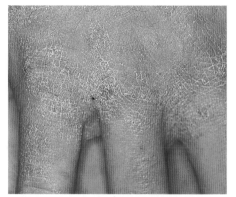

Secondary lesions result from infection or are caused by scratching. Scaling, erythema, and all stages of eczematous inflammation occur as a response to excoriation or to irritation caused by overzealous attempts at self-medication.

Differential Diagnosis

- Insect bites
- Eczema
- Impetigo
- Folliculitis
- Lymphomatoid papulosis

Treatment

- Permethrin (Elimite, Acticin) or lindane (Kwell) is applied to the entire skin surface from the neck down, including under the fingernails and toenails, and in the umbilicus. The patient should bathe after about 12 hours. This regimen should be repeated in 1 week. Lindane should be used with caution in infants because of reports of neurotoxicity.
- The head and neck are uncommonly affected, but if lesions are present here and need treatment, care should be taken to avoid the eyes and mouth.
- All clothes and bedding must be washed in hot water or put in a hot dryer at the time of application.
- There is no need for fumigation or extermination of the house.
- A single dose of oral ivermectin (Stromectol 6 mg scored tablet) (200 μg/kg) is also safe and effective for most patients. Repeating the dose 2 weeks later may provide a higher cure rate. Ivermectin and topical treatment provide a higher cure rate.
- There may be an association between the use of ivermectin and increased risk of death in the elderly. Therefore ivermectin should be used with caution in the treatment of scabies in the elderly, pending clarification of this association.
- Topical steroids may be used to control pruritus and inflammation after treatment with a scabicide.
- Persistent nodular lesions can be treated with intralesional steroids.

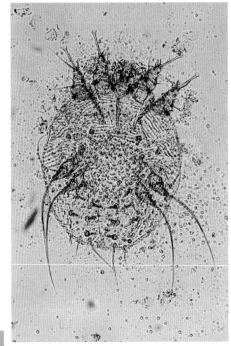

Sarcoptes scabiei in a potassium hydroxide wet mount (× 40).

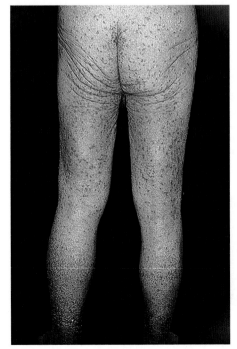

Elderly man with scabies. Infestation became much worse after treatment with topical steroids.

Pearls

- Scabies should be considered for any generalized itchy eruption unresponsive to prednisone or any pruritic rash that gets worse with steroid treatment.
- Itching that is worse at night is a cardinal feature.

- Even adequately treated scabies may continue to itch for days to weeks after treatment, and does not need to be retreated in all cases. Re-scraping should be performed.

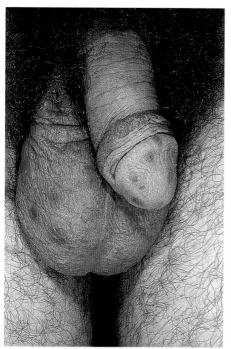

Secondary lesions. Nodules occur in covered areas such as the buttocks, groin, scrotum, penis, and axillae. Nodules on the penis and scrotum are highly characteristic of scabies.

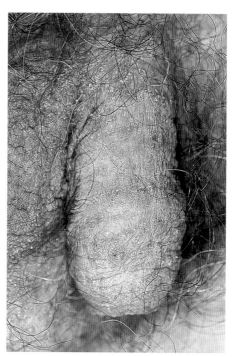

Secondary lesions dominate the clinical picture in this case. Pustules, scaling, and erythema accompany this heavy infestation of mites.

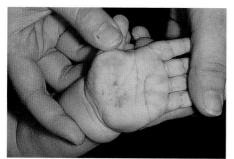

Infants can develop vesicles and pustules on the palms and soles.

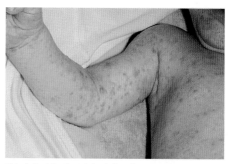

This infant had an infestation for over three months. Numerous lesions are present in all areas.

Lice (Pediculosis)

Description

- Lice are flattened, wingless insects that infest the hair of the scalp, body and pubic region.
- Each variety prefers a specific region of the body.
- Lice have three pairs of legs located on the anterior part of the body directly behind the head. The legs terminate in sharp claws that are adapted for feeding, permitting the louse to grasp and hold firmly on to hair or clothing.
- Lice attach to the skin and feed on human blood. They lay eggs on hair shafts.
- Nits are white hard oval lice eggs attached to the hair shaft.
- Rarely, lice can transmit disease, such as epidemic typhus and relapsing fever.
- An infestation by *Pediculus humanus* var. *capitis* causes head lice.
- An infestation by *Pediculosis corporis* is known as body lice.
- An infestation by *Phthirus pubis* is known as pubic lice.

Head Lice

- Head lice infestation is highly contagious.
- Direct contact is the primary source of transmission.
- Lice appear in the scalp hair more often in children.
- Lice are obligate human parasites so they cannot survive on other animals or furniture.
- The head louse does not carry any known human disease.
- Lice feed or suck blood every 3–6 hours.
- They live for about 1 month; females lay 7–10 eggs a day.
- Eggs, or nits, are firm casts cemented to the shaft, about 1 cm from the scalp surface.
- Nits hatch in 8–10 days.
- Additional information can be found at the website for the National Pediculosis Association (http://www.headlice.org).

History

- Head lice infestation is typically diagnosed by a school teacher or a school nurse.
- Girls are affected more often than boys.
- Fomite transmission via hats, brushes, or ear phones is common.
- Infestation may cause mild itching at the nape of the neck to no symptoms at all.
- Posterior cervical adenopathy is occasionally noted.
- Infestation is rare in black people.
- Infestation of the eyelashes is usually only ever seen in children.

Skin Findings

- Nits are small white eggs firmly cemented to the hair.
- Nits are sometimes easier to see than lice.
- Head lice are 3–4 mm in length. They can

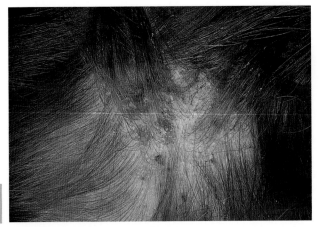

Pediculosis capitis. Head lice are most often found in the occipital areas. Nits are deposited on the shaft about 1 mm above the scalp surface. Itching in children is often intense. It is worse at night when the lice are feeding. Excoriated lesions may become infected. Serum and crust then appear with regional lymphadenopathy.

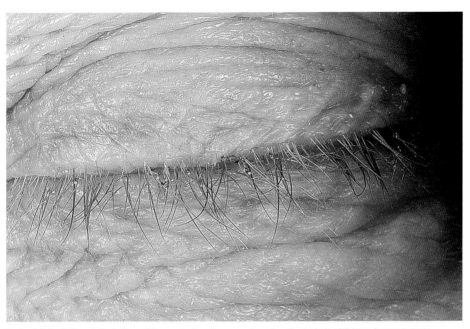

Eyelash infestation. Infestation of the eyelashes is seen almost exclusively in children. It may induce blepharitis with lid pruritus, scaling, crusting, and purulent discharge.

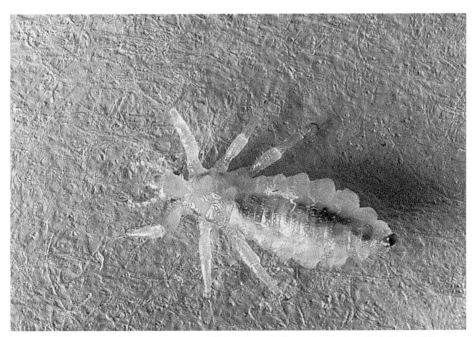

Body louse. Three kinds of lice infest humans. All three have similar anatomic characteristics. Each is a small (less than 2 mm) flat, wingless insect with three pairs of legs located on the anterior part of the body directly behind the head. The legs terminate in sharp claws that are adapted for feeding and permit the louse to grasp and hold firmly on to hair or clothing. The body louse is the largest of the three and is similar in shape to the head louse.

be seen on the hair shafts and scalp with careful observation.

- Diagnosis is usually not difficult, but may require repeated examinations.
- Head lice have an elongated body, similar to a body louse, though smaller.
- Honey-colored crusting or secondary impetigo and adenopathy occur if the papules become infected.
- Infestation may induce blepharitis with lid pruritus, scaling, crusting, and purulent discharge.
- Nits are fluorescent. School nurses use a Wood's light to screen children.

Differential Diagnosis
- Seborrheic dermatitis
- Impetigo
- Insect bites

Treatment
Standard Topical
- Permethrin rinse 1% (Nix creme rinse), an over-the-counter preparation, is often the drug of first choice.
- Synergized pyrethrin shampoos and creams (RID mousse, RID shampoo, A-200, Barc) can be purchased over the counter.
- Permethrin 5% (Elimite) is administered for treatment failures. It is left on the hair overnight under a shower cap.
- Lindane (Kwell) shampoo is left in for 5 minutes and then washed out; treatment is repeated in 1 week. It is used if over-the-counter treatment fails. Lindane-resistant lice have emerged.
- Malathion lotion 0.5% (Ovide) is rapidly pediculicidal and ovicidal. It is useful for the treatment of head lice resistant to pyrethrins and permethrin. The lotion is applied for 8–12 hours; it should be applied 7–9 days later if necessary.
- Strains resistant to synergized pyrethrins such as permethrin and lindane have emerged.
- The use of all agents should be repeated in 1 week, because younger lice may not be eradicated.
- Combing through hair with a special nit comb is also helpful in the week following treatment.
- Treatment of all close family members is controversial, but frequently recommended.

Alternative Therapies or "Home Remedies"
- Petrolatum (Vaseline), mayonnaise, or pomades applied to scalp overnight and covered with a shower cap, smother the lice. These are difficult to remove.
- Copious amounts must be used to smother all lice. This treatment does not kill nits, so it should be repeated each week for 4 weeks.
- Hair Clean 1–2–3 hairspray is an oil that kills lice in 15 minutes.
- As a last resort, shaving the scalp can be curative.

Oral Treatments
- Ivermectin (Stromectol 6 mg scored tablet), 200 µg/kg (typical adult dose is 12 mg as a single dose), is prescribed in a single oral dose and is repeated in 10 days. It attacks invertebrate nerve and muscle cells and causes paralysis and death. It has selective activity against parasites but no systemic effects on mammals.
- Trimethoprim–sulfamethoxazole (Bactrim, Septra) kills synergistic bacteria in lice. A prolonged course may be necessary.
- Antibiotics are administered for secondary infection.

Nit Removal
- Removing nits is essential.
- Combing through hair with a special nit comb (available in pharmacies) is also helpful in the week following topical treatment.
- Clear Lice Egg Remover gel applied to the hair and combed through removes eggs that survive lice killers.
- Hair saturated with a solution of 50% vinegar and 50% water, applied and removed in 15 minutes may help to "unglue" nits.

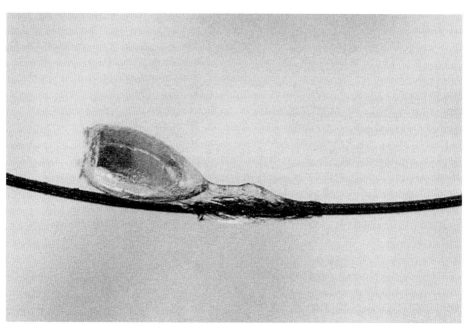

The louse egg (nit) is cemented to a hair shaft. It depends on body warmth to incubate and is therefore attached close to the scalp surface (about 1 cm above the scalp).

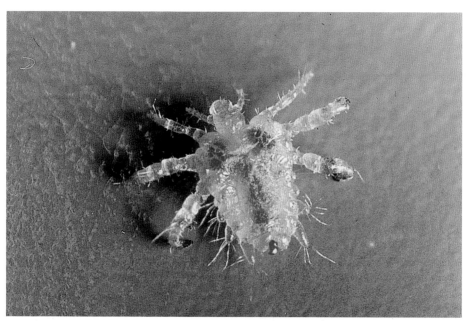

Pthirus pubis (pubic or crab louse). The crab louse is the smallest louse, with a short oval body and prominent claws that resemble those of sea crabs.

Botfly Myiasis

Description
- Myiasis is an infestation of the body tissues of animals or humans by the larval stage of non-biting flies.
- *Dermatobia hominis* causes human botfly infestation.

History
- The human botfly infestation is seen in travelers returning from Central America and South America.
- Fly larvae are deposited on the skin and penetrate to the subcutaneous tissue, where they mature into maggots.
- The larva is alive in an erythematous papule or nodule that can be mistaken as an inflamed cyst.
- Within the papule is a 1-2 mm central punctum consisting of the breathing tube of the larva.
- Many patients report discomfort and a moving sensation within the skin.
- The life cycle of the fly is unique, in that the female glues her eggs to the abdomen of a mosquito or tick, which unknowingly deposits the larvae while biting or feeding.
- At maturation, the larva exits the body and drops to the ground and matures into an adult fly.

Skin Findings
- The tender red nodule is about 2-5 mm in diameter.
- Lesions are typically found on the scalp, face or upper arms or chest.
- The larval breathing tube is mobile and can be seen opening and closing within the skin about once every minute.
- An inflamed cyst-like structure enlarges over days to weeks and is known as a "warble."

- Serous or seropurulent material can be discharged from the opening.
- Unless this nodule is inspected closely, or botfly infestation is suspected, it may be misdiagnosed.

Laboratory
- After extraction, the botfly larva appears as a juicy, white, pouch-like worm, with circular black spicules, and with a breathing tube at one end.
- There is only one larva per lesion.

Differential Diagnosis
- Inflamed or ruptured epidermal cyst
- Furuncle

Treatment
- The human botfly larva needs oxygen, so it can be forced to the surface by the application of petroleum jelly (Vaseline), Bacitracin, or bacon fat applied over the opening.
- The larva is smothered and enters the greasy trap while coming up for air. Larvae can be removed with forceps, often within 30 minutes to 3 hours after application.
- Another technique is to inject lidocaine below the larva. The pressure forces it out of the orifice.
- On occasion the opening needs to be enlarged with a #11 blade in a cross or cruciate pattern which allows easy extraction of the larvae.

Pearls
- Most cases of botfly myiasis are suspected when recent travel to Central or South America is noted.
- Another less common type of myiasis is tungiasis, caused by a red-brown sand flea called *Tunga penetrans.*
- Tungiasis is seen on the soles, toe webs, and ankles of travelers returning from Africa, or Central or South America.

A red papule 2–4 mm in diameter develops. An intense inflammatory reaction occurs in the tissue surrounding the larvae.

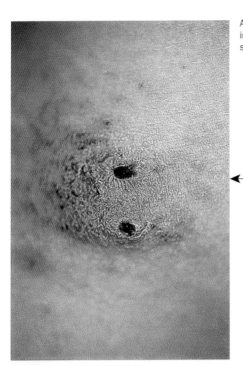

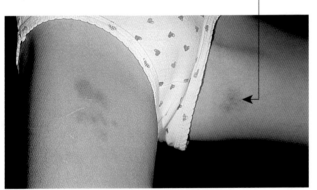

Myiasis. Lesions are found on the face, scalp, chest, arms, or legs.

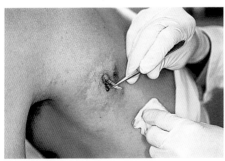

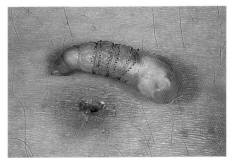

It is usually not necessary to enlarge the hole, but in this case a #11 surgical blade was used to enlarge the hole so that this very large maggot could be extracted with forceps. Xylocaine was injected into the cavity to aid in the extraction.

Bee and Wasp Stings

Description

- Honey bees are the most common source of insect stings and can cause severe allergic reactions.
- The stinger of the honey bee separates from the bee's abdomen while stinging and remains embedded in the vertebrate's tissue.
- The stingers of other bees and wasps do not detach. The detached stinger is a useful diagnostic feature for distinguishing stings of honey bees from those of other bees and wasps.

History

- The initial sharp or painful sting lasts for a few minutes and is followed by moderate burning. Symptoms resolve in a few days.
- Most reactions in children are mild.
- Children with deeper dermal reactions still have a benign course and are unlikely to have recurrent reactions.
- Severe reactions are more common in adults.
- Localized or systemic allergic reaction may develop.
- Patients sensitized by prior stings may develop large, local reactions, with edematous swelling forming hours after the sting and resolving in a few days.
- Edema is more prominent with head and neck stings.
- A toxic systemic reaction may develop hours after the sting.
- Vomiting, diarrhea, headache, fever, muscle spasm, and loss of consciousness can occur.
- Allergic anaphylactic reactions involve itching, hives, shortness of breath, wheezing, nausea, and abdominal cramps. They occur within minutes to an hour after the sting.
- Most fatal bee and wasp stings occur in a hypersensitive person older than 40 years of age and who has received a single sting on the head or neck. Deaths are caused by respiratory dysfunction or anaphylaxis.
- Delayed-onset allergic symptoms (up to 1 week after the sting) range from anaphylaxis to serum sickness.
- Multiple stings can cause death in non-allergic people.
- The median lethal dose of bee venom is estimated to be 500–1500 stings.

Skin Findings

- A hive or raised pink wheal with a central pinpoint red punctum appears minutes after the sting and lasts for about 20 minutes.
- Angioedema may occur, which is a localized reaction that appears thick, hard and edematous over an area as large as 10–50 cm.

Differential Diagnosis

- Hives
- Angioedema
- Bites from other insects

Treatment

- The stinger should be removed as fast as possible. The degree of envenomation does not differ if the stinger is scraped or pinched off. A delay of just a few seconds in removing the stinger leads to greater venom delivery.
- Localized non-allergic reactions are treated with ice and cool wet dressings, while allergic reactions may also require antihistamines.

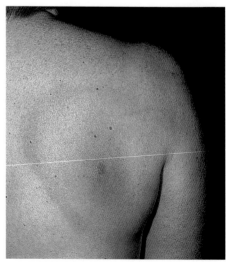

A large local allergic reaction larger than 10 cm in diameter.

- Severe generalized reactions are treated with aqueous epinephrine (adrenaline) 1 : 1000 (0.3–0.5 ml subcutaneously), which is repeated at 20-minute intervals if needed.
- If the patient is hypotensive an intravenous 1 in 10,000 dilution of epinephrine (adrenaline) can be administered.
- Intravenous methylprednisolone (Solu-Medrol) may be used for generalized reactions to reduce release of vasoactive compounds.
- Preloaded epinephrine (adrenaline) syringes kits are available (e.g. EpiPen Auto-Injector, Ana-Kit).
- An antihistamine (e.g. Benadryl) 25–50 mg can be administered orally or intramuscularly.
- Venom immunotherapy is highly effective for those with systemic reactions.

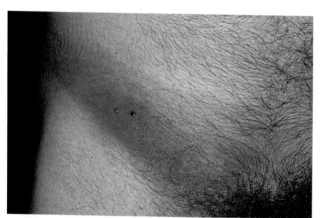

A large urticarial plaque began to occur minutes after a sting. The black spot in the center is the sting site. This lesion was intensely itching and was treated with an ice-cold wet compress.

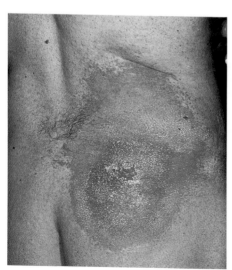

Huge urticarial plaque in a patient with a known history of bee-sting allergy.

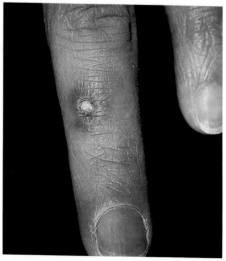

Severe local reaction with necrosis and ulceration at the site of a bee sting.

Black Widow Spider Bite

Description
- The adult female of the black widow spider (*Latrodectus mactans*) is about 3-4 cm in length and has a shiny, fat abdomen resembling a large grape.
- The black widow spider has a characteristic red hourglass-shaped marking on the ventral surface of the abdomen.
- *Latrodectus mactans* is found from the southern United States to southern New England, but related widow spiders are found in other areas of the United States and the world.
- Systemic disease is due to the envenomation of a neurotoxin. Only the females are capable of envenomation.
- The protein component of venom (alpha-latrotoxin) causes acetylcholine depletion at motor nerve endings and catecholamine release at adrenergic nerve endings, which account for the associated symptoms.

History
- The black widow spider typically encounters humans near her web in wood or lumber piles, under a log, in a crevice of a barn, or in shoes.
- This spider is not aggressive but envenomation occurs when the spider's environment is disturbed, or the spider is inadvertently trapped, or pressed against the skin.
- The initial bite reaction may be only mildly painful.
- Abdominal pain (100%), hypertension (92%), muscle complaints (75%), a target lesion (75%), and irritability or agitation (66%) are the most common symptoms.
- Migratory muscle cramps and spasm, headache, nausea, vomiting, hypertension, weakness, tremors, paresthesias, and ultimately paralysis may occur.
- Cramping abdominal pain is common and is the classic presenting complaint; it mimics an acute surgical abdomen and occurs minutes to hours after the bite.
- Symptoms may increase in severity for up to 24 hours and then slowly subside over 2-7 days.
- Residual weakness, tingling, nervousness, and muscle spasms may persist for weeks to months.
- In the young and elderly, convulsion, paralysis, and shock may occur. Death is rare.
- All symptoms are collectively known as *latrodectism*.

Skin Findings
- The clinical appearance is variable; typically, mild erythema or swelling occurs at the bite site.
- Red-brown fang marks may be seen.
- The nodes draining the bite site may become painful and enlarged.

Differential Diagnosis
- Brown recluse spider bite
- Acute surgical abdomen

Treatment
- Ice should be applied to restrict the spread of venom.
- Antivenin (*Latrodectus mactans*) for acute symptoms is given intramuscularly or intravenously. It may also be useful days (up to 90 hours) after a bite for patients with persistent symptoms (e.g. weakness, muscle cramping, orthostatic tachycardia, increased blood pressure). The severity of symptoms usually abates within 3 hours after treatment. Occasionally, retreatment is indicated.
- Calcium gluconate given intravenously for an acute abdomen acts as a muscle relaxant.
- Pain is relieved with oral or intravenous opioids and benzodiazepines.
- Muscle relaxants such as diazepam (Valium) and methocarbamol (Robaxin) may also help.

Pearls
- Patients report spider bites, especially from black widow and brown recluse spiders, much more often than they actually occur.
- When they do occur, it is the constellation of symptoms that is needed make the clinical diagnosis.
- Laboratory tests and biopsy are not helpful in confirming this diagnosis.

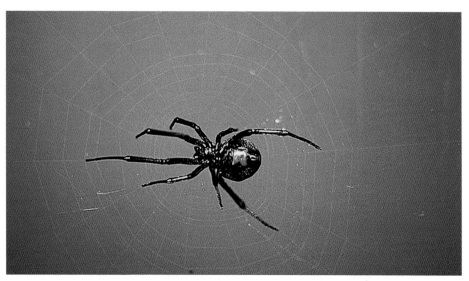

Black widow. Adult females have a total length of 4 cm and are the only spiders capable of envenomation. The female has a smooth black body, a globose abdomen that resembles an old-fashioned shoe button, long slender legs, and a red hourglass marking on the underside of the abdomen. Black widow spiders place their webs close to the ground in protected places near logs, and in dark sheltered areas such as crevices in old barns, lumber piles, and privies. They usually do not bite when away from the web because they are clumsy and need the web for support.

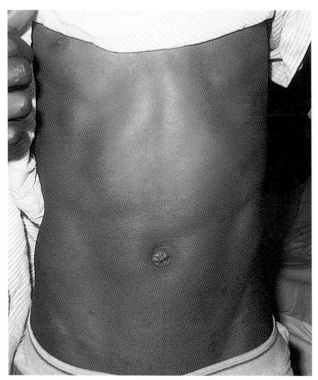

Severe muscle pain is an early sign of envenomation. Pain begins in muscles near the bite site and then occurs in large groups. Cramps and muscle contractions can occur in any muscle groups but are most severe in the abdomen. The pain can mimic appendicitis.

Brown Recluse Spider Bite

Description

■ The bite of the brown recluse spider (*Loxosceles reclusa*) may cause necrotic or dermonecrotic arachnidism.

■ The spider is yellow, tan or brown in color and can be identified by a dark brown, violin-shaped marking on its cephalothorax (hence the name the fiddle-back spider).

■ The body length is 10-15 mm, and the leg span is about 25 mm.

■ The brown recluse spider is a shy, nocturnal, non-aggressive arachnid.

■ It lives in dark areas such as woodpiles, under rocks, or in dark corners of attics, garages, or basements.

■ Most are located in the south central United States.

History

■ Humans come in contact with the spider accidentally.

■ The bite frequently goes unnoticed.

■ Localized pain, burning, and stinging occur at the bite site 6-8 hours later, as vasospasm causes local tissue ischemia.

■ Systemic symptoms—including fever, chills, nausea, vomiting, weakness, joint and muscle pain—are uncommon; they occur 12-24 hours after the bite and are not related to the extent of the local reaction.

■ Sphingomyelinase D is cytotoxic and hemolytic and is the toxin responsible for the necrosis.

■ Death rarely occurs; most patients respond well to treatment.

Skin Findings

■ The bite site may show localized hive-like reaction with minimal redness and swelling early in the course.

■ Some 10% of cases go on to develop significant necrosis.

■ A cyanotic color, followed by expanding necrosis of the skin, develops within days.

■ The most severe reaction occurs in fatty areas such as the thighs, abdomen, and buttocks.

■ The dermonecrosis can be deep and ultimately leaves an ulcer that takes weeks to months to heal.

■ Upper airway obstruction has been reported in brown recluse bites on the neck.

Laboratory and Pathology

■ Histology depends on the time the biopsy is taken.

■ Early in the course, neutrophils are present, followed by "mummified" coagulative necrosis of the epidermis, adnexae and dermis.

■ Vasculitis may occur in larger vessels, which resembles polyarteritis nodosa, and accounts for the dermonecrosis.

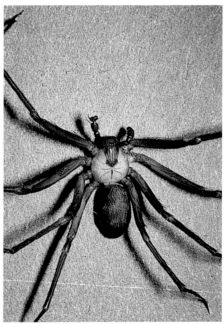

The brown recluse spider *Loxosceles reclusa* (fiddle-back spider) is small, approximately 1.5 cm in overall length. Its color ranges from yellow or tan to dark brown.

Differential Diagnosis
- Ecthyma gangrenosum
- Necrotizing vasculitis
- Necrotizing fasciitis
- Pyoderma gangrenosum
- Polyarteritis nodosa

Treatment
- The majority of bites heal with supportive care alone.
- Treat mild localized reactions with ice, cold wet dressings, elevation and mild analgesics. The cold limits the activity of sphingomyelinase D.
- Necrotic skin needs local wound and ulcer care. Surgical debridement is not usually needed.

- Antibiotics and tetanus toxoid are given when indicated.
- Dapsone 50–100 mg/day orally, may be helpful in preventing severe necrosis.
- The use of systemic steroids is controversial.

Pearls
- A high degree of suspicion is needed to make the diagnosis of brown recluse spider bite.
- Brown recluse spider bites can produce a dramatic dermonecrotic reaction that can be confused with other systemic diseases.

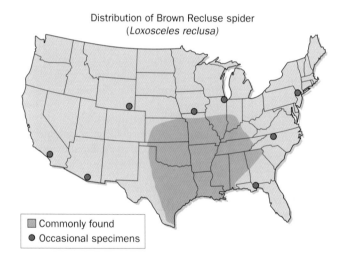

Distribution of Brown Recluse spider
(*Loxosceles reclusa*)

Commonly found
Occasional specimens

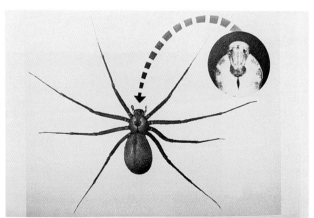

A characteristic, dark, violin-shaped or fiddle-shaped marking is located on the spider's back. The broad base of the violin is near the head, and the violin's stem points toward the abdomen.

Lyme Disease

Description
■ Lyme disease is a tick-borne disease caused by the spirochete *Borrelia burgdorferi*.
■ *Borrelia* evolves though three stages and can affect almost all organ systems.
■ The cutaneous eruption of Lyme disease is called erythema migrans.
■ In Europe there are other species of *Borrelia* which cause Lyme disease.

History
■ Like syphilis, Lyme disease affects many organ systems, occurs in stages, and mimics several other diseases.
■ Disease onset is 3–28 days after an infective tick bite.
■ The three stages may overlap or occur alone.
  ● Stage 1: there is an expanding target-like patch (erythema migrans) and influenza-like symptoms occur, including fever, headache and arthralgias.
  ● Stage 2: there are cardiac and neurologic system problems.
  ● Stage 3: arthritis and continuous chronic neurologic problems persist.

Skin Findings
■ The initial tick bite inflicts a local inflamed bite reaction. The bite may be painless and go unnoticed.
■ The tick must stay attached for at least 24 hours for infection to occur.
■ Skin changes (erythema migrans is the most characteristic) are not present in all cases.
■ Erythema migrans is a bright red expanding eruption occurring at the site of *Borrelia* inoculation.
■ It begins as a small papule with a slowly enlarging ring of erythema, which fades in 2–3 weeks leaving a normal to light blue surface.
■ The erythematous patch remains flat, blanches with pressure, and (rarely) develops vesicles. It may reach up to 10 cm or more in diameter.
■ The expanding border of erythema migrans may be slightly raised.

■ Approximately 20–50% of patients have multiple concentric rings at sites of subsequent hematogenous dissemination.

Laboratory
■ Diagnosis of Lyme disease without clinical confirmation of erythema migrans is difficult.
■ Routine laboratory studies are not helpful.
■ Serologic testing is the only practical laboratory method of diagnosing Lyme disease, but insensitivity and interlaboratory variability are frequent problems.
■ The results of serologic testing for anti-*Borrelia* antibodies by enzyme-linked immunoassay are positive at the initial presentation in 25% of infected patients and are positive in 75% of infected patients 4–6 weeks later, even with antibiotic therapy.
■ The more specific Western immunoblot test is used to corroborate equivocal or positive results obtained with the enzyme-linked immunoassay.
■ High titers of immunoglobulin G or immunoglobulin M indicates disease, but lower titers can be misleading.
■ A culture of *B. burgdorferi* is possible with tissue biopsy on modified Barbour–Stoenner–Kelly medium but this is not practical.

Differential Diagnosis
■ Tinea
■ Insect bites
■ Granuloma annulare
■ Urticaria
■ Cellulitis
■ Fixed drug eruption

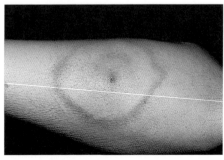

Erythema migrans. "Bull's-eye" lesion.

Treatment

- Preventing tick bites is the first line of defense.
- The patient should wear protective garments, tuck the pants into the socks, and wear closed-toed shoes.
- *N,N*-diethyl-meta-toluamide can be used on the skin, or permethrin on the clothing.
- Ticks should be detected and removed as soon as possible.
- A number of special instruments for tick removal (e.g. Ticked Off) are available.
- Adults with early Lyme disease should receive 21 days of treatment with doxycycline 100 mg twice a day, amoxicillin 500 mg three times a day, or cefuroxime axetil (Ceftin) 500 mg twice a day.
- Amoxicillin 25–50 mg/kg/day divided into three doses or cefuroxime axetil 250 mg twice a day are used for children under 8 years of age.
- Disease that has progressed to stage 2 or stage 3 may require more intensive treatment.

- Within 72 hours of discovering a deer tick that is obviously engorged, or that has been attached for more than 72 hours, on an adult from an area where Lyme disease is endemic, administer 200 mg of doxycycline as a single dose.
- Within 72 hours of discovering a deer tick that has been attached for 36–72 hours, consider 200 mg of doxycycline as a single dose.
- Where a tick has been attached for less than 36 hours, it is not necessary to treat the bite; however, some patients and physicians may prefer to treat prophylactically anyway.
- In children, the dosage and efficacy of prophylactic treatment have not been evaluated.
- Guidelines for the management of asymptomatic patients with elevated Lyme titers have not been established.

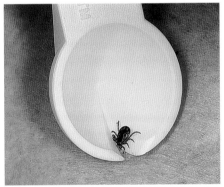

A simple plastic tool called Ticked Off removes ticks, including the mouth parts. These inexpensive tools are generally available.

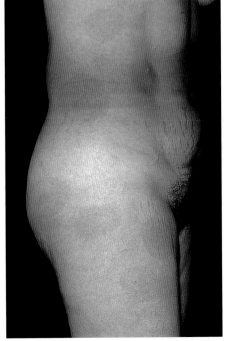

The most common configuration of the lesion is circular, but as migration proceeds over skinfolds, distortions of the configuration occur. Multiple lesions may occur.

Rocky Mountain Spotted Fever

Description

- Rocky Mountain spotted fever is a potentially lethal disease caused by *Rickettsia rickettsii*, a short Gram-negative bacillary organism.
- The infection is characterized by an acute onset of fever, a severe headache, myalgia, vomiting, and a petechial rash.
- It is transmitted by ticks, usually either *Dermacentor* or *Ixodes* species.
- Organisms disseminate via the bloodstream and multiply in vascular endothelial cells.
- This condition occurs most commonly in the South Central and Southeastern United States and Brazil, in the summer and early fall.

History

- The bite of a tick is typically painless, so the patient may not recall a recent tick bite.
- Travel to an endemic area or recent outdoor activity are helpful clues.
- The incubation period is on average 6-8 days after the bite.
- Abrupt onset of fever (95%), severe headache (90%), myalgia (85%), and vomiting (60%) occur.

Skin Findings

- The skin findings evolve and appear a few days after the fever. Signs of previous tick bite may not be found.
- The rash is discrete and macular, blanches with pressure, and becomes petechial in 2-4 days.
- It appears first on the wrists and ankles, which is characteristic.
- Hours later, the rash involves the palms and soles (75%), and then becomes generalized.
- The rash does not occur at all in about 15% of cases. Rashless or spotless disease is much more common in adults.
- The rash is difficult to see in dark-skinned patients.

Non-skin Findings

- Multiple organs are involved in severe disease

- Hepatosplenomegaly is present in 25-50% of cases.
- Neurological symptoms include seizures, meningitis, cranial nerve palsies, and paraparesis.
- Respiratory distress, abdominal pain, diarrhea, sever myalgia, myocarditis, retinal thrombosis, and edema on the dorsum on the hands and feet may occur.

Course and Prognosis

- The fever subsides in 2-3 weeks and the rash fades with residual hyperpigmentation.
- The mortality rate in treated patients is 4% and 20% in untreated patients.
- Many of those who die have a fulminant course and are dead in 1 week.

Laboratory

- The diagnosis must rely on clinical criteria (fever, rash, headache, myalgia) and tick exposure, since laboratory confirmation cannot occur before 7-14 days after the onset of illness.
- Histology has limited use in diagnosis; Giemsa stain is used but not always accurate at identifying organisms in vessels.
- Indirect fluorescent antibody tests on acute and convalescent sera are fairly accurate and can be used to confirm the diagnosis.
- Serologic evidence appears in the second week of infection. A titer greater than 1 : 128 is required.
- The leukocyte count can be high, low or normal; thrombocytopenia, an elevated serum hepatic aminotransferase level, and hyponatremia are common.

Differential Diagnosis

- Meningococcemia
- Mononucleosis, measles and other viral exanthems
- Drug eruptions
- Toxic shock syndrome
- Typhoid fever
- Vasculitis
- Kawasaki syndrome

Treatment

- Empiric treatment should be started if Rocky Mountain spotted fever is suspected.

- Doxycycline 100 mg twice a day for at least 7 days and at least 48 hours after resolution of fever is the current treatment of choice.
- Doxycycline is the most favorable agent for children younger than 9 years of age.
- Up to five courses of doxycycline may be administered with minimal risk of dental staining.
- Chloramphenicol 50 mg/kg/day is an alternative.

Pearls

- Petechial rash of the wrists and ankles, followed by involvement of the palms and soles, is characteristic.
- A therapeutic trial of doxycycline or tetracycline should be considered for any adult who has been in an endemic geographic area during the summer months and who has fever, myalgia, and headache, and who is suspected of having Rocky Mountain spotted fever.

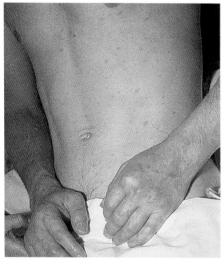

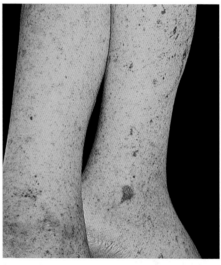

The rash is reported in 83% of cases and typically begins on the fourth day, erupting first on the wrists and ankles. Within hours it involves the palms and soles (73%) and then it becomes generalized. The rash is discrete and macular and blanches with pressure at first; it becomes petechial in 2–4 days.

A generalized petechial eruption that involves the entire cutaneous surface, including the palms and soles.

Reported cases of Rocky Mountain spotted fever, 1990

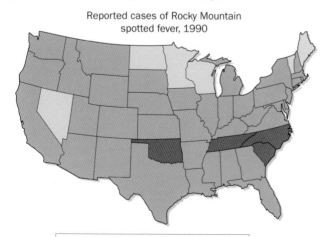

Cases per 100,000 population
☐ 0 ☐ <1.0 ■ ≥1.0 Alaska, Hawaii = 0

Flea Bites

Description
- A pruritic eruption with papules seen on the legs is typical of a flea bite.

History
- Clusters of pruritic red or purpuric papules develop on the legs; they are often grouped around the ankles.
- Pants and socks offer some protection.
- This is a self-limited, itchy eruption. Depending on the patient's sensitivity, it may subside in days to weeks.
- Flea eggs can lie dormant for over 1 year and can reactivate with vibrations from footsteps.

Skin Findings
- Initially, tiny red dots or bite puncta may be seen, often grouped around the ankles.
- Clusters of pruritic red or purpuric papules may develop on the legs.
- Red, raised urticarial lesions known as papular urticaria develop in hypersensitive patients, especially children.
- Pruritus can be intense in hypersensitive patients.
- The persistent scratching can lead to round, white scars after healing.
- Diagnosis is usually not difficult.

Description
- The flea itself is a small red-brown, hard-bodied, wingless insect.
- It is flattened laterally so that it can squeeze between the hairs of its host.

Treatment
- The bites are treated symptomatically.
- Topical antipruritics such as Sarna lotion can help.
- Infected lesions require antibiotics.
- Mild to moderately potent topical steroids are useful for treating papular urticaria.
- Fleas must be eradicated. Infested animals, animal bedding, and rugs must be treated.

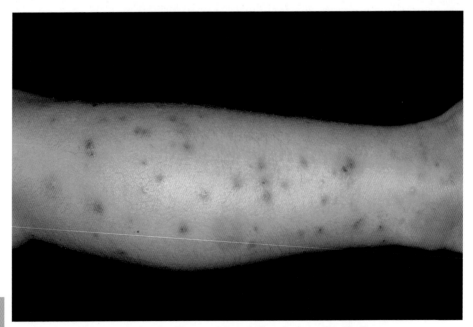

Flea bites in a child were excoriated and became infected. These lesions will heal with scars.

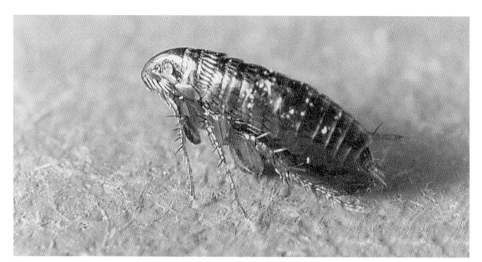

Fleas are tiny red-brown hard-bodied wingless insects that are capable of jumping approximately 60 cm. They have distinctive laterally flattened abdomens that allow them to slip between the hairs of their host. They live in rugs and on the bodies of animals, and they may jump onto humans.

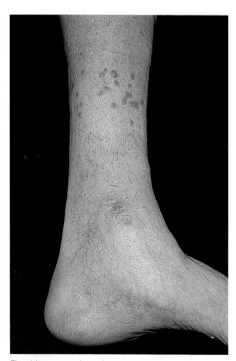

Flea bites occur in a cluster or group.

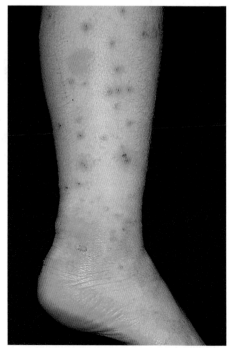

Flea bites are typically clustered about the lower leg. Fleas jump but cannot reach higher than above the calf. Children scratch bites, which causes them to persist and become infected.

Cutaneous Larva Migrans (Creeping Eruptions)

Description
- Cutaneous larva migrans is a migratory infestation most often seen on the feet.
- It is caused by the aimless wandering of the hookworm larvae within the skin.
- *Ancylostoma braziliense* is the most common species in North America.
- "Creeping eruption" is another name for this condition.

History
- The lesions typically begin about 3 weeks after a beach vacation in the Caribbean, Africa, South America, southeast Asia, or even the south-eastern United States.
- Infection can also occur in children who play in sand boxes, and in carpenters and plumbers who work under houses.
- The patient notes itchy, inflammatory, serpiginous lesions that migrate in a snake-like fashion.
- The larvae are indiscriminate, and the parasite can penetrate the skin when humans walk on moist feces-contaminated sand.
- If untreated the larvae die in 2–8 weeks, but persistence up to 1 year has been reported.
- The larvae are eventually sloughed away as the epidermis matures.
- Typically the resolution of migration and itching occurs within 2–3 days after therapy has begun.
- It may take about 1 week for the more intense allergic inflammatory response to resolve.

Skin Findings
- A local pruritic inflammatory response to the larval secretions occurs within 3 weeks of infection.
- A serpiginous red to purple lesion with a 3-mm wide tract is characteristic.
- Feet and ankles are most commonly involved, followed by buttocks, genitals and hands.
- Itching is moderate to intense, and sometimes, secondary infection and eczematous inflammation can occur.
- The worm migrates about 2 cm daily.

Non-skin Findings
- Loeffler syndrome is a possible complication of *Ancylostoma braziliense* infection and includes patchy lung infiltration and eosinophilia.

Laboratory
- Up to 30% blood eosinophil count has been reported.
- Chest x-ray may show a patchy infiltration.

Treatment
- Freezing of the leading edge of the lesion with liquid nitrogen is often ineffective.
- Ivermectin 200 µg/kg (average dose 12 mg) administered as a single oral dose is effective.
- Lesions heal within 5 days after starting ivermectin. A second round of treatment with the same dose is given for relapses.
- Albendazole (either 400 mg per day orally or 200 mg orally twice a day for 7 days) is effective and well tolerated. Its action is rapid, pruritus disappears in 3–5 days, and cutaneous lesions disappear after 6–7 days of treatment.

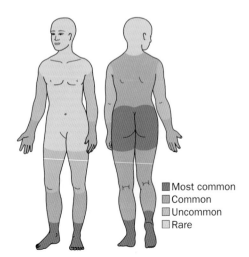

- ■ Most common
- ▨ Common
- ▧ Uncommon
- ☐ Rare

- Thiabendazole 15% in a liquid or a cream compound is applied topically three times a day for 5 days. It is applied to affected areas and 2 cm beyond the leading edge because the parasite is often located beyond the clinical lesion. The preparation is often difficult to obtain.
- Antibiotics are used for secondary infection.

- Topical or systemic steroids may be needed to treat severe pruritus.
- Typically, the resolution of migration and itching occurs within 2–3 days after therapy has begun.
- It may take a week or so for the more intense allergic inflammatory response to resolve.

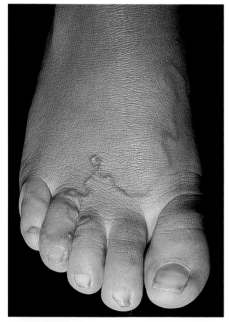

The trapped larva struggles a few millimeters to a few centimeters each day laterally through the epidermis in a random fashion, creating a tract reminiscent of the trail of a sea-snail wandering aimlessly over the sand at low tide.

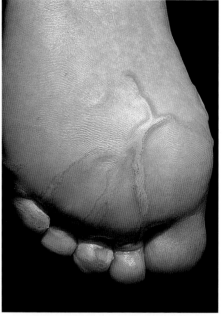

The 1-cm larva stays concealed directly ahead of the advancing tip of the wavy, twisted red to purple 3-mm tract. Any skin surface can be affected.

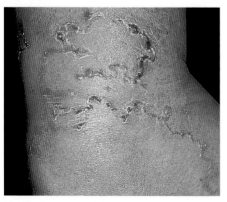

Many larvae may be present in the same area, creating several closely approximated wavy lines.

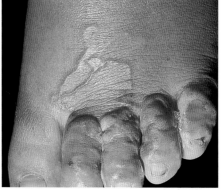

During larval migration, a local inflammatory response is provoked by the release of larval secretions. Itching is moderate to intense, and secondary infection or eczematous inflammation occurs.

Fire Ant Stings

Description

- Imported fire ants are small, colored yellow to red or black, and have large heads.
- They have prominent inward-curving jaws and stingers on their tails.
- They were imported from South America and are now established in south-eastern United States.
- They form large colonies with giant mounds.
- The bite causes a painful pustular lesion.
- Sting reactions range from local pustules and large, late-phase responses to life-threatening anaphylaxis.

History

- Initially burning and sharp pain occur at the sting site. A single ant can inflict multiple stings. The ant either runs across the skin, leaving a line of stings, or rotates around the point of mandible attachment, leaving a ring of stings.
- Children who are unaware of the danger are common victims, often receiving stings on their legs.
- An infestation of buildings with fire ants may be associated with indoor attacks.
- A systemic allergic reaction can occur, occasionally resulting in death from anaphylactic shock. This has been reported to happen with just one sting.

Skin Findings

- The classic lesion is two pinpoint red dots (the bite) surrounded by a ring of pustules (the sting).
- Edema and itching are accompanied by a wheal of 5–10 mm. Sterile vesicles form in about 4 hours, evolve into pustules in 24 hours, and resolve in 3–10 days. Lesions may scar.
- Occasionally there is a large local late-phase reaction resulting in a red, edematous, indurated, pruritic plaque which resolves in 24–72 hours.

Laboratory

- Skin testing is the most common diagnostic method for diagnosing allergy.
- A venom enzyme-linked immunoassay assay can confirm fire ant hypersensitivity.
- Imported fire ant venom-specific immunoglobulin E antibodies can be measured by radioallergosorbent assay (RAST) in patients suspected of allergic reactions.

Differential Diagnosis

- Other insect bites
- Folliculitis

Treatment

- Cool, wet dressings are helpful for comfort.
- Topical antipruritics (Sarna lotion) and oral antihistamines are usually all that are needed.
- A short course of prednisone is used only for severe local reactions.
- Immunotherapy should be considered for severe cases.

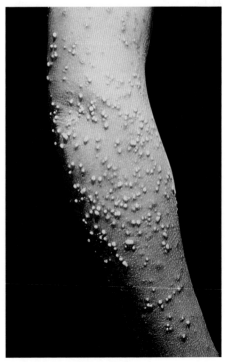

Fire ant stings. Numerous pustules occurred after a child was attacked by a large colony of ants.

Swimmer's Itch

Description

- Swimmer's itch is a pruritic inflammatory response to the larval form of non-human schistosome parasites obtained while swimming in fresh-water lakes.
- The diagnosis is often missed when this condition occurs sporadically, because of its non-specific characteristics.
- The eruption occurs in areas not covered by the swimming suit.
- It is frequently confused with sea-bather's eruption.

History

- Indiscriminate larvae (cercariae) released from a snail seek out a warm-blooded host, such as a bird or a rodent, but may accidentally penetrate human skin.
- The larvae are restricted primarily to fresh water.
- This condition occurs worldwide, but the Great Lakes area has the highest incidence in the United States.
- Cercariae die after penetration, resulting in an inflammatory skin reaction.
- The intensity of the eruption depends on the degree of sensitization.
- Initial symptoms are minor after the first exposure.
- Papules occur only after sensitization, approximately 5–13 days after the penetration.
- A typical eruption occurs with subsequent exposures.
- The eruption begins as bathing water evaporates and cercariae begin penetrating.

- Pruritus and rash reach maximal intensity in 2–3 days.
- This condition subsides without treatment in 2–3 weeks.

Skin Findings

- Itching begins in approximately 1 hour after swimming.
- It is followed hours later by discrete, highly pruritic, red, edematous, bite-like papules.
- Occasionally pustules are surrounded by erythema.
- A highly sensitive person may develop secondary urticaria, vesicles, or eczematous plaques.
- The most characteristic feature is the location of the eruption, involving areas not covered by the bathing suit.

Differential Diagnosis

- Sea-bather's eruption (occurs beneath the bathing suit) after swimming in salt water
- "Hot tub" (*Pseudomonas*) folliculitis

Treatment

- The eruption is self-limited.
- Symptoms should be relieved as the eruption fades.
- Itching is controlled with antihistamines and cool wet dressings.
- Intense inflammation is suppressed with medium-potency topical steroids.
- Antibiotics may be administered for secondary infection.
- Immediate towel drying might be effective if the eruption is anticipated, since most larvae penetrate the skin as water is evaporating.

Animal and Human Bites

History

- The type of animal, as well as the animal's behavior, should be determined.
- The patient's health status, such as immunosuppression, should be known.
- Cats have long, sharp teeth that often puncture and penetrate down to tendon and bone.
- Rabies transmission should be considered in the unprovoked attack of a wild animal or an unvaccinated domestic animal.
- Seemingly trivial bites can result in severe complications.
- Human bites from an infant or child must be distinguished from those from an adult, which may be due to child abuse.

Physical Examination and Skin Findings

- The bite site should be checked for depth and underlying injury.
- Tendon and nerve function should be tested, as well as vessel integrity.
- Body cavities and joints should be evaluated for penetration.
- Human bites from adults can be identified by the width of the dental arch, which is greater than that of toddlers (4 cm).

- Crush injury is more common in animal bites.
- Pain, erythema, purulence and swelling suggest infection.

Laboratory

- *Pasteurella* species are the most common isolates from dog and cat bites.
- Infected wounds should be cultured for aerobic and anaerobic organisms.
- Cultures taken at the time of injury are of little value.
- Crush injuries, suspected fractures, and foreign body penetrations should be examined radiographically.

Treatment

- Antibiotics are used to prevent infection.
- Cat bites with a deep puncture, wounds that require debridement, and contaminated wounds are routinely treated with antibiotics.
- Asplenic, immunocompromised elderly patients and those with diabetes are routinely treated with antibiotics.
- Empirical therapy for dog bites and cat bites should be directed against *Pasteurella* organisms, streptococci, staphylococci, and anaerobes.
- Empirical therapies include a 3–7 day course of amoxicillin–clavulanate (Augmentin); or a second-generation

cephalosporin with anaerobic activity such as cefprozil (Cefzil); or combination therapy with either penicillin and a first-generation cephalosporin such as Cefadroxil (Duricef); or clindamycin and fluoroquinolone. Longer courses are used for infected wounds.

- When given alone, azithromycin, trovafloxacin, and the new ketolide antibiotics may also be useful.
- The decision whether to close the wound is made based on the increased risk of infection versus the cosmetic benefits.
- Facial lacerations from dog or cat bites are usually closed.
- Clean wounds, or those that can be easily cleansed, are stitched immediately.
- Rabies infection is the other major consideration when dealing with animal bites.
- Wounds are irrigated with normal saline or povidone–iodine 1% solution at high pressure. Cleaning a bite with soap is as effective as cleaning with quaternary ammonium compounds in lowering the risk of transmission of rabies.
- A healthy animal should be confined and observed for 10 days.
- Any animal that behaves wildly or erratically after biting a person should be destroyed and examined histologically for rabies.
- Rabies prophylaxis is indicated if the laboratory evaluation finds that the animal was rabid or if the animal was not captured.
- Patients not previously vaccinated are given both human rabies vaccine (a series of five doses administered in the deltoid area) and rabies immune globulin (20 international units/kg). As much as possible of the rabies immune globulin should be infiltrated in and around the wound, and the remainder should be given intramuscularly at a site distant from that used for vaccine administration.
- Vaccination is prophylactic; once signs of rabies occur the chance of survival is diminished.
- Tetanus immune globulin and tetanus toxoid are given to patients who have two or fewer primary immunizations.
- Tetanus toxoid alone is given to those who have completed a primary immunization series but who have not received a booster for more than 5 years.

13 Vesicular and Bullous Diseases

Dermatitis Herpetiformis

Description
- A rare, chronic, intensely pruritic vesicular and bullous dermatosis associated with a gluten-sensitive enteropathy.

History
- It affects males and females in a ratio of 2 to 1.
- It occurs rarely in black and Asian people.
- There is increased incidence in association with human leukocyte antigens DRw3, B8, and DQw2.
- Prevalence is estimated at 11 in 100,000 to 39 in 100,000.
- Age of onset is most often between the second and fifth decades; rare in children.

Skin Findings
- Severe unremitting itching and burning.
- Clustered vesicles or excoriations are symmetrically distributed on the elbows, knees, sacrum and base of the scalp, but may be generalized.
- Intact vesicles often destroyed by scratching and are often difficult to identify.
- Although lesions are commonly vesicles, they may be erythematous papules or urticarial papules.
- Oral lesions are very uncommon.

Non-skin Findings
- Gastrointestinal involvement is usually asymptomatic.
- Changes seen with small bowel follow-through as blunting of intestinal villi.
- Small bowel biopsy shows villous atrophy.
- Less than 20% of patients malabsorb fat, D-xylose, or iron.

- The severity of skin disease does not correlate with degree of intestinal involvement.
- There is increased risk of small bowel lymphoma and non-intestinal lymphoma which is reduced with gluten-free diet.
- Hypothyroidism or thyroid disorders may be associated.

Laboratory
- Skin biopsy shows subepidermal clefting and papillary dermal tips stuffed with neutrophils and occasional eosinophils.
- An inflammatory infiltrate of neutrophils and occasional eosinophils is typical in the upper dermis.
- Direct immunofluorescence of skin biopsy is the gold standard for diagnosis.
- Biopsy is taken from adjacent normal perilesional skin.
- Granular or fibrillar immunoglobulin A deposits in dermal papillae in 90% of cases.

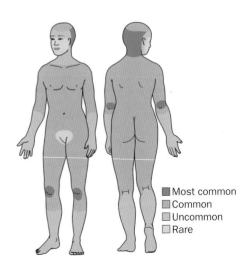

- Most common
- Common
- Uncommon
- Rare

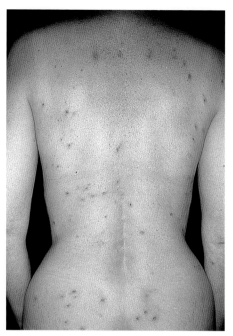

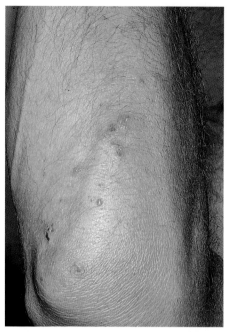

The vesicles are symmetrically distributed and appear on the elbows, knees, scalp and nuchal area, shoulders, and buttocks. The distribution may be more generalized.

Vesicles appear singly or in clusters and resemble herpes simplex. Patients scratch the vesicles to relieve itching, therefore it is often difficult to find an intact lesion to biopsy.

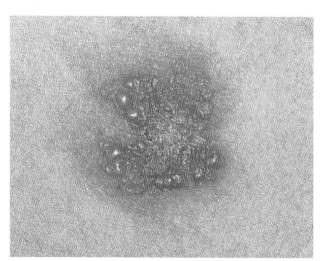

"Herpetiform" refers to the typical grouping of vesicles.

- Circulating immunoglobulin A anti-endomysial antibodies are found in the serum of 70% of patients not on a gluten-free diet.
- Serum anti-endomysial antibody titers correlate with severity of jejunal villous atrophy.

Course and Prognosis

- Typically chronic, with spontaneous remission in about a third of cases.
- Systemic iodides may aggravate dermatitis herpetiformis.
- The disease is recurrent, but usually well controlled with oral sulfones such as dapsone, or a strict gluten-free diet.

Differential Diagnosis

- Insect bites in generalized cases (usually shorter lived)
- Scabies (when excoriated, is also intensely itchy; look for burrows)
- Eczematous dermatitis prurigo

Treatment

- A gluten-free diet can control the disease alone or allow decreased requirement for oral medication.
- Strict adherence to gluten-free diet is required for many months for effective control.
- Gluten is present in all grains except rice, oats and corn. Gluten-free foods can be ordered from: ENER-G Foods Inc., 6901 Fox Ave SO, PO Box 24723, Seattle, WA 98124 0723; Tel: 1 800 331 5222.
- Motivation and dietary instruction are required for successful adherence to gluten-free diet. Gluten Intolerance Group of North America offers a newsletter and other services: PO Box 23053, Seattle, WA 98102 0353; Tel: 1 206 325 6980.
- Treatment does not alter disease duration but allows for disease control and remission.
- Oral dapsone 100–150 mg every day is the drug of choice and typically relieves itching and burning within 48–72 hours.
- Daily maintenance dose varies in the range of 25–200 mg per day.
- Obtain pretreatment glucose-6-phosphate dehydrogenase levels due to increased risk of severe hemolysis in deficient patients.
- Prudent dapsone monitoring for hemolysis, anemia, and methemoglobinemia is recommended with weekly complete blood count for 1 month and then monthly for 6 months, and semi-annually thereafter.
- Sulfapyridine 1.0–1.5 g per day is effective in some patients as an alternative to dapsone.
- Tetracycline 500 mg one to four times daily, or minocycline 100 mg twice a day and nicotinamide 500 mg two or three times a day, have been reported to be helpful in some cases.

Pearls

- Intense unremitting itching unresponsive to prednisone suggests scabies or dermatitis herpetiformis.
- Immunofluorescence confirms the diagnosis of dermatitis herpetiformis.
- Although dermatitis herpetiformis is a blistering disease, bullae are rarely seen; pruritis induces scratching, removing the vesicles and small bullae, leaving only crusted papules.

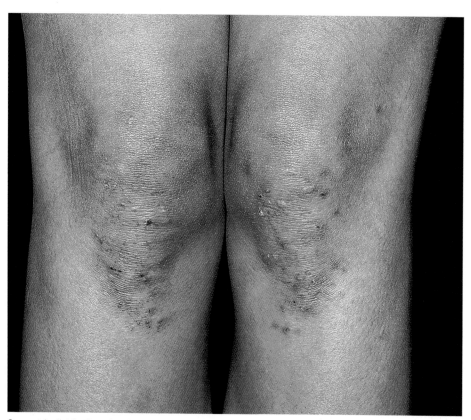

Symmetric distribution of vesicles in dermatitis herpetiformis.

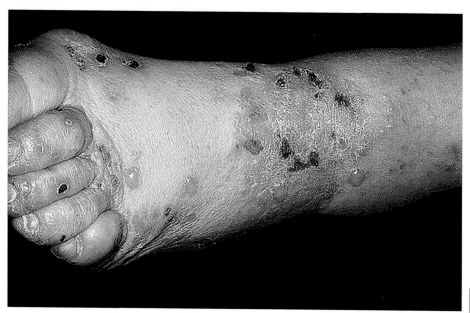

Vesicles and bullae are present in this generalized eruption.

Pemphigus Vulgaris

Description
- A rare, potentially life-threatening, autoimmune, intraepidermal blistering disease involving the skin and mucous membranes.

History
- Mean age of onset is 60 years.
- There is no gender predilection.
- Incidence is estimated at 0.5–3.2 cases per million.
- Incidence is highest in people of Ashkenazi Jewish descent.
- Oral erosions usually precede the onset of skin blisters by weeks or months.
- Itching is minimal; most patients describe tenderness or irritation.

Skin Findings
- Bullae vary from 1–3 cm in diameter.
- They appear gradually and may be localized for a considerable length of time, but become generalized if untreated.
- Bullae rupture easily because the vesicle roof, which consists of a thin portion of the upper epidermis, is very fragile.
- Application of pressure to small intact bullae causes the fluid to dissect laterally into the mid-epidermal areas altered by bound immunoglobulin G.
- Traction pressure on intact skin causes bullae formation (Nikolsky's sign).
- Exposed erosions last for weeks before healing with brown hyperpigmentation, but without scarring.
- Painful oral erosions occur in 50–70% of patients and typically precede the skin blisters by weeks or months.
- Blisters, erosions, and lines of erythema may appear in the pharynx and esophagus.

Laboratory
- Skin biopsy shows an intraepidermal bulla or acantholysis (separation of epidermal cells) and a mild to moderate infiltrate of eosinophils.
- Direct immunofluorescence is performed on two biopsies, one from the edge of a fresh lesion, and a second from an adjacent normal area.
- Immunoglobulin G and often complement C3 are found in the intercellular substance areas of the epidermis.
- Indirect immunofluorescence confirms circulating serum immunoglobulin G antibodies in 80–90% of patients with active disease.
- Antibodies are directed against desmoglein 3, an intracellular keratinocyte adhesion molecule.
- The level of antibody reflects the activity of disease.
- Periodic serum tests to detect changes in titers are helpful in evaluating the clinical course.

Course and Prognosis
- In the past, death occurred in all cases, usually from cutaneous infection. Nowadays death occurs in only 5–15% of cases, usually from complications of steroid therapy.
- Patient comorbidities—such as osteoporosis, diabetes and hypertension—undoubtedly contribute to mortality risk.

Differential Diagnosis
- Pemphigus foliaceus and paraneoplastic pemphigus (neoplasia-associated pemphigus) may be difficult to exclude without direct immunofluorescence.
- Immunofluorescence testing and dermatology referral are recommended for all bullous diseases.

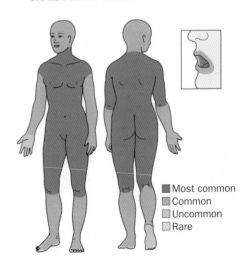

- Most common
- Common
- Uncommon
- Rare

Treatment

- Treatment is very complicated and best accomplished with the help of experts.
- The goal of treatment is to arrest blister formation.
- Prednisone with an immunosuppressive adjuvant agent such as azathioprine or cyclophosphamide is standard treatment.
- Adjuvant drugs have a "steroid-sparing" effect.
- Therapeutic choices are affected by the patient's age, and degree of involvement.
- Starting dosages of prednisone typically vary between 40 and 120 mg/day and are subsequently tapered to establish a minimum dose that controls most disease activity.
- Cyclophosphamide (1.5–2.5 mg/kg/day) or azathioprine (1.0–2.5 mg/kg/day) is initiated with or after starting corticosteroids.
- Plasmapheresis, pulse-dose intravenous corticosteroids, mycophenolate mofetil, gold, dapsone, and intralesional steroids may be more effective for selected patients than the above regimens.
- Direct immunofluorescence should be performed before therapy is discontinued.
- A negative direct immunofluorescence finding is a good indicator of remission.

Pearls

- Pemphigus vulgaris may present with only oral lesions.
- Early cutaneous finding of pemphigus vulgaris may resemble bullous pemphigoid and other immunobullous diseases.
- Mortality from pemphigus vulgaris is significant and early limited disease is easier to treat effectively.
- Strongly consider dermatology referral for suspected cases, as both diagnosis and management require specialist training.

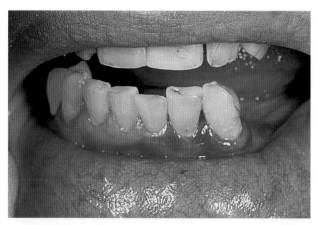

Oral erosions usually precede the onset of skin blisters by weeks or months.

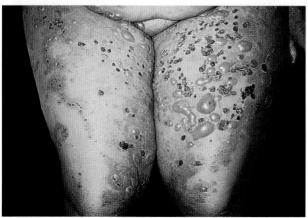

Flaccid blisters rupture easily because the roof consists only of a thin portion of the upper epidermis and is very fragile. Healing is with brown pigmentation but without scarring.

Pemphigus Foliaceus

Description
■ Pemphigus foliaceus is an autoimmune, intraepidermal blistering disease characterized by crusted patches and erosions.
■ Blister location is more superficial in the epidermis compared to pemphigus vulgaris.

History
■ The age of onset varies more widely than in pemphigus vulgaris.
■ It occurs in middle-aged and older people.
■ There is no racial predilection.
■ Pain and burning are more often reported than itching.
■ Sun or heat may worsen the signs and symptoms.

Skin Findings
■ Lesions appear in a "seborrheic distribution" on the face or first appear on the scalp, chest, or upper back.
■ Intact blisters are not usually seen.
■ The vesicle roof is so thin that it ruptures and serum leaks out and desiccates, forming localized or broad areas of crust.
■ If present, intact thin-walled blisters are sometimes seen near the edge of the erosions.
■ The upper portion of the epidermis can be dislodged with lateral finger pressure.

Non-skin Findings
■ There is increased incidence of thymoma, myasthenia gravis and other autoimmune disease.

Laboratory
■ Skin biopsy shows an intraepidermal bulla or acantholysis (separation of epidermal cells) in the upper epidermis and mild to moderate infiltration of eosinophils.
■ Direct immunofluorescence is performed on two biopsies, one from the edge of a fresh lesion and the second from an adjacent normal area.
■ Immunoglobulin G and often complement C3 are found in the intercellular substance areas of the epidermis.

■ Indirect immunofluorescence on serum confirms circulating immunoglobulin G antibodies in approximately 75% of patients with active disease.
■ Antibodies are directed against desmoglein 1, an intracellular keratinocyte adhesion molecule.
■ The level of antibody reflects the activity of disease.
■ Antibodies of pemphigus vulgaris can be distinguished from those of pemphigus foliaceus by testing on two tissue substrates.

Differential Diagnosis
■ Lesions are well demarcated and do not extend into large eroded areas as those of pemphigus vulgaris.
■ Impetigo may appear similar to pemphigus foliaceus; the two are not mutually exclusive.
■ Seborrheic dermatitis with crusting which does not clear as expected should raise suspicion of pemphigus foliaceus.
■ As with all blistering disorders, skin biopsy and immunofluorescence testing is recommended.

Course and Prognosis
■ May be localized for years or progress rapidly and become generalized evolving into an exfoliative erythroderma.

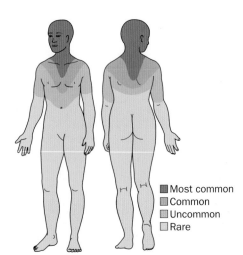

■ Most common
■ Common
■ Uncommon
□ Rare

- May last for years and may be fatal if not treated.

Discussion

- *Fogo selvagem* is Portuguese for "wild fire." It is an endemic form of pemphigus foliaceus found in certain rural areas of Brazil and Colombia.
- Pemphigus erythematosus (Senear–Usher syndrome) may be a combination of localized (face and other seborrheic areas) pemphigus foliaceus and systemic lupus erythematosus.
- Many of these patients have a positive antinuclear antibody, but few have any other signs or symptoms of lupus.
- Pemphigus foliaceus has been reported in approximately 5% of patients taking D-penicillamine or captopril.

- Most cases are mild, many showing spontaneous recovery once the drug is stopped.
- The pemphigus-like eruption is not always limited, and mortality approaches 10%.

Treatment

- Early localized disease may be managed with group I–III topical steroids.
- Active widespread disease is treated like pemphigus vulgaris.

Pearl

- Early pemphigus foliaceus may resemble seborrheic dermatitis or other papulosquamous diseases.

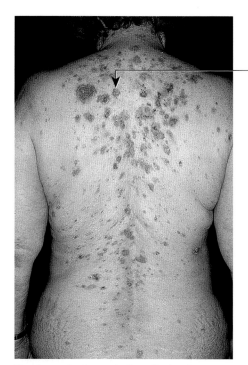

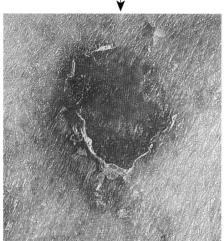

The disease begins gradually on the face in a "butterfly" distribution, or it first appears on the scalp, chest, or upper back as localized or broad continuous areas of erythema, scaling, crusting, or occasionally bullae.

The roof of the vesicle is so thin that it ruptures. Serum leaks out and desiccates, forming localized or broad areas of crust. Intact thin-walled blisters are sometimes seen near the edge of the erosions.

Bullous Pemphigoid

Description

- An uncommon, autoimmune, subepidermal blistering disease which primarily affects elderly people.

History

- Most cases occur after age 60 years.
- Childhood cases have been reported but are rare.
- There is no racial or gender prevalence.
- Immunoglobulin G autoantibodies directed against hemidesmosomal proteins are present.
- The trigger factor for the formation of autoreactive antibodies is unknown.
- Drugs including furosemide, captopril, and some non-steroidal anti-inflammatory drugs have been implicated.

Skin Findings

- The eruption is usually generalized with a predilection for skinfolds and flexural areas and dependent areas.
- Begins with a localized area of erythema or with pruritic urticarial papules coalescing into plaques.
- A diagnosis of hives is frequently made in this pre-blistering stage.
- Plaques turn dark red in 1–3 weeks as vesicles and bullae rapidly appear on their surface.
- Itching is usually moderate to severe.
- The bullae are tense with good structural integrity.
- Firm pressure on the blister will not result in extension into normal skin as occurs in pemphigus.
- Bullae rupture within 1 week, leaving an eroded base which does not spread and which heals rapidly.

Non-skin Findings

- Peripheral blood eosinophilia occurs in some patients.
- Oral blisters, if present, are mild and transient.

Laboratory

- Skin biopsy shows subepidermal bulla with an infiltrate of eosinophils within the dermis and blister cavity.

- Direct immunofluorescence of skin sampled next to a blister confirms immunoglobulin G and/or complement C3 in a linear band at the basement membrane zone in about 90% of cases.
- Direct immunofluorescence studies may be useful in following response to treatment.
- As the disease subsides, complement C3 deposits disappear.
- Indirect immunofluorescence will demonstrate circulating immunoglobulin G antibodies in the sera of approximately 70% of patients.
- Circulating autoantibody titers do not correlate well with disease activity, unlike pemphigus.

Differential Diagnosis

- Pemphigus vulgaris also affects the elderly but is even rarer and presents with fragile bullae and/or oral lesions.
- Dermatitis herpetiformis tends to have smaller vesicles and favors elbows, knees, buttocks and posterior scalp.
- Bullous drug eruptions favor the same areas as bullous pemphigoid.
- Skin biopsy with immunofluorescence is therefore recommended for all blistering diseases.
- Some blistering diseases such as epidermolysis bullosa acquisita and cicatricial pemphigoid have similar direct immunofluorescence patterns, which further require testing on salt-split skin to distinguish.

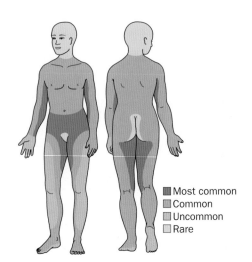

Most common
Common
Uncommon
Rare

Course and Prognosis

- Untreated bullous pemphigoid may remain localized and undergo spontaneous remission, or may rapidly generalize.
- Recurrences may be less severe than the initial episode.
- Duration varies for treated patients from 9 weeks to 17 years.
- The remission rate is 30% at 2 years and 50% at 3 years.
- Late relapse is observed after disease-free intervals of more than 5 years.
- Mortality rate at 1 year is 19%, often from treatment side effects in addition to patient comorbidities.

Discussion

- Dermatologists are trained well in bullous disorders and the biopsy techniques and tests required for an accurate diagnosis.
- Affected elderly patients often have significant comorbidities such as diabetes, osteoporosis, and hypertension.
- Management requires a team approach with a dermatologist, a primary care provider and visiting nurse care if required.

Treatment

- The goal of treatment is to arrest blistering, decrease itching, protect the skin and limit secondary infection.
- Itching is controlled with hydroxyzine 10-50 mg every 4 hours as needed.

Hydroxyzine causes sedation. Use with caution in the elderly.

- Class I topical steroids may be used to control limited disease, applied twice daily until lesions are healed and for 2 weeks thereafter.
- Prednisone is probably the treatment of choice (1.0–1.5 mg/kg/day) until blistering ceases.
- Most patients are controlled in 28 days and the dosage can be gradually tapered to 0.5 mg/kg/day at 3 months and 0.2 mg/kg/day at 6 months.
- Steroid sparing agents include tetracycline 1.0-2.5 g per day, minocycline 200 mg/day and niacinamide 1.5-2.5 g per day.
- 40% of patients respond to dapsone (100 mg per day) alone and the addition of dapsone may help to produce a remission.
- Consider adjuvant immunosuppressive therapy with cyclophosphamide or azathioprine if dapsone and prednisone fail.
- Intravenous immunoglobulin therapy has been used for patients unresponsive to conventional immunosuppressive treatment.
- Bedridden patients benefit from air mattress support and other skin protective measures.

Pearls

- Sustained remission requires gradual taper of prednisone and other agents.

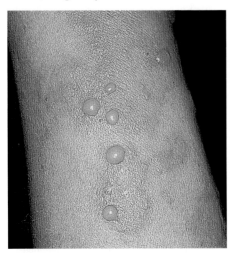

Pemphigoid begins with a localized area of erythema or with pruritic urticarial plaques that gradually become more edematous and extensive.

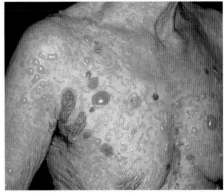

The eruption is often generalized, but the most common sites are the lower part of the abdomen, the groin, and the flexor surfaces of the arms and legs. The palms and soles are affected. The plaques turn dark red or cyanotic in 1–3 weeks, resembling erythema multiforme, as vesicles and bullae rapidly appear on their surface.

14 Connective Tissue Disease

Lupus Erythematosus

General Description

- Cutaneous lupus erythematosus is a disease with a wide spectrum of manifestations ranging from solitary chronic skin lesions in chronic lupus erythematosus, to widespread polymorphous lesions in subacute cutaneous lupus erythematosus, to multiple organ involvement in systemic lupus erythematosus. Lupus is thought to be a dysregulation of T cells causing the activation of B cells, producing a variety of autoantibodies directed against cellular antigens such as DNA, RNA, and RNA–protein complexes.

Treatment Overview

- There are many treatment options. Whether to use topical agent alone, or with the addition of a systemic agent, depends on the degree of disease extent and severity and other individual underlying medical conditions.
- Sunscreen usage and sun avoidance behavior is an essential element of therapy.
- Topical or intralesional corticosteroids, retinoids, and oral antimalarial therapy are standard treatments.
- Sun-screens should be used that block broad-spectrum ultraviolet A—especially ones that contain avobenzone (Parsol 1789), and titanium dioxide and zinc oxide.
- Sun-protective clothing is available from Sun Precautions (2815 Wetmore Avenue, Everett, WA 98201; Tel: 1-800-882-7860; http://sunprecautions.com) and from many other venders.
- Smoking cessation should be encouraged as better disease control may be achieved.
- Newer immune modulators, pimecrolimus cream (Elidel) or tacrolimus ointment (Protopic), can be effective. Both are applied twice daily to lesional skin for extended periods and may be preferred first-line topical therapy for facial lesions.
- Cyclical use of group I–II topical steroids; these are administered twice a day for 2 weeks and moisturizers are used for 1 week.
- Steroids, such as triamcinolone (Kenalog) 10 mg/ml, are injected into chronic lupus erythematosus lesions.
- Corticosteroid-impregnated tape (Cordran tape) is used for chronic lupus erythematosus lesions.
- Hydroxychloroquine 200–400 mg once daily (dose less than 6.5 mg/kg once daily) is an effective oral treatment in most cases; the onset of effect requires 4–8 weeks. Ophthalmic exams are required at baseline and every 6 months to 1 year.

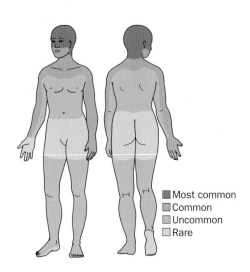

- Most common
- Common
- Uncommon
- Rare

■ Other medications for cutaneous lupus erythematosus that may be considered include: dapsone 25–200 mg once daily (especially useful for bullous lupus erythematosus, or vasculitic lesions of lupus erythematosus, or urticarial vasculitis associated with subacute cutaneous lupus erythematosus, and oral ulcerations); thalidomide 50–300 mg once daily at bedtime; sulfasalazine 1.5–2 g once daily; prednisone 0.5–1.5 mg/kg once daily; retinoids e.g. acitretin 10–50 mg once daily or isotretinoin 1 mg/kg once daily; gold (oral Auranofin or parenteral); azathioprine; methotrexate; mycophenolate mofetil; and cyclophosphamide.

■ High-dose intravenous immunoglobulin G (IVIG) 1 g/kg once daily for two consecutive days a month can be used when other agents fail; treatment is expensive, and response duration limited.

■ Monoclonal antibody infusions have been successful in treating patients with severe refractory cutaneous lupus erythematosus.

■ Skin disease often occurs with systemic disease in patients with systemic lupus erythematosus. Such patients require systemic immunosuppressive therapy to treat this form of lupus.

Chronic cutaneous lupus – scalp

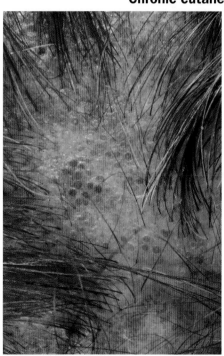

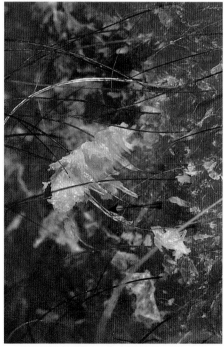

Chronic cutaneous lupus (discoid LE) of the scalp. Hyperkeratosis and inflammation occurs. Older lesions scar and show follicular plugs. Keratin accumulates and dilates the follicular orifice causing the follicular plugging.

Keratin accumulates on the surface causing scale. Keratin dilates the follicular orifice and accumulates around the hair shaft and fills the follicular canal. Elevation of the surface scale with forceps reveals the columns of scale that occupy the follicular canal. These keratin spires resemble carpet tacks, thus the name "carpet tack scale".

343

Chronic Cutaneous Lupus

Description

- Chronic cutaneous lupus is the most common form of cutaneous lupus erythematosus; lesions may be localized or widespread and consist of scaling erythematous papules and plaques, often with central atrophy and scarring.
- Chronic cutaneous lupus lesions are not always "discoid" and this term should no longer be used.

History

- Chronic lupus erythematosus is more common in women.
- It is perhaps more common in people with an African–American background.
- The peak incidence is in the fourth decade.
- Trauma and ultraviolet light may initiate and exacerbate lesions.
- Photosensitivity is present in 50% of patients with discoid lupus erythematosus.
- There is a lower incidence of systemic disease; 1–5% of cases progress to systemic lupus erythematosus. Patients with non-localized, widespread disease are at greater risk of advancing to systemic disease.
- Scarring alopecia is permanent.

Skin Findings

- Lesions may occur on any body surface, but the scalp, face, and ears are the most common areas.
- Chronic lupus erythematosus begins asymptomatically; there are well-defined, elevated, red to violaceous, 1–2 cm, flat-topped plaques with firmly adherent scaling.
- Follicular plugs are prominent; peeling the scale reveals an under-surface that looks like a carpet penetrated by several carpet tacks.
- Epidermal atrophy gives the surface either a smooth white or wrinkled appearance.
- Lesions may be hypertrophic or verrucous; they may involve the palms and soles or the oral mucosa.
- Lesions endure for months; they either resolve spontaneously or progress with further atrophy, ultimately forming smooth, white or hyperpigmented, depressed scars with telangiectasia and scarring alopecia.
- Scalp disease begins with erythema, scaling, and follicular plugging.
- Hair follicles are destroyed, resulting in irreversible, scarring alopecia. Hair loss is haphazard in distribution.

Treatment

- Treatment options include group I–III topical steroids, intralesional steroids, antimalarials (e.g. hydroxychloroquine 200 mg twice daily), dapsone, and oral corticosteroids. Difficult cases are treated with methotrexate, azathioprine, thalidomide or isotretinoin. Sunscreens are an essential aspect of therapy. Some patients may respond to tacrolimus ointment (Protopic). A broad spectrum, water-resistant sunscreen should be applied daily.

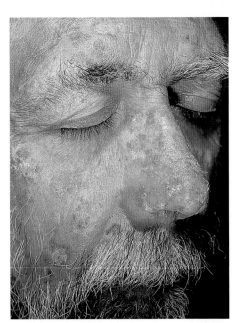

The face is the most commonly affected area. Epidermal atrophy occurs early and gives the surface either a smooth, white appearance or a wrinkled appearance.

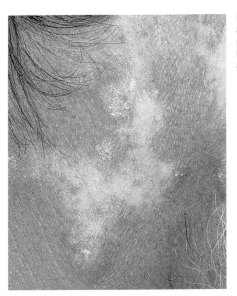

Follicular plugs may or may not be prominent. They are not present in this lesion. These lesions progress, ultimately forming smooth and white or hyperpigmented depressed scars with telangiectasia and scarring alopecia.

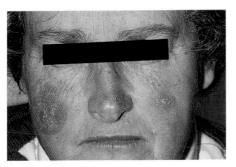

Discoid LE. Red plaques and scale. Scarring has not yet occurred.

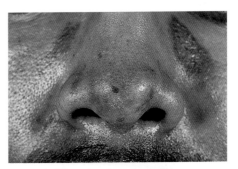

Lesions in African Americans heal with hyperpigmented or white disfiguring scars.

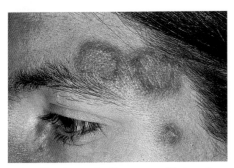

Red scaling plaques had been present for months. Plaques look like psoriasis but show follicular plugs.

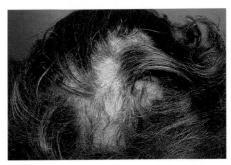

Discoid lupus is a common cause of scarring alopecia.

Subacute Cutaneous Lupus Erythematosus

Description
- Subacute cutaneous lupus erythematosus is a form of cutaneous lupus erythematosus typically characterized by non-scarring, erythematous psoriasiform lesions or annular lesions in a sun-exposed distribution.
- It is most common in white, young to middle-aged women.

History
- Often a sudden eruption after sun exposure, but often gradually progresses to involve more skin over time.
- Lesions occur on the upper trunk, nape of the neck, upper back and shoulders, extensor arms, face, and dorsal hands.
- Internal involvement is limited and less severe than in systemic lupus erythematosus; it may not be notable at all.
- Individual lesions may last for months.
- This condition tends to be chronic and recurrent, with flaring during spring and summer months, or times of high sun exposure.

Skin Findings
- There are two patterns: papulosquamous and annular polycyclic. The annular polycyclic lesions may have little scaling.
- Lesions occur most often on the sun-exposed trunk; they are rarely seen below the waist.
- Subtle gray hypopigmentation and telangiectasia are seen in the center of annular lesions; this becomes more obvious as lesions resolve. Hypopigmentation fades in several months, but the telangiectasia persists.
- Follicular plugging, adherent hyperkeratosis, scarring, and dermal atrophy are not prominent features; these are more typical of discoid lesions.
- Other signs include photosensitivity in 70–90%, periungual telangiectasia, discoid lupus erythematosus, and vasculitis.
- Variants of subacute cutaneous lupus erythematosus include annular, papulosquamous, neonatal lupus erythematosus, complement C2-deficient lupus erythematosus-like syndrome, drug-induced subacute cutaneous lupus erythematosus, and tumid lupus.

Laboratory
- The antinuclear antibody titer is elevated in 50–72% of cases.
- Anti-Ro (anti-SS-A) antibody titer is elevated in 50–100% of cases.
- Anti-La (anti-SS-B) coexists with anti-Ro (anti-SS-A) and is usually not present as a unique antibody.
- Leukopenia is present in 25–50% of patients with subacute cutaneous lupus erythematosus.

Differential Diagnosis
- Drug eruptions, especially thiazides
- Dermatomyositis
- Secondary syphilis
- Psoriasis
- Cutaneous T cell lymphoma
- Seborrheic dermatitis
- Tinea corporis

Discussion
- Patients with subacute cutaneous lupus erythematosus do not meet criteria for systemic lupus erythematosus, though involvement is not strictly cutaneous; some have renal or neurologic involvement and other systemic manifestations such as fatigue and arthralgia. Hematologic involvement with leukopenia, decreased complement levels and lymphopenia may also occur. The overall prognosis is better for subacute cutaneous lupus erythematosus than for lupus erythematosus.
- Medications associated with subacute cutaneous lupus erythematosus include hydrochlorothiazide, calcium channel blockers, and terbinafine.
- Mothers with Ro antibodies may transmit neonatal lupus; the incidence in one study was 7.6%.

Neonatal Lupus
- Neonatal lupus is acquired through transplacental maternal autoantibodies,

typically to Ro/SS-A. The infant presents with cutaneous lupus lesions at birth or within days to months after birth, or congenital heart block. Thrombocytopenia is present in 10–20%.

■ Neonatal lupus skin lesions are annular plaques with overlying fine scale; they resolve spontaneously in weeks to months and may leave residual telangiectasias, mild atrophy or pigmentary alteration. Lesional skin biopsy shows typical lupus erythematosus changes, and Ro antibodies are present in most affected neonates and their mothers.

■ Complete irreversible heart block occurs in roughly half of infants with neonatal lupus, and can cause significant morbidity and mortality.

■ A mother of a child with neonatal lupus is at high risk for having other children similarly affected; early prenatal counselling and high-risk obstetric expertise is advised.

■ Sun-protective measures are an essential element of treatment for neonatal lupus. Low-potency topical steroid or topical immune modulators tacrolimus or pimecrolimus may hasten lesion resolution.

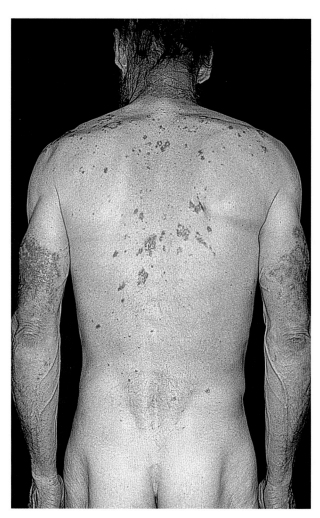

Subacute cutaneous lupus erythematosus. There are two morphologic varieties: a papulosquamous pattern and an annular polycyclic pattern. Both occur most often on the trunk; one predominates. Lesions are prominent in sun-exposed areas.

Acute Cutaneous Lupus Erythematosus

Description
■ Acute cutaneous lupus erythematosus is a serious multisystem disease.

History
■ Women are affected more often than men, in a ratio of 8 to 1.
■ It occurs most frequently in people aged 30–40 years.
■ Sunlight exacerbates acute cutaneous lupus erythematosus and may induce it.
■ Acute cutaneous lupus erythematosus is a multisystem disease; there may be fever, arthritis, and renal, cardiac, pulmonary, and central nervous system involvement.

Skin Findings
■ Superficial and indurated, non-pruritic, erythematous to violaceous plaques appear on the sun-exposed chest, shoulders, extensor arms, and backs of the hands.
■ There may be fine scaling on the surface, and obvious follicular plugging.
■ In 10–50% of patients a butterfly rash appears over the malar and nasal bridge.
■ Atrophy does not occur.
■ Nail fold capillary microscopy reveals tortuous "meandering" capillary loops.
■ The patient may have excess vellus hair at the frontal margin (lupus hair) or diffuse hair thinning.
■ Alopecia (scarring and non-scarring) occurs in 20% of cases.

Differential Diagnosis
■ Contact dermatitis
■ Rosacea
■ Erysipelas
■ Seborrheic dermatitis
■ Tinea
■ Drugs (e.g. hydralazine, procainamide, and anticonvulsants may cause a lupus-like syndrome)
■ Polymorphous light eruption
■ Parvovirus B19

Laboratory
■ Biopsy of lesional skin is obtained for routine study and for immunofluorescence.
■ Underlying systemic lupus erythematosus is screened for by using an antinuclear antibody titer, a complete blood count, a serum chemistry profile, and urinalysis.

Treatment
■ Sunscreens are an essential aspect of therapy. A broad spectrum, water-resistant sunscreen should be applied daily.

Pearls
■ The classic butterfly rash over the malar and nasal area occurs in 10–50% of patients with acute lupus erythematosus, but it is not the most common cutaneous presentation.
■ Assessing the rashes of lupus erythematosus and categorizing the process as chronic cutaneous lupus, subacute cutaneous lupus, or acute lupus is vital to effective and appropriate treatment. It involves careful attention to systemic symptoms, and hematologic, renal, and serologic evaluation.

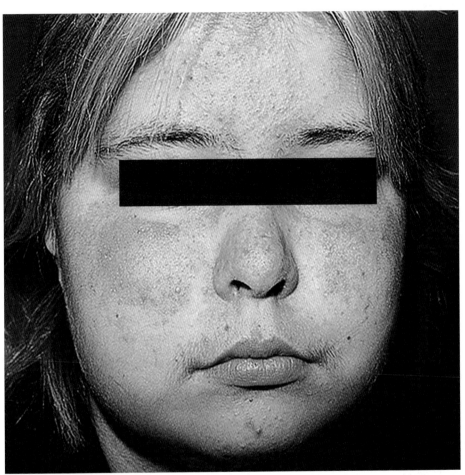

Acute lupus erythematosus. Superficial red plaques occur on sun-exposed areas. There may be fine scaling on the surface, but atrophy does not occur. Plaques last for days or weeks. Indurated plaques may last for months.

Dermatomyositis

Description

- Dermatomyositis is an acquired, idiopathic connective tissue disease characterized by proximal muscle weakness and a characteristic, violaceous skin rash prominent on the eyelids, scalp, metacarpophalangeal joints, and bony prominences.
- The condition may be associated with underlying malignancy.
- Muscle weakness is not always present.

History

- Incidence is 1 in 100,000, and females are twice as likely to develop the disease as males.
- At least 15% of cases occur in the pediatric age group.
- The disease may present with gradual onset of the typical skin findings or with a proximal muscle weakness.
- Patients with muscle disease often have difficulty combing their hair, walking up stairs, or getting up from a chair without the use of their arms. These are good screening questions.
- Cutaneous lesions often precede muscle involvement by 3-6 months.

Skin Findings

- Roughly 10% of patients have characteristic skin findings without evidence of muscle disease. The term amyopathic dermatomyositis applies to skin disease in the absence of muscle disease over 6 months; 2 years is required for confirmed amyopathic dermatomyositis.
- The heliotrope rash refers to a violaceous erythema of the eyelids.
- Pathognomonic Gottron's papules are located over bony prominences, particularly the proximal interphalangeal joints, the distal interphalangeal joints, and the metacarpophalangeal joints. The lesions are violaceous papules and plaques. Other sites include the elbows, knees, and medial malleoli.
- The shawl sign refers to the violaceous erythema over the back of the neck and posterior shoulders.

- Poikiloderma (erythema, telangiectasia, hypopigmentation and hyperpigmentation, and atrophy) is also a typical finding in affected skin of the upper chest, posterior shoulders, buttocks, and back.
- Periungual changes include ragged cuticles, erythema, and telangiectasia.
- Scalp findings are common and include alopecia, pruritus, erythema and scaling.
- Skin lesions are often pruritic.
- "Mechanic's hands" refers to scaly fissures and inflammatory changes to the hands bilaterally.
- Calcinosis is a rare but severe associated finding in dermatomyositis patients.

Non-skin Findings

- Fatigue is a common complaint; patients may not recognize muscle weakness.
- Muscle involvement is typically proximal and symmetric.
- Dysphagia occurs in 12-45%.
- Dermatomyositis may be a paraneoplastic disease; older patients are at greater risk.

Laboratory

- Skin disease findings are typical and may be supported by biopsy of affected skin.
- Elevation of serum muscle enzymes. Creatine kinase is helpful in assessing disease activity.
- A muscle biopsy may be performed; non-invasive imaging of the muscles can be done with magnetic resonance imaging.
- An abnormal electromyogram is one of the diagnostic criteria.
- Jo-1 antibody is positive in roughly 20%. It is associated with interstitial lung disease, arthritis, Raynaud's disease and a hyperkeratotic callused appearance of the thumbs and the index and middle fingers referred to as "mechanic's hand."
- Screening for malignancy is prudent with regular careful review of systems, rectal, stool guiac, pelvic and breast examination, complete blood count, serum chemistry, chest x-ray and mammogram. Consider magnetic resonance imaging and computerized tomography of the chest and abdomen. Other testing as indicated by symptoms or previous malignancy history. Screen for ovarian cancer in older women.

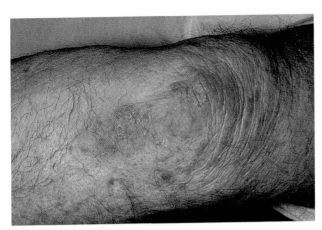

Violaceous erythema and scale appear on the extensor surfaces of the elbows. Violaceous papules in this area are called Gottron papules.

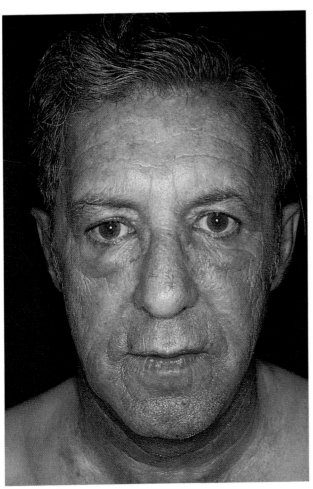

Heliotrope rash. A violaceous to dusky red rash involves the periorbital skin or only the lid margin. The "purple" skin color may be accompanied by edema.

Complications

- Untreated muscle disease can result in serious complications and chronic disability.
- Severe muscle disease may result in mortality from dysphagia, aspiration, and respiratory failure.
- Cutaneous lupus and vasculitis may overlap in some patients with dermatomyositis.

Course and Prognosis

- The disease course is variable; it may be rapid and progressive or chronic and relapsing. Spontaneous remission can also occur.
- Earlier intervention and therapy with systemic corticosteroids results in improved prognosis in patients with muscle disease.

Differential Diagnosis

- Contact dermatitis
- Lupus erythematosus
- Psoriasis
- Parvovirus B19

Pediatric Considerations

- Vascular involvement is more frequent in children and may result in cutaneous ulceration.
- Joint contractures and atrophy are more common findings affecting children.
- A source of substantial disability, soft-tissue calcification occurs in roughly 40–70% of children with dermatomyositis; treatment is difficult.
- Reduced morbidity and mortality is associated with corticosteroid treatment with or without other immunosuppression.
- Children with dermatomyositis should be treated by a specialist with particular interest in this condition.
- Malignancy is a rare association of childhood dermatomyositis.

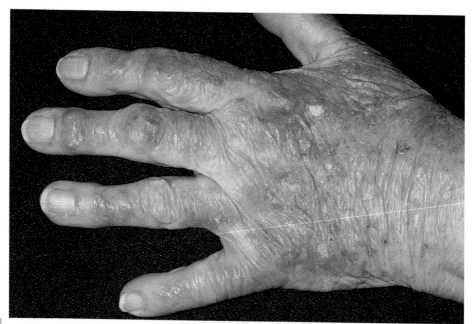

Violaceous papules over the bony prominences of the fingers are called Gottron papules. They may also be found on the elbows, knees and feet. A violaceous rash, with or without scale, may appear on the back of the hands and palms.

Treatment

- Sun protection with broad-spectrum sunscreens, protective clothing, and behaviour modification is necessary. The rash is often aggravated by sun exposure.
- Systemic corticosteroids (prednisone 0.5–1.5 mg/kg once daily) are a treatment cornerstone, though the rash may not respond.
- Hydroxychloroquine 200–400 mg once daily, alone or combined with quinacrine 100–200 mg once daily results in improvement in the skin disease but the response may not be complete.
- Steroid-sparing agents for skin disease include immune suppressive agents methotrexate 2.5–30 mg/week and intravenous immunoglobulin 2 g/kg for two consecutive days.
- Antihistamines are used for the pruritus (non-sedating during the day or sedating at night).
- Second-line agents for muscle disease treatment and steroid-sparing include: methotrexate 25–50 mg/week, azathioprine 2 mg/kg once daily, cyclosporine 5 mg/kg once daily, cyclophosphamide 2 mg/kg once daily, and intravenous immunoglobulin 2 g/kg.
- Passive range of motion exercise, rest, proper nutrition, physical and occupational therapy are all important.

Pearls

- There is no correlation between the muscle disease involvement and activity and the skin disease.
- Amyopathic dermatomyositis is more common in adults than in children.
- Findings which favor a diagnosis of dermatomyositis rather than lupus include the characteristic violaceous hue of the cutaneous lesions, eyelid involvement, frequent pruritus, and interphalangeal joint skin involvement.

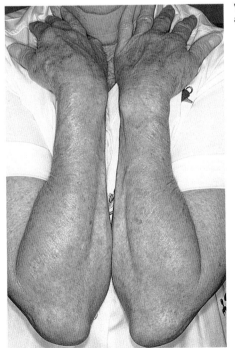

Violaceous erythema and scale may involve extensive areas of sun-exposed skin.

Scleroderma

Description

- Progressive systemic sclerosis is an idiopathic fibrosing condition which may present in a diffuse or limited form.
- Diffuse involvement can affect the entire skin surface and is associated with internal organ fibrosis and vascular abnormalities.
- A localized variant associated with CREST syndrome (**c**alcinosis, **R**aynaud's disease, **e**sophageal dysmotility, **s**clerodactyly, and **t**elangiectasia).
- The CREST syndrome is a localized variant, most commonly involving the hands and face, and follows a more indolent course.

History

- Systemic sclerosis is rare; incidence in the United States is roughly 20 cases per million population.
- Women are affected three times more often than men.
- Peak age of onset is between ages 30 and 50.
- Men, older age of onset, and Black people seem to have a worse prognosis.
- The disease may remain localized on the hands for many years.

Skin Findings

- Raynaud's phenomenon may precede the onset of progressive systemic sclerosis, and is often the first manifestation.
- Patients may complain of intense pruritus early in the disease.
- Early on, the affected skin is erythematous and swollen.
- Sclerosis occurs and the skin is smooth, yellowish, and firm. It appears tight and bound down.
- Nail folds may show capillary dilatation. Dilated, tortuous capillaries are evident in 75% of patients.
- The earliest changes may be most notable around the mouth and on the hands; there is loss of the normal facial expression lines, difficulty in opening the mouth, and the lips appear thin with radial furrowing.
- Trophic ulceration and gangrene may occur on the fingertips.
- Diffuse calcification may occur within the skin and may be apparent on radiographic exam.
- Late changes include hyperpigmentation or depigmentation, often seen on the upper chest. Hair follicles will often retain pigment while the adjacent skin is hypopigmented.
- Hair loss is evident in affected areas late in the disease. Alopecia may be partial or complete.

Non-skin Findings

- The limited form is associated with Raynaud's phenomenon, which may precede the sclerosis by years.
- In progressive systemic sclerosis, the heart, gastrointestinal tract, lungs, and kidneys may be affected.
- Scleroderma renal crisis typically occurs within the first 5 years of the disease.

Laboratory

- Antinuclear antibody patterns associated with systemic sclerosis include homogeneous, speckled, and nucleolar types. Antinuclear antibody positivity occurs in more than 90%. Nucleolar pattern is most specific.
- Antibodies to Scl-70 are associated with truncal scleroderma, and pulmonary fibrosis; renal disease in this subset is less common.
- Anticentromere antibody (speckled pattern) is highly specific for CREST syndrome.
- The homogeneous pattern is associated with PM-Scl antibodies and is a marker for polymyositis–scleroderma overlap.
- Antibodies to single-stranded DNA are associated with linear scleroderma.
- The diffuse form of the condition has protean complications; evaluation of internal organ involvement is essential, as is assessing for musculoskeletal effects, gastrointestinal, renal, and pulmonary involvement.

Differential Diagnosis

- Scleredema
- Myxedema
- Eosinophilic fasciitis (typically spares the hands and face)
- Chronic graft versus host disease.
- Occupational exposure to chemicals (polyvinyl chloride resins, epoxy resins, silica) and chronic vibration.

Complications

- Digital ulcerations and gangrene occur in roughly one-third of patients.
- Asymptomatic or symptomatic esophageal dysfunction is common.
- Gastroparesis.
- Interstitial lung disease and pulmonary arterial hypertension are two pulmonary complications; the lung involvement is the most common cause of death. Shortness of breath and dry cough are common presentations.
- Renal involvement affects 10–15% of patients. Blood pressure should be monitored regularly.

Course and Prognosis

- Progressive systemic sclerosis follows a variable and unpredictable course.
- Survival may be roughly predicted by extent of skin involvement within 1 year of diagnosis.
- The best prognosis is for patients with sclerodactyly only; truncal involvement heralds the worst prognosis, with only 21% 10-year survival.

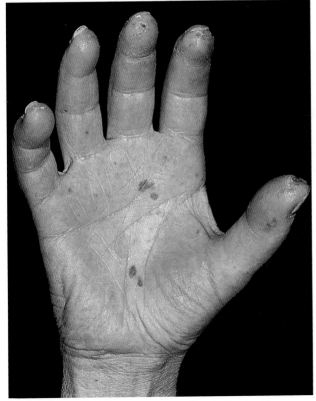

The skin is tightly bound down. The fingers are contracted. Telangiectatic mats are evident on the palms. There are fingertip ulcerations.

Treatment

- There is no reliable and effective treatment to reverse or prevent the fibrosis of systemic scleroderma; the disease is typically refractory to treatment, though angiotensin-converting enzyme inhibitors are effective in the treatment of scleroderma renal crisis.
- A multidisciplinary approach to treatment is appropriate for managing the complications of this multisystem disease. Raynaud's phenomenon may be managed with behavior modification for cold avoidance, with consideration of therapy with calcium channel blockers such as nifedipine 10 mg twice or three times daily, or amlodipine 2.5 mg once daily.
- Physical and occupational therapies are important aspects of treatment.
- For skin involvement, lubrication can help relieve pruritus. Sarna lotion or Pramosone lotion 2.5% may be tried for antipruritic effect.
- Not smoking, and prevention of trauma are key in the prevention of digital ulcerations; warm-water soaks for 20 minutes three times a day may be helpful. Meticulous wound care for ulceration is essential.
- Patient education materials may be obtained through the Scleroderma Foundation, 89 Newbury St, Suite 201, Danvers, MA 01923 or http://www.scleroderma.org.

Pearls

- Calcinosis may result in tender skin lesions and ulceration in patients with late stage scleroderma or patients with CREST syndrome. Diltiazem may be effective in some patients.
- Smoking cessation is critical, especially in patients with Raynaud's phenomenon.
- A few patients with CREST syndrome progress to systemic disease.

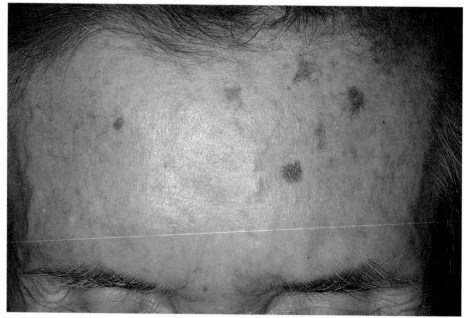

Scleroderma - an advanced case. There are no wrinkles on the forehead and the forehead cannot be wrinkled. Telangiectatic mats are present. These sharply defined, square or rectangular telangiectatic macules are found on the face, palms and lips.

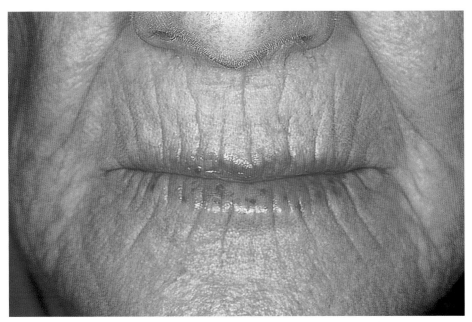

Telangiectasias are most obvious in the perioral area and neck. The skin about the mouth is drawn into furrows that radiate from the mouth.

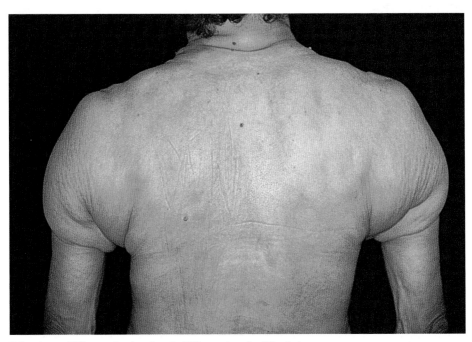

Scleroderma. Diffuse systemic sclerosis. Diffuse sclerosis of the limbs.

Morphea

Description

- An idiopathic disease which manifests as sclerotic dermal plaques with violaceous borders and central hypopigmentation.
- The condition may be localized (more than two plaques) or generalized (more than three plaques).
- The generalized form accounts for 15% of patients with morphea.
- Linear scleroderma accounts for 20% of localized scleroderma.

History

- Morphea is more common in women than in men; the ratio is 3.6 to 1.
- All ages may be affected, but the mean age of onset is 32 years.
- Incidence is 27 per million per year; prevalence of roughly 540,000 in the United States.
- Onset may be slow and insidious or rapid and progressive.

Skin Findings

- Early lesions are typically inflammatory and, thus, violaceous. Later lesions manifest hyperpigmentation, fibrosis and atrophy.
- In generalized morphea, a large area of skin may be involved; lesions are often truncal, but may involve the extremities.
- Linear scleroderma is more common on the extremities than the face.
- "En coup de sabre" is the term for linear scleroderma affecting the forehead and scalp. In the Parry–Romberg syndrome (progressive facial hemiatrophy) soft tissue and bony defects are also apparent.

Laboratory

- A skin biopsy can help confirm the clinical diagnosis; a biopsy to deep fat or fascia may be necessary if the involvement is deep. Findings include a variable degree of inflammation (typical of early lesions) and dermal sclerosis.
- Complete blood count and differential blood count. Eosinophilia is common.
- Antinuclear antibody is commonly positive in patients with generalized morphea.

Differential Diagnosis

- Systemic sclerosis (scleroderma)
- Nephrogenic fibrosing dermopathy
- Granuloma annulare
- Intramuscular injection reaction to drugs (vitamin K, pentazocine)
- Eosinophilic fasciitis

Course and Prognosis

- The natural history of the condition is unpredictable; lesions may spontaneously resolve after several years of inflammation and enlargement.
- Though lesions may soften, hyperpigmentation is often chronic and distressing to the patient.
- Patients with generalized morphea may have asymptomatic internal organ involvement; the evaluation and proper screening of such patients is presently uncertain and individualized.

Treatment

- As lesions may darken with sun exposure, sun protection is advised.
- Emollients may be comforting.
- Education of the patient regarding the disease may be all that is required, because there is no reliable effective treatment. Reassure the patient with plaque morphea that this condition is benign, and does not involve internal organs.
- Mid-potency to high-potency topical steroid cream or ointment (groups II–III) may be helpful in some cases to soften lesions and decrease pruritus.
- Inflammatory lesions can be injected with intralesional triamcinolone 5-10 mg/ml; caution is needed as intralesional steroid injection may also result in excessive atrophy.
- Calcipotriene ointment (Dovonex) twice daily can be used in adults and children; a reasonable trial of use is 8 weeks.
- For rapidly progressing symptomatic disease, consider prednisone 20–40 mg once daily for 6-8 weeks. A taper by 10 mg every other day is appropriate for

patients with lesion improvement; such treatment does not alter the natural history of the disease.

■ Hydroxychloroquine 400 mg once daily for a trial of 4 months is reasonable. If a response is obtained, a maintenance dose of 200 mg once daily is reasonable.

■ Immune-suppressing medications, such as methotrexate or cyclosporine, may be considered for a short-term therapeutic trial of 3–6 months, for inflammatory, symptomatic and/or progressive disease. Proper monitoring of such drugs is imperative.

■ Patients with linear scleroderma may benefit from surgery if there are significant contractures or leg length discrepancies. Cosmesis with autologous fat transfer can be helpful for facial atrophy.

■ Therapies with ultraviolet A1 (not widely available in the United States), systemic or bath psoralen ultraviolet A have been reported effective in small prospective uncontrolled trials.

Pearls

■ Plaque and generalized morphea are not systemic sclerosis—the patient should be reassured that the condition is benign and the lesions typically soften in time.

■ Half of patients will have lesion softening within the first 4 years.

■ Raynaud's phenomenon and sclerodactyly are associated with systemic sclerosis, and not plaque morphea.

Pediatric Consideration
• Linear scleroderma is more common in children.

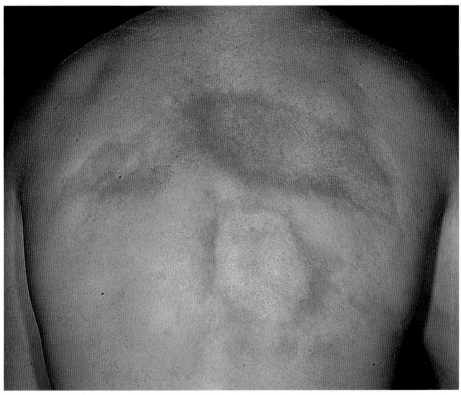

Morphea. Early lesions with a violaceous or lilac-colored active inflammatory border.

15 Light-Related Diseases and Disorders of Pigmentation

Sun-Damaged Skin, Actinic-Damaged Skin, Photoaging

Description
- Recognizable, morphologic changes in the skin as a result of years of accumulated ultraviolet radiation.

History
- Currently males appear to be affected more often than females.
- There is no known innate gender difference in susceptibility.
- Presumably traditional occupational differences are responsible.
- Persons with fair complexion (skin types I and II) are at greatest risk.
- Signs of photoaging are apparent by age 40.

Skin Findings
- The face, lateral neck and dorsal hands are the most severely affected areas. The posterior neck is equally involved in male patients.
- The skin appears older than its chronological age with all skin components affected.
- The epidermis is thinned and dry.
- Localized areas of erythema and scaling are actinic keratoses.
- Pigmentation is uneven and blotchy, solar lentigines.
- Fine wrinkles lateral to the eyes and deep furrows form on the forehead, at the angles of the mouth, and on the posterior neck.
- The skin appears loose and without resilience.
- Telangiectatic blood vessels appear on the ears and lateral cheeks.
- The skin of the dorsal hands and arms bruises with minimal trauma.

- Pilosebaceous units are prominent and dilated with retained keratin (solar comedones), especially lateral to the eyes.
- Poikiloderma describes the combination of epidermal atrophy, hyperpigmentation and hypopigmentation, and telangiectasia.
- These poikilodermatous changes are seen on sun-exposed areas of the face and lateral neck while the skin beneath the chin is unaffected.

Laboratory
- There is hyperkeratosis of the stratum corneum.
- There is flattening of the rete ridges.
- Keratinocyte atypia and dyskeratosis are seen.
- There are dermal elastosis and dilated cutaneous vessels.

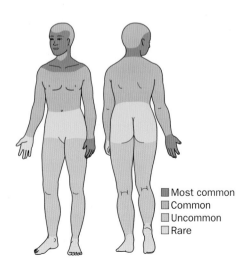

- Most common
- Common
- Uncommon
- Rare

Differential Diagnosis

- Rosacea (telangiectasia on the malar cheeks; may coexist with photoaging changes)
- Cutaneous lupus (may result in areas of atrophy and telangiectasia as well as scarring)
- Chronic use of topical steroids on the face prematurely ages the skin

Course and Prognosis

- Progressive damage from years of sun-exposure continues even after proper sun avoidance.
- Some actinic keratoses may regress completely with sun protection and time.

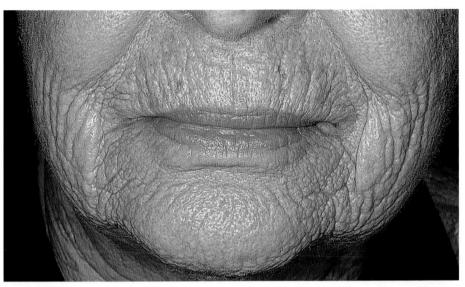

Course wrinkling occurs following loss of elastic tissue and collagen. The skin surface is firm, smooth and yellow.

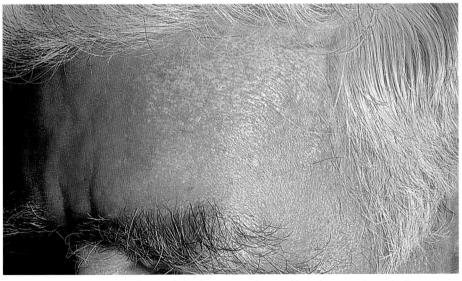

Solar elastosis is a sign highly characteristic of severe sun damage. There is coarsening and yellow discoloration of the skin.

Discussion

- A distinction is made between intrinsic aging of the skin and photoaging of the skin.

Treatment

- Topical retinoids such as tretinoin (Renova 0.01, 0.05 and tazarotene (Avage) have been shown to reverse some photoaging over several months.
- Epidermal hyperkeratosis decreases, pigmentation becomes more uniform and lighter, and new collagen is deposited within the papillary dermis.
- Improvement is dose dependent and persists as long as the retinoid is continued.
- Various peeling agents can also improve the texture and appearance of sun-damaged skin.
- Alpha-hydroxy acids reduce hyperkeratosis and promote epidermal hyperplasia.

- New collagen formation in the papillary dermis also occurs.
- Deeper peeling agents such as trichloroacetic acid (TCA) and phenol cause full-thickness epidermal damage with intentional wounding of the papillary dermis.
- Wounding causes a thin zone of scar formation (new collagen) in the papillary dermis, effectively reducing wrinkles.
- Laser resurfacing has a similar effect.
- The distinction between cosmetic and pharmaceutical has become blurred as new products continue to appear, each with claims of reversing sun-damage.
- Data may be lacking for such claims and skepticism is warranted.

Pearls

- Sun-protective measures alone improve photoaging and prevent further damage.

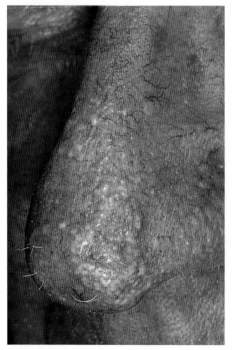

White, round 2–3 mm papules (milia) and telangiectasia occur on the face in predisposed individuals with severely sun-damaged skin.

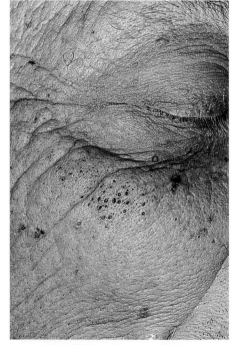

Coarse, deep wrinkles radiate from the lateral margin of the eye. Degraded collagen cannot support hair follicles. The follicles expand, accumulate sebum, and form comedones.

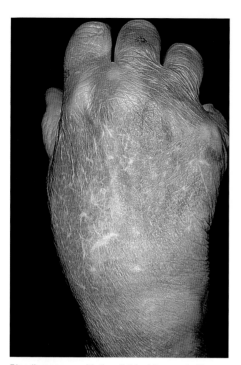

Bleeding occurs with the slightest trauma to the sun-damaged surfaces of the forearms and hands. The fragile skin tears easily and heals with criss-crossed scars.

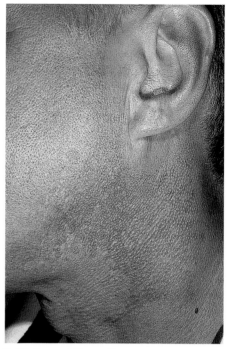

Poikiloderma of Civatte. Chronic sun exposure may cause red-brown pigmentation with telangiectasia and atrophy on the sides of the neck in predisposed individuals. The shaded area under the chin is spared.

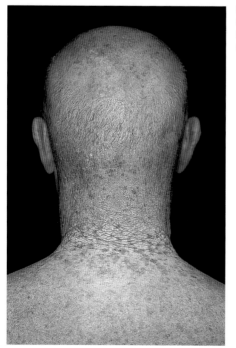

Sun-induced wrinkling on the back of the neck shows a series of criss-crossed lines. Reactive hyperplasia of melanocytes causes lentigines. Diffuse persistent erythema is prominent in fair-skinned people.

Polymorphous Light Eruption

Description
■ An idiopathic, recurrent photodermatitis that comes on acutely, usually in spring with first sun exposure.

History
■ Commonly referred to as sun poisoning or sun allergy.
■ Occurs in all races, at any age, but is most common in young women.
■ Incidence is as high as 10% in the population.
■ Occurs in northern climates where sun intensity increases in the spring, and during winter vacations while visiting southern, sunny resorts.
■ Symptoms may include pruritus, malaise, chills, headache, and nausea.
■ May only appear with first one or two exposures to sunlight in the spring.

Skin Findings
■ Lesions appear 2 hours to 5 days after sun exposure.
■ Initial symptoms are burning, itching, and erythema on exposed skin such as the upper chest, backs of the hands, extensor aspects of the forearms, and the lower legs.
■ Tends to spare the face (except in hereditary form).
■ There are several clinical types of polymorphous light eruption:
  ● The papular type is most common with small red dermal papules, disseminated or densely aggregated, on a patchy erythema.
  ● The plaque type is second most common with superficial or urticarial plaques.
  ● The papulovesicular type is least common and begins with urticarial plaques from which groups of vesicles arise.

Laboratory
■ Histopathologic changes are not specific for polymorphous light eruption.
■ Antinuclear antibodies, Ro/La antibodies, and direct and indirect

immunofluorescence help to distinguish polymorphous light eruption from cutaneous lupus.

Differential Diagnosis
■ Lupus erythematosus usually has positive antinuclear antibody and immunofluorescence.
■ Photodrug eruption can be similar in appearance; there is a history of photosensitizing drug.

Course and Prognosis
■ Lesions persist for 7–10 days.
■ Light sensitivity decreases with repeated sun exposure into the summer and recurs the next spring.
■ Patients develop the same clinical type of polymorphous light eruption each year.
■ Most have exacerbations each summer for many years.

Discussion
■ Ultraviolet A is trigger in most cases though the amount of exposure needed to trigger a flare varies.

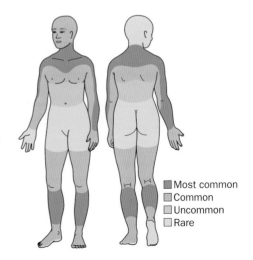

■ Most common
□ Common
□ Uncommon
□ Rare

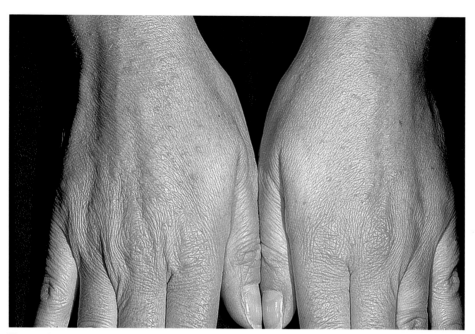

The papular type is the most common form. Small papules are densely aggregated. The back of the hands is a common site. The rash itches and is sometimes painful. Lesions persist for 7–10 days.

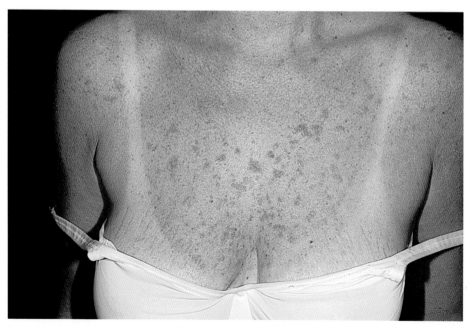

The papulovesicular type begins with urticarial plaques from which groups of vesicles arise.

- Hereditary polymorphous light eruption occurs in Inuit and Native American people.
- Autosomal dominant transmission with incomplete penetrance and variable expressivity.

Treatment

- Minimize sun exposure, especially between 10 AM and 2 PM.
- Sun-protective clothing is available from Sun Precautions (www.sunprecautions.com) and similar companies.
- Broad spectrum, ultraviolet A blocking sunscreens especially those containing avobenzone, titanium dioxide and zinc oxide.
- Using groups II–V topical steroids for 3–14 days relieves itch and fades lesions.
- Tapering off of oral steroids over 2 weeks is useful in severe cases.
- Controlled gradual exposure to sunlight or ultraviolet B or ultraviolet A can harden skin and increase one's tolerance.
- Hydroxychloroquine 400 mg/day for the first month and 200 mg per day thereafter for difficult cases.

Pearls

- Once the diagnosis is made, schedule follow-up for the next spring to plan for and avoid the next season's flare.

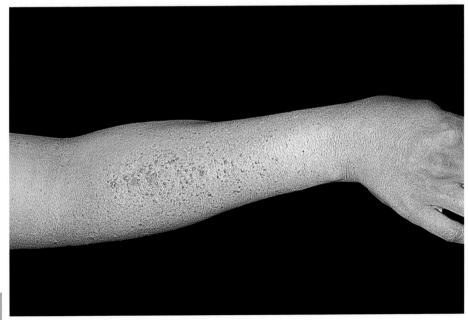

Small papules are disseminated or densely aggregated on a patchy erythema.

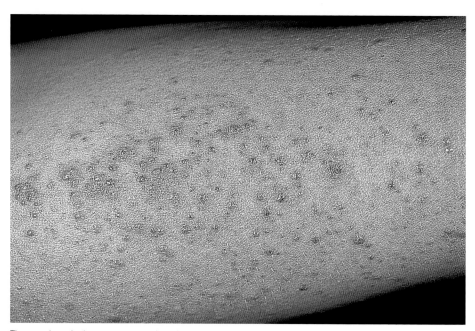

The papulovesicular type occurs primarily on the arms, lower limbs, and the V area of the chest.

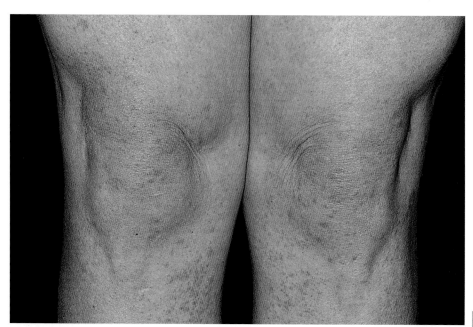

Papules are localized and symmetrically distributed. They do not occur on the entire sun-exposed areas. Itching is not a constant feature.

Porphyria Cutanea Tarda

Description
- The porphyrias represent abnormalities in the pathway for heme synthesis.
- Enzyme deficiencies along this pathway result in increased formation of metabolic intermediaries (porphyrinogens) just prior to the specific enzyme defect.
- Each type of porphyria is characterized by a specific enzyme deficiency and distinct clinical characteristics.
- The porphyrias are divided into disorders of bone marrow heme synthesis (the erythropoietic porphyrias) and disorder of hepatic heme synthesis (the hepatic porphyrias).
- Porphyria cutanea tarda is the most common form of porphyria.
- It results from a deficiency of hepatic uroporphyrinogen decarboxylase activity.
- Both acquired and familial forms exist.
- Porphyria cutanea tarda occurs when the heme biosynthetic pathway is compromised by an exogenous agent.
- The acquired "sporadic" form occurs as a complication of hepatic dysfunction or is induced by alcohol, drugs or hormones.
- Specific cutaneous changes occur in sun-exposed areas.

History
- It mostly affects middle-aged men and women, and younger women on oral contraceptives.
- There is autosomal dominant transmission in familial porphyria cutanea tarda.
- "Sporadic" porphyria cutanea tarda may be an autosomal recessive trait.
- Estimated prevalence is 1 in 25,000 in North America.
- Alcohol and estrogens are associated with more than 80% of cases.

Skin Findings
- Early changes include erythema, edema, and vesicles.
- Blisters occur in sun-exposed areas such as the face and neck, the dorsa of the hands, and forearms.
- Blisters rupture leaving erosions and ulcers that heal with scarring.
- Milia form in previously blistered sites on the hand.
- Chronic changes include facial hypertrichosis, particularly on the temples and on periorbital skin.
- Hyperpigmentation develops on the face, neck, and hands.
- Sclerotic changes and increased skin fragility on the cheeks, posterior neck, ears and fingers give the sclerodermoid pattern.

Non-skin Findings
- Liver disease occurs in association with ethanol abuse, estrogens, aromatic hydrocarbons; benign, malignant or metastatic tumors; chronic renal failure during dialysis; sarcoidosis; hepatitis C infection, hepatitis B infection and human immunodeficiency virus infection.

Laboratory
- Histopathology confirms subepidermal split and thickening of superficial dermal vascular endothelium.

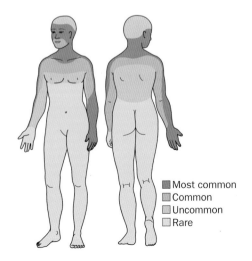

Most common
Common
Uncommon
Rare

- Direct immunofluorescence shows deposition of immunoglobulin G, immunoglobulin M, and complement C3 surrounding blood vessels in the papillary dermis.
- Fecal analysis shows elevated coproporphyrins.
- Quantitative assays of fecal, urine, and red blood cell porphyrins.
- A 24-hour urine collection contains uroporphyrin in a ratio of about 4 : 1 to the coproporphyrin fraction.

- Urine may have a red-brown discoloration—so-called port-wine urine—from high levels of porphyrin pigments and may show a bright pink fluorescence under a Wood's light.
- Order liver function tests, iron studies, renal function tests as well as human immunodeficiency virus and hepatitis viral serologies.
- Consider computerized tomography scan or ultrasound of liver to examine for tumors.

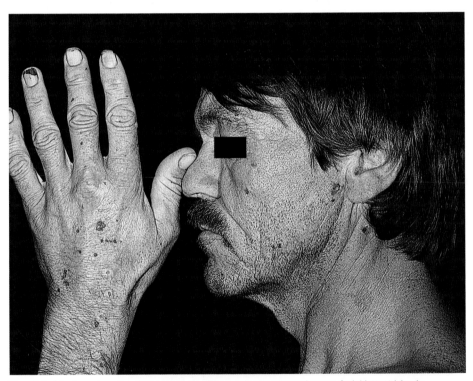

The clinical features in order of frequency are blistering in sun-exposed areas, facial hypertrichosis, hyperpigmentation, and sclerodermoid changes.

Differential Diagnosis

- Pseudoporphyria (usually due to non-steroidal anti-inflammatory drugs and is clinically indistinguishable from porphyria cutanea tarda)
- Porphyrin studies are negative
- Porphyria variegata (cutaneous signs of porphyria cutanea tarda coexist with the abdominal pain and neuropsychiatric symptoms of acute intermittent porphyria)
- Acute intermittent porphyria (skin manifestations are absent)
- Protoporphyrin and coproporphyrin are in feces
- Elevated urinary levels of gamma-aminolevulinic acid and porphobilinogen occur during attacks

Course and Prognosis

- Porphyria cutanea tarda in association with alcohol abuse tends to be chronic and relapsing until the alcohol dependence is addressed.

Treatment

- Complete elimination of alcohol and exposure to other hepatotoxins results in complete clinical clearing of bullae and skin fragility in 2 months to 2 years.
- Iron removal by phlebotomy is the treatment of choice.
- It reduces hepatic iron stores and produces remissions of several years' duration.
- One unit of blood should be removed every 2–4 weeks until the hemoglobin drops to 10 gm/dl or until the serum iron drops to 50 mg/dl.
- The average number of units of blood required for remission varies between 8 and 14.
- Chloroquine in very low dosages may also be used.
- Chloroquine causes the release of hepatic tissue-bound uroporphyrin, and subsequently it is rapidly eliminated by the plasma and excreted by the urine.
- A too-rapid release of porphyrins might severely affect liver function.
- Complete clinical and biochemical response has occurred with the use of chloroquine 125 mg twice weekly for 8–18 months.
- Remission in most patients has been for more than 4 years.
- Measuring plasma uroporphyrin is an effective way to monitor the progress of patients with porphyria cutanea tarda.
- Treatment should continue until plasma uroporphyrin drops below 10 mmol/L.
- Combined treatment with repeated bleeding and chloroquine results in remission in an average of 3.5 months.
- The time necessary for remission with chloroquine alone is 10.2 months.
- The time necessary for remission with phlebotomy alone is 12.5 months.
- Sunscreens which contain Parsol 1789 (e.g. Ombrelle) that block ultraviolet A light should be used.
- Physical sun-blockers that contain titanium dioxide are moderately effective.

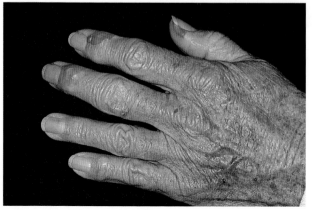

Porphyria cutanea tarda. Blisters formed on a non-inflamed base following sun exposure.

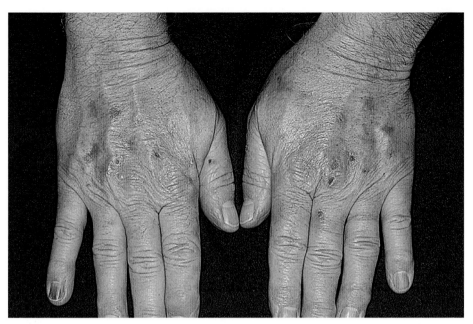

Porphyria cutanea tarda. The classic presentation with erosions, vesicles and bullae localized to the backs of the hands.

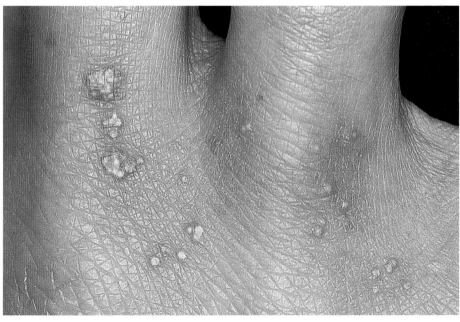

White milia form during the healing process and are permanent.

Vitiligo

Description
- A disfiguring depigmenting disease of unknown origin that causes destruction of melanocytes.

History
- 1% of the population affected and 50% begin before age 20.
- Both genders are affected equally.
- There is positive family history in 30%.
- Patients relate the first onset in the aftermath of emotional stress, illness or skin trauma such as sunburn.

Skin Findings
- There are two clinical types, types A and B.
- Type A is the more common pattern involving a fairly symmetric pattern of white depigmented 0.5–5.0 cm macules and patches with well-defined borders.
- Type B is segmental vitiligo; this is limited to one segment of body, such as one extremity.
- Type B is more common as a childhood disease.
- In type A borders may have a red halo of inflammation or rim of hyperpigmentation.
- Loss of pigmentation is not as obvious in fair-skinned people, but is easily seen in dark-skinned people.
- In type A common sites include the dorsal hands and fingers, face, body folds, axillae, and genitalia.
- Type A has a predilection for orifices including the eyes, nostrils, mouth, nipples, umbilicus, and anus.
- Vitiligo occurs at sites of trauma (Köbner's phenomenon).
- Wood's light accentuates the hypopigmented areas.

Non-skin Findings
- In type A there is an increased incidence of autoimmune thyroid disease.

Laboratory
- Skin biopsy shows an absence of melanocytes and a sparse lymphocytic inflammation.

Differential Diagnosis
- Lupus erythematosus (tends to scar as well as depigment in darker skin types)
- Pityriasis alba (hypopigmented, scaly and self-limited)
- Piebaldism (usually presents early and tends to favor ventral surfaces only)
- Tinea versicolor (scaling and a positive potassium hydroxide examination)

Course and Prognosis
- Slowly progresses over years in a highly variable course.
- Some patients have very stable disease while others progress at alarming rate.
- Segmental vitiligo develops quickly, then stabilizes, rarely spreading.
- Depigmented areas are at increased risk for sunburn and subsequent skin cancers.

Discussion
- Vitiligo can be devastating for dark-skinned people, especially if there are cultural implications.
- Every effort should be made to listen to the patient's concerns and all efforts should be made on their behalf.

Treatment
- Broad spectrum sunscreens that contain avobenzone (Parsol 1789) e.g. Ombrelle, PreSun Ultra and/or titanium dioxide or zinc oxide.

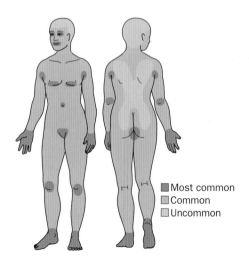

■ Most common
□ Common
□ Uncommon

- Sun-protective clothing is available from Sun Precautions (http://www.sunprecautions.com) and similar companies.
- Concealing and camouflaging agents, such as DermaBlend, Covermark, and Elizabeth Arden Concealing Cream, are effective but require some practice in application for good cosmesis.
- Suggest a local qualified cosmetic consultant as a resource for color matching.
- Sunless or self-tanning lotions darken the skin by staining and work best for skin phototypes II and III.
- Group I–V topical steroid ointments are safe and effective for limited disease.

- Apply twice daily for 6 weeks, stop for 2 weeks; repeat for two more cycles if there are no side effects.
- The face and neck respond better than other areas but avoid group I steroids on the face.
- Tacrolimus ointment 0.1% (Protopic) may be effective in some cases. Continuous application can be used with this safe topical medication.
- Pulse-dose systemic steroids may arrest or slow rapidly progressing cases, but have potential side effects and risk.
- Topical or systemic photochemotherapy with psoralen with ultraviolet A light therapy is somewhat effective but supervision by a dermatologist is needed for this office-based treatment.

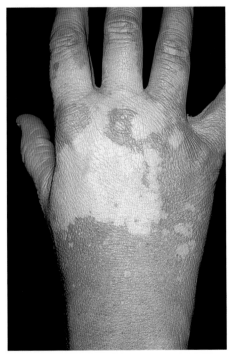

The margins of the lesions may become more hyperpigmented. The borders are sharply defined.

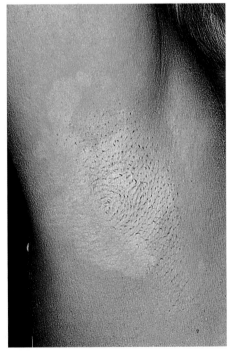

Examine the axillae, groin and anal area in all patients suspected of having vitiligo. These areas are commonly involved or may be the only areas involved.

- Potential side effects, the expense and inconvenience limit the usefulness of therapy with psoralen plus ultraviolet A.
- Narrow-band ultraviolet B light treatment may be effective.
- There are reports of laser-induced repigmentation, but this is still an evolving therapy and it is not widely available.
- Patients with involvement of more than 40% of the body surface may choose to remove the remaining normal pigment with 20% monobenzone (Benoquin cream).

- Apply monobenzone twice daily for 6–18 months to chemically destroy all melanocytes in the skin.
- Depigmentation is irreversible, requiring the patient to be informed, and subsequent close attention to sun protection.

Pearls

- Proper treatment requires a frank discussion of the patient's goals, of reasonable expectations, and risks and benefits of treatment.

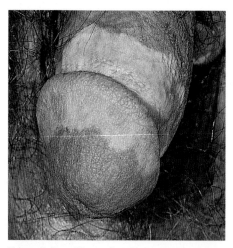

The genitalia, axillae, and anal areas may be the first or only areas affected. These sites should be examined in all patients suspected of having vitiligo.

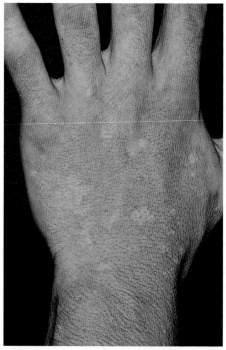

Vitiligo on the back of the hand. This area is resistant to all forms of treatment.

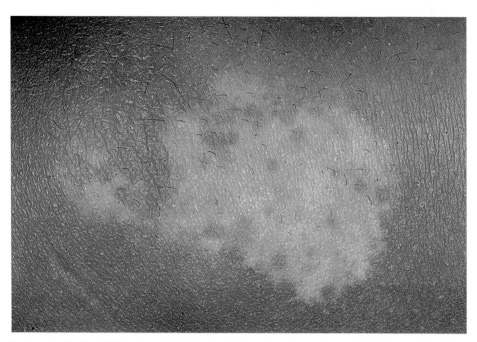

Treatment with either PUVA or topical steroids stimulates repigmentation from perifollicular areas. These areas of repigmentation enlarge and merge to produce confluent repigmentation.

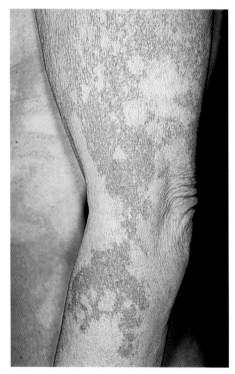

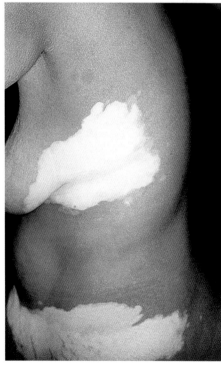

Loss of pigment may be partial or complete. Complex patterns are typical.

Several areas of depigmentation have merged to form large areas of pigment loss.

Idiopathic Guttate Hypomelanosis

Description
- Idiopathic guttate hypomelanosis is a common dermatosis of unknown etiology consisting of small white macules on the sun-exposed upper and lower extremities.

History
- Idiopathic guttate hypomelanosis occurs in middle-aged and older people.
- It is more common in women.
- There is a higher prevalence in family members; genetic predisposition is likely.
- It occurs in 50–70% of people over the age of 50.
- It is symptomatic.

Skin Findings
- Macules are white and hypopigmented, 2–5 mm, with regular borders.
- There is smooth to slight xerotic scaling.
- Macules are scattered on the exposed upper and lower extremities.
- Patients have signs of photoaging, including atrophy, lentigines, and xerosis in the same areas.

Laboratory
- Skin biopsy is not usually needed but it confirms epidermal atrophy, patchy absence of melanocytes and melanin.
- Potassium hydroxide examination of scale is negative.

Differential Diagnosis
- Vitiligo (tends to be symmetric with macules extending into patches)
- Tinea versicolor (favors upper trunk and has positive potassium hydroxide examination)
- Chemically induced hypomelanosis from occupational exposure to depigmenting agents (favors hands and forearms)
- Tuberous sclerosis (presents in childhood and adolescence along with associated neurologic signs)
- Pityriasis alba (probably represents post-inflammatory hypopigmentation; tends to resolve over several years)

Course and Prognosis
- The lesions are stable in size and remain fixed.
- The number of lesions increases with age.

Discussion
- Appearance and potential for malignancy are the major reasons for patients' concerns.
- Actinic damage has been incriminated as the major cause, but a senile degenerative phenomenon may play a role.

Treatment
- Reassurance is all that is required for most patients.
- White macules can be camouflaged with tinted makeup such as Covermark or DermaBlend.
- Self-tanning creams that contain dihydroxyacetone darken the lesions, but the appearance is speckled and not pleasing.
- A light spray with liquid nitrogen may partially fade the lesions though there is the potential for worsening the dyspigmentation.
- Intralesional triamcinolone (2.5 mg/ml) infiltrated into individual lesions may

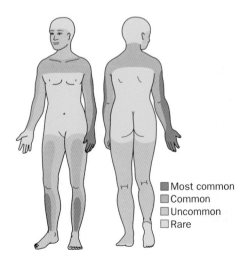

Most common
Common
Uncommon
Rare

partially cause repigmentation of lesions, though there is risk of atrophy.

■ Encourage sun protection with clothing, as sunscreens are less effective than clothing.

Pearls

■ Patients should be warned that any treatment may worsen the dyspigmentation and should be performed only by experienced providers.

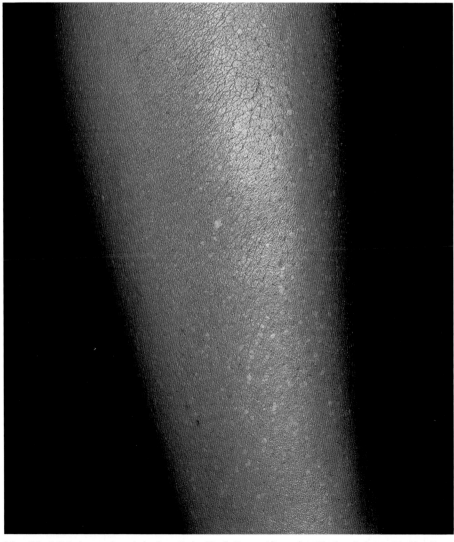

Idiopathic guttate hypomelanosis is characterized by 2–5-mm white spots with sharply demarcated borders. They are a sign of photodamage.

Lentigo (Plural Lentigines), Juvenile Lentigo, Solar Lentigo

Description
- Common, benign, brown macules occurring on sun-exposed skin of Caucasian people.

History
- Three lesions of localized hyperpigmentation occur in Caucasian people.
- These lesions are freckles (ephelides), juvenile lentigo, and solar lentigo.
- All three are similar in size, distribution and clinical appearance.
- They differ in age of onset, clinical course and relationship to sun exposure.

Freckles
- Freckles appear in childhood and occur as an autosomal dominant trait.
- They are usually confined to the face, arms and upper trunk.
- They increase in number and darken in color in response to sun exposure.
- Freckles lighten in color without sun exposure.
- They often fade completely in the winter.

Juvenile Lentigines
- Lentigines are extremely common in Caucasian people.
- Juvenile lentigines appear in childhood with a mean number of 30 lentigines in each prepubertal child.
- Lesions do not increase in number or size or darken in color in response to sunlight.
- Juvenile lentigines do not fade in the absence of sunlight.
- Juvenile lentigines also occur as a characteristic feature of certain hereditary syndromes.

Solar Lentigines
- Solar lentigines commonly occur on the skin of sun-exposed Caucasian people.
- They increase in number and size with advancing age.
- Roughly 75% of white people over the age of 60 have one or more lesion.
- They develop in response to actinic damage.

Skin Findings
- Freckles are sharply defined macules of 1-2 mm, with uniform color.
- Freckles vary from red or tan to light brown.
- The number varies from a few sparse lesions over the nose and malar cheeks to hundreds with near confluence on sun-exposed skin.
- They are usually limited to the face, arms, and upper trunk.
- Juvenile lentigines are round to oval macules, 2-10 mm in diameter.
- They are usually darker than freckles, uniformly tan or brown or black.
- Color is uniform although the pigment may have a lacy or fine-grained pattern.
- A drop of mineral oil applied to the lesion reduces surface glare and allows for evaluation of the junctional pigmentation pattern.
- Solar lentigines tend to be larger, 2-20 mm oval to geometric macules.
- Color is most often uniform though pigment may appear as fine grains.
- Lentigines may appear blotchy, though the borders should be sharply defined.

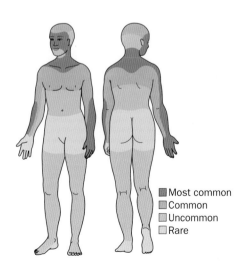

- Most common
- Common
- Uncommon
- Rare

The surrounding skin shows actinic damage.

Non-skin Findings

- Lentigines are a feature of rare autosomal dominant syndromes.
- Peutz–Jeghers syndrome consists of multiple lentigines of the oral mucosa with associated intestinal polyposis.
- The LEOPARD syndrome consists of multiple **l**entigines, **e**lectrocardiogram abnormalities, **o**cular disorders, **p**ulmonary stenosis, **a**bnormalities of genitalia, **r**etardation of growth, and **d**eafness.

- A third syndrome described by Carney is known as LAMB or NAME. This syndrome consists of lentigines, atrial and/or mucocutaneous myxomas, myxoid neurofibromas, ephelides, and blue nevi.

Laboratory

- Freckles show increased melanin within basal layer keratinocytes.
- Rete ridges are not elongated.
- Junctional melanocytes are larger but not increased in number.
- In juvenile lentigo there is an increased number of non-nested melanocytes along the dermoepidermal junction.

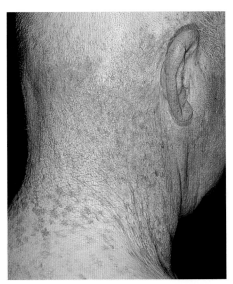

Reactive hyperplasia of melanocytes causes persistent pigmentation in the form of lentigines on the neck and upper back. These permanent lesions may occur after one bad episode of sunburn.

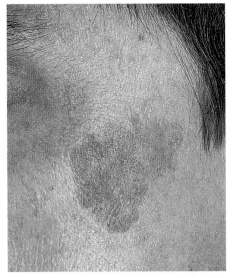

The lesions vary in size from 0.2 cm to 2 cm and become more numerous with advancing age. The lesion should be carefully examined. Seborrheic keratosis and melanoma have a similar appearance.

- The rete ridges are elongated.
- Melanin is increased within basal layer keratinocytes.
- Solar lentigines also show irregular elongation of rete ridges, basal layer keratinocyte hyperpigmentation, and increased numbers of junctional melanocytes.
- Melanophages may be present in the papillary dermis.
- Histologically similar lesions occur on the lower mucosal lip and in the nail bed.

Differential Diagnosis

- Flat seborrheic keratoses tend to have some surface hyperkeratosis.
- Spreading pigmented actinic keratosis also has epidermal hyperkeratosis and a defined border.
- Lentigo maligna is best diagnosed by skin biopsy and careful histologic review.
- When numerous lentigines are present, consider the possibility of an associated syndrome such as Peutz–Jeghers, LEOPARD syndrome, or NAME (LAMB).

Course and Prognosis

- Freckles appear in early summer and usually fade by early winter.
- Juvenile lentigo persists year-round with little change over years or may spontaneously resolve.
- Solar lentigo is usually persistent; additional lesions may appear elsewhere on sun-exposed skin.
- Lesions are asymptomatic but may be of cosmetic concern to the patient.

Discussion

- It is difficult to discern between freckles and similar juvenile lentigines.
- Freckles darken and then fade with the seasons where lentigines do not.
- Junctional nevi of similar size are also similar in appearance.
- Skin biopsy will confirm melanocyte nesting along the dermoepidermal junction in a junctional nevus.

Treatment

- Freckles do not require treatment and will fade in the winter months.
- Sunscreens appear to prevent the appearance of new freckles and seasonal darkening.
- Juvenile lentigines similarly do not require treatment.
- Solar lentigines are best prevented with sun-protective measures including sun avoidance, hats, clothing, and sunscreens.
- Monitor existing lesions for interval change. Stable lesions do not require treatment though it may be requested for cosmetic reasons.
- Hydroquinone solutions, tretinoin, azelaic acid cream, glycolic acid peels and creams are all of value in reducing hyperpigmentation over weeks to months.
- Light cryosurgery is also effective but requires some experience.

Pearls

- Any lentigo which develops a localized area of hyperpigmentation or hypopigmentation, an irregular outline, or localized thickening should be biopsied.

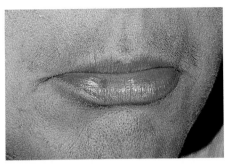

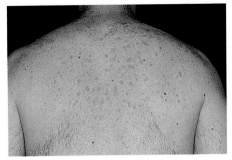

Labial lentigines (labial melanotic macule) occur on the vermilion border of the lower lip. These brown macules have a smooth border and are benign.

Solar lentigo ("liver spots") appears on the face, arms, dorsa of the hands, and upper trunk following a single episode of sunburn or after years of sun exposure. These flat brown macules increase in number and size.

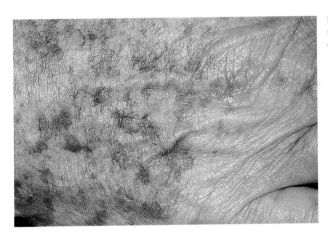

Lentigo ("liver spots") occurs in sun-exposed areas of the face, arms, and hands.

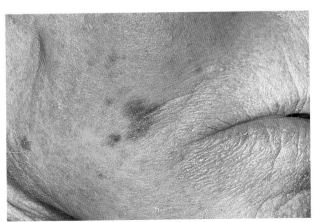

A biopsy should be taken from any lentigo that develops a highly irregular border, or where there is a localized increase in pigmentation, or localized thickening, to rule out lentigo maligna melanoma.

Melasma (Chloasma, Mask of Pregnancy)

Description

- Acquired brown hyperpigmentation of the face and neck in genetically predisposed women.

History

- This is a common complaint in women with darker skin tones.
- Around 10% of cases occur in men.
- The forehead, malar eminences, upper lip, and chin are most frequently affected.
- Pigmentation develops slowly and is more prevalent after sunlight exposure.
- It occurs during the second or third trimester of pregnancy and in some women taking oral contraceptives.

Skin Findings

- Symmetric macular eruption of brown hyperpigmentation.
- The intensity of the color varies with deeper pigmentation in darker-skinned people.
- Color is usually uniform, but may be variable.
- Edges of the lesions can be irregular but well defined.
- There are no signs of inflammation.

Differential Diagnosis

- Post-inflammatory hyperpigmentation (similar pigmentation but not usually limited to the upper face)
- Lentigines (may be clustered on the upper cheeks)

Course and Prognosis

- Usually after pregnancy or with discontinuation of contraceptives the pigment fades slowly over months.

Treatment

- Minimize sun exposure at mid-day and encourage wearing of hats.
- Sunscreens that block both ultraviolet A and ultraviolet B.
- Depigmentation with bleaching creams that contain hydroquinone.
- Over-the-counter products are at 2% concentrations (Porcelana).
- Prescription products include 3% (Melanex) and 4% (Lustra, Claripel, Eldoquin forte and Solaquin forte).
- Hydroquinone can be an irritant and a sensitizer.
- Tretinoin cream 0.025%, 0.05%, 0.1% (Retin-A) and tretinoin emollient cream 0.05% (Renova) enhance the effectiveness of hydroquinones.
- Tretinoin is also effective as monotherapy.
- Combination products containing tretinoin, hydroquinone and fluocinolone (Tri-Luma) may be more effective and more convenient. This is applied once each day for a maximum duration of 6 months.
- Azelaic acid (Finacea cream) with or without tretinoin is safe during pregnancy.
- Superficial peels with glycolic acid hasten the effects of tretinoin and hydroquinone.

Pearls

- Sun avoidance is mandatory to prevent and reduce melasma.
- Patients must be made aware that treatment requires several weeks and strict sun protection.

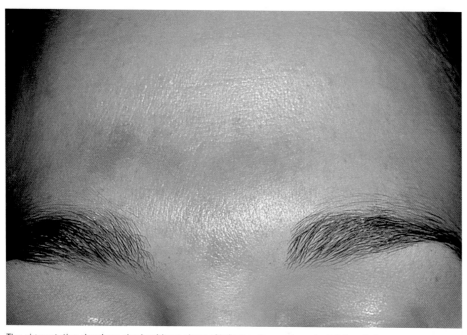

The pigmentation develops slowly without signs of inflammation and may be faint or dark.

The forehead, malar eminences, upper lip, and chin are most frequently affected.

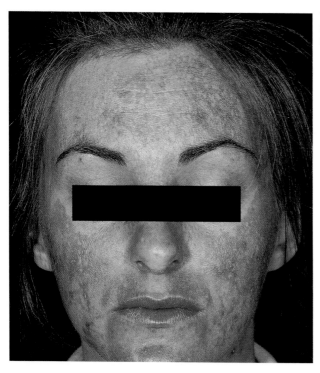

16 Benign Skin Tumors

Seborrheic Keratosis

Description
- A seborrheic keratosis is a common, benign, persistent epidermal lesion with variable clinical appearance.
- It is one of the most common benign growths seen on the skin and can be confused with cutaneous malignancies.

History
- Seborrheic keratoses are unusual before age 30.
- Most people develop at least one seborrheic keratosis in their lifetime.
- Males and females are equally affected.
- Lesions may be localized to the areola in both males and females.
- The tendency toward multiple seborrheic keratoses may be inherited.
- This condition is usually asymptomatic, but sometimes it is cosmetically bothersome.
- Depending on the location, the lesion can be subject to irritation.

Skin Findings
- There are usually multiple lesions, which can arise at any site except the lips, palms and soles.
- The size and surface appearance of the lesions vary considerably.
- Most are 0.2-2.0 cm, although larger lesions can occur.
- Lesions may be flat or raised.
- The surface may be smooth, velvety, or verrucous.
- Retained keratin cysts may be seen just under the surface within clefts.
- The color of lesions is extremely variable, including white, pink, brown and black, and the color may vary within a single lesion.
- Lesions tend to be sharply demarcated, oval, and often oriented along skin cleavage lines.
- Most have a "stuck-on" appearance and waxy texture.
- The surface tends to crumble when picked.
- Dermatosis papulosa nigra describes the seborrheic keratoses of the face seen more commonly in African–American people.
- Dermatosis papulosa nigra lesions are 1–2 mm, dark brown keratotic papules concentrated around the eyes and upper cheeks, with an incidence of 30-35% in African–American people.
- Stucco keratoses describe the small, whitish seborrheic keratoses more commonly found on the lower legs and ankles of older Caucasian people.

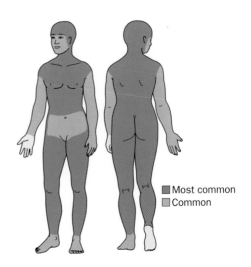

■ Most common
□ Common

Inflamed seborrheic keratosis is a clinical description for a seborrheic keratosis with clinically obvious inflammation; there may be edema, erythema and hemorrhage.

Non-skin Findings

- The sign of Leser–Trélat is the sudden explosive onset of numerous seborrheic keratoses in association with internal malignancy.

Laboratory

- Several histologic subtypes of seborrheic keratosis are recognized.
- Acanthosis, hyperkeratosis, and papillomatosis are universal features.
- The degree to which these features develop varies considerably within individual lesions and among subtypes.
- Horn cysts and pseudo-horn cysts are usually present.
- The degree of melanin pigment varies from almost none (stucco keratosis) to extreme (melanoacanthoma).
- Inflamed seborrheic keratoses show marked dermal inflammation, sometimes making the diagnosis difficult.

Course and Prognosis

- Unless disturbed, seborrheic keratoses tend to persist and grow slowly.
- Some lesions may be removed by trauma.

Discussion

- Raised or pedunculated seborrheic keratoses may be indistinguishable from skin tags and compound melanocytic nevi.
- Flat seborrheic keratoses may mimic spreading pigmented actinic keratosis or superficial spreading melanoma. If doubt exists, a skin biopsy should be performed.
- Although seborrheic keratoses have no malignant potential, there are rare reports of melanoma, basal cell carcinoma and squamous cell carcinoma developing within a seborrheic keratosis. A biopsy should be performed for a significantly changing seborrheic keratosis.

Treatment

- Treatment may be indicated for symptomatic lesions.
- Lesions in areas of friction and frequent trauma often become irritated and symptomatic.
- Removal is often requested for cosmetic reasons.
- Patients should be informed that cosmetic removal of seborrheic keratoses is not usually covered by medical insurance.
- Cryosurgery is effective for flat or minimally raised lesions.
- Thicker lesions are best removed by cautery and curettage under local anesthesia.
- Residual scarring, if any, is minimal. Applying gentle pressure to the surrounding skin often provides enough tension to allow for easy curettage of lesions.
- Hypopigmentation or hyperpigmentation are possible side effects of cryotherapy or any method of removal.

Pearls

- Seborrheic keratoses are common benign growths with multiple variants that can mimic other more worrisome skin tumors.
- Removal is not warranted unless lesions become inflamed and symptomatic.
- Some keratoses are heavily pigmented, resembling melanoma, and therefore should be biopsied.
- When dermatologists unknowingly remove melanomas, it is thought that they are seborrheic keratoses clinically in 85% of cases.

Rough Surface Keratoses

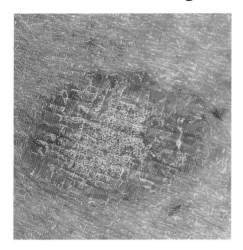 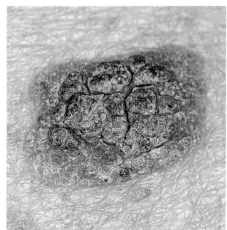

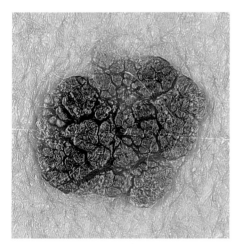 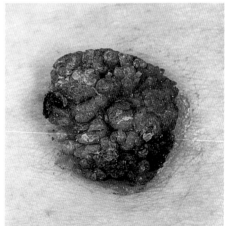

The rough-surfaced seborrheic keratoses are the most common benign skin tumor. They are oval to round flattened domes with a granular or irregular surface that crumbles when picked. Flatter lesions are found on the arms and legs. Patients often refer to these lesions as warts because of the similar appearance.

Smooth Surface Keratoses

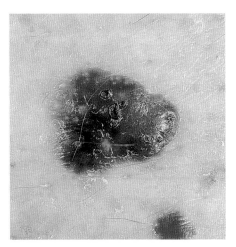 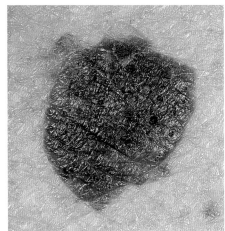

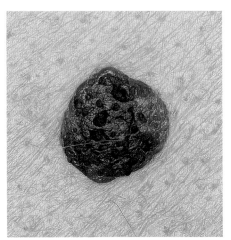 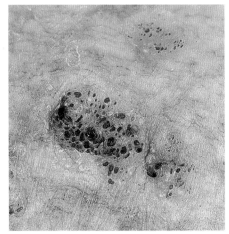

Smooth-surfaced, dome-shaped tumors have white or black pearls of keratin, 1 mm in diameter, embedded in the surface. These horn pearls are easily seen with a hand lens. Melanomas do not contain horn pearls.

Keratoses Mimicking Melanoma

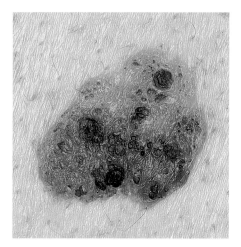
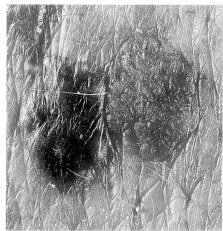

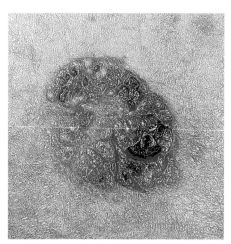
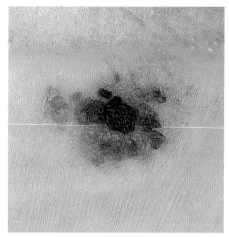

Some seborrheic keratoses may have many of the features of superficial spreading and nodular melanoma. The colors are variable, and the white areas look like areas of tumor regression. A magnified view shows several horn cysts that are typically found in seborrheic keratoses and rarely present in melanoma. A biopsy should always be performed if melanoma is suspected.

Irritated Seborrheic Keratoses

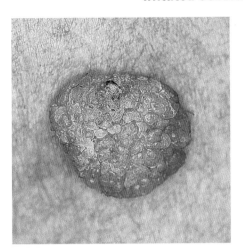 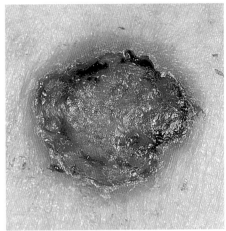

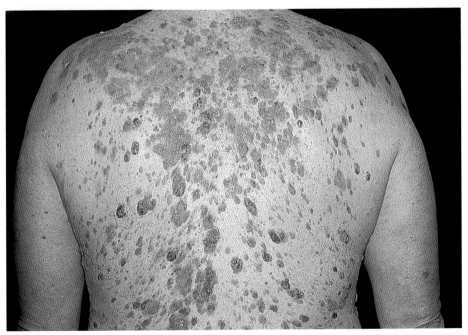

Irritated seborrheic keratoses become slightly swollen and develop an irregular, red flare in the surrounding skin. They may develop into a bright red, oozing mass with a friable surface that resembles an advanced melanoma or a pyogenic granuloma.

Seborrheic Keratoses

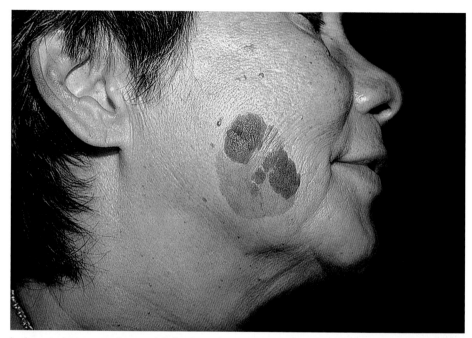

Lesions can become very large and disfiguring and resemble melanoma. Examine the surface closely with a hand lens. Look for horn pearls that are only found in seborrheic keratoses.

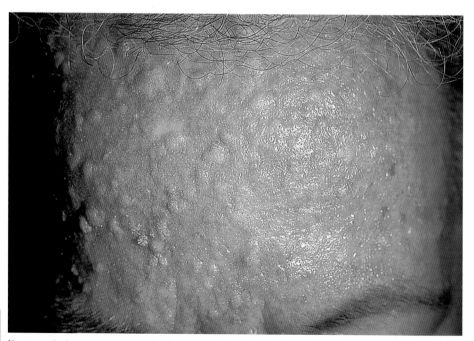

Numerous lesions may appear on the face in predisposed people.

Seborrheic Keratoses

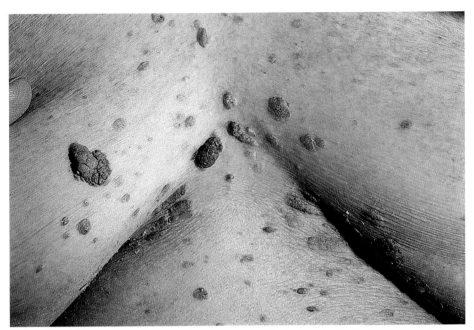

Lesions are often concentrated in the presternal area and under the breasts. Chafing from clothing or from maceration in this intertriginous area can start irritation.

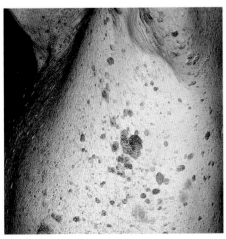

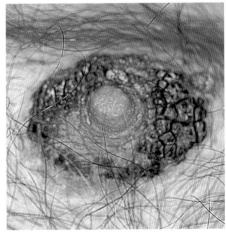

The number varies from less than 20 in most people to numerous lesions on the face or trunk.

Lesions may be localized to the areola in both men and women.

Stucco Keratoses

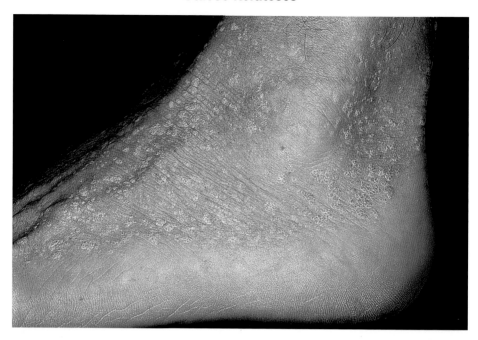

Stucco keratoses are white, papular, warty lesions occurring on the lower legs, especially around the Achilles tendon area, and the dorsum of the foot. The 1–10 mm lesions are round, very dry and stuck-on, considered by most patients to be simply manifestations of dry skin. The dry surface scale is easily picked intact from the skin without bleeding, but it recurs shortly thereafter. Cryosurgery in this area may produce excessive hyperpigmentation. Curettage of individual lesions may be the best treatment option for those few patients who request their removal.

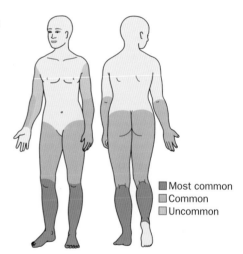

■ Most common
☐ Common
☐ Uncommon

Stucco Keratoses

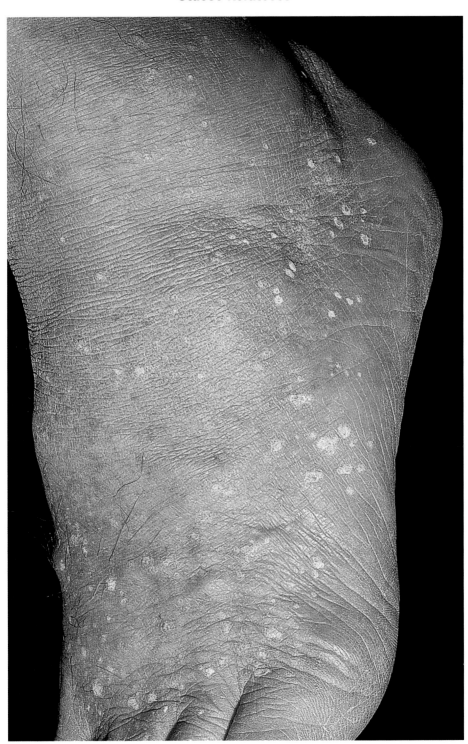

Skin Tags

Description
- Skin tags are common benign fleshy papules occurring in the skinfolds.

History
- Skin tags, or acrochordons, are uncommon before age 30 but are common thereafter.
- Women are affected more often than men.
- Roughly 25% of adults have at least one skin tag.
- The majority of patients with skin tags have only a few lesions.
- They are more common in overweight persons.
- There may be a familial tendency toward multiple skin tags.
- Undisturbed lesions are usually asymptomatic.
- As a result of their location, skin tags may become irritated by friction, jewelry or clothing.
- They may become tender when traumatized, twisted, torn, or thrombosed.

Skin Findings
- A skin tag is a skin-colored or brown 1–5 mm papule.
- Papules may be flat or filiform, although most are soft, fleshy, and pedunculated on a thin stalk.
- The axillae are the most common location, followed by the neck.
- Lesions also occur on the eyelids as well as in other intertriginous areas such as the inframammary and inguinal creases.

Non-skin Findings
- A previously reported association between skin tags and colonic polyps has not been confirmed by further studies.
- Skin tags are part of the Birt-Hogg–Dube syndrome, which also includes trichodiscomas and fibrofolliculomas of the face, neck and chest. Patients with this syndrome may have associated renal cell carcinoma, colonic adenomas, pulmonary cysts and medullary carcinoma of the thyroid gland.

Laboratory
- Skin biopsy confirms a papule with a characteristic thinned epidermis and a loosely arranged fibrous stroma with capillaries.

Course and Prognosis
- Left undisturbed, skin tags persist indefinitely.
- With torsion, skin tags may become thrombosed and tender.
- With this acute change, patients usually seek care because they are concerned about skin malignancy.
- Thrombosed skin tags often appear black, or hemorrhagic, or both.
- Any delay in seeking care allows the residual skin tag time to fall off on its own; thus no residual lesion is seen.

Differential Diagnosis
- Warts
- Nevi
- Seborrheic keratosis

Treatment
- Asymptomatic skin tags do not require treatment.
- Patients often request removal because of tenderness or for cosmetic reasons.
- Patients should be informed that medically unnecessary removal of skin

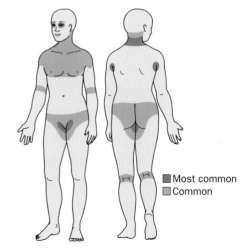

■ Most common
□ Common

tags is usually not covered by medical insurance.

- Skin tags are best treated by scissors excision with or without local anesthesia.
- Electrocautery and cryosurgery can also be used.
- The need to submit all skin tags for histologic review has been a topic of debate in recent years.

- Many dermatologists feel that histologic confirmation is usually not necessary.

Pearls

- Skin tags do not present a diagnostic dilemma.
- Skin tags around the eyelids may resemble other skin tumors and may need a biopsy for confirmation.

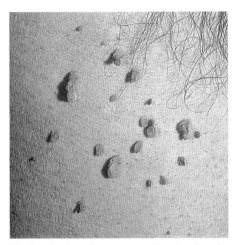

Skin tags begin as tiny, brown or skin-colored, oval excrescences attached by a short, broad-to-narrow stalk.

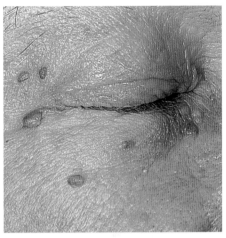

Skin tags occur around the eyes and may resemble warts.

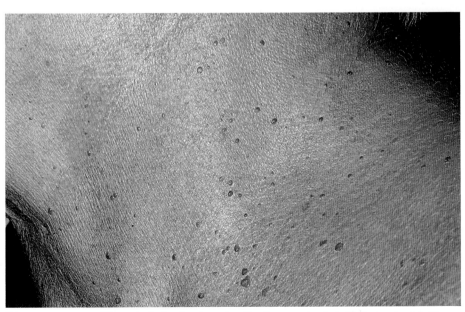

Skin tags start as small brown to flesh colored papules. They become elevated with time and eventually become polypoid and protrude from a narrow base.

Dermatofibroma

Description
- Dermatofibroma is a common, benign, indolent, dermal papule most commonly occurring on the legs of adults.

History
- Dermatofibromas arise spontaneously in adults and occasionally in children.
- The lesions occur more often in women.
- Lesions on the legs of women are subject to repeated trauma from shaving and can be annoying.
- Most are asymptomatic, but pruritis and tenderness may occur.
- The etiology is unknown.
- Controversy exists as to whether the lesion represents a spontaneous benign neoplastic process or reactive hyperplasia in response to injury.
- Most patients do not recall a specific trauma to the area.
- Some patients note itching when the lesion is first noted and attribute this to an insect bite.
- Dermatofibromas tend to persist indefinitely while remaining stable in size and appearance.

Skin Findings
- Discrete firm pink dermal papules of 3–7 mm in diameter are typical.
- Lesions larger than 3.0 cm are occasionally seen.
- Most dermatofibromas are dome shaped, although some are depressed below the surrounding skin surface.
- The lesion is fixed within the skin, but movable over the underlying subcutaneous fat.
- On palpation, the lesion feels like a firm button.
- Pinching a dome-shaped dermatofibroma between two fingers causes the lesion to dimple and retract below the level of surrounding skin.
- Dermatofibromas are typically flesh-colored to pink with a poorly defined rim of tan to brown pigmentation.
- Rarely, lesions may be blue to black as a result of hemosiderin deposition, and may resemble melanoma.
- The surface may be smooth and shiny to scaly or excoriated.
- Although dermatofibromas may arise on any cutaneous surface, most are found randomly distributed on the extremities.
- Lesions are usually solitary, however multiple lesions can occur.

Laboratory
- Skin biopsy shows a focal unencapsulated proliferation of spindle-shaped cells resembling fibroblasts, histiocytes, and collagen.

Course and Prognosis
- Dermatofibromas attain their maximum size over months to years and then persist indefinitely.
- Spontaneous involution is rare.
- Depending on location, lesions may be subject to repeated trauma from shaving or friction from boots.

Discussion
- Lesions with large amounts of hemosiderin deep within the tumor may be blue to black and suggestive of nodular melanoma or pigmented dermatofibrosarcoma protuberans. Biopsy is warranted in such cases.
- Dermatofibroma can clinically mimic melanoma with a central pink nodule and surrounding pigmentation.

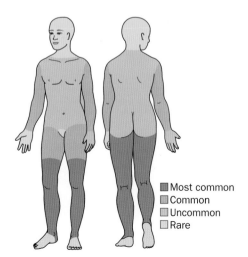

Most common
Common
Uncommon
Rare

- Dermatofibrosarcoma protuberans resembles dermatofibroma histologically and, less commonly, clinically.
- This insidious malignancy usually occurs on the trunk and presents as a slow-growing, often recurrent, poorly defined red-purple nodule or plaque.
- Overall, the histologic findings are similar to those of dermatofibroma, so a superficial biopsy may be falsely reassuring.
- Deep punch or excisional biopsy that includes subcutaneous fat confirms that dermatofibrosarcoma protuberans is more cellular than most dermatofibromas.
- Malignant cells extend into the subcutaneous fat.

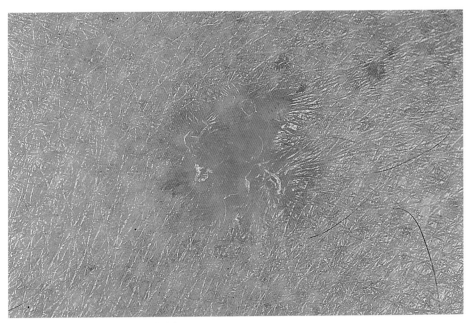

Early lesions are elevated, hard and pink.

Treatment

- Dermatofibromas are benign skin tumors that do not require treatment unless they are symptomatic, repeatedly traumatized, or cosmetically bothersome. The patient should be assured that the lesion is benign.
- Surgical excision with primary closure is the treatment of choice for symptomatic lesions.
- Caution should be used when removing lesions for cosmetic reasons, as the final appearance may be less cosmetically acceptable than the original lesion.
- If the lesion is incompletely excised by shave excision, the patient should be warned of possible recurrence.
- Intralesional corticosteroid injection has been used to flatten elevated lesions. This form of treatment produces unpredictable results and is generally not recommended.

Pearls

- Dermatofibromas should be stable in size, appearance, and color. If they are not, they should be biopsied.
- Pigmented lesions that are suspected to be traumatized should be biopsied.
- A shave biopsy is not appropriate when the diagnosis is in question. An excision is optimal so that the entire lesion, including the deep dermal component can be evaluated histologically.

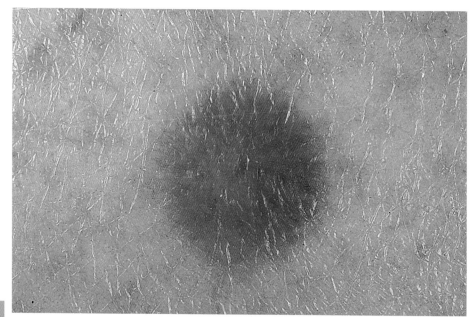

New lesions are pink and elevated. After months the border becomes tan to brown and the center retains the pink color.

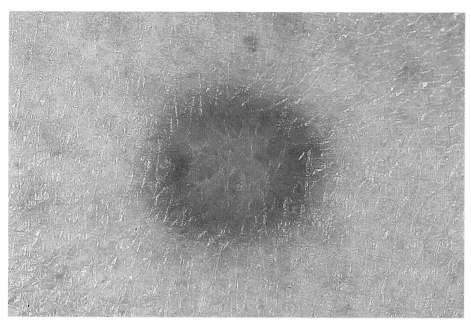

The density of the brown pigmentation increases with time and the distinction between the border and the pink becomes more apparent. Patients become concerned about melanoma with the increasing density of the pigmentation.

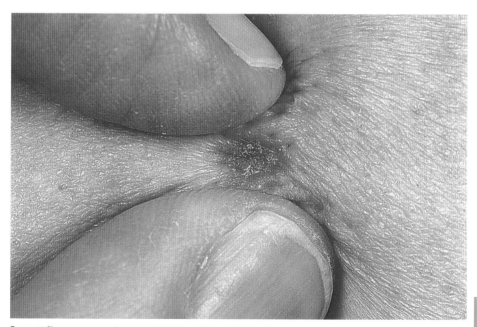

Dermatofibromas retract beneath the skin surface during attempts to compress and elevate them.

Keloids and Hypertrophic Scars

Description
■ A keloid is an exuberant scar that extends beyond the area of trauma or injury.
■ A hypertrophic scar is an inappropriately exuberant healing response to trauma or injury, occurring in a predisposed person.

History
■ Males and females are affected with equal frequency.
■ Keloids can occur at any age but tend to occur before age 30.
■ Keloids are more common in African–American people than Caucasian people.
■ Hypertrophic scars and keloids can arise at any skin site. Most occur on the chest, head and neck. The earlobe is another common site.
■ Lesions occur at sites of trauma and injury, which includes surgery, burns, piercing, acne and sites of inflammation.

Skin Findings
■ Normal scars are usually red and firm during the initial weeks of healing.
■ Itching and tenderness are common for both normal scars, hypertrophic scars and keloids.

Hypertrophic Scars
■ Hypertrophic scars have a similar color and texture compared to normal scars, but are present for a longer period of time, lasting for months.
■ They are larger and more raised than expected of scars from the injury.
■ The surface is smooth, dome-shaped and shiny with prominent vessels.
■ One portion of a scar may appear normal, and another portion may appear to be hypertrophied.
■ Unlike keloid scars, hypertrophic scars remain confined to the site of injury.

Keloids
■ By definition keloids extend beyond the area of trauma or injury.
■ Keloids are firm, red to violaceous, large tender nodules.
■ Keloids are usually hyperpigmented in African–American people and red to purple in Caucasian people.
■ Some keloids are enormous, measuring 10–20 cm or more.
■ Depending on the type of original injury, the lesion may be linear or nodular.
■ In rare instances, keloids may arise spontaneously, without preceding trauma. This usually occurs on the chest and shoulders.

Laboratory
■ A skin biopsy is usually not needed to make the diagnosis.
■ Biopsy can induce further scarring and should be used only if necessary.
■ Hypertrophic scars contain randomly dispersed fibroblasts and whorled bundles of new collagen.
■ Keloids extend beyond the wound margins and contain thick bands of eosinophilic collagen with fewer fibroblasts.

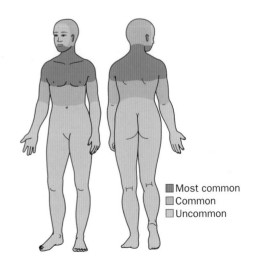

■ Most common
■ Common
□ Uncommon

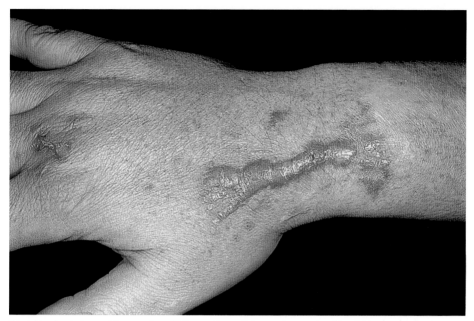

A keloid extends beyond the margins of injury and usually is constant and stable without any tendency to subside.

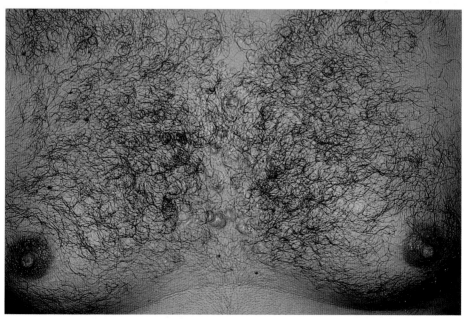

Small multiple hypertrophic scars and keloids form in predisposed people following cystic acne.

Course and Prognosis

- Hypertrophic scars tend to regress even without treatment, although it may take several years to reach a final outcome.
- Keloid scars show no tendency toward regression and tend to enlarge over time.

Differential Diagnosis

- Dermatofibrosarcoma protuberans
- Sarcoidosis (especially for facial keloids)
- Recurrence of original tumor (such as those arising in surgical scars from excision of malignancy)

Discussion

- The diagnosis of a keloid and hypertrophic scar is usually straightforward.
- There is a history of localized trauma, and the injury site is intact.
- There is no history of prior injury in dermatofibrosarcoma protuberans.
- If doubt exists, biopsy is warranted.

Treatment

- People with a history of hypertrophic or keloid scars should be discouraged from having cosmetic procedures or body piercing.
- Both types of scar are best explained as unpredictable scarring.
- Patients who require surgical procedures in areas at increased risk of abnormal scarring should be advised of this possibility in advance and should be reminded at the time of suture removal.
- Despite meticulous surgical and post-surgical care, keloid and hypertrophic scars do occur. This process is determined genetically.

- The parents of a child who has had a procedure that resulted in a keloid or hypertrophic scarring need reassurance and a management plan.
- Early abnormal scarring typically responds better than older, less active scarring; early intervention is advised.
- Intralesional corticosteroid injection is the treatment of choice.
- Triamcinolone (Kenalog) injection at concentrations of 5–20 mg/ml are given at intervals of 2–4 weeks.
- Close follow-up is needed at higher concentrations to minimize the risk of overtreatment and permanent atrophy.
- Radiation therapy and more recently pulse-dye laser therapy have been used for hypertrophic scars and keloids.
- Compression therapy and silastic sheeting are helpful but inconvenient.
- Newer topical silicon-containing gels have been marketed for the treatment of hypertrophic scars, although efficacy in all patients is questionable.
- Surgical correction of hypertrophic scars and keloids requires experience and careful monitoring. These scars tend to recur, sometimes larger, after surgical removal.
- A referral to a dermatologist or plastic surgeon with an interest in scar removal should be considered.

Pearls

- Hypertrophic scars and keloids are difficult to eradicate no matter what procedure is used.
- A patient with a family history or personal history should avoid unnecessary surgical procedures and body piercing.

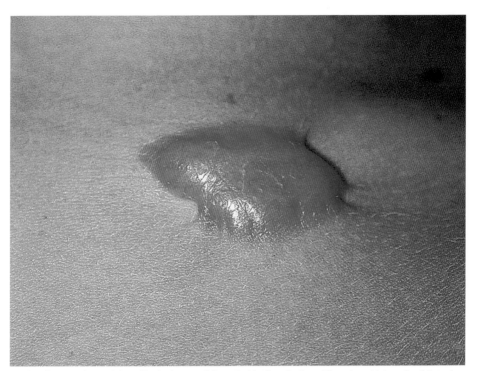

A keloid formed after an injury. The lesion was injected with triamcinolone 10 mg/cc at intervals of 4 weeks. The lesion was flat after 4 treatments. Early lesions respond better than older lesions.

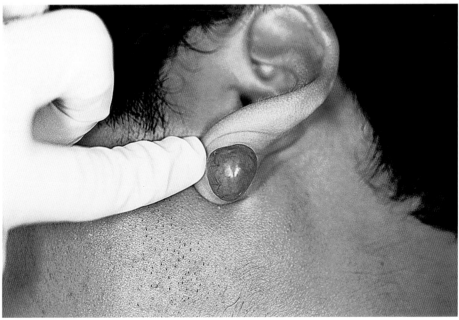

Very large keloids may form in the ear lobe after ears are pierced. African Americans are predisposed to this adverse effect.

Keratoacanthoma

Description
■ Keratoacanthoma is a rapidly growing crateriform nodule with a distinctive clinical appearance that is best regarded as a low-grade squamous cell carcinoma.

History
■ The peak incidence of keratoacanthoma is between ages 50 and 70. This tumor is rare before 40 years of age.
■ Caucasian people with fair complexions (skin types I and II) are more often affected.
■ Typical locations include the face, neck, dorsal hands and sun-exposed extremities.
■ Keratoacanthoma does not occur on the palms or soles.
■ The lesion erupts rapidly and is often tender.
■ Chemical exposure and human papillomavirus have been implicated as a cause in animal models, although the role of human papilloma virus in humans is controversial.

Skin Findings
■ Solitary flesh-colored to dull red, crateriform nodules, measuring 0.5–2.0 cm.
■ A central keratotic plug or depression conceals a deep keratinous cavity.
■ This plug or depression gives the nodule its characteristic volcano-like shape.
■ The nodule is firm, tender to palpation or pressure, and can grow rapidly.
■ Keratoacanthoma nearly always appears on sun-damaged skin.
■ Three growth phases are described:
  ● In the proliferative phase, a solitary papule appears suddenly and then rapidly grows to its maximum size over 2–4 weeks.
  ● In the mature phase, the lesion is stable in size and appearance for weeks to months; it may appear crateriform if the core has been partially removed.
  ● In the resolving phase, the base becomes indurated, the central core is expelled, and the base resorbs, leaving a pitted scar. Resolution may take several months.

Non-skin Findings
■ Rare cases of multiple keratoacanthomas have been reported, both as an eruptive (Grzybowski) form and as a familial adolescent (Ferguson–Smith) form.
■ Patients with Muir–Torre syndrome develop sebaceous adenomas. Sometimes keratoacanthomas are present. Such patients should also be evaluated for visceral malignancy and gastrointestinal malignancy.
■ Patients on immunosuppressive therapy after organ transplant are at increased risk of developing keratoacanthomas and invasive squamous cell carcinoma. Examination for enlarged lymph nodes should always be performed in this patient population.

Laboratory and Pathology
■ The epidermis is expanded with atypical keratinocytes.
■ The keratin core is composed of eosinophilic, glassy appearing, atypical, prematurely keratinized cells.

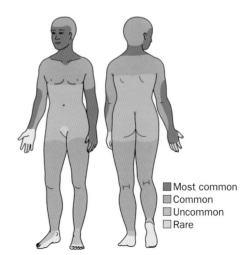

Most common
Common
Uncommon
Rare

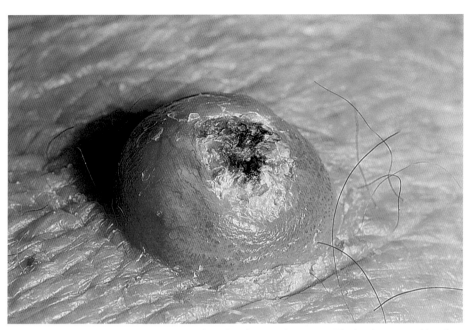

Keratoacanthoma begins as a smooth, dome-shaped, red papule that may rapidly develop a central keratin-filled crater. Lesions grow rapidly. Squamous cell cancers ar usually slow growing tumors.

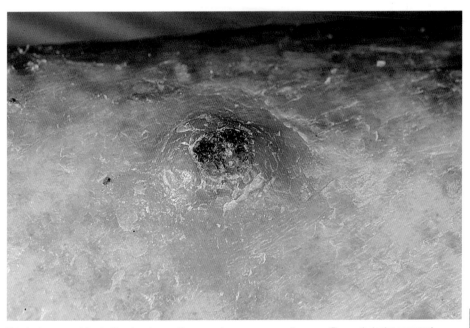

This lesion resembles both a keratoacanthoma and a squamous cell cancer. The pathologist reported features of both tumors. Therefore it was treated as a squamous cell cancer with a wide excision.

Course and Prognosis

- Left undisturbed, keratoacanthomas may resolve spontaneously or progress into invasive squamous cell carcinoma.
- Although a keratoacanthoma has been historically described as a regressing or absorptive lesion, today, most agree that it should be treated as a squamous cell carcinoma.
- Depending on location, the resultant pitted scar that occurs after spontaneous resolution may be cosmetically unacceptable.
- Rarely keratoacanthomas will attain a size of up to 10 cm and are locally destructive.
- Subungual keratoacanthomas are especially painful and locally destructive.
- Because not all keratoacanthomas regress, they should be regarded as squamous cell carcinomas.

Differential Diagnosis

- Squamous cell carcinoma
- Giant molluscum contagiosum
- Warts

Discussion

- Keratoacanthoma cannot be reliably distinguished from invasive squamous cell carcinoma clinically or histologically.

Treatment

- It is best to presume a diagnosis of squamous cell carcinoma pending biopsy results and clinical follow-up.
- An excisional biopsy or shave biopsy should be performed.
- It is important to biopsy deep enough to evaluate the dermis for possible invasion.
- Treatment options include complete excision with margins and electrodesiccation and curettage.

Pearls

- Keratoacanthomas characteristically grow rapidly and resemble volcanic craters.
- Radiation therapy is considered for tumours in areas where excisional surgery might result in deformity.
- Intralesional methotrexate and topical 5-fluorouracil have been successful.

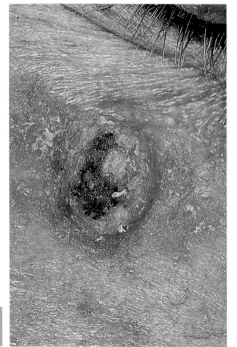

Keratoacanthomas are dome-shaped tumors with a central crust. The history of sudden appearance and rapid growth supports the diagnosis. Squamous cell carcinoma may have a similar appearance but these tumors usually enlarge slowly over many months.

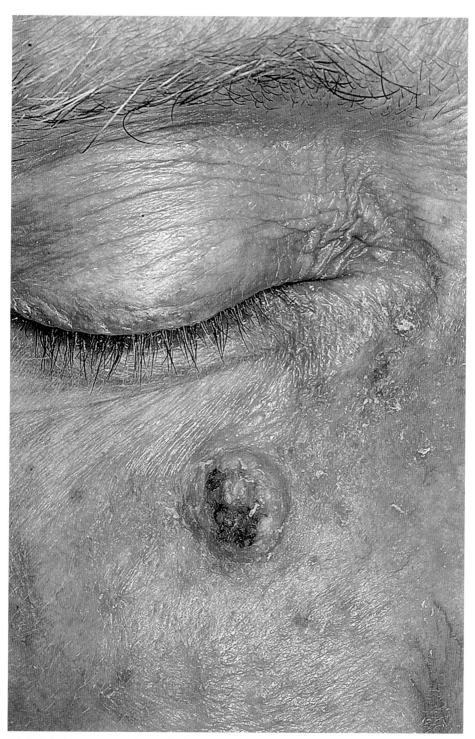

This large lesion was present for months. It grew quickly, formed the typical central crust, and stopped enlarging.

Nevus Sebaceus

Description

- Nevus sebaceus is a distinctive congenital lesion of the head (usually scalp), composed of skin and appendageal components.

History

- Nearly all nevus sebaceus lesions are present at birth or appear in early childhood.
- Lesions change clinically and histologically with age.
- Not all lesions may be noticed at birth.
- At puberty nevus sebaceous lesions tend to enlarge, and they may be noticed for the first time at this point.

Skin Findings

- Nevus sebaceus occurs most commonly on the scalp, forehead, or postauricular areas.
- Usually only a single lesion is present.
- A linear to oval, yellowish to flesh-colored plaque usually measuring 1-3 cm in diameter appears.
- The lesion evolves in three stages corresponding to sebaceous gland maturation through childhood, puberty, and adulthood.
- In childhood, the plaque is barely raised and has a velvety surface, is hairless, is pink to tan, and is asymptomatic.
- Around puberty, the plaque tends to thicken, become larger and more verrucous, and has a yellow-white and pink speckled appearance. Lesions at this stage are easily traumatized and may be tender.
- The third stage of evolution occurs during adulthood. Approximately 20% of lesions undergo neoplastic change and may develop either benign or malignant tumors of the skin. Such a change is seen as a new nodule or erosion developing within a previously stable nevus sebaceus.
- The malignancies are low grade and show little tendency to become invasive.

Non-skin Findings

- A triad of nevus sebaceus, epilepsy, and mental retardation can occur but is very rare.
- This appears to overlap clinically with the linear epidermal nevus syndrome.

Laboratory

- The histopathologic characteristics vary depending on the age of the patient at the time of biopsy.
- In the first few months of life, the sebaceous glands are well developed as a result of maternal hormonal stimulation, although surrounding hair structures are incompletely differentiated.
- Thereafter, and through the rest of childhood, the sebaceous glands are small in size and number; incompletely developed hair structures may be seen.
- With puberty, hormonal influences bring about diagnostic changes. Sebaceous glands mature and increase in size and density. Hair structures remain undifferentiated, and papillomatous epidermal hyperplasia develops. Ectopic apocrine glands may also be found deep within the underlying dermis.

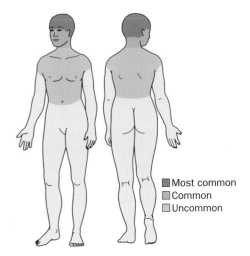

Most common
Common
Uncommon

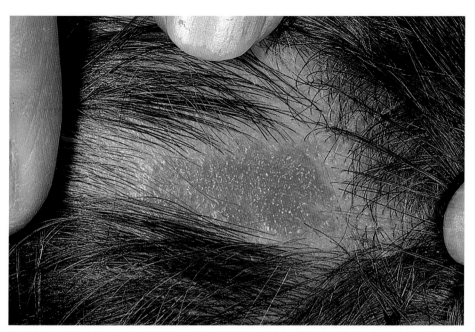

This 12-year-old boy has reached puberty and the lesion has become thicker. This change at puberty is expected and represents, in part, sebaceous gland and epithelial hyperplasia.

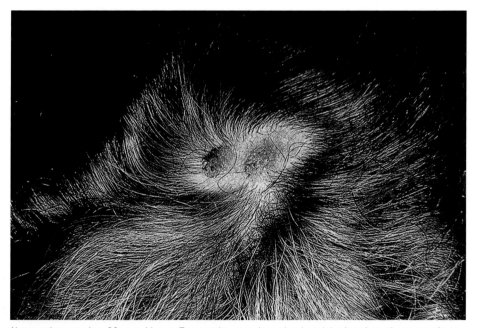

Nevus sebaceous in a 30-year-old man. Two papular areas have developed. Lesions have the propensity to develop many different tumors. This lesion should be excised.

Appendageal tumors may develop later in life within nevus sebaceus. Each such tumor has its own histologic pattern. The most common tumor is syringocystadenoma papilliferum, a benign apocrine tumor seen in up to 20% of lesions. Basal cell carcinoma is the second most common tumor and most common malignancy that develops in nevus sebaceus; it occurs in roughly 7% of lesions.

Course and Prognosis

- Nevus sebaceus remains stable throughout childhood and undergoes predictable change at puberty.
- Depending on location, nevus sebaceus can be disfiguring.
- Neoplastic change occurs during adulthood with enough frequency to warrant prophylactic excision at puberty in some children.

Differential Diagnosis

- Linear epidermal nevus (may share some histologic features)

Treatment

- Excision of the entire lesion is recommended.

Pearls

- During puberty, there is a massive proliferation of sebaceous glands.
- The nevus develops a verrucous or velvety surface irregularity.
- Nevus sebaceus has a tendency to develop basal cell carcinoma within the nevus after puberty.
- Surgical invasion of a sebaceous nevi should be considered in infancy for certain lesions (e.g. large scalp sebaceous nevi).
- A larger lesion may be excised in stages without any concern of inducing malignant change.
- Large defects on the scalp are easier to repair during infancy.

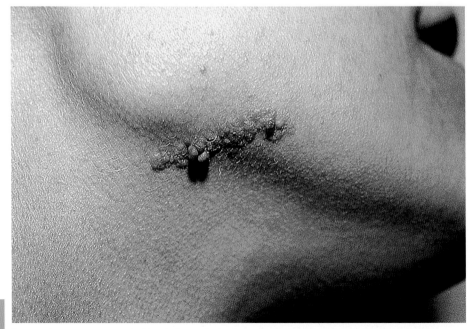

Nevus sebaceus occurs most often on the scalp. Lesions are also found on the face, neck and trunk.

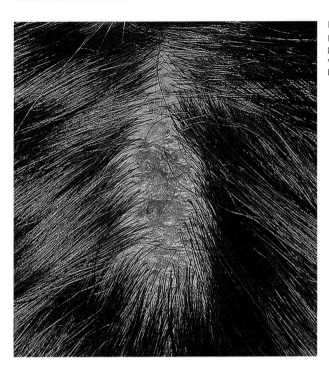

Hormonal changes during puberty stimulate sebaceous gland growth. This causes the velvety smooth surface to become verrucous and nodular.

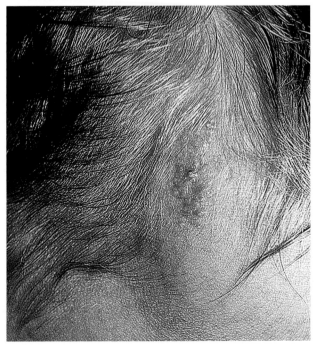

Lesions are found on the scalp, face, behind the ear and on the neck and trunk.

Chondrodermatitis Nodularis Helicis

Description
- Chondrodermatitis nodularis helicis is an inflammatory condition of the helical ear cartilage.
- It is an exquisitely tender papule on the most lateral edge of the helix or anti-helix.

History
- Usually occurs in those over the age of 40 and the incidence increases with age.
- Men are affected more often than women.
- The helix is involved more commonly in men.
- Lesions on the anti-helix are more common in women.
- These variations may relate in part to historical differences among men and women in sun-exposure patterns, occupation, recreational activities, and hairstyles.
- Gender differences in ear structure may also play a role.
- As a rule, most patients are in the habit of sleeping on the affected side.
- Pressure from resting on a pillow causes pain, forcing the patient to alter sleeping position and affecting the ability to sleep comfortably.
- This condition is less symptomatic during the daytime.

Skin Findings
- The primary lesion is a firm, tender, red to pink, papule of 2–4 mm with a central keratotic punctum.
- The punctum has firm, adherent crust or scale, resembling a small cutaneous horn.
- The surrounding skin shows actinic damage with atrophy and telangiectasia.
- Occasionally there is more than one lesion and, rarely, they occur bilaterally.
- The universal symptom is pain described as stabbing and sharp. Papules are quite tender to palpation.

- This condition is classically found on the most prominent and lateral portion of the auricle.

Laboratory
- Skin biopsy reveals both acute and chronic inflammation.
- The epidermis is thinned, with compacted parakeratotic scaling, and often shows central erosion or ulceration.
- There is dermal necrosis with surrounding granulation tissue.
- A deep biopsy may contain underlying degenerated cartilage.

Course and Prognosis
- The etiology of chondrodermatitis nodularis helicis is unclear, although is believed to be related to focal dermal necrosis due to repetitive trauma.
- Over many years, dermal injury may result from actinic damage, physical pressure, or a combination of both.
- The vascular supply to this tissue is tenuous, and damage is slow to heal.
- Inflammation and granulation tissue reflect attempts at healing the damaged collagen.
- Without treatment, the lesions persist indefinitely.
- Recurrences are common, even after aggressive therapy.

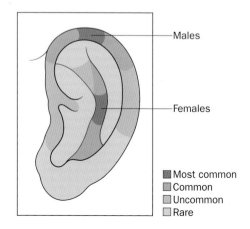

Males
Females

■ Most common
□ Common
□ Uncommon
□ Rare

Differential Diagnosis

- Squamous cell carcinoma (closely resembles chondrodermatitis nodularis helicis)
- Basal cell carcinoma (closely resembles chondrodermatitis nodularis helicis)

Discussion

- Chondrodermatitis nodularis helicis tends to be painful, and is dull red with poorly defined border.
- Basal cell carcinomas tend to be better defined and have a translucent or pearly appearance.
- Squamous cell carcinomas as a rule tend to be larger, more necrotic and less tender than chondrodermatitis nodularis helicis lesions.
- Skin biopsy should be performed, which is diagnostic.

Treatment

- Any therapy must include efforts to relieve pressure on the affected area to allow for healing.
- Patients who are able to sleep on the back should be encouraged to do so.

- Pillows should be positioned to minimize pressure on the ear.
- Topical therapy is rarely successful.
- Intralesional steroids can be effective in a minority of cases.
- Patients should expect some residual discomfort after injection.
- Surgical removal of the lesion along with the inflamed cartilage can be curative.
- Shave excision is directed at removing all the inflamed tissue, thus exposing the underlying cartilage.
- Curettage and light electrodesiccation of the base is performed, and the wound is allowed to heal by secondary intention.
- Definitive therapy involves surgical resection of the involved cartilage of the pinna.
- Recurrences are common after any of the above therapies.

Pearls

- Squamous cell carcinoma closely resembles chondrodermatitis nodularis helicis and a biopsy to distinguish the two should be performed.
- A deep shave removal biopsy can be both diagnostic and curative.

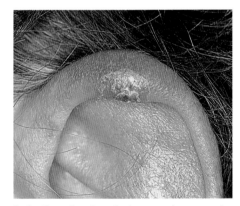

During the active stage the base may become red and swollen; pain is constant.

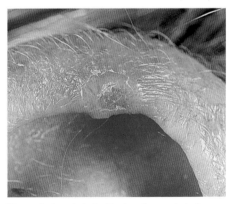

The central scale lacks the keratinous plug of a keratoacanthoma. Removal of the scale reveals a small central erosion.

Epidermal Cyst

Description

■ An epidermal cyst is a firm, subcutaneous, keratin-filled cyst originating from true epidermis, most often from a hair follicle.

History

■ Epidermal cysts arise spontaneously, usually after puberty.
■ They occur most commonly on the trunk, postauricular fold and on the posterior neck.
■ Cysts frequently develop in areas of friction.
■ Lesions are usually solitary.
■ Unlike pilar cysts, the epidermal cyst wall is fairly delicate and prone to rupture.
■ Rupture is followed by an acute foreign body reaction to keratin extruded into the dermis and acute inflammation. Such lesions appear to be infected.
■ Although bacteria can be isolated from the cysts, they usually contain normal skin flora.

Skin Findings

■ The firm, dome-shaped, pale yellowish intradermal or subcutaneous cystic nodules range from 0.5–5.0 cm in size.
■ Cysts are somewhat mobile but are tethered to the overlying skin through a small punctum that often appears as a comedo.
■ This punctum represents the follicle from which the cyst developed.
■ Inflamed epidermal cysts are warm, red and boggy, and tender on palpation. Furuncles have a similar appearance.
■ Sterile, purulent material and keratin debris often point towards and drain to the surface.
■ If the inflammatory response is brisk enough to destroy the cyst wall, then it is unlikely the cyst will recur.
■ More often than not the inflammation subsides, and the cyst recurs.
■ Scarring often follows, which makes the cyst more difficult to remove.

Non-skin Findings

■ Multiple epidermal cysts occurring on the face, scalp, and back should raise suspicion of Gardner syndrome. This rare, autosomal dominant condition is associated with colonic polyposis and adenocarcinoma of the colon.

Laboratory

■ The epidermal cyst is lined with squamous epithelium that appears thinned and flattened.
■ The cyst cavity is filled with characteristic layers of cornified lamellated keratin.

Course and Prognosis

■ Epidermal cysts grow slowly to a maximum size and tend to persist indefinitely.
■ Depending on location, epidermal cysts may be subject to repeated external trauma, inflammatory changes, and rupture.

Treatment

■ Epidermal cysts on the face may rupture and lead to scarring. The cosmesis of elective surgical excision must be weighed against scar from rupture.
■ Such lesions are far more difficult to remove once they have ruptured.
■ Asymptomatic epidermal cysts occurring elsewhere do not require treatment.

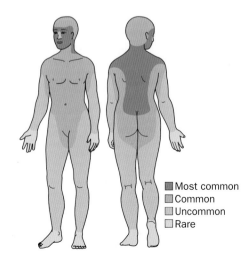

■ Most common
□ Common
□ Uncommon
□ Rare

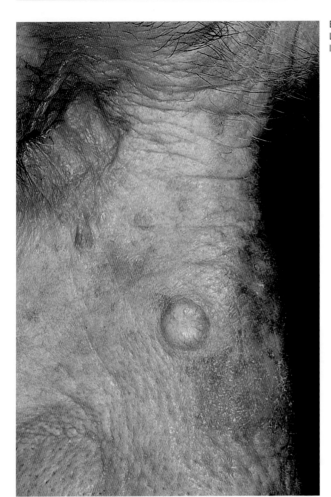

Epidermal cysts vary in size. Lesions of this size will show little tendency to rupture.

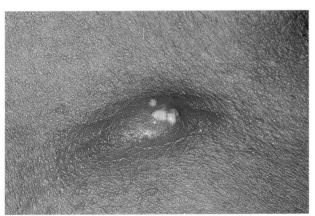

Ruptured cysts that are close to the skin surface will "point" and the cyst contents will exude onto the skin surface.

- Symptomatic or recurrent epidermal cysts should be removed.
- Ruptured, inflamed epidermal cysts should be incised and drained under local anesthesia.
- Attempts should be made to remove the cyst lining either by curettage or blunt dissection with scissors and forceps.
- Very large cyst cavities may then be packed with a wick to aid further drainage.
- Epidermal cysts that have not previously ruptured can be excised easily and completely under local anesthesia.
- Recurrent epidermal cysts that have previously ruptured and scarred are best excised along with the surrounding scar once the inflammation has subsided.

Pearls

- Inflammation after rupture of an epidermal cyst is often suspected and misdiagnosed as infection, but cultures are usually sterile.
- Epidermal cysts occur in areas where sebaceous glands are large and numerous, including such areas as the labia and posterior auricle.
- Incision and drainage with curettage do not always completely eradicate epidermal cysts.
- Complete surgical excision with narrow margins is curative.

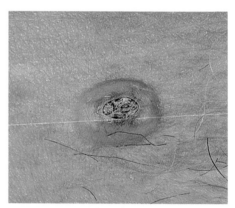

Giant comedones are variants of epidermal cysts. They have a large orifice and are easily removed by incision and drainage. The cyst wall must be removed to ensure the lesion does not recur.

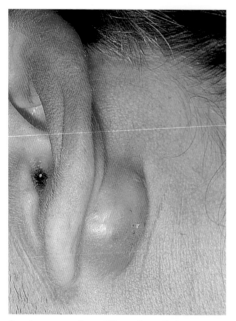

Spontaneous rupture of the wall results in discharge of the soft yellow keratin into the dermis. A tremendous inflammatory response ensues.

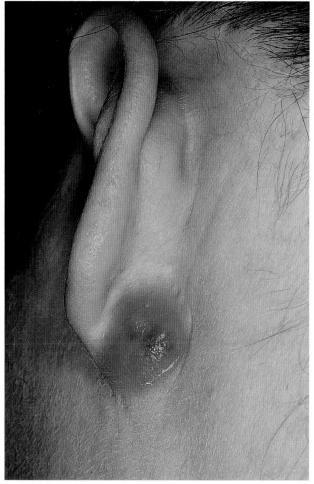

Epidermal cysts occur commonly on the back of the ear. This cyst spontaneously ruptured and stimulated an intense inflammatory reaction. Incision and drainage relieves the pain and hastens healing. The cyst appears infected but the inflammation is a foreign body reaction to cyst contents.

Pilar Cyst (Wen)

Description

- A pilar or trichilemmal cyst is a firm, subcutaneous, keratin-filled cyst originating from the outer root sheath of the hair follicle. It is most commonly found on the scalp.

History

- Pilar cysts are less common than, but otherwise similar to, epidermal cysts.
- Roughly 90% of pilar cysts are found on the scalp, with the remaining 10% occurring on the face, neck, back, and scrotum.
- Pilar cysts develop from epithelial cells of the outer root sheath of the hair follicle.
- This epithelium undergoes a different form of keratinization than cutaneous epithelium.
- Pilar cysts almost always develop after puberty.
- The tendency to develop pilar cysts often has an autosomal dominant inheritance.
- Pilar cysts are multiple in 70% of patients who have them.
- Pilar cysts persist indefinitely and slowly grow to a stable size unless they rupture.
- Pilar cysts rupture less frequently than epidermal cysts, presumably because the pilar cyst possesses a thicker wall.
- Rupture usually results from external trauma to the head, thus releasing cyst contents into the surrounding dermis.
- A brisk foreign body inflammatory reaction follows and can be painful and resembles a furuncle.

Skin Findings

- Pilar cysts are clinically indistinguishable from epidermal cysts, differing only in pattern of distribution.
- Both present as a firm, mobile subcutaneous nodule ranging from 0.5–5.0 cm.
- No central punctum is seen over a pilar cyst—as is found over an epidermal cyst.
- When such a cyst is surgically dissected, the pilar cyst possesses a tough, white-gray wall that is more resistant to tearing than the wall of an epidermal cyst.

- The pilar cyst wall separates easily and cleanly from the surrounding dermis.
- If a pilar cyst ruptures the area becomes inflamed, red and tender, and boggy on palpation.

Laboratory

- The histologic characteristics of the pilar cyst are distinct from those of the epidermal cyst.
- The cell wall shows a palisade arrangement of epithelial cells, with pale cytoplasm but no granular layer.
- The cyst contains concentric layers of homogeneous eosinophilic keratin.

Discussion

- Large cysts may be cosmetically objectionable.
- Some cysts are so large and tender that they may interfere with wearing hats and helmets.
- Acute inflammation after rupture is often misdiagnosed as infection.
- Antibiotics are of little value in such cases.
- Incision and drainage under local anesthesia improve comfort and limit scarring.
- Elective excision before rupture prevents this complication.

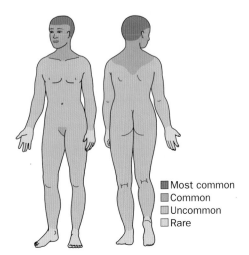

■ Most common
□ Common
□ Uncommon
□ Rare

Treatment

- Pilar cysts are easily removed under local anesthesia.
- An incision is made over the cyst, exposing the cyst's glossy white external surface.
- The cyst wall is freed easily from the surrounding connective tissue by blunt dissection.
- At this stage, smaller cysts may be expressed intact up through the incision by steady, firm pressure on each side of the incision.
- Larger cysts which cannot be expressed in this manner should be incised, and their contents removed by curettage.
- The incised cyst wall is clamped and (through a combination of gentle traction and pressure on each side of the incision) the now smaller, partially emptied cyst is delivered through the incision.
- If sutures are needed, they are placed and removed in 7–10 days.

Pearls

- The term "sebaceous cyst" has been incorrectly applied to this common lesion.
- Pilar cysts are usually multiple and on the scalp.
- They are easily removed via surgical excision.

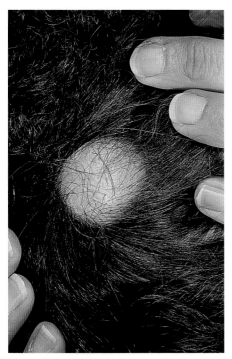

Pilar cysts occur in the scalp and are freely movable.

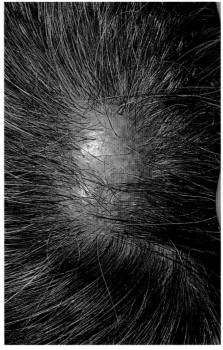

This large pilar cyst has exerted pressure against the skin and has destroyed hair follicles.

Sebaceous Hyperplasia

Description
- Sebaceous hyperplasia is a common benign condition consisting of prominently enlarged sebaceous glands on the face.

History
- Sebaceous hyperplasia occurs in both men and women.
- Papules rarely appear before age 30 but become increasingly more common with advancing age.
- Roughly 80% of patients over age 70 have at least one such lesion.
- Most lesions represent a single, hypertrophied sebaceous gland with multiple lobules arranged around a central enlarged sebaceous duct.
- Lesions occur in all skin types but are more easily seen in lighter skin.
- The etiology of sebaceous hyperplasia is unknown. Genetic inheritance almost certainly plays a role.
- Sun damage has been suggested as a contributing factor.
- The lesions are entirely asymptomatic, but are persistent.
- Papules can become disfiguring and are mostly of cosmetic concern.
- Older patients are typically concerned that the lesions represent basal cell carcinoma.

Skin Findings
- The lesion begins as a 1–2 mm, soft, pale yellow to skin-colored minimally elevated papule.
- With time the lesion attains a maximum size of 3–4 mm and develops a central umbilication.
- Mature papules possess a distinctly yellow-orange color and are more sharply defined from the surrounding skin.
- Papules may be solitary but are more commonly multiple and scattered randomly on the forehead, nose, and cheeks.
- An orderly array of fine telangiectasias may radiate outward and between the

papules from the umbilication toward the periphery of the papule.
- Because of the smooth surface, sebaceous hyperplasia papules can be misdiagnosed as basal cell carcinoma.

Laboratory
- Skin biopsy confirms the presence of multiple sebaceous lobules of a single sebaceous gland arranged around a central sebaceous duct.
- This duct corresponds to the central umbilication seen clinically.

Discussion
- Individual lesions may be confused with basal cell carcinoma, small keratoacanthoma or molluscum contagiosum.
- Lesions of sebaceous hyperplasia have an orderly radial arrangement of telangiectasias in contrast to the haphazard distribution of telangiectasias on the surface of a basal cell carcinoma.

Treatment
- Treatment is not required but may be requested for cosmetic reasons.

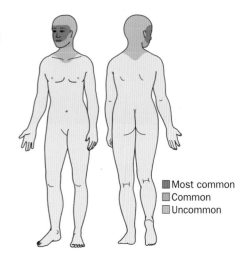

Most common
Common
Uncommon

- Carbon dioxide laser, shave excision, electrodesiccation with curettage, and trichloroacetic acid are all effective ablating procedures.
- The sebaceous lobules located within the superficial dermis must be destroyed for the treatment to be successful.
- Overtreatment causes scarring.
- Reassurance is often all that is needed.

Pearls

- Sebaceous hyperplasia papules can be confused with basal cell carcinoma.
- Clues to the diagnosis of sebaceous hyperplasia are the umbilicated center, radial orderly arrangement of telangiectasias and the presence of multiple lesions.

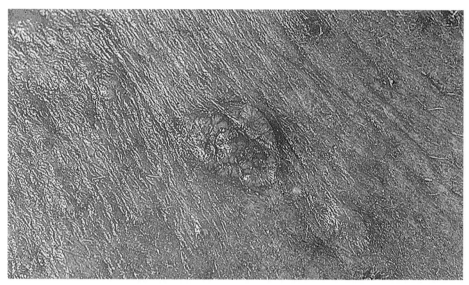

Individual lesions are made up of a cluster of yellow-white globules. There may or may not be a depressed central pore. Small vessels are found in the valleys between the globules.

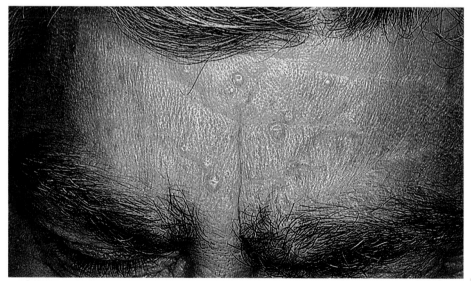

Yellow-white papules are commonly found on the forehead and cheeks. The central pore is an almost constant feature. Individual lesions may be mistaken for basal cell carcinoma. The vessels in basal cell carcinoma course randomly over the surface.

Syringoma

Description
■ Syringomas are small, firm, skin-colored papules occurring most commonly in women around the eyelids, upper chest and on the vulva.

History
■ Syringomas are the most common tumor of the intraepidermal eccrine sweat glands.
■ Small, benign, appendageal tumors develop after puberty and increase in number throughout young adulthood.
■ Women are affected more than men.
■ Syringomas most commonly present as multiple small papules around the eyes.
■ Lesions are asymptomatic, stable in size and appearance, and are persistent.
■ The autosomal dominant inheritance of multiple syringomas is well established.
■ Syringomas occur with increased frequency in persons with Down syndrome or trisomy 21.
■ Facial lesions are of cosmetic concern, and most patients request removal of larger lesions.
■ The patient may be concerned that the lesions are cancerous.
■ Women seeking evaluation of vulvar lesions may be concerned that the lesions are genital warts.

Skin Findings
■ Multiple, skin-colored to yellow, barely raised papules of 1-2 mm.
■ Papules are most commonly found on the lower eyelids.
■ They also occur on the malar cheeks, axillae, anterior chest, abdomen, umbilicus, and vulva.
■ Papules are usually symmetrically distributed and asymptomatic.

Laboratory and Pathology
■ Increased numbers of dilated, epithelium-lined eccrine ducts are encased in a fibrous stroma.
■ These ducts resemble "tadpoles" when cut in cross section.

Course and Prognosis
■ Syringomas persist indefinitely and remain small.
■ These lesions have no potential for malignancy.

Differential Diagnosis
■ Seborrheic keratoses
■ Sebaceous hyperplasia
■ Common warts
■ Flat warts
■ Xanthelasma
■ Sarcoidosis
■ Other appendageal tumors (such as trichoepithelioma)

Discussion
■ Trichoepithelioma is a benign appendageal tumor with differentiation toward hair follicle.
■ Like syringomas, trichoepitheliomas also appear after puberty and occur most commonly on the face.
■ Multiple lesions can be inherited in autosomal dominant fashion.
■ Sebaceous hyperplasia tends to be umbilicated and yellowish, and is scattered about the face rather than grouped around the eyes.
■ Flat warts occur on the face as small, flat, skin-colored or pink papules.

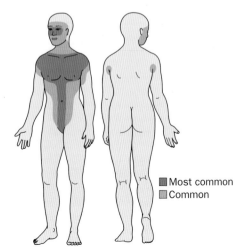

■ Most common
■ Common

- Xanthelasma occurs on eyelid skin, especially upper eyelids, and represents cholesterol deposition within dermal macrophages.
- If doubt exists, biopsy should be performed.

Treatment

- Syringomas may be removed for cosmetic purposes.
- Electrodesiccation and curettage, laser surgery, and trichloroacetic acid may be used.
- Sharp dissection or scissor excision of lesions is easily performed under local anesthesia.

- All of these procedures can lead to scarring, so care and precision are warranted.
- Cryosurgery is not recommended as it is rarely effective.

Pearls

- Syringomas are clinically subtle and can be confused with other dermatoses initially; a biopsy may be needed for confirmation.
- Removal, by any procedure, must be weighed against the risk of scarring.

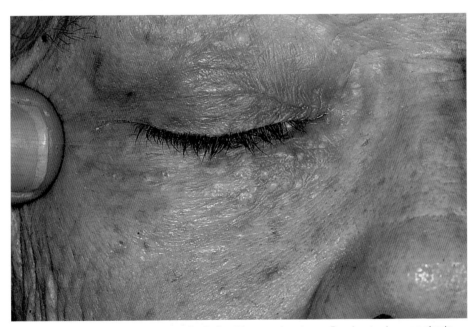

The lower lids are the most common area for finding this appendage tumor. Prominent sebaceous glands may have the same appearance. Lesions may be removed with curved scissors to improve the appearance.

17 Premalignant and Malignant Non-Melanoma Skin Tumors

Basal Cell Carcinoma

Description
- Basal cell carcinoma is the most common cutaneous malignancy in humans.
- It is locally invasive and destructive, and is usually slow growing, but rarely metastasizes.

History
- It may occur at any age but is more common after the age of 40.
- The highest incidence occurs in people with fair skin (types I and II). It is less common in Asian–American people and is rare in African–American people.
- Cumulative sun exposure and prior ionizing radiation are risk factors.
- Tumors occur most commonly on the sun-exposed skin of the face, scalp, ears, and neck, but less often on the trunk and extremities, and rarely on the dorsal hands.
- Several clinical variants of basal cell carcinoma are recognized; these include nodular basal cell carcinoma, pigmented basal cell carcinoma, superficial basal cell carcinoma, micronodular basal cell carcinoma, and morpheaform basal cell carcinoma. Each varies in terms of clinical appearance, histology and aggressiveness.

Skin Findings
- Nodular basal cell carcinoma is the most common variant.
- The lesion is a pearly-white, almost translucent, dome-shaped papule with overlying telangiectasias.
- The papule or nodule enlarges slowly, may become flattened in the center or may develop a raised, rolled, and translucent border.
- Tumors frequently ulcerate, bleed, and become crusted in the center.
- Basal cell carcinomas may contain melanin that imparts a brown, black, or blue color through all or part of the lesion.
- It may present as a papule or nodule on the ear that resembles squamous cell carcinoma.
- Curettage demonstrates the characteristically soft texture of the tumor as compared to the surrounding normal skin.

Nodular Basal Cell Carcinoma
- The lesion begins as a pearly white or pink, dome-shaped papule.
- The center frequently ulcerates and bleeds and subsequently accumulates crust and scale.
- Telangiectatic vessels become prominent as the lesion enlarges. The growth pattern is irregular, forming an oval, multilobular mass.

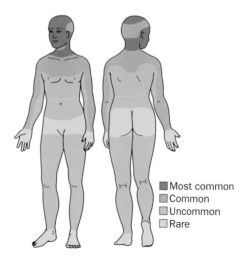

■ Most common
■ Common
■ Uncommon
□ Rare

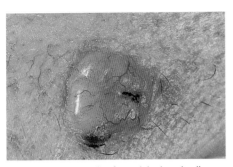

The classic presentation for nodular basal cell carcinoma. A dome-shaped pearly tumor with telangiectasias meandering randomly over the surface.

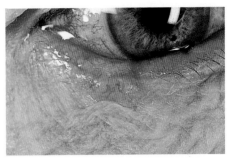

This nodular basal cell carcinoma was initially diagnosed as a nevus. The lesion enlarged and ulcerated. A biopsy confirmed the diagnosis and it was removed by Mohs micrographic surgery.

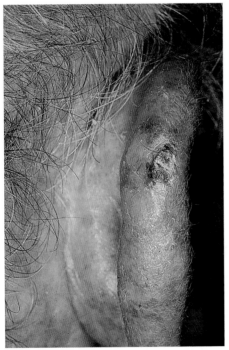

Basal cell carcinoma may appear on the ear. These lesions are often imbedded in the skin and are not appreciated until they become large. Squamous cell carcinoma may have an identical appearance.

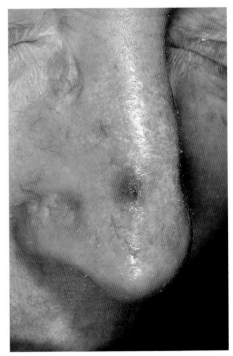

Nodular basal cell carcinomas are common on the nose. This lesion ulcerated and then began to heal. Nasal tumors are best treated by Mohs micrographic surgery.

Pigmented Basal Cell Carcinoma

- This is equivalent to nodular basal cell carcinoma, except that there is also melanin pigment.
- It may resemble malignant melanoma, and therefore must be biopsied.

Superficial Basal Cell Carcinoma

- This is the least aggressive form of basal cell carcinoma; it is found more commonly on the trunk and extremities.
- There may be multiple lesions; patients tend to develop this type of tumor earlier in life than those with nodular basal cell carcinoma.
- The lesions are flatter and not as deeply invasive as the lesions of nodular basal cell carcinoma. The borders are less distinct but have the same pearly quality. Stretching the skin may accentuate the raised border.
- The tumor spreads peripherally, sometimes for several centimeters, and invades after considerable time.
- Areas within the tumor may show healing with scarring.
- The circumscribed, round to oval, red, scaling plaques resemble those of eczema, psoriasis, extramammary Paget's disease, or Bowen's disease (squamous cell carcinoma in situ).

Micronodular Basal Cell Carcinoma

- Micronodular basal cell carcinoma resembles nodular basal cell carcinoma clinically, but microscopically there are islands of tumor cells extending beyond the clinical margins.
- Because this histologic variant extends beyond the suspected clinical borders, it recurs more frequently after traditional treatment.

Morpheaform and Sclerosing Basal Cell Carcinoma

- Morpheaform and sclerosing basal cell carcinoma is the most subtle and least common variant of basal cell carcinoma; it is also the most difficult to eradicate.
- Lesions resemble scar tissue clinically; they are pale-white to yellow, and waxy on palpation.

- Because of the innocuous appearance of this variant, biopsy and diagnosis are often delayed.
- The margins are indistinct, and tumor cells may extend more than 7 mm from the clinical lesion; thus, unlike the nodular variant, it is more likely to recur after narrow excision.
- Both the morpheaform and sclerosing forms are more aggressive, tend to recur more often and should be followed more closely.

Non-skin Findings

- Basal cell nevus syndrome is an autosomal dominant condition of multiple basal cell skin cancer and multiple possible associated anomalies of the skeleton, skin, and central nervous system.
- Skeletal anomalies include odontogenic cysts, frontal bossing, hypertelorism, bifid ribs, kyphoscoliosis, and shortened fourth metacarpals.
- Skin anomalies include multiple basal cell carcinomas appearing in childhood, and palmoplantar pitting.
- Central nervous system anomalies include calcification of the falx cerebri and medulloblastoma.

Laboratory and Pathology

- Nests of basaloid tumor cells are in close approximation to a distinctive stroma in nodular and pigmented basal cell carcinomas.
- Superficial basal cell carcinomas appear as multifocal extensions of the basal layer of the epidermis into the superficial dermis.
- In nodular basal cell carcinomas, there are larger islands of tumor cells within the dermis; tumor islands may be solid or may contain cystic cavities.
- Pigmented basal cell carcinoma is similar to nodular basal cell carcinoma but differs in that tumor islands contain melanin pigment.
- In morpheaform or sclerosing basal cell carcinomas innumerable scattered fine strands of tumor cells are embedded within a fibrous stroma.

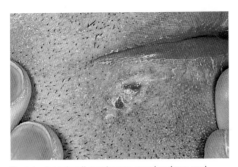

Nodular basal cell carcinoma may be deep and subtle. Stretching the skin accentuates the pearly nodular tumor.

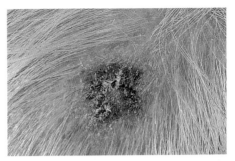

Pigmented basal cell carcinoma is a nodular basal cell carcinoma that contains melanin. It has the typical pearly appearance with surface telangiectasia found in nodular basal cell carcinoma. Melanoma is in the differential diagnosis.

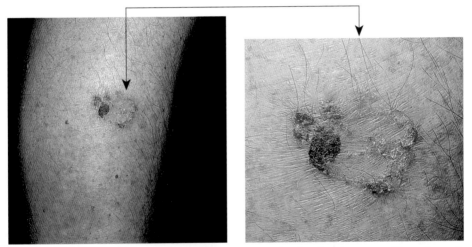

Superficial basal cell carcinoma. The circumscribed, round-to-oval, red scaling plaque resembles a plaque of eczema, psoriasis, extramammary Paget's disease, or Bowen's disease. The superficial basal cell carcinoma spreads peripherally, sometimes for several centimeters, and invades after considerable time.

Course and Prognosis

- Without treatment basal cell carcinomas persist, enlarge, ulcerate and invade and destroy the surrounding structures.
- In large lesions focal areas of spontaneous healing with scarring may appear.
- Inadequately treated basal cell carcinomas recur, often underneath areas of scarring—which leads to delay in detection.
- In patients who develop one basal cell carcinoma, the annual risk of developing another basal cell carcinoma is 5–8%.

Discussion

- Basal cell carcinomas are rarely—if ever—life threatening; metastases virtually never occur, unless the patient is immunocompromised.
- Depending on tumor location, local destruction of normal tissue by the tumor can result in significant impairment. Inadequately treated tumors may extend undetected to destroy wide areas of the face.

Treatment

- The goal of treatment is eradication of the tumor and return of normal anatomic form and function.
- The treatment of basal cell carcinoma is determined by the size and location of the tumor, by the histologic variant, and the patient's concerns.
- Clinical aggressiveness correlates with histologic pattern.
- Electrosurgery involves electrodesiccation and curettage of obvious tumor.
- It is usually performed for well-defined, small nodular basal cell carcinomas and superficial basal cell carcinomas.
- The 5-year cure rates for curettage can approach 92% for primary tumors but is only 60% for recurrent tumors.
- Office excision is preferred for well-defined nodular basal cell carcinomas.
- Office excision allows confirmation of surgical margins and may result in a more acceptable scar than that caused by electrosurgery.

- The 5-year cure rates approach 90% for primary tumors and 83% for recurrent tumors.
- Mohs micrographic surgery is a highly specialized, tissue-sparing method of excision used for difficult tumors with contiguous growth, especially basal cell carcinomas.
- Mohs micrographic surgery is used for recurrent basal carcinomas, for histologically aggressive forms of basal cell carcinomas, and for tumors in anatomically important locations (such as around the eyes, nasal ala, mouth and ears), and tumors with a high risk of recurrence. It is the treatment of choice for morpheaform basal cell carcinoma.
- Obvious tumor is debulked, and then excision is performed in stages. Excision is guided by sequential frozen-section mapping in three dimensions.
- This allows for histologically confirmed removal of the tumor with the smallest of surgical margins and surgical defect.
- The 5-year cure rates for Mohs excision approach 99% for primary tumors and 96% for recurrent tumors.
- Mohs micrographic surgery is useful when tissue sparing is required because of anatomic location, recurrent tumors and basal cell carcinomas with indistinct borders.
- Nonsurgical options are increasing. These include radiation therapy, photodynamic therapy, and topical immune modulators.
- Radiation therapy may be useful for tumors that are difficult to treat surgically, such as those on the eyelids, and for patients who are unwilling or unable to tolerate surgery.
- Improvements in computerized treatment models now allow the radiation oncologist to precisely treat a localized tumor with high-dose radiation in fractional doses over several weeks.
- The 5-year cure rate is roughly 90% for both primary and recurrent tumors.
- Cosmesis can be excellent, although expected long-term radiation changes in the treated skin may limit the use of this modality to elderly patients.

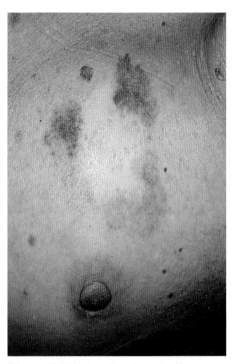

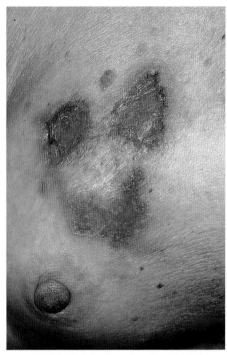

This superficial basal cell carcinoma had been previously treated by desiccation and curettage. Months later it recurred at the periphery.

The superficial basal cell carcinoma on the left was treated with imiquimod cream (Aldara) applied every other day. Intense inflammation occurred and treatment was stopped. The lesion healed and there have been no recurrences.

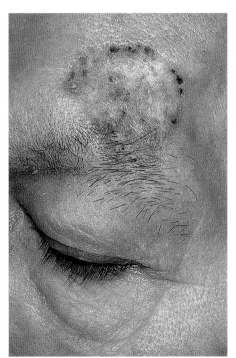

Superficial basal cell carcinoma may be mistaken for eczema, psoriasis or ringworm. It bleeds and heals in cycles just like a nodular basal cell. The lesion may increase in size to cover very wide areas before the diagnosis is made. Lesions tend to remain superficial but may eventually penetrate deep into the dermis or subcutaneous tissue. A biopsy showed that tumor cells were superficial and the lesion cleared with every other day application of imiquimod cream (Aldara).

■ Topical Imiquimod (Aldara) 5% cream is an immune response modifier shown to be 85% effective, or better, for superficial basal cell carcinomas. It is not yet approved for this indication by the Food and Drug Administration. Daily application by the patient at home for 6 weeks results in complete eradication in most cases. Inflammation at the treatment site limits its use; rest periods may be needed.

■ Aldara for nodular basal cell carcinoma is controversial; it is less effective for nodular basal cell carcinomas compared to superficial basal cell carcinomas.

■ All patients with basal cell carcinomas require follow-up to monitor for the development of new tumors and for recurrence at the treated site, regardless of which treatment is used.

Pearls

■ The patient should know that basal cell carcinomas are neither life-threatening nor trivial. Patients must be followed after treatment.

■ Basal cell carcinomas may present as non-healing ulcers and may appear on any body surface, including the genitalia and legs.

■ Morpheaform or sclerotic basal cell carcinoma is a firm, flat to slightly raised, pale to white papule which may resemble a scar; it may be missed clinically, but confirmed histologically. It is more aggressive than other basal cell carcinoma variants and frequently recurs without adequate treatment. If it is on the face, or if it is recurrent, referral for Mohs surgery is recommended.

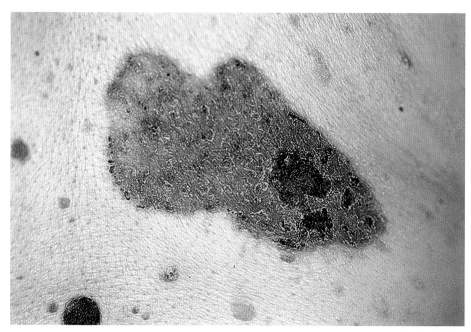

The back is a common place to find superficial basal cell carcinoma. The patient was not aware of the lesion. The sharp border is characteristic. Eczema has a less distinct border. This lesion lacks the silvery scale of psoriasis. The surface of these tumors is often crusted. This lesion was treated with imiquimod cream (Aldara).

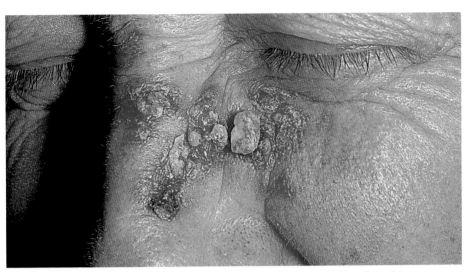

The cycle of growth, ulceration, and healing continues as the mass extends peripherally, and deeper. Lesions of enormous size may be attained.

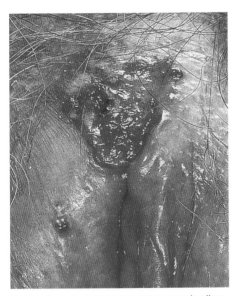

Basal cell carcinomas may present as non-healing ulcers and may appear on any body surface, including the vulva.

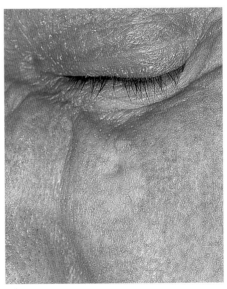

Morpheaform basal cell carcinoma is waxy, firm, flat or slightly raised, and either pale white or yellowish, and it resembles localized scleroderma.

Actinic Keratosis

Description

- Actinic keratoses are common, persistent, keratotic lesions with malignant potential.
- Lesions are most commonly found in the sun-exposed areas of elderly patients with fair skin types who have had significant sun exposure in their lifetime.

History

- Years of cumulative sun exposure and keratinocyte damage lead to the formation of actinic keratoses.
- Individual lesions become progressively more common after age 40.
- Multiple lesions are common in people with skin types I and II.
- The slight variation in the distribution of lesions among men and women may relate to either the absence of hair or to hairstyle.
- Spontaneous regression is reported, although most lesions persist without treatment.
- About 10–20% of actinic keratoses progress to invasive squamous cell carcinoma over several years.
- Transplant patients with actinic keratosis must be followed closely.
- Progression of lesions to squamous cell carcinoma is much more common in these patients.

Skin Findings

- Actinic keratoses are found along with other signs of chronic sun exposure, such as uneven pigmentation, atrophy or thinning, and telangiectasias.
- Lesions are found predominantly on the face, head, neck, and dorsal hands.
- Actinic keratoses initially present as a poorly defined area of redness or telangiectasia.
- Over time, the lesion becomes more defined and develops a thin, adherent, yellowish or transparent scale. At this stage, lesions are sometimes easier to detect by palpation than by observation. One may find a discrete change in skin texture associated with minimal erythema. Patients frequently point out these areas to the physician.
- With time, the adherent scale becomes progressively thicker and yellow in color.
- Retained scale may form an elongated keratinous structure or a cutaneous horn.
- Such advanced lesions may be difficult to distinguish from invasive squamous cell carcinoma without skin biopsy, and probably should be treated as such.
- "Spreading pigmented actinic keratosis" describes actinic keratoses with fine reticulated pigmentation and minimal scaling; they may mimic a solar lentigo or melanoma in situ.
- Lentigo maligna (melanoma in situ) also occurs most frequently on sun-damaged skin. Skin biopsy will establish the correct diagnosis.
- Actinic cheilitis is a sun-induced keratinocyte atypia of the lower lip. There is focal crusting and scaling along with blurring of the vermilion border, which appears whitish or gray.
- Actinic lesions in this location can be quite subtle clinically and behave aggressively.
- Like its cutaneous counterpart, actinic cheilitis may progress to overt squamous cell carcinoma of the lip.

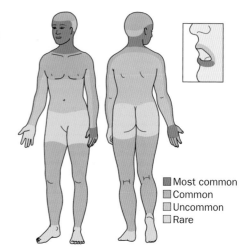

- Most common
- Common
- Uncommon
- Rare

Actinic keratosis. An early lesion with dilated vessels and minimal scale.

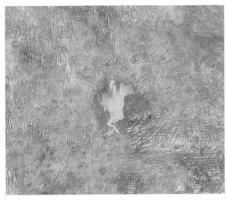

Actinic keratosis. An early lesion. Scale is yellow, sharp and tightly adherent.

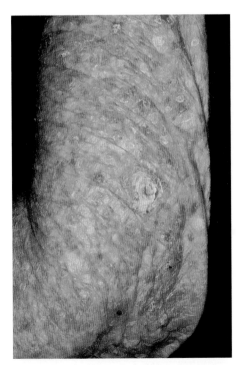

Actinic keratosis. Numerous lesions are present on the arm. The single dense lesion was excised. The other lesions cleared after a 7-week course of topical 5-fluorouracil.

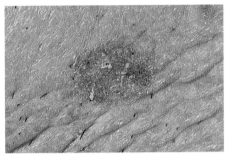

Pigmented actinic keratosis has all of the features of actinic keratosis. There is sharp adherent surface scale and subtle to dense brown pigmentation.

Laboratory and Pathology

- Biopsy is often helpful for distinguishing advanced actinic keratoses and actinic cheilitis from invasive squamous cell carcinoma.
- The histologic hallmark is a disordered epidermis with keratinocyte atypia.
- By definition, invasion into the dermis of atypical keratinocytes is not seen with actinic keratoses.
- Similarly, the lesions of spreading pigmented actinic keratosis show keratinocyte atypia with increased pigmentation, whereas atypical melanocytes are seen in lentigo maligna.

Course and Prognosis

- As a rule untreated actinic keratoses persist and grow slowly.
- A small percentage of lesions spontaneously regress with continued sun protection, however, other populations of actinic keratoses progress to squamous cell carcinoma.
- The behavior of an individual lesion cannot be predicted.
- It has been estimated that 20% of patients with multiple actinic keratoses develop squamous cell carcinoma in one or more lesions.
- Squamous cell carcinomas that develop on the ear, the scalp, or at the vermilion border are more likely to metastasize than squamous cell carcinomas at other skin sites.

Discussion

- Inflammatory disorders involving the head and neck, such as seborrheic dermatitis and rosacea, can limit detection of actinic keratoses. Adequate control of these disorders helps in the prompt recognition and treatment of actinic keratoses.
- Actinic keratoses of the lower legs are frequently multiple, hyperkeratotic, and distributed over a large area.

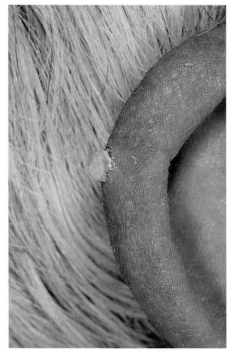

Actinic keratosis may accumulate dense scale on the surface and become a cutaneous horn. These lesions are excised. Squamous cell carcinoma has an identical appearance.

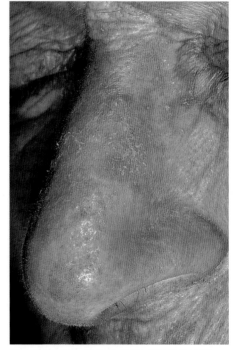

Almost the entire surface of the nose is covered with scale. This broad-based actinic keratosis is best treated with topical 5-fluorouracil.

- Numerous lesions may form on the dorsal hand; these lesions have the potential to develop into squamous cell carcinoma.

Treatment

- The patient with multiple actinic keratoses requires at least annual follow-up.
- Visible or detectable lesions represent a fraction of the total number of atypical keratinocytes actually present.

- Most of the atypia is scattered within sun-damaged skin and below the level of clinical detection.
- These patients will almost certainly develop more clinically apparent lesions with time.
- Adequate sun avoidance with sun-protective clothing and sunscreens should be encouraged to limit further damage.
- Application of liquid nitrogen (cryotherapy) to solitary superficial lesions is the most common method of removal.

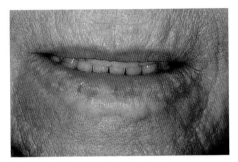

Actinic cheilitis presents with erythema and scaling. There is a loss of lip lines and the skin becomes smooth and eroded.

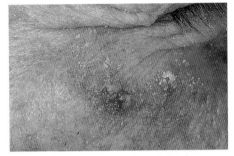

This actinic keratosis had been present for over 3 years. The central area has eroded and degenerated into an invasive squamous cell carcinoma. Typical features of an actinic keratosis are found at the periphery.

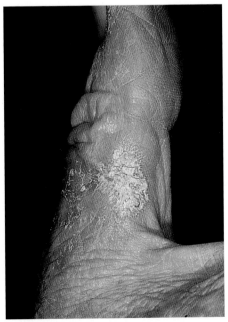

This actinic keratosis covers a wide area. It was treated in segments and cleared after three treatment sessions with cryospray.

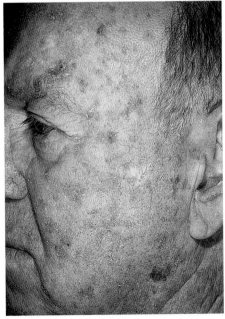

Topical chemotherapy with 5-fluorouracil. Lesions become inflamed during the first week of treatment.

- Patients with significant photodamage, or multiple and recurrent lesions present difficult treatment problems.
- Topical 5-fluorouracil 5% cream or solution is useful in reducing the number of atypical keratinocytes and has been the standard in topical, non-surgical treatment of actinic keratoses. In recent years, other, non-surgical options have increased.
- Treatment should be tailored for specific areas of the skin, in terms of concentration of the cream, the number of applications per day, and the duration.
- 5-Fluorouracil is available as a cream of 0.5% (Carac), 1% (Fluoroplex), and 5% (Efudex) and as a 1% (Fluoroplex) and 2% (Efudex) solution.
- Although treatment of all sun-damaged areas may be appropriate, it is rarely practical to treat large areas at one time. It may instead be convenient to treat limited areas on a rotating basis.
- Treatment with 5-fluorouracil involves application of medication twice a day for 3–5 weeks, or longer.
- Erythema will appear if actinic keratoses are present. This is followed by burning and oozing. Treatment may be stopped prior to completing the 3-week course if intense inflammation, crusting or discomfort occurs.
- Patients should be evaluated during the treatment period for discomfort and other complications.
- Imiquimod 5% cream has been shown to effectively treat multiple actinic keratoses when applied three to five times weekly for up to 4 weeks.

- Inflammatory changes similar to those with 5-fluorouracil occur with Imiquimod.
- Electrodesiccation and curettage are also effective for hypertrophic lesions.
- All destructive methods ablate the epidermis with minimal effect on the dermis. All have some risk of post-procedure hypopigmentation and scar formation, especially in people with darker skin. This should be clearly explained to the patient before treatment.
- Carbon dioxide laser vermilionectomy is the preferred treatment for extensive actinic cheilitis, but 5-fluorouracil and Imiquimod can also be used on the mucosa (with extreme caution). Application of 5-fluorouracil and Imiquimod on the oral mucosa should be less frequent and for a shorter duration.
- Carac is applied daily; other 5-fluorouracil preparations are usually applied twice daily.

Pearls

- Invasive squamous cell carcinoma can develop from actinic keratosis, especially with thicker lesions, or lesions not responding to treatment, or lesions of the lower lip.
- A biopsy should be considered in any patient who does not respond appropriately to treatment and in those actinic keratoses that are recurrent or hypertrophic.
- Some patients may require two or three visits per year to adequately treat the numerous actinic keratoses present and prevent progression to squamous cell carcinoma.

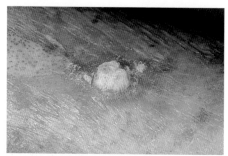

A clinical diagnosis of squamous cell carcinoma was made on this thick lesion. Biopsy, however, showed that this was an actinic keratosis with all of the atypical cells confined to the epidermis.

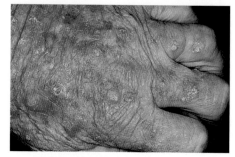

Actinic keratosis on the back of the hands and forearms is often very thick. Differentiating an actinic keratosis from invasive squamous cell carcinoma by inspection may be difficult.

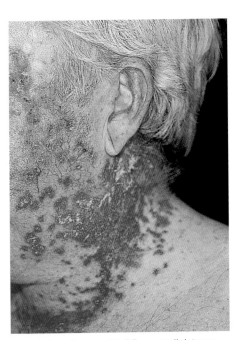

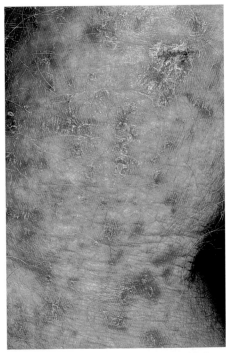

Topical chemotherapy with 5-fluorouracil. Intense inflammation is induced. Thick indurated lesions become inflamed.

Actinic keratosis 3 weeks after treatment with 5-fluorouracil cream. Lesions are inflamed but have not reached the lesion disintegration phase. Treatment was stopped 1 week later when the lesions eroded.

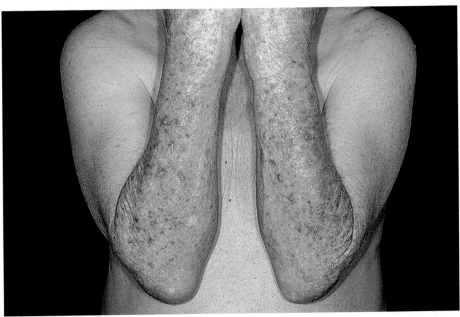

Actinic keratosis 4 weeks after starting treatment with 5-fluorouracil cream. Lesions on the arms are usually thicker and more resistant to treatment. They may require 6–7 weeks of treatment to reach the lesion disintegration phase.

Squamous Cell Carcinoma

Description

■ Cutaneous squamous cell carcinoma is an invasive, primary cutaneous malignancy arising from keratinocytes of the skin or mucosal surfaces.

■ It is most commonly found on the head, neck, or hands of elderly patients.

■ Lesions may develop from precursor actinic keratoses or may arise de novo.

History

■ Squamous cell carcinoma is the second most common form of skin cancer.

■ It comprises 20% of all primary cutaneous malignancies.

■ The lifetime risk of developing a cutaneous squamous cell carcinoma is estimated to be between 4% and 14%.

■ More than 100,000 new cases of primary cutaneous squamous cell carcinoma are diagnosed in the United States each year.

■ Approximately 2500 deaths occur annually from squamous cell carcinoma arising in the skin.

■ The incidence of squamous cell carcinoma doubles with each 8° to 10° decline in latitude.

■ Primary cutaneous squamous cell carcinomas usually occur on sun-exposed skin from years of accumulated actinic damage.

■ Nearly 90% of cutaneous squamous cell carcinomas in men and nearly 80% of such tumors in women occur on the head, neck, and hands.

■ Squamous cell carcinoma on the leg occurs more often in women than in men.

■ Caucasian people with fair complexions (skin types I and II) are at greatest risk.

■ Although the majority of squamous cell carcinomas are caused by ultraviolet light exposure, other extrinsic factors can play a causal role.

■ Such factors include other forms of radiation; chemicals such as hydrocarbons and arsenic; tobacco; chronic infections such as osteomyelitis; chronic inflammation; burns (Marjolin's ulcer); and human papillomavirus infection.

■ Historically, squamous cell carcinoma has been considered as a low-grade tumor with a metastatic rate of less than 1%.

■ With the current epidemic of all primary cutaneous malignancies and recent epidemiologic attention, it is clear that squamous cell carcinoma is far more aggressive than previously believed.

■ "Conduit spread" refers to the perivascular or perineural extension of tumor cells.

■ Ultimately the tumors may metastasize, usually via the lymphatics, to local lymph nodes.

Skin Findings

■ As with actinic keratoses, squamous cell carcinomas typically occur on sun-exposed areas.

■ Tumors are found within a background of sun-damaged skin with atrophy, telangiectasias, and blotchy hyperpigmentation.

■ Actinic keratoses are aggregates of atypical keratinocytes contained within the epidermis.

■ At the very least, actinic keratoses represent squamous atypia, if not squamous cell carcinoma in situ.

■ Unlike the lesions of Bowen's disease, which show full-thickness involvement, actinic keratoses show partial epidermal cellular atypia.

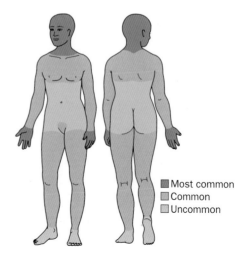

■ Most common
■ Common
■ Uncommon

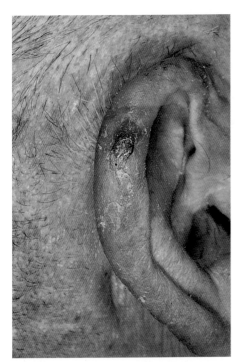

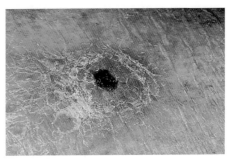

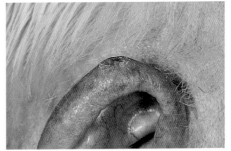

Differentiating actinic keratosis from squamous cell carcinoma can be difficult. Excisional biopsy demonstrated invasion of atypical squamous cells into the dermis and proved the diagnosis of squamous cell carcinoma.

Squamous cell carcinoma is commonly found on the ears. The thick smooth mass had been present for over a year. The patient sought help after the surface eroded.

This large mass had been slowly growing for 2 years. Patients are often not concerned until the skin breaks down and ulcerates. Basal cell carcinoma may have an identical appearance.

Squamous cell carcinoma retains surface scale. The lesion is called a cutaneous horn if it accumulates a large amount of scale.

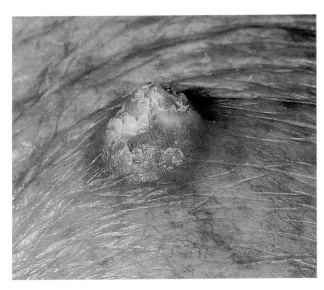

- Early invasive squamous cell carcinoma may have the appearance of a hypertrophic actinic keratosis.
- The lesion has a red, poorly defined base and an adherent yellow-white scale.
- The diagnosis is made by skin biopsy.
- The untreated lesion becomes larger and more raised, developing into a firm, red nodule with a necrotic crusted center.
- Squamous cell carcinoma may arise de novo, appearing as a sharply defined, smooth, dull red, firm, dome-shaped nodule with a crusted center.
- Removal of the crust reveals a central cavity filled with necrotic keratin debris, often with a foul odor.
- Keratoacanthoma is now considered a variant of invasive squamous cell carcinoma. Most authors consider keratoacanthoma to be a low-grade squamous cell carcinoma.
- Diagnosis is based on histology.
- Bowen's disease represents full-thickness squamous cell carcinoma in situ.
- A slow-growing and barely raised red plaque with adherent dry scale appears.
- If untreated, invasion ultimately occurs within a lesion of Bowen's disease.
- When this occurs, the area of invasion develops the dull red nodular thickening of squamous cell carcinoma.
- Similarly, erythroplasia of Queyrat (squamous cell carcinoma in situ of the penis) may also become invasive.
- Nodular or ulcerated areas should suggest invasion and thus warrant biopsy.
- Many lesions may appear on the sun-exposed bald scalp.
- Squamous cell carcinomas arising from actinic keratosis may have a thick, adherent scale.
- Actinic keratosis may become thick, indicating progression into squamous cell carcinoma.
- Cutaneous horns may begin as actinic keratosis and progress into squamous cell carcinoma.

Non-skin Findings

- As previously discussed, squamous cell carcinomas have metastatic potential.
- Metastases are usually to the regional lymph nodes and are detected within 2–3 years.
- Palpable regional lymph nodes suggest metastatic disease.

Laboratory

- Skin biopsy should be performed for all suspected squamous cell carcinomas.
- Biopsy should include the dermis so that invasion can be assessed.
- Malignant keratinocytes are confined to the epidermis in both actinic keratoses and Bowen's disease.
- In actinic keratoses, malignant cells are usually few in number, are well demarcated, and possess overlying parakeratosis.
- In Bowen's disease, malignant cells are greater in number, are found at all levels of the epidermis, and extend into the epithelium of adnexal structures.
- In invasive squamous cell carcinomas, malignant cells breach the dermoepidermal junction and invade the dermis.
- Tumor cells vary in their degree of differentiation.
- The surgical margins of excised lesions should be examined carefully to ensure complete excision.
- Lesions should be graded as to their degree of differentiation, their depth of invasion, and the presence of perineural invasion.

Course and Prognosis

- The long-term prognosis for adequately treated, non-metastatic squamous cell carcinoma of the skin is excellent.
- Such patients are at increased risk of developing additional primary skin malignancies, so periodic follow-up is warranted in all patients.
- The metastatic rate of squamous cell carcinomas arising on sun-exposed skin is now estimated to be between 2% and 6%.

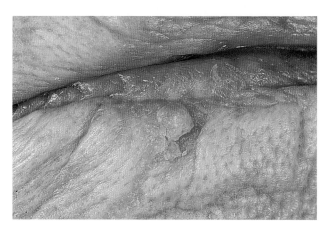

This lower lip tumor appears to be a superficial actinic keratosis. Palpation revealed a large firm mass in the dermis. Biopsy showed squamous cell carcinoma.

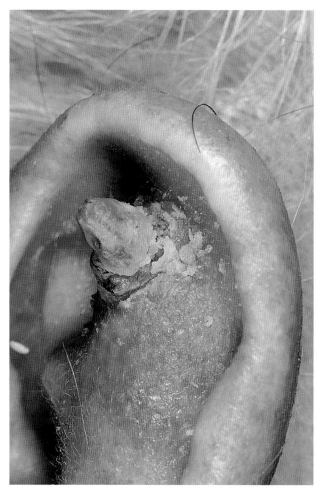

The clinical diagnosis of cutaneous horn is made for any lesion that has accumulated thick scale. The differential diagnosis includes actinic keratosis, squamous cell carcinoma, and wart. Biopsy showed that this lesion was a squamous cell carcinoma.

- Risk factors for metastasis include the following:
  - Tumor larger than 2.0 cm in diameter, invasion deeper than 0.4 cm, or both
  - Decreased degree of differentiation of tumor cells
  - Recurrent lesions
  - Perineural invasion
  - Adenoid-producing or mucin-producing variant of squamous cell carcinoma
  - Immunosuppressed host
  - Tumor arising in a scar or a chronic wound
- The risk of metastases is also higher for tumors at specific anatomic sites.
- The metastatic rate for squamous cell carcinomas arising on the lip or ear is estimated at 10–20%.
- The 5-year mortality rate is similar to that of other head and neck tumors.
- Half of such patients ultimately die as a result of metastatic disease.
- Tumors arising within scar tissue have a metastatic rate as high as 30%.

Complications

- Patients on immunosuppressive therapy after organ transplantation are at higher risk for cutaneous malignancy, including squamous cell carcinoma.
- Tumors arise with increasing frequency between 5 and 10 years after transplantation.
- Such patients must be followed closely and their tumors treated aggressively.

Treatment

- The treatment of primary squamous cell carcinoma of the skin involves wide local excision with histologic confirmation of margins.

- Mohs micrographic surgery may be useful for specific sites where tissue sparing is of importance.
- Cure by Mohs technique assumes contiguous tumor growth such as that seen in basal cell carcinoma.
- Squamous cell carcinoma can have skip areas (noncontiguous growth), and this renders Mohs technique somewhat less effective for squamous cell carcinoma.
- Palpation of regional lymph nodes is mandatory for all invasive squamous cell carcinoma patients.
- Lymph node biopsy is indicated for suspected nodal disease.
- The role of elective node dissection for high-risk lesions is currently under investigation.
- Imaging studies may be warranted for high-risk tumors.
- Radiation therapy may be considered when surgical resection is not feasible.
- Careful follow-up at regular intervals is recommended for all squamous cell carcinomas. Follow-up should include the following:
  - Skin examination and biopsy of new lesions suspicious for malignancy
  - Visual inspection and palpation of the excision scar for nodularity and other evidence of skin recurrence
  - Careful examination of the regional lymph node with node biopsy, if indicated, to detect early metastatic disease
- The sun-exposed lower lip is a common site. Palpation may reveal a deep nodular mass. Squamous cell carcinomas originating on the lip, ear and scalp tend to be more aggressive and metastasize to the regional lymph nodes and beyond.

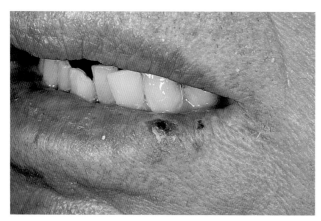

The diagnosis of actinic keratosis was made after observation of minimal surface scale. A large firm mass was then palpated below surface scale. Biopsy showed squamous cell carcinoma.

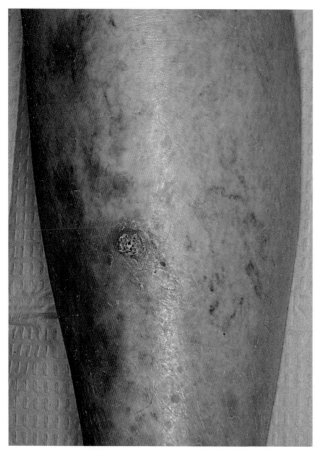

Squamous cell carcinoma of the lower leg. This lesion evolved from an actinic keratosis that was not adequately treated with cryosurgery.

Bowen's Disease

Description
- Bowen's disease is an intraepidermal (in situ) cutaneous malignancy arising from keratinocytes of the skin and mucosal surfaces.
- It is a superficial variant of squamous cell carcinoma.

History
- Bowen's disease may arise in sun-exposed and sun-protected areas.
- There are multiple etiologies, including ultraviolet light (actinic), other forms of radiation, chemicals (arsenic), and human papillomavirus.
- Lesions within sun-protected areas suggest a past history of arsenic exposure or relation to human papilloma virus.
- The onset is insidious; lesions are persistent and slowly enlarge over months to years. Slow progression may ultimately lead to invasion.
- Lesions are minimally symptomatic, and patients often delay seeking care.

Skin Findings
- A solitary, barely raised, red plaque with adherent dry scaling appears.
- At first glance, the plaque suggests a single plaque of psoriasis or eczema.
- On closer inspection the surface scaling is irregular, fissured, and adherent.
- Focal areas of pigmentation are often present and suggest superficial basal cell carcinoma.
- The border is slightly elevated, but usually is not raised or rolled.
- Little if any inflammation is present.
- If untreated, the plaque extends laterally over many years, eventually becoming invasive squamous cell carcinoma.
- Unlike actinic keratoses (partial thickness) Bowen's disease represents full-thickness replacement of the epidermis with tumor cells.
- Erythroplasia of Queyrat (penile Bowen's disease) is also squamous cell carcinoma in situ occurring on the glans under the foreskin of the uncircumcized penis.

These lesions are strongly defined red plaques with a moist, glistening surface.
- Analogous lesions occur on the vulva.

Non-skin Findings
- Patients with plaques in sun-protected areas may have a history of arsenic exposure.
- Those with a confirmed history of arsenic exposure are at increased risk of lymphoreticular and gastrointestinal malignancies.

Laboratory and Pathology
- Malignant keratinocytes are seen at all levels within the epidermis (full thickness) in a "windblown" pattern.
- Atypical cells extend down along the adnexal epithelium well below the skin surface.
- Atypical cells do not breach the dermoepidermal junction.

Course and Prognosis
- Bowen's disease is similar to actinic keratoses in that both are intraepidermal lesions containing malignant keratinocytes. However, Bowen's disease is a less common and potentially more aggressive lesion.

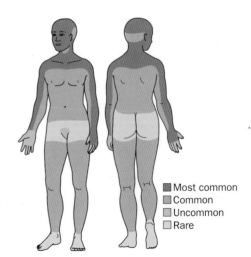

- Most common
- Common
- Uncommon
- Rare

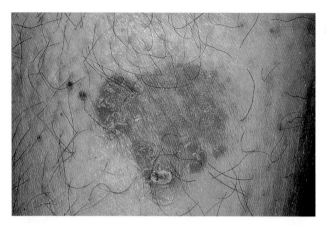

Bowen's disease is a slowly growing lesion with intraepidermal atypical squamous cells. This plaque looks like psoriasis.

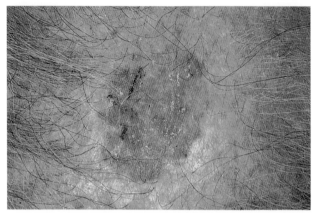

The diagnosis of Bowen's disease is often not made until after biopsy. This plaque looks like an actinic keratosis.

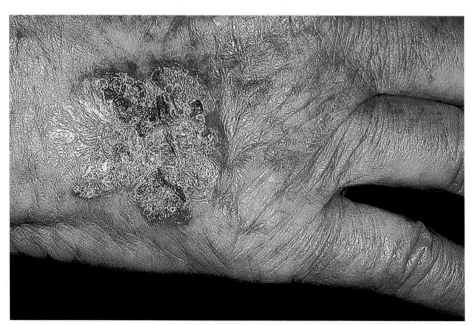

A plaque of Bowen's disease had been present for years. The lesion recurred after cryotherapy and has developed into invasive squamous cell carcinoma.

- Lesions are full-thickness, extend in continuity with epithelium of adnexal structures, and predictably become invasive.
- Erythroplasia of Queyrat has a greater tendency toward invasion and metastases, estimated at 10–30%.

Differential Diagnosis
Clinical
- Psoriasis
- Localized chronic eczematous dermatitis
- Superficial basal cell carcinoma
- Seborrheic keratosis

Histologic
- Mammary and extramammary Paget's disease
- Amelanotic melanoma

Discussion
- Skin biopsy might be needed to confirm the clinical diagnoses.
- Special stains may be required to discriminate between the histologic differential diagnoses.

Treatment
- Treatment with excision, curettage, cryosurgery, topical 5-fluorouracil or Imiquimod.
- Follow at regular intervals after treatment.
- Recurrences occur from cells deep in follicular structures and ill-defined lateral margins.
- Any areas suspicious for recurrence should be biopsied or excised without delay.
- Biopsy or excise areas suspicious for recurrence.

Pearls
- The borders of Bowen's disease lesions are well defined, and lesions closely resemble psoriasis, chronic eczema and seborrheic keratosis.
- Some patches of Bowen's disease may be treated with steroids for suspected eczematous dermatitis. Therefore "eczema" that does not respond to steroids may be Bowen's disease.
- Bowen's disease of the penis (erythroplasia of Queyrat) is a moist, slightly raised, well-defined, red, and smooth or velvety plaque.

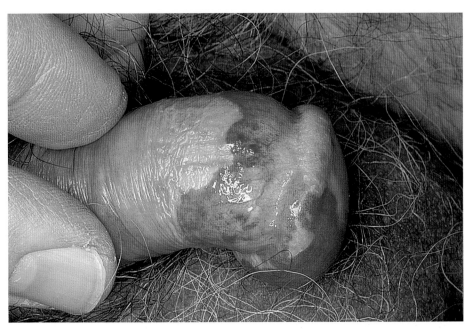

Bowen's disease of the penis (erythroplasia of Queyrat) is a moist, slightly raised, well-defined, red, smooth or velvety plaque.

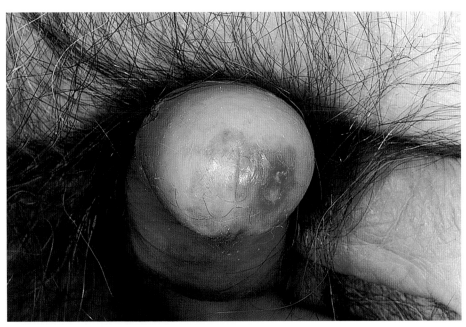

Analogous to Bowen's disease of the skin, erythroplasia of Queyrat grows very slowly and has the potential for degeneration into squamous cell carcinoma.

Leukoplakia

Description

- Leukoplakia is a descriptive clinical term reserved for white patches or plaques occurring on the mucosal surfaces pending definitive diagnosis.
- Diagnostic possibilities range from benign hyperkeratosis to squamous cell carcinoma.

History

- Leukoplakia is a common, sometimes chronic, condition of the oral mucosa.
- It occurs more frequently in men than in women.
- It usually appears after age 40, and the prevalence approaches 8% after age 70.
- Most lesions are asymptomatic.
- More than 80% of people with leukoplakia use some form of tobacco.

Skin Findings

- Leukoplakia begins as a single small, well-defined, translucent to white, slightly elevated papule.
- Individual lesions may resolve completely, recur, or progress.
- Multiple papules may coalesce into larger plaques over time.
- Uneven hyperkeratosis or small erosions may develop.
- Focal red areas or discreet papules termed *erythroplakia* may develop within plaques, giving a speckled appearance.
- Lesions may occur anywhere on the oral mucosa but are most commonly found on the buccal mucosa and lower lip.

Laboratory and Pathology

- The clinical appearance is often more striking than the histologic characteristics.
- Varying degrees of hyperplasia and hyperkeratosis may occur in the mucosa.
- There is a sparse, mixed inflammatory infiltrate in the submucosa.
- Squamous cell carcinoma in situ is the most common malignancy seen.

Course and Prognosis

- "Leukoplakia" is a descriptive clinical term, not a definitive diagnosis. The term is often misused to designate a premalignant condition.
- "Premalignant" implies epithelial dysplasia, and impending conversion to a true malignancy.
- Thus "leukoplakia" is best used to describe a chronic, whitish, oral plaque in which dysplasia has yet to be shown by biopsy.
- There is always a risk of malignant transformation with time. This is especially true for lesions on the ventral tongue and floor of the mouth.
- Factors that favor or promote malignant transformation include tobacco, alcohol, ultraviolet light, and some human papilloma virus infections.
- When malignant change is demonstrated histologically, a definitive diagnosis of squamous cell carcinoma is made.
- Invasive squamous cell carcinoma of the mucosa has a much greater risk of metastasis than squamous cell carcinoma arising in skin.

Differential Diagnosis

- Candidiasis (thrush)
- Oral hairy leukoplakia
- Frictional hyperkeratosis
- Lichen planus
- White sponge nevus
- Squamous cell carcinoma

Discussion

- Oral candidal lesions are less adherent; this diagnosis is confirmed by potassium hydroxide examination.

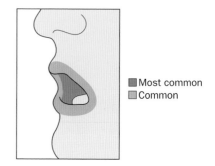

■ Most common
□ Common

- The presence of *Candida* organisms does not exclude the possibility of an underlying condition.
- Oral hairy leukoplakia occurs in patients with advanced disease caused by the human immunodeficiency virus. White patches occur most commonly on the lateral aspect of the tongue. Epstein–Barr virus is the causal agent.
- Frictional hyperkeratosis results from surface trauma, dental appliances or bite abnormalities.
- Lesion location correlates with the source of the trauma.

Treatment

- Patients who use tobacco products should be encouraged to stop.
- Any area of change, especially areas of erythroplakia, should be biopsied.

- Localized areas of epithelial dysplasia may be treated by cryosurgery, electrocautery, or topical 5-fluorouracil. Combinations of these therapies are sometimes used.
- Areas demonstrating squamous cell carcinoma, either in situ or invasive, are best treated with surgical excision. Close clinical follow-up, including lymph node examination, is required.
- Indefinite clinical follow-up is required after treatment to detect recurrence. This includes inspection of other areas of the oral mucosa as well as regional lymph node examination.

Pearls

- One cannot overstate the importance of close clinical follow-up and oral biopsy.

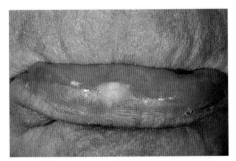

Leukoplakia. The white papules are slightly elevated, well demarcated and show little tendency to extend peripherally.

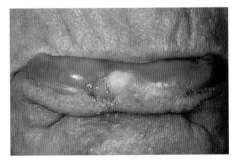

Leukoplakia 2 weeks after treatment with topical 5-fluorouracil.

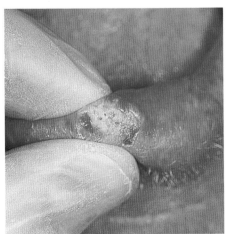

Degeneration to carcinoma develops in less than 20% of all patients with leukoplakia and takes 1 year to 20 years. All lesions should be palpated; a firm mass indicates squamous cell carcinoma.

Cutaneous T cell lymphoma

Description

- Cutaneous T cell lymphoma, also known as mycosis fungoides, is a distinct helper-T cell lymphoma of the skin.
- It may eventually invade the lymph nodes, peripheral blood, and internal organs.
- The disease most often evolves through several stages: from early or pre-mycosis fungoides, patch, plaque, and tumor stages. Some patients may have only one stage present or may have all four stages present simultaneously at the time of diagnosis.
- Sézary syndrome is the leukemic form of cutaneous T cell lymphoma; it develops de novo or may evolve from classic plaque/patch cutaneous T cell lymphoma, or from what appears to be chronic eczema.

History

- There are 0.5 cases per 100,000 people.
- Men are affected twice as often as women.
- Most cases are diagnosed in the fifth and sixth decade of life.

Skin Findings

- "Parapsoriasis" is a term that some use to describe the pre-mycosis fungoides phase of cutaneous T cell lymphoma. Clinically, this entity looks similar to patch stage cutaneous T cell lymphoma, but is not diagnostic of cutaneous T cell lymphoma histologically. Some feel this is a precursor stage of cutaneous T cell lymphoma. This early or pre-mycosis fungoides stage may not respond to repeated courses of topical steroids and may persist for months or years.
- Patch stage cutaneous T cell lymphoma can be confused with eczema, but one sees a sharply demarcated red to pink, scaly, atrophic, mottled, telangiectatic eruption.
- In the plaque stage, dusky red to brown, slightly elevated patches and plaques are seen. The disease in this form is often located on the "bathing trunk" area—the buttocks, hip, and upper thighs. The inner aspects of the upper arms and legs are often involved early. The shape of the individual plaques is variable; round, oval, arciform, or serpiginous patterns occur, occasionally with central clearing. The extent varies from a few isolated areas to a major portion of the skin.
- In the tumor stage, red-brown expanding nodules proliferate; they are variable in size, and ulceration may occur.
- In Sézary syndrome, erythroderma and generalized scaling occur; the palms and soles may be thickened; alopecia and ectropion are common. Infiltration of the entire skin produces a red, thickened skin with increased scale (exfoliative dermatitis) or without scale (erythroderma). Peripheral node enlargement and generalized pruritus are also common with Sézary syndrome.

Non-skin Findings

- The initial workup should include clinical evaluation for peripheral lymphadenopathy and hepatosplenomegaly.

Laboratory

- Despite new and improved laboratory diagnostic methods, recognition of the physical signs of the disease by the clinician is still the most sensitive method of detection.

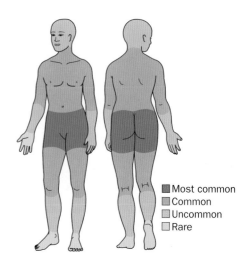

■ Most common
■ Common
□ Uncommon
□ Rare

- Baseline laboratory tests include complete blood count with a peripheral smear examination for Sézary cells, liver function tests, blood urea nitrogen levels, creatinine level, and chest x-ray. The results are usually normal in the patch and plaque stages. The CD4/CD8 count and ratio are done in generalized patch/plaque disease and in higher stage disease.

- Histologically, cutaneous T cell lymphoma lesions exhibit a superficial and deep, band-like and perivascular lymphocytic infiltrate with collections of lymphocytes (Pautrier's microabscesses) within a thickened epidermis. The infiltrate becomes mixed, with lymphocytes, eosinophils, and plasma cells, as the plaque stage progresses. Some lymphocytes are atypical, having a large hyper-convoluted or cerebriform nucleus (Sézary cells).

- Multiple large biopsies may be necessary.

- Molecular studies may be diagnostically helpful in the early stages or in clinically

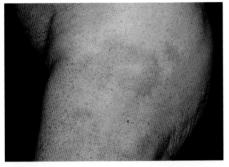

Early lesions are red with subtle scale or fine wrinkles. They persist for months with little peripheral extension and are often diagnosed as eczema and treated with topical steroids.

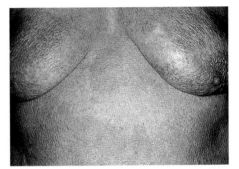

Infiltration of the entire skin produces a thickened red hide with scale (exfoliative dermatitis) or without scale (erythroderma).

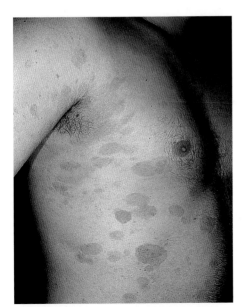

Lesions tend to remain fixed in location and size, and the margins are sharply delineated.

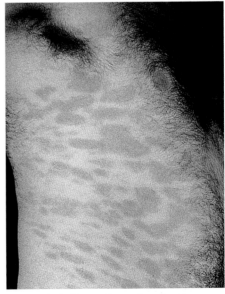

A red psoriasis-like eruption and an atrophic, mottled, telangiectatic surface, referred to as large-patch parapsoriasis or poikiloderma vasculare atrophicans, occur.

atypical cases; polymerase chain reaction and Southern blotting may reveal T cell receptor gene rearrangement, indicating the presence of a clonal population of cells.

Differential Diagnosis
- Atopic dermatitis
- Eczematous dermatitis
- Allergic contact dermatitis
- Psoriasis
- Drug eruption

Treatment
- Treatment is stage related.
- A referral to a dermatologist or oncologist is recommended for staging and treatment.
- In the patch and plaque stages, topical steroids, topical chemotherapy (nitrogen mustard, carmustine), psoralen plus ultraviolet A, ultraviolet B, total-body electron beam therapy, interferon, denileukin, topical or oral retinoids, or a combination of these therapies are used.
- In the tumor stage, spot radiation and interferon and combinations of the above treatments can be effective.
- In erythroderma or Sézary syndrome, extracorporeal photopheresis, interferon, oral retinoids, methotrexate, prednisone, and cyclophosphamide (Cytoxan) or combinations of these therapies are used, along with supportive care if needed.

Course and Prognosis
- In general, the course and prognosis relate to the stage of the disease.
- The early cutaneous T cell lymphoma and patch stages can last for many years without progression to tumor development, adenopathy, or internal organ involvement.
- Some patients simply have smoldering inflammatory changes resembling eczema that are kept under control with topical steroids; at the other end of the spectrum is progression to the plaque and tumor stage, and visceral organ infiltration.
- Necrosis and ulceration of plaques and tumors are common in progressive cases.

- Cutaneous T cell lymphoma may eventually infiltrate the lymph nodes and viscera; if there is no response to treatment, cutaneous T cell lymphoma can be fatal.

Pearls
- Early-stage (or pre-mycosis fungoides) and patch-stage cutaneous T cell lymphoma closely resemble eczema.

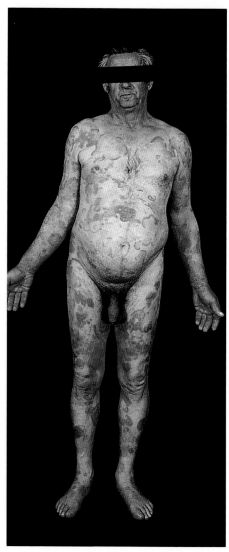

Necrosis and ulceration of plaques and tumors are common.

■ Eczematous dermatitis that does not respond to traditional therapy or that is recurrent may not be eczema, but may represent early or pre-mycosis fungoides.

■ A biopsy can be diagnostic of cutaneous T cell lymphoma with appropriate clinical correlation. However, multiple biopsies (three to six) over several months may be needed to confirm this diagnosis.

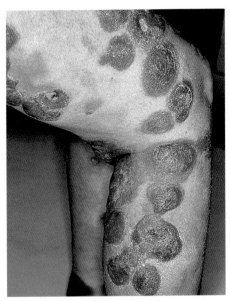

Tumors develop from pre-existing plaques or erythroderma, or they may originate from red or normal skin.

Tumors vary in size. Some become huge.

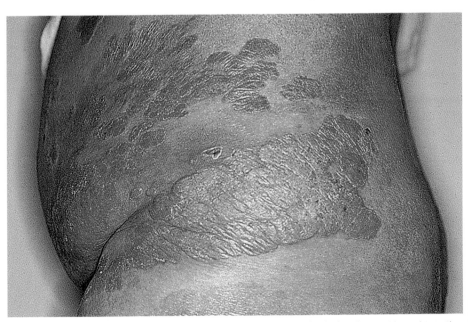

The plaques vary in shape, and the extent of involvement varies from a few isolated areas to a major portion of the skin.

Paget's Disease of the Breast

Description
- Paget's disease of the breast is a rare, distinctive cutaneous presentation of intraductal carcinoma of the breast.

History
- Paget's disease is the most common cutaneous presentation of breast cancer.
- However, it represents less than 5% of all cases of breast cancer.
- It occurs almost exclusively in women.
- The incidence increases with age, reflecting the incidence of breast cancer.
- It has an insidious onset, lasting months to years, usually in the fourth to sixth decades of life.
- It may be asymptomatic, and when it is symptomatic patients complain of localized itching, irritation, and discomfort.
- It is often misdiagnosed as "nipple eczema."
- Paget's disease should be suspected in cases of "nipple eczema" that do not improve after the use of topical corticosteroids.
- Patient denial or delay in seeking care results in a delay in the biopsy, diagnosis and treatment.

Skin Findings
- The lesion is a pink-to-red, sharply demarcated, irregular-shaped, scaly patch or plaque.
- The process appears eczematous, but will not respond to topical steroids. The plaque is indurated and has sharp margins, which remain relatively fixed for weeks.
- Malignant cells migrate through the epidermis, and the disease becomes initially apparent on the areola and, at a much later date, on the surrounding skin.
- The nipple, areola, and surrounding skin may be involved.
- Most often it is unilateral, but it can be bilateral.
- Initially induration is minimal.
- Over time induration, infiltration, and nodularity develop.
- An underlying breast mass is palpable in roughly 50% of cases.

- Eventually there is local destruction of the nipple and areola with retraction.

Non-skin Findings
- Underlying intraductal carcinoma is found in the affected breast.
- The contralateral breast should also be examined.
- The risk of cancer in the second breast is increased in patients who already have cancer in one breast.
- The regional lymph nodes are rarely palpable unless a palpable breast mass or superficial ulceration is present.

Laboratory and Pathology
- Skin biopsy confirms the presence of Paget's cells, which are large, round, pale, mucin-producing cells within the epidermis.
- Paget's cells are scattered among the normal-appearing keratinocytes, often displacing cells along the basal layer.
- Unlike keratinocytes, Paget's cells lack intracellular bridges, and are positive for periodic acid–Schiff and carcinoembryonic antigen.
- These special stains help distinguish mammary Paget's disease from melanoma and Bowen's disease.
- Deep biopsy may show continuity with an underlying intraductal carcinoma.

Course and Prognosis
- Mammary Paget's disease is caused by the intraepidermal spread of malignant cells from an underlying intraductal carcinoma of the breast.
- The prognosis is determined by breast cancer staging and therapy.
- The 5-year survival rate exceeds 90% when neither a breast mass nor regional lymph nodes are palpable.
- The 5-year survival rate is roughly 40% when an underlying breast mass is palpable.

Differential Diagnosis
- Nipple eczema
- Erosive adenomatosis of the nipple
- Bowen's disease
- Superficial basal cell carcinoma
- Tinea and candidal infections
- Contact dermatitis and other causes of eczematous dermatitis

Discussion

- Eczematous dermatitis is usually pruritic and should respond to topical corticosteroids.
- Adenomatosis of the nipple is a benign condition best confirmed by biopsy.
- Yeast and fungal infections should be confirmed by potassium hydroxide examination and should improve with topical antifungal therapy.
- The presence of yeast or a fungus does not exclude the possibility of Paget's disease.
- Skin biopsy should be performed for lesions of the nipple and areola that do not respond to topical therapy.

Treatment

- Breast and nodal examination is indicated for all patients with Paget's disease of the breast.
- Skin biopsy should be performed to confirm the diagnosis.
- Mammography should be performed.
- A referral to a breast cancer surgeon should be made for further evaluation of any palpable breast mass.

Pearls

- Skin biopsy should be performed for all dermatoses involving the nipple that do not respond to topical therapy or that persist for more than 1 month.

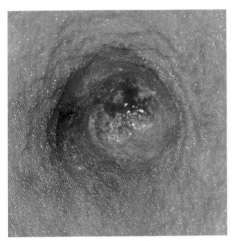

The disease begins insidiously in one breast, with a small area of erythema on the nipple that drains serous fluid and forms a crust.

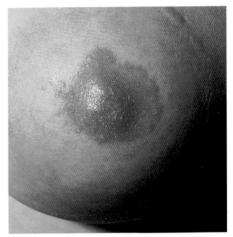

Malignant cells migrate through the epidermis, and the disease becomes initially apparent on the areola and, at a much later date, on the surrounding skin.

The process appears eczematous, but the plaque is indurated and has sharp margins, which remain relatively fixed for weeks.

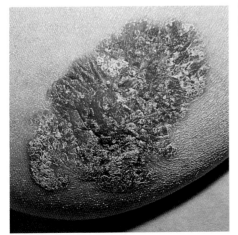

Extramammary Paget's Disease

Description

■ Extramammary Paget's disease is a rare, easily overlooked, intraepidermal malignancy involving the anogenital or axillary skin.

History

■ Extramammary Paget's disease is an intraepidermal adenocarcinoma.
■ It occurs in areas where apocrine glands are found.
■ It may be divided into two groups based on the source of the underlying primary adenocarcinoma.
■ The majority of cases represent adenocarcinoma in situ with extension of primary adenocarcinoma in situ from adnexal structures.
■ A minority of cases reflect an intraepidermal spread of tumor cells from non-cutaneous adenocarcinomas, via local or lymphatic spread.
■ Urogenital and rectal carcinomas are the most common origins of non-cutaneous adenocarcinoma associated with extramammary Paget's disease.
■ These include transitional cell cancer of the urethra and bladder, as well as carcinomas of the cervix, vagina, Bartholin's glands, and the prostate.
■ Local contiguous or regional lymphatic spread of these carcinomas leads to intraepidermal invasion.
■ Extramammary Paget's disease is rare before age 40.
■ It occurs more often in women than in men.
■ It most commonly occurs on the vulva and perineum in older women.
■ In men, the scrotum, penis, anal and perianal skin are most commonly affected.
■ It may extend to involve the lower abdomen, inguinal folds, buttocks, and thighs.
■ Other rare sites include the axillae, ears, and eyelids.
■ The patient may complain of itching and irritation, but rarely pain.
■ The lesion slowly and relentlessly increases in size.

Skin Findings

■ A red to white-gray plaque with a velvety or scaly surface is typical.
■ The plaque is sharply demarcated and has irregular borders.
■ The lesion may appear eczematous or lichenified.
■ Scaling, erosion, and serous exudate may occur.
■ It is most often unilateral.

Non-skin Findings

■ Depending on site of origin, the non-cutaneous primary adenocarcinoma may be visible and palpable.
■ Regional lymph nodes are usually not palpable early in the course of the disease.

Laboratory and Pathology

■ The histologic features of extramammary Paget's disease are identical to those of mammary Paget's disease.
■ Deep biopsy reveals an underlying adnexal adenocarcinoma or Paget's cells within the lymphatics.
■ Like mammary Paget's disease, extramammary Paget's disease stains positive to periodic acid–Schiff and carcinogenic antigen.

Course and Prognosis

■ Unlike Bowen's disease, in extramammary Paget's disease dermal invasion and regional metastases appear to occur earlier in the disease course.
■ Therefore, once the diagnosis is made, aggressive treatment and close follow-up are indicated.
■ Less than 25% of all patients with extramammary Paget's disease have an underlying non-cutaneous malignancy.
■ Of those patients with extramammary Paget's disease and underlying malignancy, 25% eventually die from the underlying malignancy.
■ The most common sites of metastases are the inguinal and pelvic lymph nodes, followed by the liver, bone, the lungs, the brain, the bladder, the prostate, and the adrenal glands. Regional and widespread

metastases may develop from any one of the primary sites.

■ The prognosis depends on site of the primary adenocarcinoma, its clinical stage, and therapy.

Differential Diagnosis

Clinical

■ Eczematous dermatitis
■ Lichen simplex chronicus
■ Intertrigo
■ Candidiasis
■ Tinea
■ Bowen's disease

Histologic

■ Bowen's disease
■ Melanoma

Treatment

■ The surrounding, clinically normal appearing skin may also be involved.
■ Local excision with obvious clear margins of the involved areas is standard.
■ Although the lesion appears to be sharply defined clinically, histologic confirmation of margins is vital.
■ There is a high recurrence rate, even after excision with apparently appropriate margins.
■ There may be benefit from Mohs micrographic excision, as an initial procedure or for recurrences.
■ Dissection of palpable regional lymph nodes may be warranted.
■ Radiotherapy is also an option for difficult cases or recurrent disease.

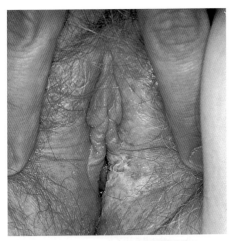

A white eroded plaque with ill-defined borders on the labia.

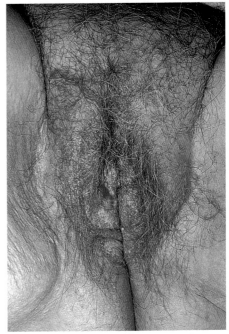

The disease appears as a white-to-red, scaling or macerated, infiltrated, eroded, or ulcerated plaque most frequently observed on the labia majora and scrotum.

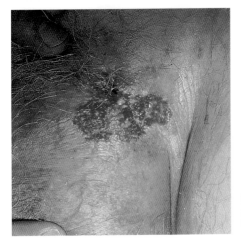

Three biopsies were taken before malignant cells were demonstrated at the periphery of this chronic ulcer at the base of the scrotum.

Cutaneous Metastasis

Description

■ A cutaneous metastasis is an uncommon, often overlooked sign of underlying malignancy.

History

■ Cutaneous metastases occur in 0.7–9.0% of all cancer patients.

■ Detection of cutaneous metastases may alter disease staging and therapy.

■ Cutaneous metastases presenting as the first sign of underlying occult malignancy are uncommon but occur most frequently with tumors of the lung, kidney, and ovary.

■ More commonly cutaneous metastases are a sign of extranodal disease in people with known underlying malignancy.

■ Cutaneous metastases may herald recurrence in a patient with a prior history of malignancy.

■ Excluding lymphomas, the origin of primary tumors metastasizing to skin reflect the underlying gender differences of primary tumors.

■ Common primary sites of men and women with cutaneous metastases are shown in the table opposite.

Metastases to the skin occur via lymphatic or hematogenous spread.

Skin Findings

■ About 75% of skin metastases in male patients occur on the head and neck, anterior chest, and abdomen.

■ About 75% of skin metastases in female patients occur on the anterior chest or abdomen.

■ The abdominal wall is the most common site for tumors presenting as metastatic disease.

■ Scalp metastases in men tend to be from the lung or kidney and present early in the disease.

■ Scalp metastases in women tend to be from the breast and present late in the disease.

■ Facial metastases tend to be from oral squamous cell carcinoma, renal cell carcinoma, lung and breast cancer.

■ Eyelid metastases tend to be from the breast or melanoma.

■ Neck metastases are more often a direct extension from deep nodes from the lung, oral squamous cell carcinoma, or breast carcinoma.

■ Most cutaneous metastases do not have a distinct clinical appearance.

■ Most present as a cluster of discrete, firm, painless nodules.

Breast Cancer

■ About 70% of all cutaneous metastases in women are related to breast cancer.

■ Skin involvement occurs in 24% of breast cancer cases.

■ It is the presenting sign 3.5% of the time.

■ The most common representation of cutaneous breast metastasis is an aggregate of discrete, firm, non-tender, skin-colored nodules that appear suddenly, grow rapidly, attain a certain size (often 2 cm), and remain stationary.

■ Several other distinct clinical patterns of metastatic breast cancer are recognized.

■ Inflammatory metastatic carcinoma resembles erysipelas in the anterior chest but without fever or tenderness. Redness is caused by capillary congestion; there is no inflammatory infiltrate.

■ *En cuirasse* metastatic carcinoma is a diffuse morphea-like induration of skin ("encasement in armor") that begins as scattered, firm, lenticular papulonodules that coalesce. Local lymphatic spread is possible.

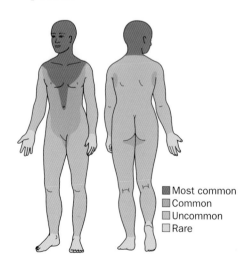

■ Most common
☐ Common
☐ Uncommon
☐ Rare

- In telangiectatic metastatic carcinoma, the violaceous papulovesicles resemble lymphangioma circumscriptum; there is local lymphatic spread. It may be pruritic and may resemble vasculitis.
- In nodular metastatic carcinoma, multiple firm papules or nodules appear on the anterior chest. They may be ulcerated and may suggest melanoma or pigmented basal cell carcinoma.
- Alopecia neoplastica has asymptomatic, non-inflammatory, circular areas of alopecia. There is distant hematogenous spread.
- In Paget's disease of the breast, there is a sharply defined plaque of erythema and scaling on the breast, suggestive of eczema, but the eruption is persistent. It is usually unilateral but may be bilateral. This represents a direct spread from underlying breast cancer.

Colon and Rectal Carcinoma

- Colon and rectal carcinoma is the second most common source of skin metastases in both genders.
- It usually presents late in the disease course.
- The abdomen and perineum are the most common sites.
- It may present as inflammatory metastatic carcinoma of the inguinal folds or as a chronic cutaneous fistula.

Melanoma

- Melanoma is the third most common cause of metastasis to the skin.
- Melanoma typically invades the liver, lungs and brain, but may also show up at distant cutaneous sites.
- Skin is the most common primary site of melanoma, followed by ocular and mucosal sites.

Common Primary Sites of Origin for Men and Women with Cutaneous Metastases		
Site of Origin	**Percentage of Metastases**	
	Women	Men
Breast	69%	2%
Colon	9%	19%
Melanoma	5%	13%
Lung	4%	24%
Connective tissue sarcoma	2%	3%
Cervix	2%	3%
Pancreas	2%	2%
Oral cavity squamous cell carcinoma	1%	12%
Bladder	1%	2%
Ovary	4%	—
Prostate	—	1%
Salivary glands	2%	2%
Skin squamous cell carcinoma	—	1%
Kidney	—	6%
Thyroid	—	1%
Stomach	—	6%
Liver	—	1%

- There are cases of systemic or metastatic melanoma without a primary cutaneous melanoma.

Lung Carcinoma
- Historically, lung carcinoma is more common in men than women.
- There is a localized cluster of cutaneous non-specific nodules, most often on the anterior chest or abdomen.

Renal Cell Carcinoma
- Renal cell carcinoma comprises 6.8% of all cutaneous metastases.
- It presents on the head and neck region most commonly.
- A well circumscribed, bluish nodule with prominent vascularity appears.

Oral Squamous Cell Carcinoma
- Oral squamous cell carcinoma usually occurs in men with a known primary tumor.
- It presents as multiple nodules on the head and neck region.
- It may be difficult to discern metastatic disease from primary squamous cell carcinoma of the skin.

Neuroblastoma
- Neuroblastoma is the most common neonatal tumor.
- About 30% of patients with congenital neuroblastomas have subcutaneous and cutaneous metastases.
- It presents on the skin as multiple firm, mobile, blue subcutaneous nodules that blanch when stroked and may show a "blueberry muffin" appearance.
- The neoplasm also metastasizes to the liver, lymph nodes and bone marrow.

Lymphomas
- Cutaneous metastases occur in 6.6% of all patients with lymphoma.
- A skin lesion is the presenting sign in 5% of patients and the first sign of extranodal disease in 7.6% of patients.
- These are firm, raised, smooth, red-to-violaceous nodules and plaques which may ulcerate.
- It may be difficult to discern primary lymphoma arising in skin from metastatic disease.

Leukemia Cutis
- Leukemia cutis appears as macules, papules, ecchymoses, palpable purpura, or ulcers.
- It often precedes or is concurrent with a diagnosis of systemic leukemia.
- Lesions are seen in 25–30% of infants with congenital leukemias and may precede other manifestations of leukemia by up to 4 months.
- Myeloblastomas may occur in acute myelocytic leukemia. The greenish color of chloromas is due to myeloperoxidase within the lesions.
- Mucocutaneous involvement is more common in monocytic leukemias, with involvement ranging from papules to plum-colored nodules and gingival infiltrations.
- Adult T cell leukemia involves the skin in 75% of patients.

Non-skin Findings
- The primary tumor site and potentially other non-cutaneous metastases are usually detectable by imaging studies.

Laboratory
- Skin biopsy confirms malignant cells of primary tumor origin.
- Tissue-specific immunohistochemical stains may be of value in cases in which the primary site is not obvious.
- Fresh, unfixed specimens are optimal for specialized immunohistochemistry and molecular studies.

Course and Prognosis
- The prognosis is determined by the tumor type, extent of disease, and available treatment options for the primary tumor.
- In general, metastatic disease has a poor prognosis.

Discussion
- In some cases, excision of symptomatic or disfiguring skin metastases can significantly improve a patient's quality of life.

Treatment
- Therapy is directed by the underlying malignancy.

Pearls

- Biopsy should be performed for any new nodule in an old scar or any new nodule in a new scar if a malignancy was the reason for excision.

- Besides discreet nodules or plaques, the second most common pattern of cutaneous metastasis is inflammation with erythema, edema, warmth, and tenderness.

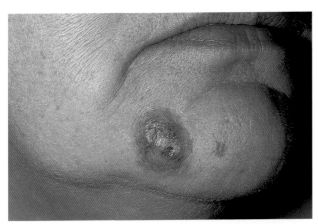

The most common representation of cutaneous metastasis is an aggregate of discrete, firm, non-tender, skin-colored nodules that appear suddenly, grow rapidly, attain a certain size (often 2 cm), and remain stationary.

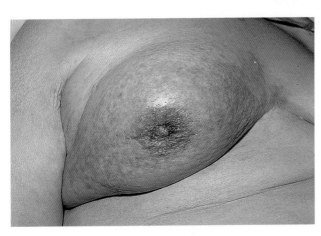

The second most common pattern of cutaneous metastasis is inflammation with erythema, edema, warmth, and tenderness.

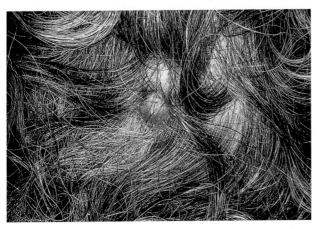

Biopsy of this hard nodule showed metastatic adenocarcinoma.

18 Nevi and Malignant Melanoma

Nevi, Melanocytic Nevi, Moles

Description

■ Nevi are benign skin tumors composed of melanocyte-derived nevus cells, classified by age of onset and the arrangement of nevus cells.

History

■ Nevi are ubiquitous in humans and equally common among males and females.
■ Those present at birth or that appear during early infancy are termed congenital nevi.
■ The incidence of acquired nevi reach a peak incidence during adolescence; fewer nevi are acquired after age 30.
■ Nevi appearing or changing after age 30 should be regarded as suspicious.
■ Sun exposure appears to be a stimulus for cell growth of nevi.
■ Most acquired nevi appear on sun-exposed skin.
■ Acquired nevi appearing in sun-protected areas should be considered suspicious.
■ Most adults have between 12 and 20 nevi; larger numbers of nevi may be a familial trait.
■ Existing nevi may increase in size and become more heavily pigmented during puberty or during pregnancy.
■ Nevi are usually asymptomatic though may on occasion be irritated by clothing or external trauma.

Evolution of Lesions

■ Acquired nevi first appear as flat, round, uniformly colored papules.
■ During this growth phase, nevi expand laterally while remaining flat and symmetric.
■ Nevi may be slightly darker in color and slightly raised in the center, and they remain stable in size and appearance for several years.
■ Over many years, nevi continue to become more elevated and uniformly lighter in color.
■ Eventually the nevus appears as a skin-colored papule or may completely disappear in older years.
■ Residual nevi are rare after age 70.

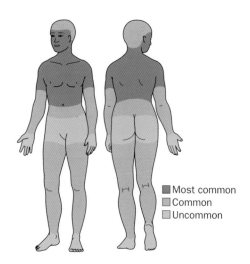

■ Most common
■ Common
■ Uncommon

Skin Findings

- Melanocytic nevi are composed of organized clusters of nevus cells arranged at various levels in the skin.
- Nevi are classified by the location and arrangement of nevus cells within the skin.

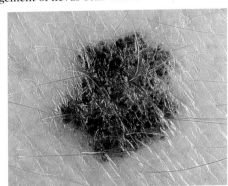

Junctional Nevi

- Junctional nevi are flat or slightly raised brown to tan macules.
- Skin markings are preserved in the surface of the nevus.
- They are most commonly found in children.
- Nests of nevus cells cluster at the dermoepidermal junction.
- Nevi of palms, soles, genitalia, and mucosa are usually junctional nevi.

Compound Nevi

- Compound nevi are slightly or markedly raised pigmented papules.
- Nests of nevus cells are found both at the dermoepidermal junction and within the dermis.
- Compound nevi can have an irregular border but are symmetric.
- The surface may be smooth or slightly papillomatous.
- The center tends to be more heavily pigmented than the periphery.
- They tend to increase in thickness and pigmentation in late childhood and adolescence.

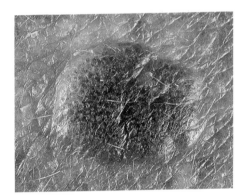

Intradermal Nevi

- Intradermal nevi are papules which are most commonly elevated, fleshy, and slightly or moderately pigmented.
- They vary in color from dark brown to normal skin color.
- Pigmentation may be arranged in flecks.
- Course, dark, terminal hairs may grow from the nevus.
- Intradermal nevi are seen mainly after adolescence.
- Nests and cords of nevus cells are found within the dermis; they may extend into the subcutaneous fat.
- Melanocytic cells are pale and fairly uniform in size and are found in cords or clusters surrounded by collagen bundles.

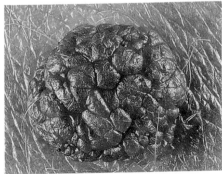

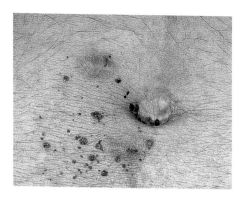

Nevus Spilus

- Nevus spilus is a sharply defined tan to brown background patch similar to a café-au-lait spot; it also contains several small monomorphic slightly raised dark brown nevi.
- Nevus spilus does not have increased coarse hairs.
- Sun exposure does not seem to play a role in the development.
- Lesions usually develop before adulthood and follow a benign persistent course.

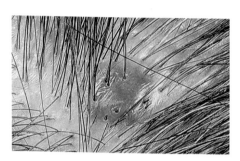

Blue Nevi

- Blue nevi are solitary bluish macules or papules most commonly found on the head and neck or buttock.
- Coloration is attributed to intensely pigmented melanocytes in the deep dermis.
- They commonly present in early childhood or at birth.
- They tend to slowly enlarge and persist for 10–15 years.
- Spindle-shaped, heavily pigmented nevus cells are located in the mid to lower dermis.

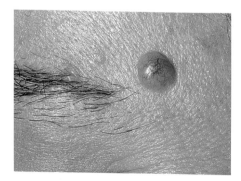

Spitz Nevus

- Spitz nevus, or spindle cell nevus, is usually a reddish pink, dome-shaped, smooth papule.
- It most often occurs on the face, scalp or legs of pre-adolescent children.
- Skin biopsy reveals overall architectural order with nested spindle-shaped nevus cells and areas with large pleomorphic nevus cells.
- Such changes would be worrisome for melanoma in an adult.
- The lesion and its biologic course are benign.
- Most dermatologists favor complete excision of Spitz nevi to minimize the risk of recurrence and associated pleomorphism.

Halo Nevi

- Halo nevi occur primarily during adolescence.
- A pre-existing nevus develops a surrounding rim of hypopigmentation that heralds the gradual disappearance of the nevus over several months.
- Skin biopsy shows a junction or compound nevus surrounded by a dense infiltrate of lymphocytes.
- Halo nevi appear to be a host response directed against the nevus cells.
- Focal atypical nevus cells may be seen though the majority of the pre-existing nevi are benign.
- The halo usually eventually re-pigments over a few years.
- Wood's light accentuates the halo.
- Halo nevi also occur in the setting of vitiligo and may develop in patients with melanoma.
- People with halo nevi should have a full skin examination to look for vitiligo and also as a screen for melanoma.

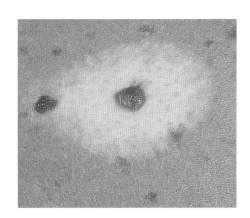

Recurrent Nevi

- Recurrent nevus phenomenon may occur at the site of a previously partially removed nevus.
- Randomly distributed pigmentation along with scar can be quite suspicious for melanoma.
- The biopsy may also be indistinguishable from melanoma.
- The history of previous biopsy and a review of the original specimen are critical to the correct diagnosis.

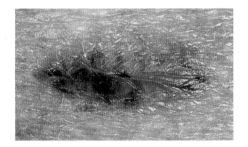

Laboratory

- Nevus cells tend to cluster or nest in discrete areas of the skin.
- Junctional nevi have nested nevus cells at the dermoepidermal junction.
- Intradermal nevi have nests and cords of nevus cells within the dermis, sometimes extending into fat.
- Compound nevi have nested nevus cells at the junction and also in the dermis.
- The term "combined nevus" is used to designate a benign nevus with typical compound or junctional nevus features and a deeper blue nevus component.

Course and Prognosis

- The vast majority of melanocytic nevi are benign and follow the course of maturation over years as described above.
- Nevi which deviate from this pattern are suspicious and biopsy is warranted.

465

- Junctional nevi are rare in adults.
- Unless known to be present since childhood, any biopsied junctional melanocytic lesion on an adult should be regarded as atypical if not melanoma in-situ.

Differential Diagnosis

- Melanocytic nevi:
  - Dysplastic nevi
  - Melanoma (careful histologic review needed by a qualified dermatopathologist)
- Spitz nevi:
  - Hemangioma
  - Pyogenic granuloma
  - Juvenile xanthogranuloma

Discussion

- Great care must be taken to minimize the risk of misdiagnosis of melanocytic lesions.
- The clinician should provide the dermatopathologist with the patient's age, location and clinical history of the lesion, any previous biopsy specimen, and the clinical differential diagnosis.
- An adequate biopsy specimen should be submitted.
- Similarly, it is the clinician's responsibility to correlate the pathologist's findings with the clinical diagnosis.

Treatment

- All nevi should be assessed.
- With the exception of the dysplastic nevus syndrome, most people produce nevi with a fairly uniform pattern and appearance.

- There is little variability from one nevus to another on a given person.
- The ABCDs of melanoma are a useful guide (see table on page 472).
- Most benign nevi are symmetric, with a well-defined, regular border, and a uniform color (perhaps with subtle variation in the hues of the dominant color), with a maximum diameter of less than 6 mm.
- Nevi that appear different from other nevi on the same patient should be regarded with suspicion.
- Suspicious nevi should be biopsied.
- Consider referral to a dermatologist.
- The current epidemic of skin cancers has prompted many patients to seek a screening examination.
- Such an opportunity for early detection and treatment, as well as for patient education, should not be missed.
- An examination of the entire cutaneous surface should be encouraged.
- Patients need to be educated on how to perform self-examination of the skin and should be encouraged to do so on a regular basis.
- Combine the teaching of self-examination techniques with the screening skin examination.
- Review the changes to watch for, including symptoms of itching and tenderness, with the patient.
- The patient should feel comfortable in seeking care for any future changes or concerns.

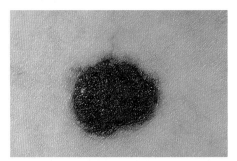

A dermal nevus with horn pearls on the surface. It is stuck onto the surface and has the consistency of a seborrheic keratosis. It can be easily removed with a curette.

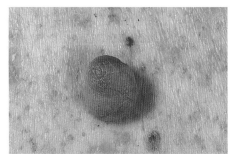

A dome-shaped smooth-surfaced papule. This common presentation for a dermal nevus occurs on the face and trunk. Patients are often more concerned with elevated lesions than with flat dark lesions.

- Sun awareness and regular use of sunscreens and sun-protective clothing should be also encouraged.

Pearls

- Benign nevi have a uniform appearance and a predictable life-cycle.

- Nevi which deviate from this pattern are suspicious and should be biopsied.
- Dermatoscopy can be helpful when evaluating nevus patterns. This requires familiarity and experience with the technique and findings.

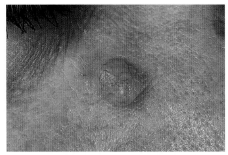

A common presentation for a dermal nevus on the face. The dome-shaped papule has telangiectasias on the surface and resembles a basal cell carcinoma. The lesion has remained stable for years.

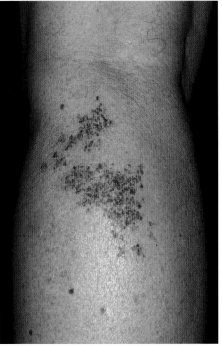

Speckled lentiginous nevi are common hairless brown lesions, dotted with darker brown to black specks. This special form of nevus is benign.

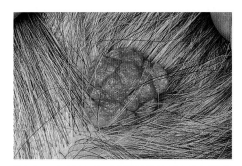

This is a common presentation for scalp nevi. There is no pigment and the surface is lobulated.

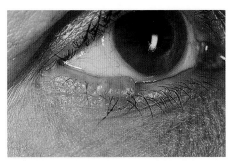

A dermal nevus with no pigment. Patients commonly think that all moles are pigmented. This smooth white papule had remained unchanged for years.

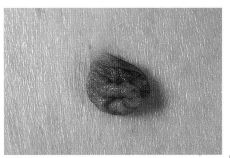

This dermal nevus has the consistency of a wrinkled sack. Biopsy showed an abundance of connective tissue and very few nevus cells.

Atypical Mole Syndrome (Dysplastic Nevus Syndrome, B–K Mole Syndrome)

Description

- Atypical mole syndrome consists of multiple clinically atypical nevi, together with an increased risk of melanoma. It occurs as a familial syndrome and also sporadically.

History

- First described in 1978 by Clark and colleagues as B–K mole syndrome.
- There are large irregular nevi with a variegated color and a palpable dermal component.
- It was found in increased numbers in the six families studied by Clark in 1978, among whom multiple family members had a history of melanoma.
- The nevi were considered to be a phenotypic marker for family members at increased risk for developing melanoma.
- The syndrome is now known as familial atypical mole to melanoma syndrome.
- Inheritance is thought to be autosomal dominant with variable expressivity.
- These clinically and histologically distinctive melanocytic nevi occur as solitary lesions, as multiple lesions in sporadic cases, and as multiple lesions in the familial syndrome.
- In all three settings, atypical nevi are considered to be precursors for melanoma, most often the superficial spreading type.
- More than 90% of patients with familial melanoma have atypical nevi.
- Nomenclature and criteria have evolved over time and are confusing.
- Currently the term atypical nevus is favored.
- Depending on criteria used, atypical nevi are common, with prevalence estimated at 5–20%.
- While solitary atypical nevi are common, the familial syndrome is uncommon.
- The incidence of sporadic (non-familial) occurrence of multiple atypical nevi is unknown.

- Males and females are equally affected.
- Atypical nevi are not present at birth and begin to appear during early childhood.
- The characteristic features of atypical moles are present at the time of puberty.
- Unlike common acquired melanocytic nevi, which stop appearing after age 30, atypical nevi continue to appear well into adulthood.
- While sun exposure does appear to favor the appearance of atypical nevi, lesions develop in both sun-exposed and sun-protected areas.
- Atypical nevi are best considered as part of a spectrum between benign nevi and melanoma.
- In such patients with multiple atypical nevi, the number of nevi varies.
- Most affected people have more than 50 melanocytic nevi, some of which are atypical in appearance.
- There is striking variability from one nevus to another.
- Nevi are usually asymptomatic.

Skin Findings

- Atypical nevi differ from common acquired melanocytic nevi.
- Atypical nevi are usually larger, ranging from 6 mm–15 mm in diameter.
- The border is irregularly outlined, indistinct, and fades imperceptibly into the surrounding skin.

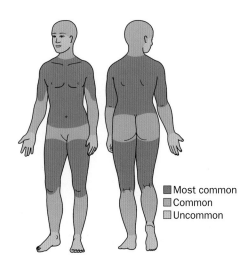

■ Most common
▨ Common
▤ Uncommon

- Color is variegated with a haphazard mixture of pink, tan, brown, and black.
- The surface is irregular, often with a central or eccentric papule surrounded by a prominent macular component.
- Atypical nevi can appear anywhere in the skin but occur most commonly on the trunk and upper extremities.
- Affected persons often have nevi in sun-protected areas, such as the scalp, groin, buttocks, the breasts in women, and the palms and soles.
- The presence of nevi in these unusual locations in prepubertal children may be the first clinical sign of the syndrome.

Non-skin Findings
- Affected people may be at increased risk of ocular melanoma.

Laboratory
- The nomenclature and histologic criteria for the diagnosis of atypical nevi remains controversial.

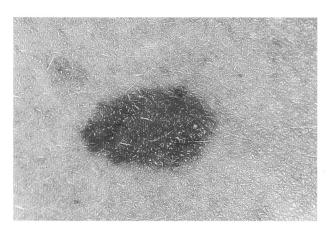

Atypical nevi have variations in pigmentation with both papular and macular components. Differentiating them from melanoma can be difficult.

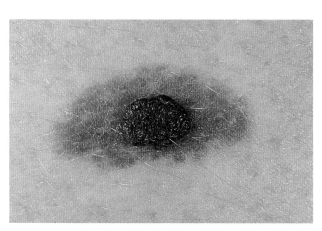

The "fried egg" pattern for an atypical nevus. The center is dark and raised. The macular periphery has pigmentation that fades into the surrounding skin.

There is general agreement on the following features.
- Architectural disorder with asymmetry.
- Intraepidermal melanocytes extend beyond the main dermal component of subepidermal fibroplasia.
- Lentiginous melanocytic hyperplasia with spindle or epithelioid melanocytes.
- Nevus cell nests are of variable size and form bridges between adjacent rete ridges.
- Variable degrees of melanocyte atypia.

Differential Diagnosis

- Atypical nevi are best regarded as part of a continuum between benign and malignant melanocytic neoplasms.

Course and Prognosis

- The likelihood of an individual atypical nevus subsequently developing into melanoma cannot be estimated, although the risk of an individual person with atypical nevi can be estimated.
- The lifetime risk of melanoma for the population born in the year 2000 is estimated at 1.3%.
- The lifetime risk of melanoma for persons with atypical nevi, but without family history of melanoma, has been estimated at 6%.
- This risk increases to 15% in patients with atypical nevi and a family history of melanoma.
- Persons with the familial atypical mole to melanoma syndrome have a 150-fold greater risk of developing melanoma by age 70 than the general population.
- This risk increases to a 500-fold greater risk if the patient has already had a melanoma.
- Thus the lifetime risk approaches 100% by age 70 in patients with the familial atypical mole to melanoma syndrome.

Treatment

- Patients with atypical nevi should have routine skin examinations, beginning around puberty.
- Consider dermatologic referral for regular monitoring of nevi.

- Consider referral to a pigmented lesion clinic for patients with numerous atypical nevi and family history of melanoma.
- The frequency of follow-up examinations depends on personal or family history of melanoma and the number of atypical nevi.
- Follow-up examinations are usually performed every 3–12 months.
- Examination should not be limited to exposed areas and should include careful inspection of the scalp, genitalia, and acral regions.
- A baseline ophthalmologic examination should be obtained since patients may also be at increased risk for developing intraocular melanomas.
- Appropriate ophthalmologic follow-up as warranted.
- Family members should also be examined.
- Photography can be extremely useful in identifying changes in nevi.
- Baseline cutaneous photographs with close-up views of the most clinically atypical moles are taken during the initial examination.
- Any lesion with documented change should be removed in its entirety and sent for histopathologic examination.
- Nevi in which the patient has noted a change should also be removed.
- Patient education and awareness can not be overemphasized.
- Patients should start by becoming familiar with their own skin and by performing monthly self-examinations.
- Sunlight has been implicated in the pathogenesis of malignant melanoma and the induction of melanocytic nevi in patients with atypical moles.
- Sun avoidance and sun-protective clothing are recommended to minimize ultraviolet exposure.
- Patients are also advised to use sunscreens with a protection factor of 15 or greater every day, even on overcast or cloudy days.
- Re-application of sunscreens every 2–3 hours should be strongly encouraged—particularly after swimming or exercising.

Pearls

- Atypical nevus syndrome represents a distinct, easily recognized clinical phenotype at increased risk of developing melanoma, particularly if there is a family history of melanoma.

- Management of such patients should focus on patient education, self-examination, and routine complete skin examinations.

Atypical Nevi

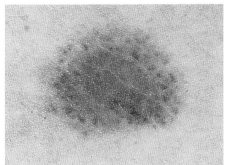 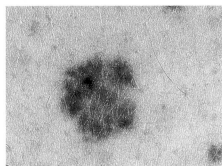

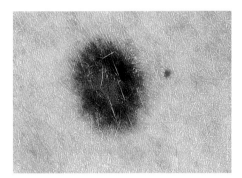 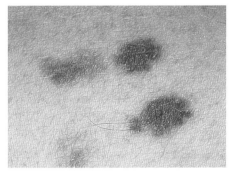

These moles are larger than common moles. They have a mixture of colors, including tan, brown, pink, and black. The border is irregular and indistinct and often fades into the surrounding skin. The surface is complex and variable, with both macular and papular components. A characteristic presentation is a pigmented papule surrounded by a macular collar of pigmentation ("fried egg" lesion).

Malignant Melanoma, Lentigo Maligna

Description

■ Melanoma is an increasingly common malignancy of melanocytes, most often arising in the skin.

■ It is potentially curable with early detection and treatment.

■ Late diagnosis of melanoma carries a poor prognosis.

History

■ Melanoma represents 4% of all cancers in men and 3% of all cancers in women.

■ Currently the most common malignancy in women aged 25–29 years and second only to breast cancer in women aged 30–35.

■ Incidence of melanoma continues to rise at a faster rate than that of any other human cancer, and the increase in its mortality is second only to that of lung cancer.

■ In 2003 there will be 92,000 new cases in the United States and an estimated 7600 deaths from melanoma.

■ The projected lifetime risk of melanoma for Americans born in the year 2000 is 1 in 75.

■ Factors that increase one's risk of developing melanoma include:
  - Fair skin (skin types I and II)
  - Presence of atypical nevi in both sun-exposed and sun-protected areas
  - Personal history of melanoma
  - Family history of atypical nevi or melanoma
  - History of blistering sunburn
  - Congenital nevi (the risk increases proportionally with increasing size)

■ The most common early signs include an increase in size, change in color or shape.

■ The most common early symptom is itching, but most are asymptomatic.

■ Later symptoms include tenderness, bleeding, and ulceration.

■ Pigmented lesions may change slowly over months to years or abruptly change.

Skin Findings

■ It cannot be over-emphasized that melanomas vary considerably in appearance—no single color or change is diagnostic.

■ Fortunately, there are clinical clues that increase the index of suspicion and warrant biopsy.

■ 30% of melanomas develop within a pre-existing nevus while the remaining 70% develop de novo.

■ The following well-known guidelines are helpful in deciding which lesions are suspicious for malignant change.

■ When melanoma develops in a pre-existing lesion, there is usually a focal area of color change.

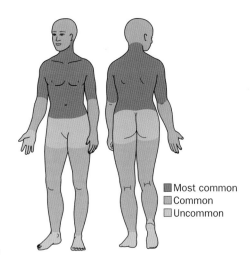

■ Most common
□ Common
□ Uncommon

The ABCDs of Malignant Melanoma Recognition	
Asymmetry	One half of the lesion does not look like the remaining half
Border irregularity	The borders is scalloped or has focal "pseudopod" extension into the surrounding skin
Color variegation	Varying hues, varying colors
Diameter > 6 mm	The longest axis of the lesion is measured

■ It is the distinction in color from the remainder of the lesion—not necessarily the color itself—that is the clinical clue.

■ Not one specific color is by itself diagnostic but should raise one's index of suspicion.

■ Slate gray, to black or deep blue may indicate melanin pigment deep within the dermis.

■ Pink or red may indicate localized inflammation.

■ White may indicate regression or scarring.

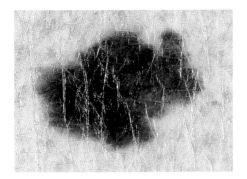

Major Subtypes of Melanoma

■ Four major clinical subtypes of melanoma are recognized, defined by clinical appearance, progression, anatomic site, and histologic appearance.

Superficial Spreading Melanoma

● This is the most common subtype, accounting for 70–80% of all melanomas.

● Of melanomas arising in a pre-existing lesion, most are superficial spreading.

● Slightly more common in females than males, usually affecting Caucasian people.

● Any cutaneous site but most often on the trunk and extremities.

● Lesions tend to be greater than 6 mm in diameter, flat and asymmetric with varying coloration.

● Lesions appear and tend to spread laterally within the skin over a few years, before nodules develop within the lesion.

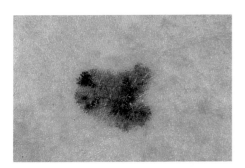

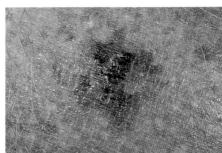

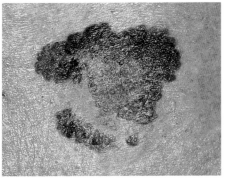

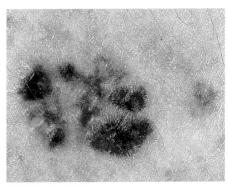

Superficial Spreading Melanoma

Nodular Melanoma

- These account for roughly 10–15% of all melanomas.
- They are equally common in males and females.
- They affect any cutaneous site, but are more often found on the extremities.

- Lesions tend to be raised, brown to black, rapidly appearing and rapidly growing papules.
- They may suggest a vascular lesion clinically; they may have focal hemorrhage.
- Lesions appear and evolve over months and tend to extend vertically in the skin.

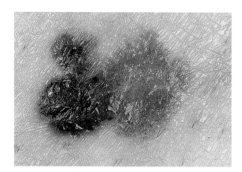

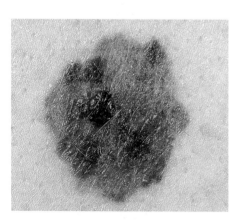

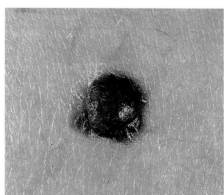

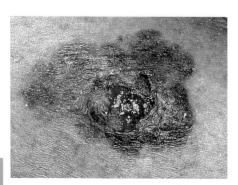

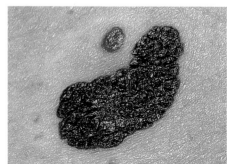

Nodular Melanoma

Lentigo Maligna and Lentigo Maligna Melanoma

- These account for about 5–10% of all melanoma.
- Lentigo maligna represents in situ (intraepidermal) melanoma.
- Progression to invasive lentigo maligna melanoma occurs in 5% of patients.
- They are equally common in males and females, usually in older people.
- They develop over years or decades on sun-exposed Caucasian skin, most often affecting the face, neck or dorsal arms.
- Lesions tend to be flat and irregularly outlined.
- The color is usually brown with some variation in epidermal pigment density.
- Lesions tend to look mottled or washed out, may contain areas or normal pigmentation.
- Wood's light often reveals irregular pigmentation extending well beyond the clinical lesion.
- Nodules and ulceration may indicate local invasion.

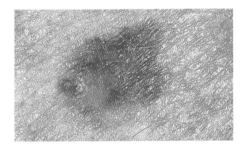

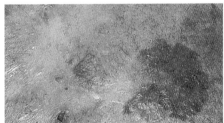

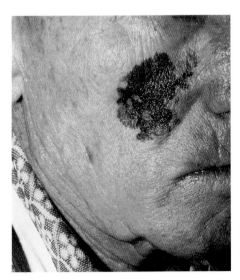

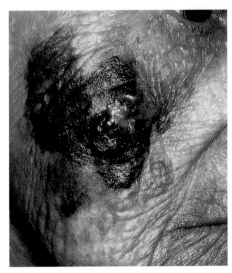

Lentigo maligna and lentigo maligna melanoma

Acral Lentiginous Melanoma

- This accounts for 7% of all melanomas.
- Acral lentiginous melanoma is more common in males than females, and usually occurs in older people.
- It occurs primarily on the hands and feet, including nails of people with darker skin types (IV–VI).
- Similar lesions also occur on the modified skin around the mouth, anus and genitalia.
- This is the most common form of melanoma in the skin of Asian and Black people, accounting for more than half of melanomas in these groups.
- It is the least common form of melanoma in Caucasian people.
- Other than location, the lesion is similar in appearance to lentigo maligna and lentigo maligna melanoma—a flat slowly expanding macule with a fairly uniform, mottled coloration.
- It appears and evolves over years.
- Amelanotic melanoma is a descriptive term for a non-pigmented melanoma; any subtype may be amelanotic.
- 2% of all melanomas are amelanotic.
- Biopsy and diagnosis are often delayed.
- Malignant cells produce little (if any) melanin pigment.
- The lesion is an innocent-appearing, enlarging, pink-red papule—like an insect bite.

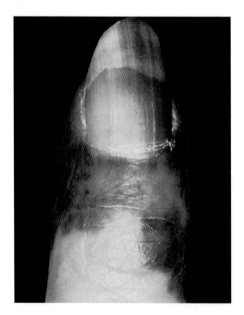

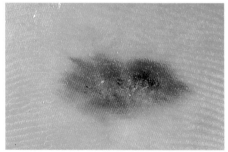

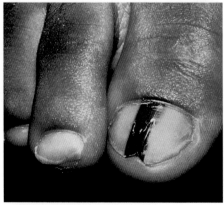

Acral lentiginous melanoma

Non-skin Findings
- Palpate the regional nodes prior to biopsy and document the findings.
- Post-biopsy inflammation may enlarge regional nodes temporarily.
- Any suspicious nodes should be evaluated by nodal biopsy.
- This could be performed at the time of excision of the primary melanoma, with or without lymphatic mapping.

Laboratory and Pathology
- All suspect lesions warrant biopsy to confirm the presence of malignant melanocytes.
- Biopsy report should state the diagnosis, anatomic site, Breslow level, and whether biopsy margins are involved.
- Breslow level is the measured vertical thickness of the melanoma and is the single most important prognostic factor.
- Ulceration or regression, if present, raises the possibility that the Breslow level may be underestimated.
- Clark level, or anatomic level of invasion, is also helpful, especially for thin melanomas occurring on thin skin areas such as the eyelid, ear and genitalia.

Biopsy
- Consider doing a sentinel node biopsy.

Differential Diagnosis
- Superficial spreading melanoma:
  - Benign nevi (moles)
  - Atypical (dysplastic) nevus
  - Seborrheic keratoses
  - Solar lentigo
- Nodular melanoma:
  - Pigmented basal cell carcinoma
  - Angiokeratoma
  - Hemangioma
  - Traumatized nevus or acrochordon
  - Pyogenic granuloma
- Lentigo maligna:
  - Spreading pigmented actinic keratosis
  - Bowen's disease
  - Solar lentigo
- Biopsy and histologic review distinguish melanoma from other tumors.

- All nevi which are removed for diagnostic or cosmetic purposes should be submitted for histologic review.
- Incomplete excision or biopsy of nevi can lead to recurrence with epidermal hyperplasia of atypical appearing melanocytes.
- This recurrent nevus phenomenon can be clinically and histologically indistinguishable from superficial spreading melanoma.
- The original excision or biopsy must be available for review to exclude a diagnosis of melanoma.

Course and Prognosis
- In general, the thinner the melanoma, the better the prognosis.
- Localized disease has a far better prognosis than metastatic disease.
- Female patients and younger patients tend to have a more favorable prognosis.
- A melanoma on an extremity has a more favorable prognosis than a melanoma on the trunk, head or neck.
- Melanoma on the scalp has a worse prognosis than melanoma elsewhere on the head or neck.

Discussion
- The ABCDs of melanoma are a useful aid to one's clinical suspicion.
- Do not overlook the patient's symptoms as well—especially itching.
- The risk of biopsy is far lower than the risk of missing a melanoma.
- Dermatology referral should be considered.
- All pigmented lesions should be examined at regular intervals by both the patient and the provider.
- This is especially true of patients at increased risk of melanoma.
- The exact location, color, size, and pattern should be recorded.
- Photography can be extremely useful as a tool for recording such data though is only as useful as the photograph resolution allows.
- Epiluminescence microscopy allows one to examine dermal pigmentation patterns within lesions, though its value is operator dependent.

Treatment

- All suspect lesions warrant biopsy.
- Remember to palpate the regional nodes prior to biopsy and document the findings.
- The only "perfect" biopsy technique is complete excision of the entire lesion into subcutaneous fat.
- This allows for accurate measurement of Breslow depth of invasion in a melanoma and avoids sampling error (a false negative result).
- Shave biopsy is not recommended for suspected melanoma.
- Shave biopsy specimen may not demonstrate the full Breslow depth of the lesion—the most important data for management and prognosis.
- Shave biopsy is also subject to sampling error.
- An incisional or punch biopsy extending into subcutaneous fat may be considered when the clinical suspicion is low, for large lesions or lesions in cosmetically important areas.
- The most clinically suspicious areas should be included in the biopsy.
- Incisional biopsy is still subject to sampling error and false negative biopsies are possible.
- More importantly, the maximum Breslow depth of invasion has not been permanently lost, even if not captured on the incisional biopsy.
- Incisional biopsy does not appear to increase the risk of metastases.
- When the lesion is highly suspicious for melanoma, then excisional biopsy is preferred.
- Re-excision of biopsy confirmed melanoma with appropriate surgical margins determined by Breslow depth is required.
- Melanoma in situ requires a re-excision margin of 0.5 cm.

Survival Rates		
Stage	**Disease Characteristics**	**5-year Survival Rate**
IA	Breslow ≤ 1.0 mm, Clark II/III, without ulceration	95%
IB	Breslow ≤1.0 mm, Clark IV/V, with ulceration Breslow 1.01–2.0 mm without ulceration	89–91%
IIA	Breslow 1.01–2.0 mm with ulceration Breslow 2.01–4.0 mm without ulceration	77–79%
IIB	Breslow 2.01–4.0 mm with ulceration Breslow > 4.0 mm without ulceration	63–67%
IIC	Breslow > 4.0 mm with ulceration	45%
IIIA	Tumor any thickness without ulceration and 1–3 positive lymph nodes with micrometastases	63–70%
IIIB	Tumor any thickness with ulceration and 1–3 positive lymph nodes with micrometastases Tumor any thickness without ulceration and 1–3 positive lymph nodes with macrometastases Tumor any thickness with ulceration and in-transit metastases or satellites without involved regional lymph nodes	46–59%
IIIC	Tumor any thickness with ulceration and 1–3 positive lymph nodes with macrometastases Tumor any thickness and ≥ 4 involved regional lymph nodes, or matted nodes, or-in transit metastases or satellites with involved regional lymph nodes	24–29%
IV	Presence of distant metastases regardless of tumor thickness or status of regional lymph nodes	7–19%

- Lentigo maligna tends to extend microscopically beyond the clinical lesion, even under Wood's light.
- For stage IA disease, surgical intervention might be the only necessary therapy with a 1.0-cm margin.
- Re-excision with a 1.0-cm margin is recommended for tumors up to 2.0 mm thick and a margin of 2.0 cm is recommended for tumors up to 4.0 mm thick.
- Ulceration increases the risk of a lesion as the Breslow level can be underestimated.
- Sentinel node biopsy should be considered for stage IB and all stage II patients.
- The number of involved regional nodes is a stronger predictor of survival than the size of involved nodes.
- Sentinel lymph node status predicts both the risk of recurrence and mortality as shown in the table on page 478.
- The therapeutic benefit of lymph node biopsy and thus removal of microscopic metastases is currently under study.
- For stages IIB, IIC and III, adjuvant treatment is often recommended with high-dose interferon-2α.
- Low-dose interferon-2α has not shown significant improvement in relapse-free time or overall survival.
- Oncology referral and/or tumor board review should be considered.
- Melanoma vaccine trials are underway for extracutaneous melanoma.
- Follow-up examination should be performed at regular intervals and include the following:
  - Visual inspection and palpation of the excision site and surrounding skin
  - Visual examination of the entire cutaneous surface
  - Palpation of regional and distant nodes
  - Palpation of the liver
  - Baseline chest x-ray and baseline computerized tomography scan of head, chest, and abdomen
- Liver function tests are rarely revealing but are often obtained at baseline.
- First degree relatives should be offered full skin examination for screening and educational purposes.

Pearls

- Full skin examination at regular intervals, especially of people at increased risk of melanoma favor early detection and treatment of this serious health problem.
- The thinner the melanoma at the time of diagnosis (thin Breslow depth) the better the prognosis. Patients with melanomas greater than 1 mm in histologic depth (Breslow depth) should consider a sentinel node biopsy.

Follow-up Guidelines (in months)				
Year from Diagnosis	Primary Tumor Thickness			
	< 0.76 mm	0.76–1.5 mm	1.5–4.0 mm	> 4.0 mm
First	12	6	3	2
Second	12	6	3	2
Third	12	6	4	3
Fourth	12	12	4	3
Fifth	12	12	6	6
Subsequent	12	12	12	12

Melanoma Mimics

Description
- A variety of melanocytic and non-melanocytic skin lesions which may bear clinical and/or histologic resemblance to melanoma.

History
- Specific subtypes of benign melanocytic nevi may suggest melanoma.
- Benign melanocytic nevi are classified as junctional, compound, or intradermal based on the location of nevus cells within the skin.
- Most benign nevi are symmetric, sharply defined, less than 6 mm in greatest diameter, usually have one dominant color, and are usually asymptomatic.
- Roughly 30–50% of melanomas arise in pre-existing melanocytic lesions.
- Nevi that develop symptoms and change in appearance are suspicious.
- Atypical nevi are often larger than 6 mm in greatest diameter, tend to have indistinct borders, and variegated pigmentation.
- It may not be possible to distinguish visually atypical nevi from melanoma.
- This discussion focuses not on changing nevi or atypical nevi, but rather on specific subtypes of benign nevi that may mimic melanoma.

Skin Findings
Blue Nevi
- Blue nevi are benign melanocytic nevi with nevus cells located deep within the dermis.
- Their blue to black coloration may suggest melanoma.
- Blue nevi are sharply defined, uniform in color, and are stable in size or appearance over many years.

Combined Nevus
- Combined nevus refers to the combination of a blue nevus deep in the dermis associated with an overlying benign junctional, compound or intradermal nevus.
- Combined nevi are usually solitary and are often asymmetric with focal dark pigmentation.
- This presentation suggests melanoma though the patient has not noted any change in the lesion's appearance.

Traumatized Nevi
- Traumatized nevi may be partially avulsed and/or have hemorrhagic crusting suggesting ulceration.
- Patients are usually aware of the trauma.
- Nevi which have been previously partially removed either by trauma or biopsy can develop recurrent nevus phenomenon over several weeks to months.
- Melanocyte hyperplasia develops superficial to the scar resulting in uneven pigmentation and irregular outlines as pigment extends into the surrounding skin—quite suggestive of melanoma.
- Recurrent nevus phenomenon can resemble melanoma histologically, too.
- The history of trauma or biopsy along with review of the original biopsy helps exclude a diagnosis of melanoma.

Pigmented Basal Cell Carcinoma
- Pigmented basal cell carcinoma contains melanin pigment but is otherwise equivalent to nodular basal cell carcinoma.
- The amount of melanin and its distribution is variable.
- Pigmented basal cell carcinoma can be mostly pink, with focal blue to gray pigment or jet black.
- The surface has a pearl-like quality but may be ulcerated.
- The appearance may suggest nodular melanoma.

Seborrheic Keratoses
- Seborrheic keratoses are benign keratinocyte tumors which also contain varying amounts of melanin pigment.
- Pigmentation can be uneven and asymmetric within a single lesion.
- Seborrheic keratoses appear after age 30 and can grow quite rapidly.
- Lesions vary from flat to verrucous, and are white to pink to jet black.

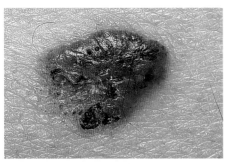

Darkly pigmented smooth-surfaced seborrheic keratosis with horn pearls imbedded in the mass.

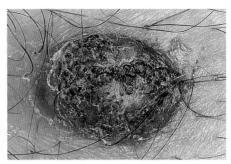

Inflamed seborrheic keratosis with a crusted surface and red border.

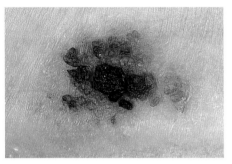

Rough-surfaced seborrheic keratosis with an irregular border.

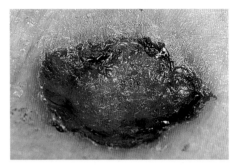

Inflamed seborrheic keratosis with a crusted surface and red border.

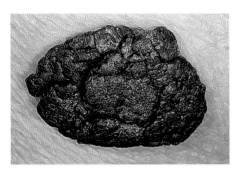

Darkly pigmented rough-surfaced seborrheic keratosis.

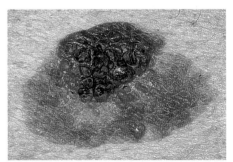

Rough-surfaced seborrheic keratosis with an asymmetric border.

Flat seborrheic keratoses may suggest lentigo maligna.

Raised lesions may suggest superficial spreading melanoma.

Spreading Pigmented Actinic Keratosis

Spreading pigmented actinic keratosis displays fine reticulated pigmentation and thin scale.

Lesions appear on sun-damaged skin and simulate lentigo maligna melanoma.

Hemangiomas

Mature hemangiomas are often dark purple in color and can mimic nodular melanoma.

Angiokeratoma

Solitary angiokeratoma can be black to red.

Trauma such as friction injury to the heel (talon noir) or injury to a nail unit may produce hemorrhage.

Hemosiderin may be present in these lesions suggesting melanin pigment.

Dermatofibromas

Dermatofibromas often contain hemosiderin, occasionally itch or are tender, and can resemble melanoma.

Any questionable lesion should be biopsied to confirm the diagnosis.

Laboratory and Pathology

Lesions which may mimic melanoma clinically are usually discriminated from melanoma histologically.

Histologic mimics of melanoma may require the use of special stains for accurate diagnosis.

Melanoma, Bowen's disease, and Paget's disease may all show malignant cells within the epidermis.

Special stains reveal the tissue of origin of the malignant cells in each disorder: melanocyte in melanoma; squamous cell in Bowen's disease; and adenocarcinoma in Paget's disease.

Similarly, special stains are useful in spindle cell tumors to confirm the origin of the malignant cells.

The nevus cells of Spitz nevus may be pleomorphic and virtually indistinguishable from melanoma cells on histologic grounds.

The overall architecture of the lesion and age of the patient help discern Spitz nevus from melanoma.

Similarly, recurrent nevus phenomenon may show highly pleomorphic cells consistent with melanoma.

The history of previous biopsy and review of the original specimen establish the diagnosis.

Lentigo maligna can be quite subtle and can resemble benign junctional nevi histologically.

As a rule, junctional nevi are lesions of childhood.

Any melanocytic lesion from an adult read as junctional nevus should be considered suspicious.

Course and Prognosis

The clinical course and complications relate to the individual diagnosis.

Discussion

Suspicious and atypical lesions should be biopsied.

Histology often discerns melanoma from lesions clinically suspicious for melanoma.

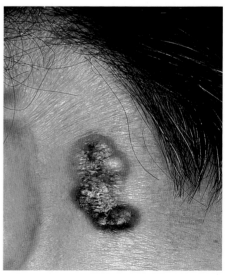

A pigmented basal cell carcinoma with a lobular surface and an irregular border.

- Histologic mimics of melanoma include malignancies derived from non-melanocytic cells.
- Special stains reveal the origin of the malignant cells.
- Melanocytic lesions which mimic melanoma histologically, such as Spitz nevus or recurrent nevus, require clinicopathologic correlation.

Treatment

- Management and follow-up are dependent on diagnosis.

Pearls

- It is the responsibility of the clinician to correlate the histologic findings with the clinical impression.

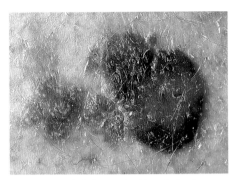

Smooth seborrheic keratosis with variation in pigmentation and an irregular border.

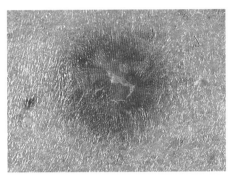

Dermatofibroma with a brown, irregular border and central clearing.

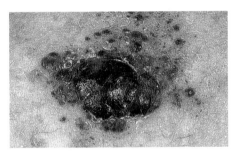

Hemangiomas vary in size and color. This complex lesion resembles a nodular melanoma.

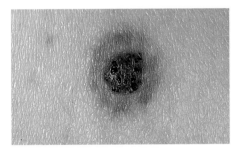

A bizarre surface pattern occurred following infarction of some of the vessels in this hemangioma. The black surface papules look like nodular melanoma.

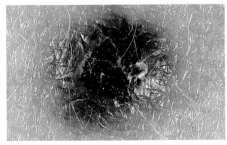

Blue nevus.

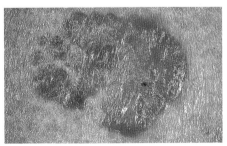

A pigmented basal cell carcinoma with areas of regression.

483

Congenital Melanocytic Nevi

Description

- Congenital nevi are benign skin tumors composed of melanocyte-derived nevus cells, present at birth, or appearing by age 2 years.
- They are considered to be a type of birthmark, of which there are many variants.

History

- Any melanocytic nevus present at birth or appearing within early infancy is considered to be a congenital melanocytic nevus.
- Roughly 1% of newborns have at least one melanocytic nevus.
- They may increase in size and become more heavily pigmented during puberty.
- They are usually asymptomatic, though they may on occasion be irritated by clothing or external trauma.

Skin Findings

- Congenital melanocytic nevi are usually dark brown and raised, with an irregular verrucous surface. Most have increased terminal hairs.
- Congenital melanocytic nevi vary greatly in size.
- Depending on their location, large lesions may be disfiguring.
- Congenital dermal melanocytosis (Mongolian spot) are poorly defined patches colored blue-black to gray.
- Congenital melanocytic nevi in newborns of dark-skinned origin are more commonly seen in the sacral region.

Non-skin Findings

- Occasionally benign nevus cells may be found within regional lymph nodes draining areas with congenital melanocytic nevi or congenital dermal melanocytosis.
- Such findings are unusual but are not necessarily indicative of melanoma.

Laboratory

- Congenital nevi are usually compound nevi with nested nevus cells at the junction and also in the dermis.
- Nevus cells may extend into fat and invest adnexal structures and blood vessels.
- Congenital dermal melanocytosis is equivalent to blue nevi histologically, with heavily pigmented spindle-shaped nevus cells located deep in the dermis.

Course and Prognosis

- The vast majority of congenital melanocytic nevi are benign and follow the course of maturation over years as described above.
- Nevi which deviate from this pattern are suspicious and biopsy is warranted.
- Congenital dermal melanocytosis often fades in early childhood, but may persist into adulthood.
- Such lesions are believed to represent incomplete migration of melanocytes to the epidermis.
- The risk of malignant degeneration occurring in congenital melanocytic nevi is controversial.
- There is general agreement that risk of malignant change is increased in giant congenital melanocytic nevi with diameters greater than 20 cm. Lifetime risk is estimated at 5–8%.
- The lifetime risk of melanoma developing in smaller congenital nevi is unclear, but may be increased in those larger than 2 cm.
- Nevus cells in congenital nevi often extend into subcutaneous fat, therefore such malignant change may not be easily detected.
- For this reason, some dermatologists favor elective excision of congenital nevi when feasible, usually around the time of puberty.

Discussion

- The clinician should provide the dermatopathologist with the patient's age, location and clinical history of the lesion, any previous biopsy specimen, and the clinical differential diagnosis.
- An adequate biopsy specimen should be submitted.
- Similarly, it is the clinician's responsibility to correlate the pathologist's findings with the clinical diagnosis.

Treatment

- All of a patient's nevi should be assessed.
- Most benign nevi are symmetric, with a well-defined, regular border, uniform in color (with perhaps subtle variation in the hues of the dominant color).
- Congenital nevi should increase in size in proportion to the patient's growth through adolescence.
- The pattern of pigmentation should remain uniform.
- Photography is helpful for following nevi over time.
- Suspicious nevi should be biopsied.
- Consider referral to a dermatologist.
- Large congenital nevi may be disfiguring depending on location and removal may be technically feasible.
- Plastic surgery referral should be considered for giant congenital nevi.
- Removal may require serial procedures with tissue expanders.
- The current epidemic of skin cancers has prompted many patients to seek a screening examination.
- Such an opportunity for early detection and treatment, as well as parent and patient education, should not be missed.
- An examination of the entire cutaneous surface should be encouraged.
- Patients and parents need to be educated on how to perform self-examination of the skin and should be encouraged to do so on a regular basis.
- Combine the teaching of self-examination techniques with the screening skin examination.
- Review the changes to watch for, including symptoms of itching and tenderness, with the patient.
- The patient and parent should feel comfortable in seeking care for any future changes or concerns.
- Sun awareness and the regular use of sunscreens and sun-protective clothing should be also encouraged.

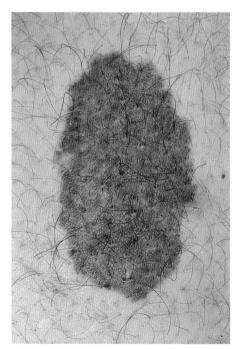 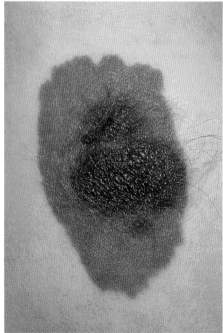

Congenital nevi with uniform surface characteristics and light pigmentation have little chance of degenerating into melanoma. Those with dense pigmentation or irregular pigmentation like the lesion on the right are considered for excision.

19 Vascular Tumors and Malformations

Hemangiomas of Infancy

Description
- Hemangiomas of infancy are benign red, purple or blue vascular neoplasms occurring within the first year of life; they exhibit endothelial cell hyperplasia.
- Terms such as strawberry hemangioma and cavernous hemangioma should be discarded since they have been used to describe both vascular growths and vascular malformations.

History
- Hemangiomas of infancy are the most common vascular tumor of infancy, occurring in 1–3% of newborns and 10% of 1-year-olds.
- 30% of these hemangiomas are noticeable at birth, and most are detected within the first 3 weeks of life. Deeper lesions may be noted later, but usually within the first month of life.
- They occur with increased frequency in girls and premature infants and have a predilection for the head and neck.

Skin Findings
- Onset and rate of growth, as well as depth in the skin, determine when they become noticeable.
- Nascent hemangiomas of infancy (early) may appear flat and pale white with a few telangiectasias and large dilated blood vessels.
- During the growth phase they are seen as bright red (superficial) or blue (deep) and feel firm and rubbery. The surface color of deeper lesions can be very subtle.
- As hemangiomas of infancy begin to involute, they become slate-gray and begin to soften.
- A small percentage of hemangiomas of infancy ulcerate and bleed. Ulcerations are painful and can lead to infection.

- Hemangiomas of infancy appear at any anatomic site, including the oral and genital mucosa.
- Most infants have a single lesion; 15–20% have multiple hemangiomas.
- Multiple cutaneous hemangiomas may be associated with visceral hemangiomas (diffuse neonatal hemangiomatosis); however, infants can have visceral involvement without cutaneous involvement.

Non-skin Findings
- Hemangiomas of infancy near the eyes, ears, and mouth can threaten the function of those organs.
- Hemangiomas of infancy located near or on the mandible ("beard" distribution) can be associated with glottic hemangiomas.
- Hemangiomas of infancy that are located in the midline can be associated with underlying cranial or vertebral anomalies.
- Large segmental facial hemangiomas of infancy can be associated with malformations of other organs (PHACES syndrome is a constellation of posterior

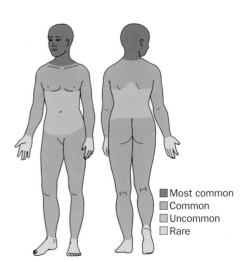

■ Most common
■ Common
■ Uncommon
□ Rare

fossa malformations, **h**emangioma, **a**rterial anomalies, **c**oarctation of the aorta and **c**ardiac defects, **e**ye anomalies and **s**ternal defects).

Laboratory and Pathology

- Skin biopsy is not usually required to make the diagnosis of hemangioma of infancy.
- Skin biopsy can be helpful for more difficult lesions.
- At a microscopic level, proliferating lesions show well-defined masses of plump endothelial cells and pericytes forming small lumina with red blood cells; regressing lesions show flattened endothelial cells in a connective tissue stroma.

- Hemangiomas of infancy express glucose transporter-1, which is thought to be a specific marker for hemangioma of infancy.
- An imaging study (an ultrasound, computerized tomography scan or magnetic resonance imaging) should be done in infants with midline lumbar and segmental facial hemangiomas, since they can be associated with a tethered spinal cord and Dandy–Walker malformation, respectively.

Superficial Hemangioma

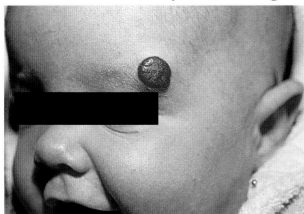

Most are small harmless birthmarks that proliferate for 8–18 months and then slowly regress over the next 5–8 months.

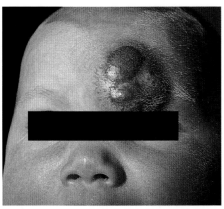

Superficial and deep hemangioma. Vital structures can be compressed, and rapidly growing areas may ulcerate.

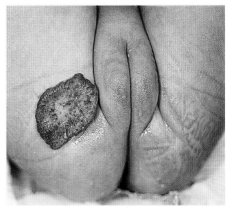

This hemangioma is undergoing spontaneous involution.

487

Infants with multiple hemangiomas and physical signs of visceral involvement (hepatosplenomegaly, pallor, tachycardia) should have a complete blood count including platelets, abdominal ultrasound and/or computerized tomography scan.

Differential Diagnosis

- Vascular growths (pyogenic granuloma and cherry angioma)
- Rare tumors of infancy (fibrosarcoma, tufted angioma)
- Vascular malformations
- Congenital hemangiomas involute quickly and do not stain with glucose transporter-1.

Course and Prognosis

- Hemangiomas follow a predictable clinical course of growth for 6 months to a year. Then they stabilize, and involute at a rate of 10% per year.

- Initial growth is rapid over weeks, and this phase is followed by a stable phase lasting for months and then slow involution with residual fibrosis and lightening in color over years.
- Lesion size, depth and location do not affect the rate of involution.
- A lesion that does not show signs of regression by age 6 years is unlikely to resolve completely.
- Ulceration occurs in 5–13% of lesions and produces recurrent bleeding and pain.
- Superficial infection can occur, but is rarely a serious problem.
- After involution the overlying skin may appear normal, but in some instances there is some degree of atrophy or residual fibrosis.

Treatment

- Most hemangiomas of infancy should be followed closely to assure that they are following a benign course and to

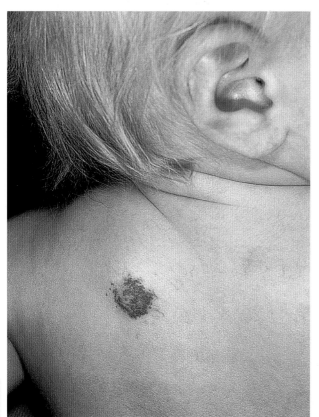

Deeper lesions are skin-colored, or red or blue masses that are ill defined.

re-assure the parents ("active non-intervention").

■ Hemangiomas of infancy should be actively treated if they are life threatening, or if they may compromise vital functions, or have potential to create permanent disfigurement (nasal tip hemangiomas). Procedures that cause scarring should be avoided, when possible.

■ For ulcerations, local measures should be used in combination to remove necrotic tissue, to keep the wound moist and prevent infection.

■ The wound should be gently cleansed with mild soap and a soft cloth.

■ A thin layer of a topical antibiotic such as Mupirocin 2% ointment (Bactroban), metronidazole gel (MetroGel), or bacitracin ointment should be applied.

■ The wound should be covered with an air permeable, barrier dressing such as polyurethane film dressing, Tegaderm, and OpSite.

■ Barrier creams such as zinc oxide 20% ointment, Desitin ointment, A&D

ointment can be used for the perineum and other sites not amenable to topical dressings.

■ Pulsed dye laser has been used successfully for ulcerations, but in a small percentage ulcerations may actually worsen.

■ Systemic prednisone or prednisolone 2–3 mg/kg orally given as a single morning dose is a widely used therapy for complicated lesions.

■ Other medical therapies include intralesional and topical corticosteroids, interferon-α (although its use is limited because of spastic diplegia in 10–20%), vincristine, and cyclophosphamide.

■ Embolization, surgical resection and radiation are sometimes used for complicated hemangiomas.

When to Refer

■ Treatment of complicated lesions should be done in consultation with specialists. Some centers have multidisciplinary clinics staffed by dermatologists, pediatric surgeons, oncologists, and radiologists who specialize in hemangioma management.

Pearls

■ Photographic documentation is helpful to follow the course of hemangiomas of infancy and is re-assuring to parents.

■ Early referral to a specialist is essential for all complicated hemangioma of infancy.

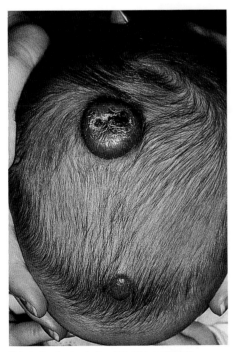

This lesion is growing rapidly. The surface is ulcerated and crusted.

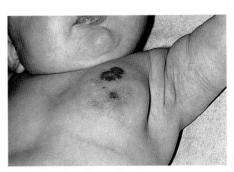

A very large, deep hemangioma.

Vascular Malformations

Description

■ Vascular malformations are anomalies of blood and lymphatic vessels due to abnormal development and morphogenesis. Unlike hemangiomas they exhibit normal endothelial cell turnover.

History

■ By definition, cutaneous vascular malformations are present at birth, but they may not become noticeable for months, sometimes years.
■ Vascular malformations are classified by vessel type (capillary, venous, arterial, lymphatic, mixed (common) and arteriovenous) and flow characteristics (slow flow and fast flow).

■ Most vascular malformations grow in proportion to the patient.
■ Most vascular malformations are sporadic and not inherited. Venous malformations can be inherited, such as multiple glomuvenous malformation and blue rubber bleb nevus syndrome (both are autosomal dominant).

Skin Findings
Capillary Malformations (Slow Flow)

■ Macular staining occurs commonly on the eyelids ("angel kiss"), forehead, and nuchal area ("stork bite"). These stains tend to resolve in early childhood, however nuchal stains commonly persist into adulthood.
■ Capillary malformations can be more substantial and involve a segment and/or

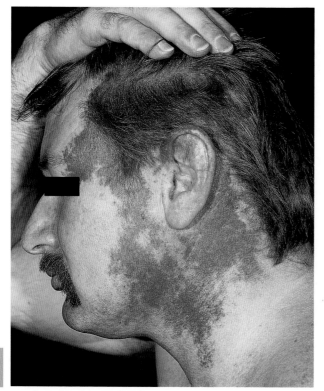

Venous malformations appear at birth as flat, irregular, red to purple patches. Later, they may become papular, simulating a cobblestone surface.

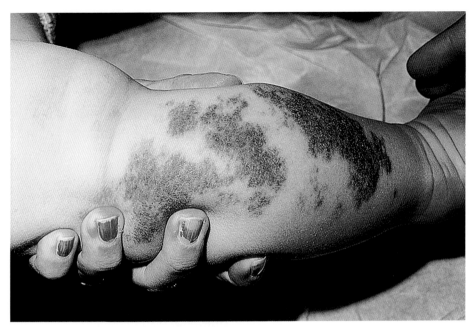

A venous malformation covering much of the lower extremity.

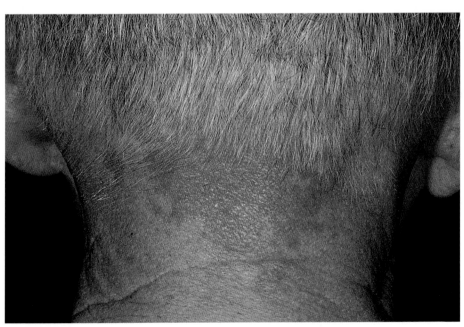

This capillary hemangioma has remained stable for years. These common lesions on the nuchal area are referred to as "stork bites".

segments of skin innervated by the trigeminal nerve (V1–V3).

Venous Malformations (Slow Flow)
■ Venous malformations usually are blue and spongy appearing; they tend to enlarge with Valsalva maneuver, and can be painful.
■ Phleboliths (small calcified nodules) commonly form and are felt as hard nodules.

Lymphatic Malformation (Slow Flow)
■ Lymphatic malformations are composed of small channels (microcystic) or large channels (macrocystic) and can be localized or diffuse.
■ Lymphangioma circumscripta is a microcystic lymphatic malformation consisting of small (1–5 mm) discrete, clear to blood-tinged papules that look like vesicles ("frog spawn").
■ Cystic hygroma is a macrocystic (large lymphatic channels) lymphatic malformation that commonly occurs in the cervicofacial region.

Arterial Malformations (Fast Flow)
■ Arterial malformations (aneurysm, stenosis, arteriovenous malformation) can cause minimal skin signs (pink stain) or they can produce massive swelling, ulceration and necrosis.
■ Arteriovenous malformations can be quiescent for years, only to cause disability through blood shunting in puberty.
■ Arteriovenous malformations are most common in the head and neck region.

Non-skin Findings
■ 10% of infants with large facial capillary malformations, especially involving trigeminal nerve V1 (forehead and upper eyelid) are at risk for underlying eye and central nervous system involvement; this triad is known as the Sturge–Weber syndrome.
■ In Sturge–Weber syndrome patients can develop glaucoma (30–70%), seizures (70–80%), and overgrowth of the underlying facial bones.
■ Large cervicofacial lymphatic

malformations can cause airway compromise.
■ Arteriovenous malformations can cause cardiac failure due to shunting; head and neck arteriovenous malformations can cause seizures and focal neurologic deficits.

Laboratory and Pathology
■ Neurologically normal infants with large facial capillary malformations may not show leptomeningeal involvement during the first year of life. Imaging of the central nervous system should be delayed until after infancy, unless the child has neurological symptoms.
■ Skin biopsy can be helpful to evaluate lesions that are difficult to characterize and will show the architecture and cell type of the corresponding malformation.

Differential Diagnosis
■ Transient macular staining (must be differentiated from capillary malformations)
■ Deep hemangiomas of infancy (but venous malformations do not have the characteristic growth pattern)
■ Nevus anemicus (irregularly outlined patch, commonly occurring on the upper chest, which is due to local vasoconstriction of the blood vessels; the border can be obscured with diascopy)

Course and Prognosis
■ Capillary malformations can darken with age and develop a cobblestone appearance.
■ Extensive venous and arterial malformations can involve deeper structures such as muscle, and can be a source of local or disseminated coagulopathy.
■ Vascular malformations may cause alterations in underlying bone and soft tissue, resulting in functional disability.
■ Lymphatic malformations can be complicated by pain, swelling, intralesional bleeding, and infection.

Treatment
■ Capillary malformations involving the forehead and lateral neck usually

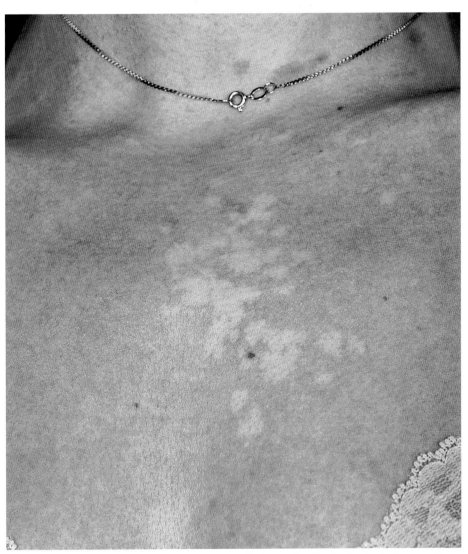

Nevus anemicus is a rare congenital lesion most frequently observed on the chest or back of women. The lesion usually consists of a well-defined white macule with an irregular border, often surrounded by smaller white macules beyond the border of the major lesion. See differential diagnosis on p. 492.

respond well to pulsed dye laser, whereas central facial, trigeminal nerve V2 and extremity lesions can be more difficult to treat.

■ Coagulopathies associated with venous malformations have been treated with compression stockings, low molecular weight heparin, hydrotherapy, massage, and physical therapy.

■ Laser surgery, surgical resection, embolization, and sclerosis are used alone or in combination to treat complicated vascular malformations.

When to refer

■ Infants with large facial capillary malformations should be evaluated by a dermatologist, an ophthalmologist and a neurologist.

■ Treatment should be performed in a multidisciplinary setting by physicians experienced with vascular malformations.

Pediatric Considerations

● Early hemangiomas of infancy and vascular malformations appear similar at birth.

● Vascular malformations can become more pronounced at puberty.

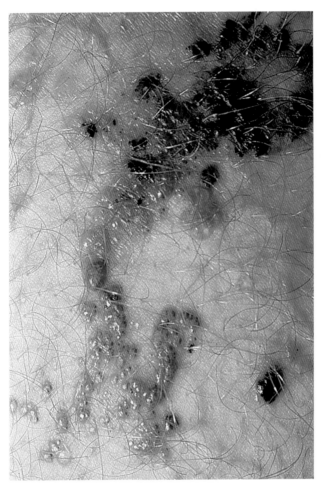

Lymphangioma circumscriptum. These hamartomatous malformations consist of grouped translucent or hemorrhagic vesicles on a dull red or brown base. Their appearance has been compared to a mass of frog's eggs ("frog spawn").

Cherry Angioma

Description

- Cherry angioma is a distinct, benign vascular neoplasm found in nearly all people older than 30 years of age.

History

- Lesions appear gradually in adulthood and are asymptomatic.

Skin Findings

- Lesions are discrete 0.5–5.0 mm, smooth, dome-shaped to polypoid papules.
- Early smaller lesions are cherry red and deeper larger lesions are maroon.
- They mostly occur on the trunk, but can be found on the head, neck, and extremities.
- The number of lesions may range from a few to hundreds.

Non-skin Findings

- Multiple eruptive cherry angiomas have been associated with bromide exposure, sulfur mustard gas, and the glycol ether solvent 2-butoxyethanol.
- The sudden appearance of such lesions may warrant a search for occult malignancy, especially for small tumors capable of hormone production (those in the pancreas, small bowel, and respiratory system).

Laboratory and Pathology

- Skin biopsy is rarely needed but demonstrates a sharply defined, benign proliferation of dilated capillaries, and post-capillary venules within the papillary dermis.
- Larger lesions show flattening of the overlying epidermis and a collarette of epithelium at the periphery.

Differential Diagnosis

- Telangiectasia
- Melanoma
- Pyogenic granuloma
- Bacillary angiomatosis

Course and Prognosis

- Undisturbed cherry angiomas persist indefinitely.
- Superficial trauma may produce bleeding.
- Isolated reports of patients with hundreds of cherry angiomas arising in association with pregnancy, and also in patients with elevated prolactin levels, suggest that hormonal factors may play a role.

Treatment

- Cherry angiomas may be ablated by electrocautery, laser surgery, cryosurgery or by simple scissor excision.
- There is a slight risk of scarring and dyspigmentation with treatment.

Pearls

- The *presence* of numerous lesions should not prompt a search for malignancy, although the *explosive appearance* of such lesions should raise concern.

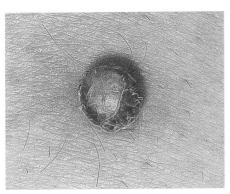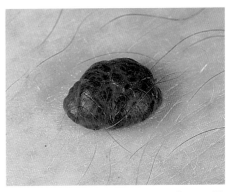

Cherry angioma. These smooth, firm, deep red papules of 0.5–5 mm occur in virtually everyone after age 30 and numbers increase with age.

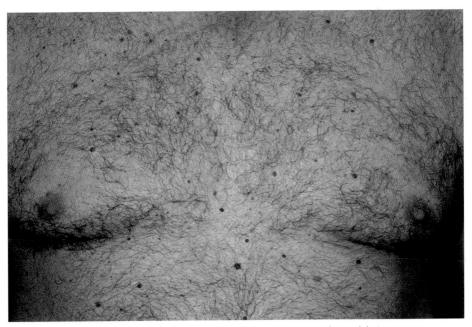

Cherry angiomas increase in number with age. They are frequently seen on the trunk but may occur anywhere on the skin. They present as small red macules and papules. Some people have hundreds of lesions. They are benign and can be removed for cosmetic purposes.

Angiokeratoma

Description

■ Angiokeratomas are scaly papules, colored red to purple, formed by dilatation of superficial blood vessels and epidermal thickening.

History

■ Angiokeratomas are common and most often seen as multiple lesions restricted to specific body sites.
■ There are four clinical variants determined by location and age of onset.

Angiokeratoma of Fordyce (Most Common)

■ Asymptomatic multiple angiokeratomas symmetrically distributed on the scrotum and vulva.
■ They appear in mid-life and persist indefinitely.
■ Scrotal angiokeratomas may be associated with inguinal hernia, varicosities of the leg, or varicocele, thus increased venous pressure is thought to play a role.
■ Vulvar angiokeratomas may develop at a younger age in pregnant woman or with use of oral contraceptives.

Solitary or Papular Angiokeratomas

■ Solitary or papular angiokeratomas occur equally in both sexes.
■ They commonly occur as a single lesion on the legs of young adults; they may be multiple and occur in any location.
■ Papular angiokeratomas are larger than the other variants and easily traumatized.

Angiokeratoma of Mibelli

■ Angiokeratomas of Mibelli are symmetric, grouped, multiple angiokeratomas occurring on the backs of the fingers and toes.
■ They appear during childhood and adolescence and continue to increase in number.
■ Because of their location, lesions may be frequently traumatized and painful.
■ Lesions are more common in females and may be associated with chilblains or pernio.

■ Angiokeratoma of Mibelli is inherited in an autosomal dominant manner.

Angiokeratoma Corporis Diffusum

■ Fabry's disease is an X-linked recessive inborn error of metabolism caused by a deficiency of the lysosomal enzyme α-galactosidase A; this defect leads to deposition of glycophospholipids in the skin (and other organs), leading to the formation of angiokeratomas.
■ Other lysosomal enzyme deficiencies (galactosidase β1-fucosidase, β-mannosidase, and neuraminidase) can produce similar symptoms to those of Fabry's disease.
■ Boys are more severely affected than girls.
■ Around puberty multiple angiokeratomas form symmetrically in the bathing-trunk area.

Skin Findings

■ Angiokeratoma is a deep red to maroon, or blue to black, sharply defined papule of 0.5–1.0 cm.

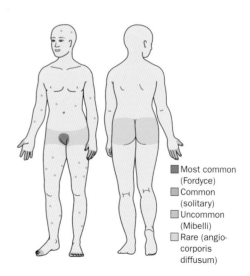

■ Most common (Fordyce)
■ Common (solitary)
■ Uncommon (Mibelli)
■ Rare (angio-corporis diffusum)

Angiokeratoma of Fordyce

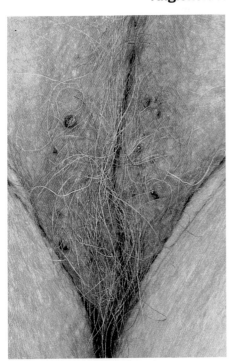

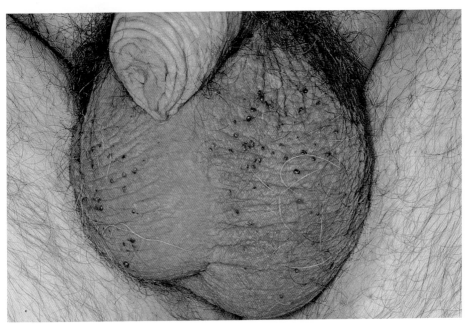

Angiokeratomas of Fordyce occur on the vulva and scrotum. Increased venous pressure, such as occurs with pregnancy and hemorrhoids, may be implicated.

- Early lesions are lighter in color, are soft, and are more easily compressed.
- Older lesions are darker, firmer, and more raised with surface scale.

Non-skin Findings

- Angiokeratoma corporis diffusum (Fabry's disease).
- In childhood and adolescence, boys develop episodic bouts of fever associated with severe pain in the extremities and abdomen; these crises can precede the angiokeratomas and are brought on by exercise and changes in temperature.
- Girls can experience minor symptoms.
- The brain (transient ischemic attacks and stroke), heart (myocardial infarction), and kidney (renal failure) can be affected.
- Men usually die by age 50.
- Most males and many carrier females develop distinctive corneal opacities; this sign can be useful to detect mildly affected males and carrier females.

Laboratory and Pathology

- Skin biopsy shows dilated blood vessels in the superficial dermis with overlying hyperkeratosis.
- All angiokeratoma subtypes have similar appearances microscopically.
- Biochemical, molecular and prenatal testing is available for Fabry's disease and other similar lysosomal storage diseases.

Differential Diagnosis

- Solitary angiokeratomas may look like malignant melanoma.
- Other lesions that may resemble a solitary angiokeratoma include

thrombosed common wart, Kaposi's sarcoma, pyogenic granuloma, pigmented basal cell carcinoma, and squamous cell carcinoma.
- Other lysosomal storage diseases can mimic Fabry's disease.

Course and Prognosis

- Undisturbed angiokeratomas persist indefinitely.
- Surface trauma often results in bleeding, but not resolution, of the lesions.

Treatment

- Cosmetically concerning lesions, or ones susceptible to trauma, can be treated with excision, electrosurgery, and laser surgery.
- Ophthalmologic and neurologic consultation should be considered in cases of angiokeratoma corporis diffusum.

When to Refer

- Children with symptoms of Fabry's disease should be referred to a dermatologist and geneticist for diagnosis, treatment and genetics counselling.
- Patients with Fabry's disease should be seen by an eye specialist, and a neurologist; other specialists such as a cardiologist and a nephrologist may need to be consulted.
- Women with a family history of Fabry's disease should be referred for prenatal diagnosis.

Pearls

- Patients with angiokeratomas of Fordyce should be re-assured that the lesions are not sexually transmitted.

Angiokeratoma Corporis Diffusum

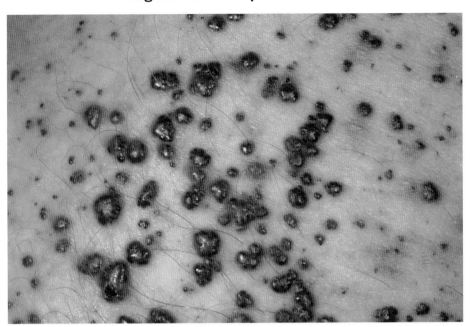

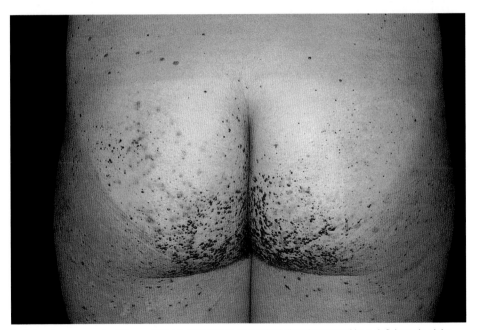

Angiokeratoma corporis diffusum (Fabry's disease) is an X-linked disorder caused by a deficiency in alpha-galactosidase A, a lysosomal enzyme. This leads to the accumulation of glycosphingolipids in most tissues. Patients have cutaneous angiokeratomas, severe pain in the extremities, paresthesias, corneal opacities, renal failure, and many heart, gastrointestinal, and central nervous system abnormalities.

Venous Lake

Description
▦ A venous lake is a dilated vein that occurs on sun-damaged skin and appears as a small blanchable dark blue-to-purple papule.

History
▦ Venous lakes are common on the sun-exposed skin of elderly patients, especially in Caucasian men.
▦ Acquired sun damage and subsequent loss of dermal elasticity (solar elastosis) cause venous lakes.

Skin Findings
▦ A venous lake is an asymptomatic dark blue-to-purple, soft papule of 2–10 mm that blanches with pressure.
▦ Multiple lesions may be present on the mucosal surface of the lip, especially the lower lateral vermilion border.
▦ Lesions may also be found on the ears.
▦ Raised lesions and lesions subject to trauma (like the mucosal surface of the lip) can be itchy and sore, suggesting thrombosis.
▦ Traumatized lesions bleed easily and form a hemorrhagic crust.

Laboratory and Biopsy
▦ Skin biopsy shows a dilated, thin-walled venule located high in the dermis or submucosa.

Differential Diagnosis
▦ Venous lakes can resemble pigmented lesions such as blue nevi and malignant melanoma; venous lakes completely blanch with diascopy.
▦ Traumatized venous lakes can become crusted and look like herpes labialis.
▦ Patients with Kaposi's sarcoma associated with human immunodeficiency virus can develop multiple blue-to-purple nodules on mucosal surfaces that resemble venous lakes.

Course and Prognosis
▦ Venous lakes are persistent and may increase in size with time.

Treatment
▦ Re-assurance of the patient is often all that is needed for venous lakes.
▦ Frequently traumatized or cosmetically concerning lesions and lesions that interfere with eating or speaking should be treated, although recurrence is common.
▦ After anesthetizing with local or regional anesthesia, the venous lake is unroofed with iris scissors and cauterized.
▦ Lasers are also effective for removing venous lakes.

When to refer
▦ Rapidly changing lesions should be referred to a dermatologist.

Pearls
▦ Frequently, patients with venous lakes are concerned about malignancy.
▦ Venous lakes with thrombosis can be tender.
▦ Lesions resemble a varicosity occurring in sun-damaged skin.

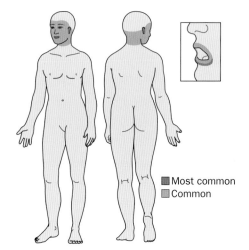

▦ Most common
▦ Common

502

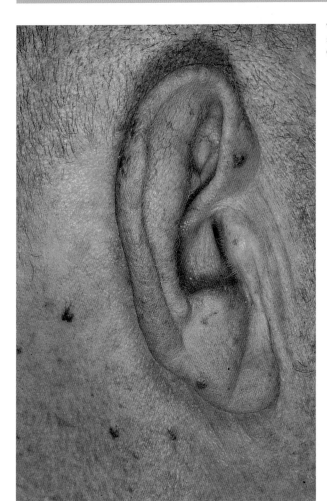

Venous lakes occur on sun-exposed surfaces of the ears, face, neck and lips.

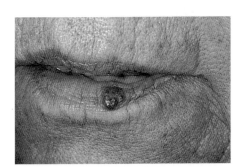

Venous lakes are dark, and patients are concerned about malignancy. The lesion should be firmly depressed to force the blood out and blanch the lesion.

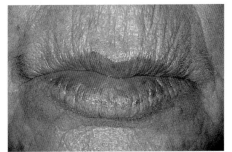

Venous lakes are common on sun-exposed surfaces of the vermilion border of the lip. Venous lakes are dark blue, slightly elevated, 0.2–1-cm dome-shaped lesions composed of a dilated blood-filled vascular channel. Several lesions may occur.

503

Pyogenic Granuloma

Description
- Pyogenic granuloma is an exophytic dome-shaped papule made up of proliferating capillaries separated by thick fibrous bands and surrounded by an epithelial collarette.
- The term pyogenic granuloma is a misnomer, since it is neither infectious nor granulomatous; many pathologists use the term lobular capillary hemangioma.

History
- Pyogenic granulomas occur more frequently in children and young adults and are less common in the elderly.
- The cause is unknown; skin trauma and hormones are thought to be important factors because pyogenic granulomas can occur at sites of injury and during pregnancy.
- Pyogenic granuloma-like lesions can be seen in acne patients who are treated with isotretinoin.

Skin Findings
- Pyogenic granulomas are yellow to deep red, glistening, dome-shaped to polypoid, papules of 3–10 mm.
- Lesions grow rapidly, bleed profusely and can be covered with yellow crust and surrounded by a collarette of scale.
- Usually lesions do not get larger than 1 cm. They can "fall off" only to re-grow.
- Gingival lesions occurring during pregnancy are referred to as epulis gravidarum.
- Lesions are more common on the head and neck and fingers.

Laboratory and Pathology
- A sample of the lesion should be sent for routine histology on all suspected pyogenic granulomas that are surgically treated.
- Skin biopsy shows lobules of proliferating endothelial cells, intersected by dense fibrous septi, and surrounded by an epithelial collarette.
- Often the epidermis is thinned with superficial erosion and exposed capillaries; secondary inflammatory changes are common.

Differential Diagnosis
- Usually the diagnosis is straightforward, especially with single lesions.
- Spitz nevi (in children)
- amelanotic malignant melanoma, squamous cell carcinoma, basal cell carcinoma (in adults; can present as a weeping, rapidly growing nodule)
- angiosarcoma (in the elderly, especially if it occurs on the head and neck; this malignancy also occurs in the setting of chronic lymphedema (Stewart–Treves syndrome) and after radiation therapy)
- bacillary angiomatosis and Kaposi's sarcoma (in patients with human immunodeficiency virus infection)

Course and Prognosis
- Pyogenic granulomas arise suddenly, attain a stable size, and persist without treatment, although some lesions spontaneously regress within 6 months.
- Larger deep-seated lesions may recur with treatment.
- Rarely, multiple satellite lesions can occur.

Treatment
- Pyogenic granulomas are best treated by biopsy followed by electrodesiccation and curettage of the base and border of the lesion.

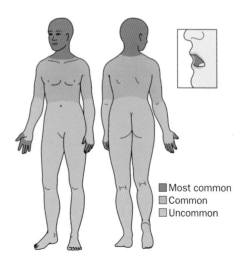

Most common
Common
Uncommon

- Most resolve with a single crateriform scar; recurrences occur in a few patients.
- Rarely, multiple satellite lesions develop at and around the site of a previously treated pyogenic granuloma. This occurs most often on the shoulder and trunk in younger patients.

When to refer

- Patients with recurrent or multiple pyogenic granulomas should be referred to a dermatologist for management.

- Infants and toddlers should be referred to a specialist, especially if the clinician is not experienced in diagnosing and treating young children with pyogenic granulomas.

Pearls

- Patients and parents should be advised of the possibility of recurrence after treatment.
- Children will typically have the new lesions covered with a dressing (the "band aid" sign) because of the bleeding.

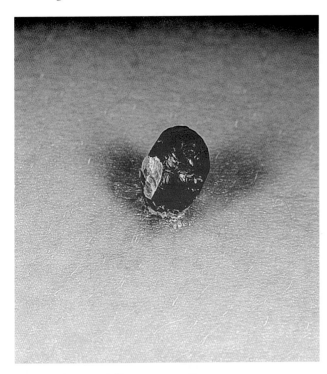

Pyogenic granuloma is a small, rapidly growing, yellow to bright red, dome-shaped fragile protrusion that has a glistening, moist to scaly surface.

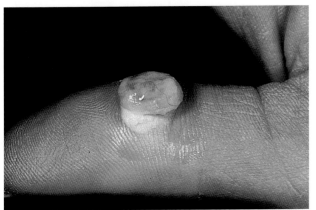

Pyogenic granuloma may bleed profusely if traumatized. The smooth dome-shaped papule with a glistening surface is highly characteristic.

Kaposi's Sarcoma

Description

- Kaposi's sarcoma is a malignancy of lymphatic endothelial cells associated with a gamma herpes virus, human herpes virus 8 (Kaposi's sarcoma-associated herpes virus).
- Kaposi's sarcoma can be divided into four clinical and epidemiological subsets: classic, endemic, immunosuppression-associated or transplant-associated, and epidemic or AIDS associated.

History

- Classic Kaposi's sarcoma is sporadic and slowly progressive and occurs predominantly in 50–70-year-old men of Eastern European or Mediterranean descent.
- In endemic regions (especially eastern and southern Africa), up to 50% of all childhood soft tissue tumors are due to Kaposi's sarcoma, and children can develop an aggressive lymphadenopathic form.
- People receiving immunosuppressive therapy for a variety of conditions— especially organ transplant recipients— are at risk for Kaposi's sarcoma.
- Patients of Mediterranean and Eastern European descent appear to be at increased risk for immunosuppression-associated Kaposi's sarcoma— supporting the theory of genetic predisposition.
- Epidemic-associated Kaposi's sarcoma is the most common AIDS-associated cancer and is 20 times more common in homosexual men, than in those who acquired human immunodeficiency virus by another means (for example, through hemophilia).

Skin Findings

- The skin lesions of Kaposi's sarcoma have a variety of morphologies (macules/patches, papules/plaques, nodules) and the lesions can vary depending upon the clinical variant.
- Classic Kaposi's sarcoma starts with purple patches on the distal lower extremities that progress proximally and become multifocal; individual lesions darken and thicken, eventually becoming brown and verrucous.
- Lesions on the lower legs can look eczematous and ulcerate.
- Early Kaposi's sarcoma nodules can feel soft; older nodules can feel firm.
- Endemic Kaposi's sarcoma (within Africa) involves the lymph nodes in people with localized nodular lesions. It occurs most commonly in men and children.
- Immunosuppression-associated Kaposi's sarcoma is morphologically similar to classic Kaposi's sarcoma; lesions typically improve and sometimes resolve with cessation of immunosuppressive therapy.
- Lesions in AIDS-associated Kaposi's sarcoma have a predilection for the face (especially the nose, eyelids, and ears), the torso and oral mucosa (especially the hard palate).

Non-skin Findings

- Besides the skin, the most commonly affected organs are the lymph nodes, the gastrointestinal tract and the lungs.

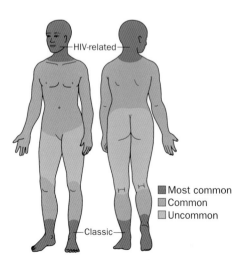

HIV-related

Classic

■ Most common
□ Common
□ Uncommon

Patients with AIDS-related Kaposi's sarcoma often have systemic involvement, particularly of the gastrointestinal tract (stomach and duodenum).

Fever, night sweats, and weight loss may be present.

Laboratory and Biopsy

Skin biopsy is indicated to confirm the diagnosis, and shows neoplastic spindle-shaped cells that form clefts and vascular channels.

The CD4 count in AIDS-related cases is often less then 200 cells/ml.

Differential Diagnosis

Early single lesions may look like pyogenic granuloma, malignant melanoma, bacillary angiomatosis

Multiple lesions may look like stasis dermatitis, progressive pigmented purpura, cutaneous T cell lymphoma

Treatment

Classic Kaposi's Sarcoma

For patients with single lesions, surgical excision can be adequate.

For multiple lesions localized to one area, radiation is the treatment of choice.

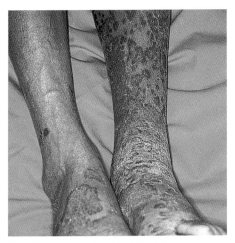

Kaposi's sarcoma related to acquired immunodeficiency syndrome occurs as a multifocal and widespread disease. It begins as violaceous macules and papules and progresses to plaques with multiple red to purple nodules.

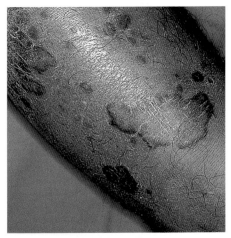

Classic Kaposi's sarcoma begins as purple patches and plaques that involve the lower extremities.

507

■ For extensive or recurrent lesions, combination therapy with surgery, radiation and chemotherapy often is needed.

Endemic Kaposi's Sarcoma
■ Radiation and chemotherapy are used.

Immunosuppression-associated Kaposi's Sarcoma
■ Usually modification or discontinuation of the immunosuppressive therapy produces regression of Kaposi's sarcoma.
■ Radiation and chemotherapy are useful for patients whose Kaposi's sarcoma does not resolve when the immunosuppressive drugs are altered.

AIDS-associated Kaposi's Sarcoma
■ Radiation therapy is very effective, especially for large, localized, and/or ulcerative lesions.

■ Cryosurgery done in 3-week intervals improves superficial Kaposi's sarcoma and is a good cosmetic treatment.
■ Intralesional vincristine has been used with success.
■ Patients can be given antiretroviral therapy alone or in combination with radiation or systemic therapy, such as cytotoxic drugs and interferon-α, directed against Kaposi's sarcoma.

Pearls
■ AIDS-associated Kaposi's sarcoma (especially facial lesions) is extremely distressing to most patients.
■ Oral Kaposi's sarcoma is not uncommon in AIDS patients and may be the presenting sign of infection with human immunodeficiency virus.

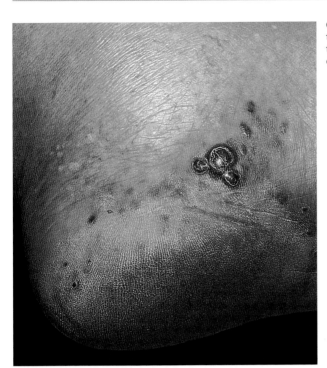

Classic Kaposi's sarcoma typically appears as nodules on the lower legs. These enlarge into dome-shaped tumors.

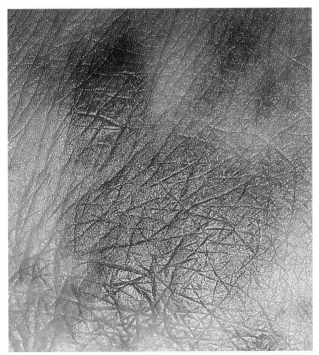

AIDS-related Kaposi's sarcoma. Flat, deep purple plaques are the initial presentation. These will become elevated and evolve into nodules.

Telangiectasias

Description

■ Telangiectasias are common asymptomatic, dilatations of capillaries, venules and arterioles within the sub-papillary plexus.

History

■ Telangiectasias occur in a variety of clinical settings.

■ Although there is little variation in the appearance of individual telangiectasias from one disorder to another, the age of onset, their distribution, and progression vary among disorders.

■ Recognition of this along with other associated clinical findings helps discern between the various disorders associated with telangiectasias.

■ It is useful to distinguish between disorders in which telangiectasias are a primary pathologic feature, and disorders in which telangiectasias arise secondarily.

Primary Telangiectasias

Hereditary Hemorrhagic Telangiectasia (Osler–Rendu–Weber Syndrome)

■ Hereditary hemorrhagic telangiectasia is an autosomal dominant condition in which telangiectasias are found on the mucosae, skin, and internal organs.

■ The earliest sign of the disorder is recurrent epistaxis in childhood.

■ Characteristic telangiectasias do not appear until early adulthood.

■ Telangiectasias are prominent on the tongue, palate, nasal mucosa, palms, soles, and nail beds.

■ Most affected people have a normal life span but are at risk of life-threatening hemorrhage.

Hereditary Benign Telangiectasia

■ Hereditary benign telangiectasia is an autosomal dominant condition.

■ Widespread telangiectasias are found on the skin but not on the mucosa and internal organs.

■ There is no associated bleeding diathesis.

Ataxia Telangiectasia (Louis Bar Syndrome)

■ Ataxia telangiectasia is an autosomal recessive condition with progressive cerebellar ataxia, telangiectasias, and immune dysfunction.

■ The earliest sign—ataxia—is evident when the child begins to walk and usually by the age of 3 years.

■ Telangiectasias appear on the conjunctivae, face, neck, and upper trunk by age 5.

■ Café-au-lait macules, skin ulcerations, poikiloderma, premature gray hair, dry skin, sclerodermatous skin changes, eczema and hirsutism may also occur.

■ People affected by ataxia telangiectasia have defective DNA repair of chromosomal breakages, Kaposi's sarcoma, and an increased sensitivity to ionizing radiation.

Generalized Essential Telangiectasia

■ Women are affected more often than men.

■ Telangiectasias first appear on the legs and then gradually, progressively, and symmetrically extend to involve the trunk and arms.

■ The pathogenesis is unknown.

Unilateral Nevoid Telangiectasia

■ There is a unilateral dermatomal distribution of fine telangiectasias.

■ The trigeminal and the IIIrd and IVth cervical nerves are the most commonly affected dermatomes.

■ This condition may be congenital or acquired.

■ The congenital form affects males more often, whereas the acquired form is seen more often in females.

■ Estrogen may play a role in the acquired form since it can begin during puberty and pregnancy, and resolve in adulthood and after delivery.

Secondary Telangiectasias

■ Telangiectasias are seen in basal cell carcinoma, rosacea, collagen vascular disorders, corticosteroid atrophy, and chronic graft-versus-host disease.

■ Secondary telangiectasias occur in the setting of altered dermal connective tissue as a result of injury or chronic inflammation.

- Damage may be from ultraviolet radiation (actinic damage), ionizing radiation, or treatment with topical or intralesional corticosteroids.
- Telangiectasias occur in scleroderma and the CREST syndrome.
- Telangiectasias in scleroderma and the CREST syndrome appear as discrete, 5-mm macular clusters—referred to as telangiectatic mats—on the face, lips, neck, upper trunk, and dorsal and palmar aspects of the hands.

- The skin of the fingers feels waxy, and Raynaud's phenomenon, cutaneous calcinosis, and ulceration may be present.

Skin Findings

- The lesion is a dilated dermal vessel with a diameter of 1 mm or less. It is not palpable and is easily blanched with diascopy.
- Lesions may appear as discrete vessels or clustered as telangiectatic mats.
- The distribution of lesions varies according to the underlying condition.

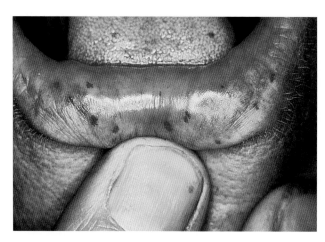

Hereditary hemorrhagic telangiectasia is an autosomal dominant inherited malformation of blood vessels. Few to numerous lesions occur primarily on the lips, the tongue, the nasal mucosa, forearms, hands and fingers, and throughout the gastrointestinal tract.

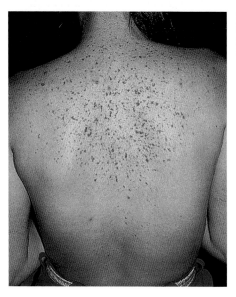

Generalized essential telangiectasia is seen primarily in women. The telangiectasias slowly progress over years and are not accompanied by associated systemic problems.

Non-skin Findings

- In hereditary hemorrhagic telangiectasia syndrome, the telangiectasias and arteriovenous fistulas may involve the gastrointestinal tract, liver, brain, and lungs; bleeding from the gastrointestinal tract may present as melena, or more insidiously as anemia.
- Patients with ataxia telangiectasia develop progressive cerebellar ataxia and severe respiratory tract infections, and are at risk for lymphoreticular malignancy.
- Telangiectasias can occur in the setting of occult liver disease.

Laboratory and Pathology

- Skin biopsy reveals a thin-walled vessel in close approximation to the overlying epidermis.
- A sparse infiltrate of lymphocytes is often seen surrounding the vessels in hereditary hemorrhagic telangiectasia.
- Depending on the clinical setting and suspicion, diagnosis-specific testing may be indicated.
- Imaging studies of the brain and internal organs should be considered for hereditary hemorrhagic telangiectasia.
- Specific serologic testing is indicated when scleroderma is suspected.
- Autoantibodies directed against centromere proteins are found in a high number of patients with the CREST syndrome; and autoantibodies to DNA topoisomerase type I are found in a high number of patients with diffuse scleroderma.

Differential Diagnosis

- Diagnosis is usually straightforward.
- Petechiae may resemble small telangiectasia.

Discussion

- Telangiectasias are easily overlooked; lesions occur in a wide range of disorders.
- Distinguishing between primary and secondary disorders narrows the differential diagnosis.

Treatment

- Cosmetically objectionable telangiectasias may be ablated with laser surgery or pinpoint electrocautery.
- Individual lesions may require several treatments.

Pearls

- Careful attention of the distribution, age of onset, and clinical progression of telangiectasias is needed, as these may provide useful diagnostic clues to underlying disease.

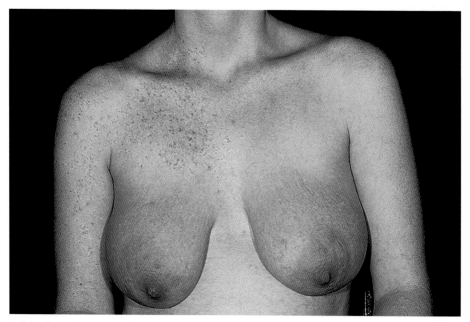

Unilateral nevoid telangiectasia syndrome. Telangiectasias appear in a segmental distribution. The acquired form begins with states of increasing estrogen blood levels: 1) at puberty in females, 2) during pregnancy, or 3) with alcoholic cirrhosis.

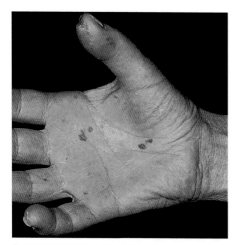
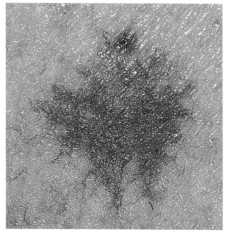

The telangiectasias of CREST syndrome and scleroderma occur as flat (macular) 0.5-cm rectangular collections of uniform tiny vessels; these are the so-called telangiectatic mats.

Spider Angioma (Nevus Araneus)

Description
■ Spider angioma is an asymptomatic blanchable pink papule due to a central dilated arteriole and very fine radial branches.

History
■ Spider angiomas are found in 10–15% of normal adults and children.
■ Lesions represent dilatations of a previously existing vessel rather than a neoplasm.

Skin Findings
■ There is a central, slightly raised, bright red vascular papule from which fine blood vessels radiate.
■ Firm pressure easily blanches the radiating vessels, whereas the central papule is less easily blanched.
■ Pulsation of the central papule with this technique confirms the arteriolar nature of the papule.
■ Spider angiomas are most commonly found on the face, and also on the neck, upper trunk, and upper arms in adults.
■ In children, lesions are also frequently seen on the hands and fingers.

Non-skin Findings
■ Spider angiomas occur with increased frequency in pregnancy and in the setting of chronic liver disease.
■ It has been suggested that spider angiomas occur in a state of relative estrogen excess.
■ Lesions arising during pregnancy tend to resolve after the birth.
■ Those found in patients with liver disease are persistent. Other stigmata of chronic liver disease such as gynecomastia, testicular atrophy, palmar erythema, ascites—and perhaps icterus—may also be present.

Laboratory and Biopsy
■ Skin biopsy is rarely indicated, but shows a central arteriole ascending into the papillary dermis, giving rise to a subepidermal ampulla.

■ Thin-walled arterioles radiate outward into the surrounding papillary dermis and branch into delicate capillaries.
■ If chronic liver disease is suggested by clinical examination, laboratory studies to assess hepatic function may be warranted, including viral hepatitis serologies.

Differential Diagnosis
■ Small basal cell carcinomas (in adults)
■ Telangiectasias (although similar in color and size, they lack the central papule and radiating vessels of spider angiomas)

Course and Prognosis
■ Spider angiomas arising during pregnancy and those occurring in children tend to disappear spontaneously over a period of 3–4 years.

Treatment
■ The patient should be re-assured that spider angiomas are common, benign lesions that usually resolve without treatment.

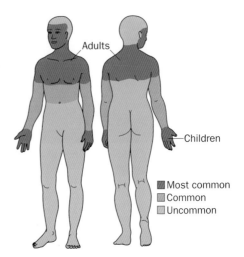

Adults

Children

■ Most common
■ Common
■ Uncommon

- If the lesion is persistent and cosmetically bothersome, it may be treated with either pulsed dye laser or electrocautery.
- The patient should know that treatment is a cosmetic procedure, that there is a slight risk of dyspigmentation and scarring, and that lesions may recur.

- Consultation with a specialist in laser treatment should be considered.

Pearls

- The association between spider angiomas and chronic liver disease is overstated.

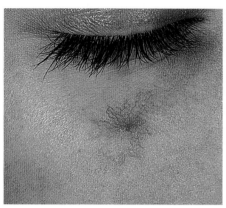

There is a central vessel with radiating smaller vessels. Firm pressure on the central vessel forces blood out and blanches the lesion.

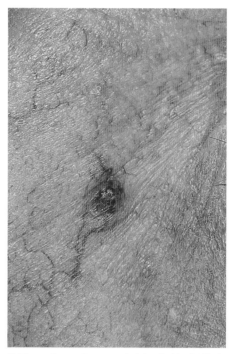

Spider angiomas form as arterioles (spider bodies) become more prominent near the surface of the skin and radiate capillaries (spider legs). They blanch with firm pressure. They are most common on the exposed surfaces of the face and arms. They increase in number with liver disease and during pregnancy and are probably stimulated by higher-than-normal concentrations of estrogen.

515

20 Hair and Nail Diseases

Androgenic Alopecia (Male Pattern Baldness)

Description
■ Androgenic alopecia is premature loss of hair of the central scalp.

History
■ Alopecia is a physiologic reaction induced by androgens in genetically predisposed men.
■ The pattern of inheritance is probably polygenic.
■ It can begin any time after puberty and usually is fully expressed by the time the patient is in his 40s.

Skin Findings
■ Terminal hair follicles are transformed into vellus-like follicles.
■ Terminal hair is replaced by fine light vellus hair, which is shorter and has a reduced diameter.
■ With time further atrophy occurs, leaving the scalp shiny and smooth. The follicles disappear.
■ It begins with bitemporal thinning that then progresses to an M-shaped recession. Then there is a loss of hair focally in the crown of the scalp, which extends to total hair loss in the central scalp.
■ There is increased growth of secondary sexual hair (that on the chest, in the axillae, and in pubic and beard areas).

Course and Prognosis
■ The progression and various patterns of hair loss have been classified by Hamilton. Triangular frontotemporal recession occurs normally in most young men (type I) and women after puberty. The first signs of balding are increased frontotemporal recession accompanied by mid-frontal recession (type II). Hair loss in a round area on the vertex follows, and the density of hair decreases, sometimes rapidly, over the top of the scalp (types III–VII).

Treatment
■ Minoxidil (Rogaine) is a topical 2% or 5% solution that is available over the counter.
  ● It is applied to a dry scalp twice a day.
  ● Ideal candidates are men under 30 years.
  ● Re-growth takes 8–12 months.
  ● It may help stop further loss but must be used continually to preserve growth.
■ Finasteride (Propecia) 1 mg is an oral prescription medication, taken daily.
■ The drug works by blocking 5α-reductase in the scalp.
■ It must be used daily and chronically to stabilize or reverse balding.
■ Decreased libido and erectile dysfunction occur in less than 2% of men taking the drug.
■ It is contraindicated for women.
■ Hair transplants have been used successfully for years to permanently restore hair.
■ Hair weaves have been refined in a process whereby strands of human hair are applied to a thin nylon filament anchored to the scalp with the patient's own hair.
■ An anteroposterior elliptic excision of bald vertex scalp with primary closure can provide an instant hair effect.

Pearls

- Both finasteride and minoxidil need to be used lifelong for continued efficacy.
- Both finasteride and minoxidil are more likely to be effective if usage begins at the earliest onset of hair loss.
- Presently there is limited efficacy of current medical treatments for hair loss. Though the risks of such treatments are minimal, the continued costs may outweigh the benefits.

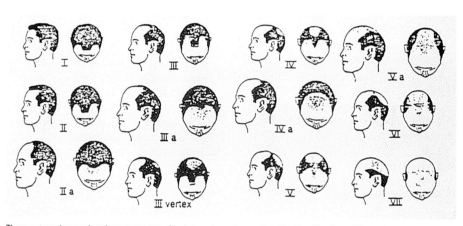

The progression and various patterns of hair loss have been classified by Hamilton. Triangular frontotemporal recession occurs normally in most young men (type I) and women after puberty. The first signs of balding are increased frontotemporal recession accompanied by midfrontal recession (type II). Hair loss in a round area on the vertex follows, and the density of hair decreases, sometimes rapidly, over the top of the scalp (types III–VII).

Androgenetic Alopecia in Women (Female Pattern Hair Loss)

Description

■ Androgenetic alopecia in women is a common hereditary, central, diffuse hair thinning that begins at a relatively early age. This is in contrast to postmenopausal hair loss that begins in women in their 50s, 60s, or 70s.

■ Affected scalp hairs have a shortened anagen cycle and progressive miniaturization of hair follicles.

History

■ Inheritance of androgenetic alopecia is poorly understood, though clearly there is genetic predisposition to pattern hair loss.

■ The true prevalence is unknown but may affect 6–25% of premenopausal women.

■ Women rarely become completely bald like men.

■ Hereditary hair thinning begins in the woman's teenage years, or 20s or 30s, and is usually fully expressed by the time they are in their 40s. There are two peaks of onset, in the 20s and the 40s.

■ Hair loss is gradual, not abrupt or massive.

■ Menses is normal and regular. Heavy menses causes iron deficiency and increased hair shedding. Pregnancies are normal, and there is no infertility or galactorrhea.

■ Certain drugs cause hair thinning. Hair re-grows when the drug is stopped.

Skin Findings

■ Most women experience a gradual loss of hair on the central top of the scalp, with retention of the normal hairline without frontotemporal recession, and the scalp becomes more visible.

■ There is increased spacing between hairs, often pencil-eraser-sized areas lacking visible hairs.

■ There are a variety of hair diameters in the central scalp. Many of the hairs are miniaturized (thin and short). Hairs along the frontal hairline are normal.

■ Hair diameters become thinner over time. This is noticed when the hair is gathered into a ponytail.

Laboratory

■ Biopsy is sometimes performed to rule out the diffuse form of alopecia areata or telogen effluvium.

■ Most patients do not require hormonal evaluation. Most women have no signs of hyperandrogenemia and have normal serum androgen levels.

■ Dehydroepiandrosterone sulfate, serum free or total testosterone, and prolactin levels should be determined if one or more of the following is present: irregular menses, hirsutism, virilization, cystic acne, galactorrhea, or infertility. A subset of women may have polycystic ovarian disease and insulin resistance.

■ The level of thyroid-stimulating hormone should be determined to rule out a treatable thyroid disease.

■ Patients with heavy menses should have the following tests: serum iron determination, total iron binding capacity, and ferritin level. Replacement of low iron state may be helpful.

■ Scalp biopsy is performed in patients suspected of having a scarring alopecia.

Treatment

■ The term "female pattern baldness" should be avoided. Instead, the term "female pattern hair loss" should be used when talking to patients.

■ 2% topical minoxidil solution (Rogaine) may be effective in some women. It is applied twice a day for a trial of 6 months. If effective, it must be continued for persistent effect. If there is no response the 5% solution may be tried twice daily. The 5% solution is approved for use in men.

■ Patients with abnormal laboratory studies can be referred to an endocrinologist or a gynecologist.

■ There are no restrictions on frequency of washing, combing, hair coloring, or permanents.

■ Estrogen is not usually prescribed to treat women for androgenetic alopecia.

- Though finasteride is helpful in men, in women a dose of 1 mg daily was not beneficial in a 1-year study of 137 postmenopausal women.
- Women with androgenetic alopecia who desire an oral contraceptive should use a progestin with little androgenic activity—such as norgestimate or ethynodiol diacetate.

Pearls

- Hair loss is a common complaint in women and can be emotionally devastating.
- Widening of the part is often the earliest visible change. Hair loss is often most obvious in the frontal scalp.
- The "Christmas tree" pattern of loss is evident with hair loss of the frontal scalp exceeding loss of the occiput.

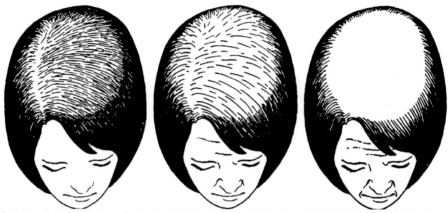

Evolution of the female type of androgenetic alopecia. (From Montagna W, Parakkal PF (1974) *The Structure and Function of Skin*, 3rd ed. New York: Academic Press.)

Telogen Effluvium

Description

- Telogen effluvium is a non-scarring, non-inflammatory, diffuse hair loss (alopecia) which is typically sudden in onset and occurs 3–5 months after a systemic stress, such as childbirth, a severe medical illness, surgery, high fever, and occasionally in response to medication.

History

- Telogen effluvium may be acute or chronic. The acute form occurs abruptly after a specific trigger, and is of less than 12 months duration.
- Chronic telogen effluvium may or may not have an identifiable inciting stressor; it may be acute or slow in onset and greater than 12 months duration.
- The hair loss is often most noted by the patient as clumps of hair coming out in the shower or in the hairbrush.
- The quantity of hair lost each day is often dramatic, very noticeable and distressing to the patient, however, such loss may not be easily detected on direct inspection by others.
- The hair loss typically occurs 3 months after the inciting stressor since the loss is a result of anagen (growing phase) hairs shifting abruptly into catagen (the apoptotic stage), and then into telogen (resting phase) when the hair is lost.
- Not all anagen hairs undergo this phase shift; the quantity of hairs shifting stage determines the amount of loss.
- The most common form of telogen effluvium results from *early conversion of hairs to telogen phase*, as noted due to systemic stress such as surgery, major illness, and crash dieting. The hair loss is 3–5 months after the major stress.
- Telogen effluvium can also be caused by a *delayed anagen release*, where affected hairs are delayed in their conversion to telogen hairs; this type of telogen effluvium occurs after childbirth. When delayed anagen release occurs, hairs cycle into telogen and are shed 3–5 months later.
- Chronic telogen effluvium is believed to be caused by a short anagen cycle. Affected patients are typically middle-aged women with thick hair prior to onset of shedding.
- Hair loss in infants occurs between birth and 4 months; re-growth is typical by 6 months.

Skin Findings

- The scalp hairs are primarily affected; the density of hairs is variably reduced. Early on, the reduction in hair density may be undetectable by the clinician.
- The hair density as manifest by the part width is similar at the occiput and at the crown.
- Pull test is positive: gentle pulling of hair clumps in multiple regions of the scalp will yield more than two or three telogen (club) hairs per pull.
- Bitemporal thinning may be observed.

Non-skin Findings

- The fingernails may show horizontal ridges (Beau's lines) that indicate a similar growth arrest occurring several months previously.

Laboratory

- Hair pluck is an uncomfortable test where at least 10 hairs are plucked from the scalp. Examination of the hair bulbs using light microscopy will yield an increased telogen to anagen ratio above the normal ratio of 1 to 10. This test is rarely required for diagnosis and is uncomfortable for the patient.
- Biopsy is not typically indicated if the clinical findings and history are supportive. Biopsy shows no inflammation, no miniaturization of hair follicles, and an increased number of telogen and catagen follicles, but no inflammation or miniaturization of hair follicles. A 4 mm punch biopsy for horizontal sectioning should show between 25 and 50 hairs; more than 12–15% of the hairs would be in telogen.
- Consider the ratio of iron to total iron-binding capacity. Ferritin may be low in anemia, vegetarianism, or if there is a history of heavy menstrual cycles.
- Anorexia, crash dieting, or dramatic weight loss may manifest as low ferritin, albumin, and total protein.

Thyroid function tests are indicated if symptoms or signs of thyroid disease are present.

Course and Prognosis

- This form of hair loss does not affect all hairs; thus the loss of hairs is never total.
- Re-growth of hairs occurs in 95% by 12 months; there is no scarring or permanent loss.
- Sometimes re-growth occurs during a time when the affected patient also is experiencing hair loss due to miniaturization of hairs as occurs in androgenetic alopecia; in this case re-growth of hair may not appear as complete.
- The course of chronic telogen effluvium is unpredictable. It is often waxing and waning, and may last several months to several years.

Differential Diagnosis

- Androgenetic alopecia
- Diffuse form of alopecia areata (biopsy may be necessary)
- Loose anagen hair syndrome (the pull test should yield some anagen hairs)

Treatment

- Spontaneous re-growth is the rule.
- No treatment is likely to shorten the course, or hasten re-growth.
- If medications are responsible, they should be discontinued if possible.
- The most important aspect of treatment is an emotionally supportive relationship during the evaluation, diagnosis, and follow-up.
- Education of the patient regarding hair cycle dynamics, the short arrest in growth due to a specific stressor, and the likelihood of re-growth are helpful and reassuring details to discuss.
- Minoxidil 5% solution applied twice daily may be helpful for chronic telogen effluvium.

Pearls

- Understanding the hair cycle is important for understanding the dynamics of telogen effluvium. Hair loss is emotionally traumatizing; support and reassure the patient that this form of hair

loss has an excellent prognosis for complete re-growth.
- Weekly hair collection may also be very reassuring by demonstrating that the hair loss is diminishing with time.
- Ask the patient to collect all hairs lost in the shower, on the pillow and hair brush once weekly in the morning. The hairs are put in a labeled plastic bag and the quantity is compared over time.
- Medications associated with telogen effluvium include amphetamines, captopril, coumarin, carbamazepine, cimetidine, enalapril, etretinate, lithium, metoprolol, and propranolol.

Hair Facts and Hair Cycle Dynamics

- Human hair growth is dynamic; the growth of hairs on the scalp is mosaic (hairs are cycling through anagen, catagen and telogen phases; the growth cycle phase of individual hairs is variable).
- Anagen phase is the growing phase. Approximately 85–90% of all hairs are in anagen, and it lasts roughly 3 years.
- Catagen phase is the transitional, apoptotic phase. Roughly 3–5% of hairs are in catagen. It lasts roughly 1–2 weeks.
- Telogen phase is the resting phase, in which 5–10% of hairs are in telogen. The duration is roughly 3 months.
- The normal number of scalp hairs is 100,000.
- The average number of hairs shed per day is 100–150.
- The normal anagen to telogen ratio in a "hair pluck" is 9 to 1.

Scalp Biopsy Mechanics

- Scalp biopsy for alopecia should be taken from near the edge of the affected region. A punch biopsy should be taken on an angle parallel to hair growth. One punch biopsy can be submitted whole for standard transverse sectioning. A second punch biopsy, 4-, 5- or 6-mm punch can be bisected horizontally about 1 mm above the dermal–subcutaneous junction. Each piece is then embedded cut-side down by the pathologist. Serial horizontal sections can then be performed and are best read by a pathologist who is experienced in reading horizontal scalp biopsies.

Alopecia Areata

Description

- Alopecia areata is a non-scarring hair loss, typically of rapid onset in a sharply defined, usually round or oval area.
- The loss may be diffuse or patchy, or band-like at the margins of the scalp.
- It is likely to be due to an immunologic phenomenon.

History

- Alopecia areata is most common in children and young adults.
- There is a sudden occurrence of one or several areas of hair loss of 1–4 cm.
- The eyelashes and beard may be involved, and—rarely—other parts of the body.
- Total hair loss of the scalp (alopecia totalis) is seen most frequently in young people; it may be accompanied by cycles of growth and loss.
- Total hair loss of the body (alopecia universalis) is very rare.
- Stress is frequently cited as the cause, but there is little evidence that it plays a role.
- Re-growth begins in 1–3 months and may be followed by loss in other areas.
- The prognosis for total permanent re-growth in cases with limited involvement is good, but it is poorer for patients with more involvement.

Skin Findings

- A wide spectrum of involvement is seen. The most common pattern is patchy. Other patterns include the ophiasis pattern (a band-like loss at the scalp margins), and the ophiasis inversus pattern (spares the periphery of the scalp while involving the crown).
- The diffuse pattern is the least common, in which there is decreased hair density throughout the scalp.
- The skin is typically very smooth, or may have short stubs of hair.
- The hair shaft is poorly formed and breaks on reaching the surface. Tapered hairs resembling exclamation points may be best seen at the margin of an area of loss.
- New hair is usually the same color and texture, but may be fine and white.

Non-skin Findings

- Structural and functional abnormalities of the thyroid may occur.
- Diffuse fine nail pitting occurs in up to 30% of cases.

Laboratory

- Biopsy of affected scalp may be performed if the clinical presentation is not typical. Biopsy findings include peribulbar lymphocytes, miniaturized follicles, a telogen vellus hair ratio of 1.5 to 1, and increased telogen and catagen follicles. The presence of eosinophils in a biopsy is a helpful diagnostic sign in cases that are difficult to diagnose.
- Alopecia areata may be associated with thyroid disease, pernicious anemia, Addison's disease, vitiligo, lupus erythematosus, ulcerative colitis, diabetes mellitus, and Down syndrome.
- Tri-iodothyronine, thyroxine, thyroid-stimulating hormone, antithyroglobulin, and antimicrosomal antibody testing should be considered, especially for children.

Differential Diagnosis

- Trichotillomania
- Tinea capitis
- Syphilis
- Telogen effluvium
- Androgenic alopecia

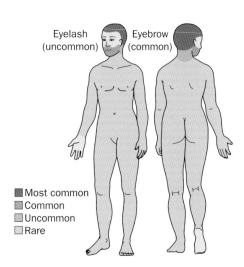

Eyelash (uncommon)   Eyebrow (common)

■ Most common
□ Common
□ Uncommon
□ Rare

Treatment

- In most areas hair re-grows and no treatment is needed.
- Group I topical steroids applied twice a day are minimally effective. They should be used in cycles, such as 2 weeks of treatment and 1 week of no treatment.
- Intradermal injection of triamcinolone acetonide (Kenalog) 2.5–10 mg/ml is effective.
  - Injections may be repeated at 4-week intervals.
  - Atrophy is the major side effect.
  - This treatment should be reserved for patients with a few small areas of hair loss.
- Anthralin (Drithocreme 1%, 0.5%, 0.25%, or 0.1%), applied once a day in concentrations high enough to induce a visible dermatitis, is occasionally effective.
- Squaric acid dibutyl ester is used by some specialists; sensitization is generally with a 2% concentration to an area of 4 cm, waiting 2 weeks for sensitization, followed by application of 0.001% in children and 0.01% in adults applied to affected areas, three or four times a week. Such contact allergy can be severe, however.

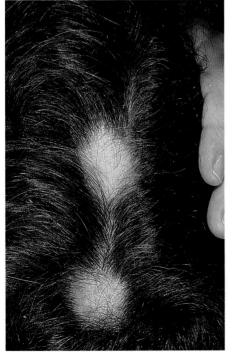

Alopecia areata is characterized by the rapid onset of total hair loss in a sharply defined, usually round area. The duration and extent of loss varies greatly. Most cases are asymptomatic but a few patients complain of burning. The skin feels smooth.

- An intravenous pulse of methylprednisolone may be effective in patients with rapidly progressing extensive multifocal alopecia areata.
- Oral corticosteroid therapy does not prevent the spread or relapse of severe alopecia areata, and when re-growth is obtained, it is rarely maintained off therapy.
- A hair prosthesis should be considered and encouraged for patients with diffuse loss when emotional distress is high.
- A network of support groups across the country is available to help patients cope: Alopecia Areata Foundation (http://www.alopeciaareata.com).

Pearls

- Patients with a diffuse pattern of alopecia areata are panicked by the marked diffuse hair shedding, which is rapid and progressive. Gentle hair pull in these patients reveals more than 10 hairs per pull, consisting of dystrophic anagen hairs or telogen hairs.

Pediatric Considerations

- Hair loss at any age is emotionally distressing, but is particularly challenging and upsetting for children. Emotional support and encouragement are essential.
- Most children with localized alopecia areata will re-grow hair in the affected regions within 1 year.
- If intralesional injections are used in children, they should be for limited areas of loss only, of low strength (2.5–5 mg/ml Kenalog intralesionally). EMLA topical anesthetic can be applied 2 hours prior to injection of the affected area to diminish the pain of injection.

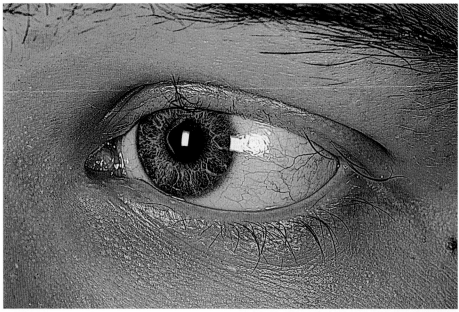

Alopecia areata may involve the eyelashes. Some patients manually extract their lashes. This is called trichotillomania.

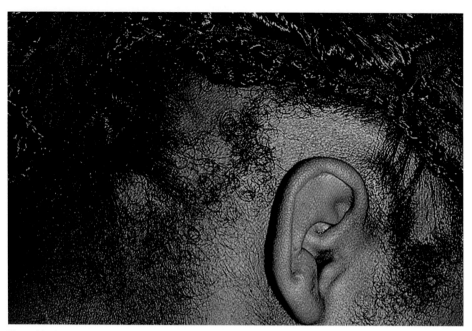

The ophiasis pattern occurs when hair loss occurs on the sides and lower back of the scalp. This pattern is associated with a poor prognosis for regrowth. Other indicators of a poor prognosis are onset at a young age, extensive loss, family history of alopecia areata and nail dystrophy.

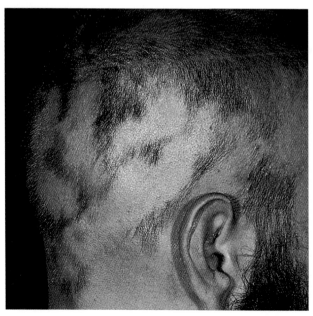

Alopecia areata. A wide spectrum of involvement is seen. The majority of patients report the sudden occurrence of one or several 1–4-cm areas of hair loss on the scalp.

Trichotillomania

Description
- Trichotillomania is the recurrent pulling of one's hair, that results in significant hair loss. The urge to pull hair is overwhelming; after hair pulling, anxiety is relieved temporarily.
- It may involve many hours each day of pulling the hair—or thinking about pulling it.
- Often the "puller" does not admit to this habit.

History
- Trichotillomania is a habit tic most commonly found in young children.
- It is also seen in adolescents and adults.
- The female to male ratio is 2.5 to 1.
- Hair is twisted around finger, pulled, and rubbed until it is extracted or broken.
- Favorite sites are the easily reached areas—the frontoparietal scalp, eyebrows, and eyelashes.
- It first manifests during inactive periods, perhaps while watching television, or before falling asleep.
- Parents seldom notice the behavior.
- It is often associated with underlying anxiety, depression, and low self-esteem.
- It can be a chronic problem, and it often resolves spontaneously.

Skin Findings
- There is a patch of hair loss with an irregular, angulated border.
- The hair density is greatly reduced; the involved area is not completely bald and smooth like in alopecia area.
- Short broken hairs of varying lengths are randomly distributed in the involved site.

Laboratory
- Potassium hydroxide test rules out non-inflammatory tinea capitis.
- Plucked hair shows no telogen hair roots (100% in the active growing anagen phase).
- Gentle hair traction produces no more hair loss.
- Skin biopsy reveals a marked increase in catagen hairs.

Differential Diagnosis
- Alopecia areata
- Tinea capitis
- Syphilis

Treatment
- Treatment is often delayed, or not sought, because of embarrassment.
- Response is best to combination therapy including psychopharmacology, psychotherapy, and behavior modification (such as habit substitution), rather than psychotherapy alone.
- The child's attention should be diverted when hair is being pulled.
- The parents and physician should be accepting and supportive rather than judgmental and punitive.

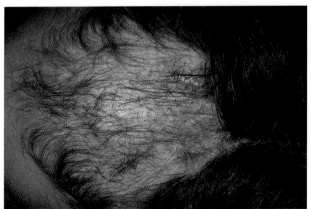

The favorite site is the easily reached frontoparietal region of the scalp, but any scalp area, or the eyebrows and eyelashes, may be attacked.

- Extensive involvement or persistence requires psychiatric evaluation. Psychotherapy can be helpful.
- Trichotillomania shares features with obsessive-compulsive disorder, including response to medication.
- Clomipramine (Anafranil), fluoxetine (Prozac), and pimozide (Orap) can be effective; however, not all patients respond fully to psychopharmacology alone.

Pearls

- The favorite site is the easily reached frontoparietal region of the scalp, but any scalp area or the eyebrows and eyelashes may be attacked.
- The affected area has an irregular angulated border, and the density of hair is greatly reduced, but the site is never bald as in alopecia areata.

- Multiple visits to providers and specialists seeking a diagnostic answer is typical for this condition; a biopsy can be helpful and supportive of this diagnosis.

Pediatric Considerations

- This condition is most commonly seen in children. A careful social history seeking sources of distress or emotional difficulties is advised.
- Discussion with an understanding physician or parent is most helpful for the affected child. Referral for psychiatric evaluation and consideration for behavioral and pharmacologic therapy may be delicate but is highly recommended.

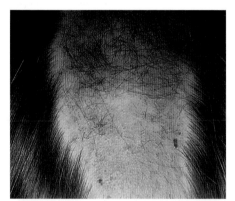

The affected area has an irregular angulated border and the density of hair is greatly reduced, but the site is never bald, as in alopecia areata.

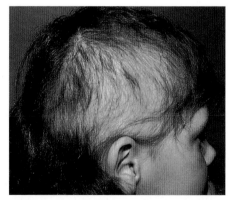

Several short broken hairs of varying lengths are randomly distributed in the involved site. Hair that grows beyond 0.5–1 cm can be grasped by small fingers and extracted.

Nail Diseases

Anatomy

- The nail plate is hard, translucent, dead keratin.
- The nail fold includes the skin surrounding the lateral and proximal aspects of the nail plate. The proximal nail fold overlies the matrix. Its keratin layer extends onto the proximal nail plate to form the cuticle.
- The matrix synthesizes 90% of the nail plate. The lunula (white half-moon), which is visible through the nail plate, is the distal aspect of the nail matrix.
- The nail bed extends from the distal nail matrix to the hyponychium. The nail bed consists of parallel longitudinal ridges with small blood vessels at their base. Bleeding induced by trauma or vessel disease occurs in the depths of these grooves, producing the splinter hemorrhage pattern.
- The hyponychium is a short segment of skin lacking nail cover; it begins at the distal nail bed and terminates at the distal groove.

Growth rates

- Fingernails grow at a rate of 0.5–1.29 mm per week. It takes approximately 5.5 months for a fingernail to grow from the matrix to the free edge.
- Toenails take 12–18 months to be replaced.

- A reduction in the rate of matrix-cell division occurs during systemic diseases such as scarlet fever, causing thinning of the nail plate (Beau's lines).
- Nail growth rate decreases with age and poor circulation.

Nail biopsy

- Nail biopsies are usually performed by specialists.
- Nail biopsies are used to diagnosis tumors, inflammatory disease, and infections.
- The ideal ungual biopsy is performed after avulsion of the plate. This allows clear visualization of the matrix and bed.
- A punch or excisional biopsy technique is chosen, which provides a sufficient amount of tissue and produces a minimal amount of scarring.

Ridging and Beading

- Longitudinal ridging is a common aging change that is occasionally seen in young people.
- Beading occurs at all ages but is more common in the elderly. The beads cover part or most of the plate surface and are arranged longitudinally.
- Patients may sand or buff the nail to smooth the surface. Elon nail conditioner (http://www.ilovemynails.com) prevents dryness and cracking.

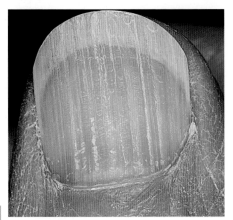

Longitudinal ridging is an aging change. It also occurs as a normal variant in young patients.

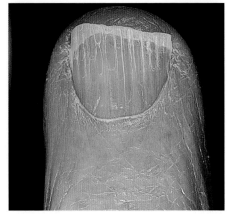

Ridging and beading is an aging change. Both beads and ridges appear in this nail.

Onycholysis

■ Onycholysis is the separation of the nail from the nail bed. It is more common in women with long nails. Vigorous cleaning under the nail accelerates the process.

■ Separation begins at the distal end and slowly progresses proximally.

■ The non-adherent portion of the nail is white, yellow, or green tinged.

■ Causes include psoriasis, trauma to long nails, *Candida* or *Pseudomonas* infections, internal drugs, contact with chemicals, maceration from prolonged immersion, and allergic contact dermatitis (e.g. to nail hardener or adhesives).

■ Screen patients with unexplained onycholysis for hyperthyroidism and asymptomatic thyroid disease.

■ Treat by cutting the separated portion of the nail. This promotes dryness and discourages infection. Do not soak the fingertip.

■ Avoid exposure to contact irritants.

■ Yeast grows in the space between the nail and nail bed. Use liquid topical agents (e.g. fungoid tincture that contains miconazole). Use oral fluconazole (Diflucan) for resistant cases. A short course of fluconazole (e.g. 150 mg every day for 5–7 days) may have to be repeated as the nail grows out.

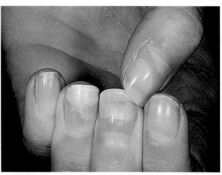

Onycholysis occurring in a woman with long nails. The separated nails appear yellow or white. Patients think they have a fungal nail infection.

Habit-tic Deformity

■ Biting or picking a section of the proximal nail fold of the thumb with the index fingernail is a common habit. Other nails can be affected.

■ Linear bands of horizontal grooves extend up the nail surface. Nail rippling from chronic eczema of the proximal nail fold causes a similar appearance.

■ Patients who can stop this habit will eventually re-grow normal nails.

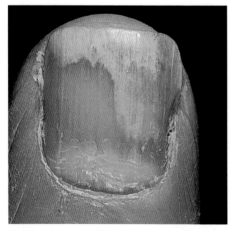

Onycholysis is separation of the nail plate from the nail bed. It is common in women with long nails. Low-grade repeated pressure on the distal plate lifts the nail.

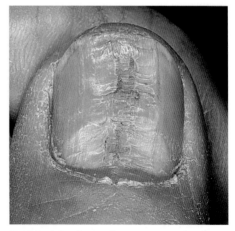

Habit tic deformity usually appears as a sharply defined band of rippling down the center of the nail plate. Here the rippling is uneven and the process was incorrectly interpreted as a fungal infection.

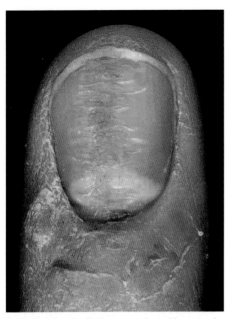

Habit-tic deformity. Erythema, scale and hypertrophy of the proximal nail fold may occur with habitual picking.

- Subungual scaly debris may accumulate under the distal nail plate. The yellow-white debris elevates the distal nail. This also is commonly mistaken for nail fungus infection.
- Surface distortion of the nail plate occurs when psoriasis affects the nail matrix.
- Oil spot lesions are yellow-brown spots seen through the nail surface. Psoriasis of the nail bed causes serum and scaling debris to accumulate under the nail plate.
- Treatment of skin disease with systemic agents such as cyclosporin, methotrexate or acitretin will improve the nails.
- Many topical agents (Calcipotriol, tazarotene, and anthralin) have been tried but results are discouraging. Intralesional injections at monthly intervals into the matrix and lateral nail folds are effective but are painful. Triamcinolone acetonide (Kenalog) 2.5–5 mg/ml is delivered with a 30-gauge needle. The procedure is painful and most patients do not continue.

Psoriasis

- The incidence of nail involvement in psoriasis varies from 10% to 50%.
- Nail involvement may be the only sign of psoriasis but it usually occurs simultaneously with skin disease. One or several nails may be involved.
- Pain may restrict activities.
- Pitting is the most common finding. There may be a few or many and they are haphazardly distributed on the surface.
- Onycholysis is separation of the nail from the nail bed. Separation begins at the distal groove or under the nail plate and may involve several nails. The separated nail appears yellow and is often misinterpreted as a fungal infection.

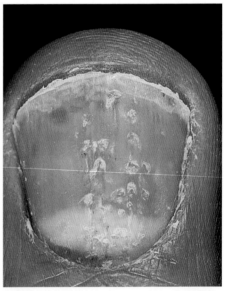

Pitting is the most characteristic sign of psoriasis of the nail plate. Look at all of the other nails for other signs of psoriasis. Patients with nail psoriasis may have no skin disease.

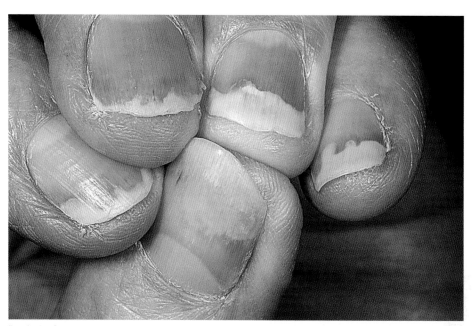

Psoriasis. Separation of the distal nail plate and the accumulation of subungual debris is a common finding in psoriasis of the nail unit. The same changes may occur with traumatically induced onycholysis. A diagnosis of tinea is often incorrectly made.

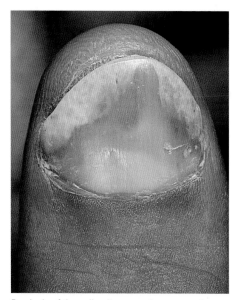

Psoriasis of the nail unit can produce a complex picture. Here there is subungual debris, and separation of the nail from the nail bed. Accumulation of serum under the nail bed creates a light brown spot called an oil spot lesion.

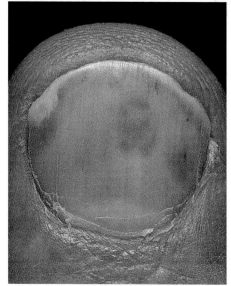

Psoriasis (oil spot lesion). Psoriasis of the nail bed under the nail plate causes serum to accumulate. This brown stain can be seen through the nail plate and resembles an oil spot.

531

Acute paronychia

- Bacterial infection of the proximal and lateral nail fold causes the rapid onset of pain and swelling.
- Trauma and manipulation is the cause or it may occur spontaneously.
- Pus accumulates behind the cuticle or deeper in the lateral nail folds.
- Pus is drained by inserting the pointed end of a comedone extractor or similar instrument between the nail fold and the nail plate. Pain is abruptly relieved.
- Deeper infections may require incision to drain the abscess.
- Small confined abscesses may respond to just drainage. Larger abscesses with surrounding erythema are treated with antistaphylococcal antibiotics.

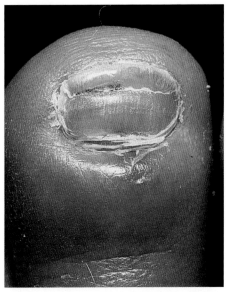

Acute paronychia. Acute onset of erythema and swelling occurred when the cuticle was manipulated.

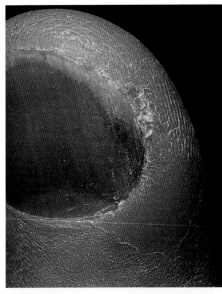

Acute paronychia. Intense erythema, swelling and pain developed in 24 hours. Purulent material drained when a blunt instrument was inserted between the nail and proximal nail fold.

Chronic Paronychia

- Contact irritant exposure is the major cause. Bakers, dish washers, surgeons and dentists are at risk.
- Many or all fingers are involved. There is tenderness, erythema and mild swelling about the proximal and lateral nail folds.
- The cuticle disappears leaving the space between the proximal nail fold and the nail plate exposed to infection. Manipulation of the cuticle accelerates the process.
- Both bacteria and yeast grow in the warm moist space under the proximal nail fold. A small quantity of pus can be expressed from under the proximal nail fold.
- Chronic inflammation causes the nail plate to be distorted but it remains uninfected.
- Psoriasis may have an identical appearance.
- Goals of treatment are to avoid irritation and suppress inflammation and infection.
- Vinyl gloves, and wearing a cotton glove underneath, affords protection (http://www.allerderm.com).

- Group V topical steroids and not oral antibiotics are the mainstay of treatment.
- Fungoid tincture (miconazole) is applied twice daily to the proximal nail fold and allowed to flow into the space created by the absent cuticle. The cuticle may never re-form in patients with longstanding inflammation.
- Fluconazole (150 mg/day) for 1–2 weeks may control treatment-resistant cases. Short courses of fluconazole may have to be repeated as the infection recurs.

Pseudomonas infection

- Separation of the nail plate (onycholysis) exposes a damp, macerated space between the nail plate and the nail bed.
- *Pseudomonas* thrives in this warm moist space and stains the under surface of the nail plate a green-black color. There is little discomfort or inflammation as occurs with subungual hematoma.
- Apply a few drops of a bleach mixture (one part chlorine bleach to four parts water) under the nail three times a day. Vinegar (acetic acid) may also be used.
- Cut unattached nail to eliminate the damp space under the nail.

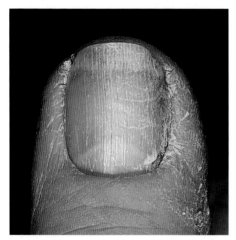

Chronic inflammation of the nail folds will eventually cause the nail plate to be discolored and to fragment. This appears to be a fungal infection but a potassium hydroxide examination and biopsy were negative.

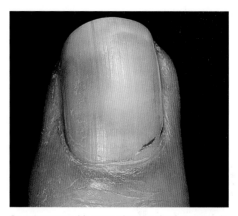

Pseudomonas with green pigmentation has grown in this space created by the separation of the nail from the nail plate.

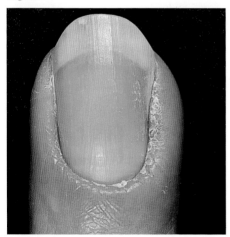

Chronic paronychia occurs in people whose hands are repeatedly immersed in water. The cuticle disappears and the lateral and proximal fail folds are tender and swollen.

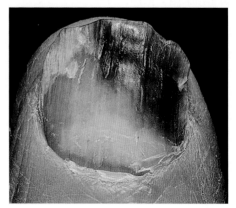

Chronic *Pseudomonas* infection under the nail plate has caused deep green pigmentation of the full thickness of the nail plate.

Hangnail

- Triangular strips of skin may separate from the lateral nail folds, particularly during the winter months.
- Attempts at removal may cause pain and extension of the tear into the dermis.
- Separated skin should be cut before extension occurs. Constant lubrication of the fingertips with thick skin creams (e.g. Aquaphor ointment) and avoidance of repeated hand immersion in water is beneficial.

Ingrown toenail

- Ingrown nails are caused by lateral pressure of poorly fitting shoes, by improper or excessive trimming of the lateral nail plate, or by trauma.
- They occur most often on the large toe. The first signs are pain and swelling.
- The nail pierces the lateral nail fold and enters the dermis, where it acts as a foreign body.

- The area of penetration becomes purulent and edematous as granulation tissue grows alongside the penetrating nail.
- Treatment involves removing the penetrated nail with scissors and curetting the granulation tissue. Small areas of granulation tissue can simply be treated with silver nitrate sticks.
- Cellulitis may occur and need treatment with oral antibiotics.
- Cool wet dressings suppress inflammation and treat swelling.
- Podiatrists treat chronic recurrent ingrown nails by destroying the lateral nail matrix with phenol.

Subungual hematoma

- Trauma to the nail plate may cause immediate bleeding and pain.
- Bleeding may cause separation and more pain.
- Puncture the nail surface with a red-hot paperclip tip to drain the blood.
- Trauma to the proximal nail fold causes hemorrhage that may not be apparent for days. The nail plate may emerge from the nail fold with bloodstains and mimic melanoma.

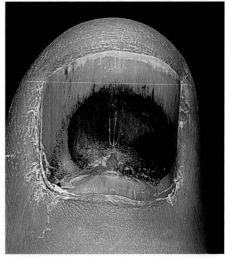

Ingrown nail. The nail plate has penetrated the lateral nail fold. Erythema and swelling occurred. Granulation tissue has appeared at the distal lateral fold.

Trauma to the nail causes bleeding in the closed space under the nail. Blood turns dark brown or black and takes months to disappear. Melanoma can have a similar appearance. The history is important.

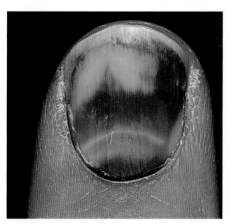

Accumulation of blood occurs under the nail plate following trauma. Trauma occurred weeks ago in this patient. The blood has lysed but the staining will persist until the nail grows out.

Nail hypertrophy

- Gross thickening of the nail plate may occur with tight-fitting shoes or other forms of chronic trauma. Pressure on the nail from shoes causes pain with every step.
- Thick nails are often misdiagnosed as a fungal infection.
- The nail plate may be reduced with sandpaper or a file, or the nail can be removed and the nail matrix permanently destroyed with phenol so that the nail will not re-grow.

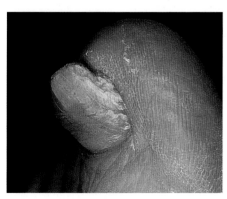

Onychomycosis. Nails become thick from constant pressure or from infection with fungi.

White spots or bands

- White spots in the nail plate are common and probably are a result of repeated low grade trauma.
- The spots or bands eventually grow out and disappear.
- Patients often misinterpret this finding as a fungal infection.

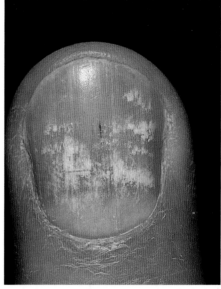

White bands are a common finding and are probably caused by low grade trauma to the proximal nail fold.

Distal Plate Splitting

- Brittle nails and splitting is found in 20% of adults.
- The splitting into layers or peeling of the distal nail plate resembles the scaling of dry skin.
- Nails—like the skin—dry in the winter. Repeated water immersion encourages the process. Vinyl gloves protect during wet work.
- Rehydrate the nail by soaking in water. Then apply a thick lubricant such as Aquaphor ointment or Elon nail conditioner (http://www.ilovemynails. com). These are found in some pharmacies.
- The B-complex vitamin, biotin, (2.5 mg/day) may improve nail plate thickness and integrity.

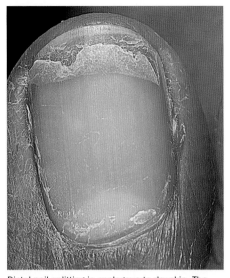

Distal nail splitting is analogous to dry skin. The distal plate separates into layers and peels away. Wetting the hand repeatedly exacerbates the problem.

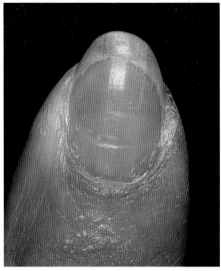

Beau's lines are transverse nail plate grooves caused by an acute change in nail plate growth. This patient had two treatment sessions with a chemotherapeutic agent.

Beau's lines

■ Beau's lines are transverse depressions or ridges of all of the nails that appear at the base of the lunula weeks after a stressful event has temporarily interrupted nail formation.

■ The lines progress distally with normal nail growth and eventually disappear at the free edge.

■ They develop in response to high fevers, scarlet fever, hand, foot, and mouth disease, among many other diseases, and in patients taking chemotherapeutic agents.

Digital Mucous Cysts

■ Digital mucous cysts are focal collections of mucin lacking a cystic lining.

■ These dome-shaped, pink-white structures occur on the dorsal surface of the distal phalanx of middle-aged and elderly people.

■ A clear, viscous, jelly-like substance exudes when the cyst is incised.

■ Cysts on the proximal nail fold compress the nail-matrix cells and induce a longitudinal nail groove.

■ Lesions are often painful and should be treated. The easiest method is to incise the cyst with a #11 blade and firmly express the clear viscous material. This can be repeated if the cyst recurs.

- Cryosurgery of the base may be effective. Remove the cyst roof with scissors and expel the gelatinous contents. Conservatively freeze the base. The treated site becomes edematous and exudative, and a bulla develops in most cases. Healing is complete in 4–6 weeks. Retreatment is often necessary.
- Surgical excision, intralesional steroid injections, and unroofing of the cyst followed by electrodesiccation and curettage have a high recurrence rate.

Nevi and Melanoma

- Junctional nevi can appear in the nail matrix and produce a brown pigmented band. Brown longitudinal bands are common in black people but are rare in white people
- Melanoma of the nail can occur anywhere around or under the nail.
- Melanoma of the nail is rare.
- The lesion may present as a pigmented band that increases in width.
- The spontaneous appearance of such a band is noteworthy to most physicians, who promptly require a biopsy.
- Benign subungual nevi are rare in white people, so subungual nevoid lesions should be regarded as malignant until proved otherwise.
- Hutchinson's sign is the periungual extension of brown-black pigmentation from longitudinal melanonychia onto the proximal and lateral nail folds. It is an important indicator of subungual melanoma.

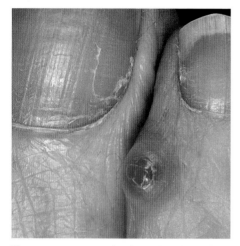

Mucous cysts occur on the dorsal distal finger. They cause the nail plate to develop a depression if they are located over the nail matrix.

Mucous cyst. A large amount of clear viscous material exudes when the surface is punctured with a #11 surgical blade. Lesions may disappear after recurrent lesions are repeatedly punctured and drained.

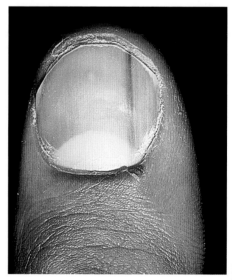

A junction nevus appeared in the nail matrix and produced a longitudinal band.

537

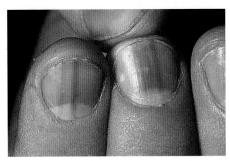

Nail bands occurred in several nails after long-term treatment with minocycline.

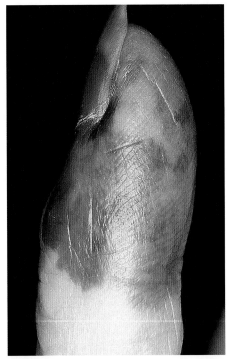

Hutchinson's sign. Extension of pigmentation onto the nail folds is a classic sign of subungual melanoma.

Fungal Nail Infections

Description

- Tinea of the nails is a fungal infection of the finger or toenail plate.
- It is caused by many different species of fungus.
- Once established, it persists. It causes social embarrassment and pain if the nail plate is distorted.

History

- The incidence of fungal nail infections increases with age.
- These infections occur in 15–20% of the population between 40 and 60 years of age.
- They are life long; there is no spontaneous remission.
- Trauma from tight-fitting shoes that are too short predisposes to infection.
- A large mass composed of a thick nail plate and underlying debris may cause discomfort with footwear.

Skin Findings

- There are four distinct patterns of nail infection. Several patterns may occur simultaneously in the nail plate.
- Distal subungual onychomycosis is the most common pattern. Fungi invade the distal area of the nail bed. The distal plate turns yellow or white as an accumulation of hyperkeratotic debris causes the nail to rise and separate from the underlying bed.

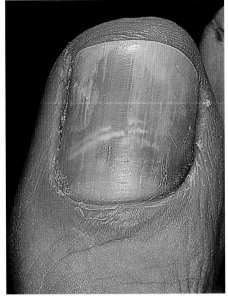

Distal subungual onychomycosis occurs when fungal hyphae invade below the distal nail plate. Proximal extension under and through the nail then follows.

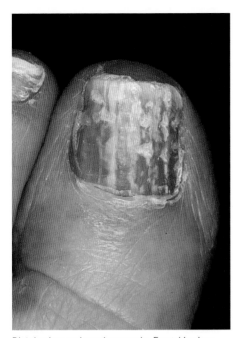

Distal subungual onychomycosis. Fungal hyphae entered the nail plate from the distal groove and have invaded the entire nail plate.

■ White superficial onychomycosis is caused by surface invasion of the nail plate, most often by *Trichophyton mentagrophytes*. The nail surface is soft, dry, and powdery and can easily be scraped away. The nail plate is not thickened and remains adherent to the nail bed.

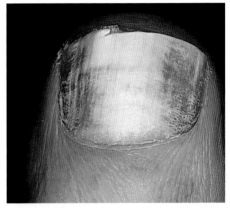

White superficial onychomycosis occurs when fungal hyphae invade the surface of the nail plate.

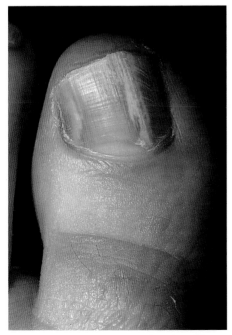

Distal subungual onychomycosis. Invasion of the plate may occur down longitudinal channels. This is a characteristic sign of distal nail plate invasion.

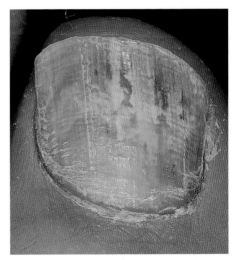

Distal subungual onychomycosis. Wide longitudinal channels are seen in the center of the nail.

- In proximal subungual onychomycosis, microorganisms enter the area of the posterior nail fold cuticle and invade the nail plate from below. The surface remains intact. Hyperkeratotic debris causes the nail to separate. *Trichophyton rubrum* is the most common cause. This is the most common pattern seen in patients with infection of the human immunodeficiency virus.

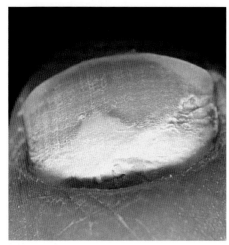

Proximal subungual onychomycosis. Fungal infection of the proximal plate occurs from invasion of fungal hyphae under the proximal nail fold.

- In candidal onychomycosis, nail plate infection caused by *Candida albicans* is seen almost exclusively in chronic mucocutaneous candidiasis—a rare disease. It generally involves all of the fingernails. The nail plate thickens and turns yellow-brown.
- Nail infection may occur with hand or foot tinea or may occur as an isolated phenomenon.

- All nails and the skin are examined to rule out other diseases that mimic onychomycosis.

Etiology

- The dermatophytes *T. rubrum* and *T. mentagrophytes* are responsible for most fingernail and toenail infections.
- *Aspergillus, Cephalosporium, Fusarium,* and *Scopulariopsis* species, considered to be contaminants or non-pathogens, can also infect the nail plate.
- Multiple pathogens may be present in a single nail.

Laboratory

- There is a tendency to label any process involving the nail plate as a fungal infection, but many other cutaneous diseases can change the structure of the nail. Some 50% of thick nails are not infected with fungus.
- In a potassium hydroxide wet mount, the subungual debris and nail plate are examined for hyphae.
- The species of fungus is identified before oral antifungal treatment is started. A culture is performed to establish the presence of dermatophytes—organisms susceptible to itraconazole (Sporanox), terbinafine (Lamisil), and fluconazole (Diflucan).
- There are no clear guidelines for monitoring patients treated with terbinafine, itraconazole, or fluconazole. A prudent approach would be to order a complete blood count and liver function tests before and 6 weeks into treatment. Laboratory monitoring is not required in patients treated with itraconazole (Sporanox) pulse dosing.

Histologic study of a nail clipping is performed if the results of the potassium hydroxide examination and culture are negative but clinical suspicion is high. The results of the histologic tests and periodic acid–Schiff staining are highly reliable for establishing the diagnosis.

Differential Diagnosis

- Psoriasis is most commonly confused with onychomycosis (the two diseases may coexist). Psoriatic nail disease may present as an isolated phenomenon without other cutaneous signs. The single distinguishing feature of psoriasis—pitting of the nail plate surface—is not a feature of fungal infection.
- Leukonychia (the occurrence of white spots or bands that appear proximally and proceed outward with the nail, probably caused by minor trauma).
- Eczema or habitual picking of the proximal nail fold (the nail plate too becomes wavy and ridged).
- Onycholysis (very common in women with long fingernails). It is caused by separation of the nail plate from the nail bed. The yellow or opaque separated nail looks like tinea.

Treatment

- Topical antifungal creams are of little value.
- Oral therapy has the highest success rate in fingernail and nail infections in young persons.
- Prolonged use of topical antifungal agents, such as Penlac Nail Lacquer, after clinical response of onychomycosis to an oral agent, may prevent re-infection.
- Systemic therapy is 50% to over 80% effective. The relapse rate is approximately 15–20% in 1 year.

- Indications for treatment include pain with thick nails, functional limitations, secondary bacterial infection, and appearance.
- Terbinafine (Lamisil) 250 mg/day is administered for 6 weeks for infection of the fingernails and 12 weeks for infection of the toenails. Terbinafine may provide the highest cure rates and longest remission. It is not effective for some candidal species.
- Itraconazole (Sporanox) 200 mg/day is prescribed for 6 weeks for fingernail infection and 12 weeks for toenail infection. Pulse dosing with 200 mg twice a day for 1 week on and then 3 weeks off is also an option. Fingernail infection requires two or three pulses; toenail infection requires three or four pulses.
- Griseofulvin may be effective at very high doses if used for many months but the other drugs are superior.
- Patients are monitored at 6 weeks and at the end of oral therapy. The infected nail plate is debrided at each visit.
- In most cases, nails do not appear clear at 12 weeks. Patients are reassured that the drug remains in the nail plate for months and will continue to kill fungus.
- Ciclopirox topical solution 0.8% (Penlac Nail Lacquer) has been approved for topical treatment of fingernails and toenails without lunula involvement. Penlac may increase the cure rate when used in combination with systemic antifungal agents.
- Nail clippers with pliers handles may be used to remove substantial amounts of hard, thick debris. The pointed tip of the instrument is inserted as far down as possible between the diseased nail and the nail bed.
- Removing the infected nail plate provides higher cure rates and longer remissions.

21 Neonatal Disease

Erythema Toxicum Neonatorum

Description
■ Erythema toxicum neonatorum is a common benign transient pustular eruption seen in the newborn period.

History
■ Erythema toxicum neonatorum occurs more commonly in healthy term infants than in premature and low birth weight infants.
■ The cause of erythema toxicum neonatorum is unknown.

Skin Findings
■ Erythema toxicum neonatorum lesions appear as "blotchy" macules that develop into superficial pink papules and pustules, taking on a "flea-bitten" appearance.
■ Macules can coalesce to form large pink patches studded with only a few to hundreds of pustules.
■ Erythema toxicum neonatorum can occur anywhere on the skin, but the face, arms, buttock, and torso are most frequently involved. The palms and soles are rarely affected.
■ Overall, erythema toxicum neonatorum can wax and wane with individual lesions appearing to occur in crops.

Individual lesions can disappear in hours or last for up to 2 weeks.

Non-skin Findings
■ There are no signs of systemic illness.

Laboratory and Biopsy
■ A smear (Wright's or Giemsa stain) of pustule fluid shows abundant eosinophils with relatively few neutrophils.
■ For atypical cases a skin biopsy can be done, showing subcorneal pustules with eosinophils.

Differential Diagnosis
■ Bacterial infection (*Staphylococcus aureus*, group B *Streptococcus, Pseudomonas aeruginosa, Listeria monocytogenes, Haemophilus influenzae, Klebsiella pneumoniae*)
■ Fungal infection (*Candida*)
■ Viral infection (herpes simplex, varicella)
■ Transient neonatal pustular melanosis
■ Scabies

Course and Prognosis
■ Erythema toxicum neonatorum resolves within 3 weeks of life, without any adverse sequelae.

Treatment
■ No required treatment.
■ Parents should be reassured.

Miliaria

Description

■ Miliaria is the term describing clear to red papules (miliaria crystallina, miliaria rubra, miliaria profunda) that result from obstruction of the eccrine sweat duct.

History

■ Miliaria is very common in newborns and infants who are "bundled" or placed in warm environments.

■ In newborns, miliaria crystallina is the most common type and is due to obstruction of the eccrine duct at the level of the stratum corneum. Warming lights and tight bundling can produce miliaria crystallina.

■ Miliaria rubra ("prickly heat" or "heat rash") is due to obstruction of the intraepidermal eccrine duct, producing leakage of sweat around the duct, and release of local inflammatory mediators. Miliaria rubra affects infants older than 1 week of age.

■ Miliaria profunda is due to eccrine duct obstruction at the dermal–epidermal junction and is rarely seen in newborns.

■ The cause of miliaria is not known, although a polysaccharide produced by certain strains of *Staphylococcus epidermidis* may play a role in obstruction of the eccrine duct.

Skin Findings

■ Miliaria crystallina and miliaria rubra show marked involvement of intertriginous areas such as the neck folds. Other common sites include the face (especially the forehead) and trunk.

■ Miliaria crystallina is characterized by multiple subtle "dew drop" vesicles. These vesicles are very superficial and break easily with gentle friction.

■ Miliaria rubra is characterized by non-follicular pustules and vesicles.

■ Miliaria profunda is characterized by small non-erythematous papules and pustules, occurring on the trunk and extremities.

Non-skin Findings

■ Febrile infants are at risk for developing miliaria.

Laboratory and Biopsy

■ Generally, skin biopsy is not necessary.

Differential Diagnosis

■ Erythema toxicum neonatorum
■ Candidiasis
■ Insect bites

Course and Prognosis

■ Miliaria lasts for hours or days.

Treatment

■ No treatment is necessary other than a cool bath and avoidance of tight bundling.

Cutis Marmorata

Description

■ Cutis marmorata is a transient benign mottling of the skin that resolves with re-warming.

History

■ Cutis marmorata is a common and normal vascular reaction pattern that is seen in both full-term and preterm infants.

■ Infants with Down syndrome, trisomy 18, hypothyroidism, neonatal lupus, and septic shock can develop vascular mottling that does not resolve with re-warming.

■ Cutis marmorata is thought to be due to an exaggerated vasomotor response to decreased core body temperature.

Skin Findings

■ Cutis marmorata manifests as blanching mottled or lace-like erythema that resolves with re-warming.

■ It occurs on the trunk and extremities.

Laboratory and Biopsy

- No laboratory testing or biopsy is required.

Differential Diagnosis

- Cutis marmorata telangiectatica congenita is a rare vascular malformation, showing a reticulated vascular pattern with dermal atrophy.

- Livedo reticularis is the cutis marmorata-like pattern seen in neonatal lupus.

Treatment

- Re-warming results in complete resolution of the erythema.
- Parents should be reassured.

22 Cutaneous Manifestations of Internal Disease

Acquired Cutaneous Paraneoplastic Syndromes

Description
- Acquired cutaneous paraneoplastic syndromes involve cutaneous findings attributed to internal malignancy.
- Some cutaneous signs are specific enough to warrant a search for occult malignancy.
- This chapter will discuss pruritus, the sign of Leser–Trélat, dermatomyositis, Sweet's syndrome, paraneoplastic pemphigus, carcinoid syndrome, and glucagonoma syndrome.

Pruritus
History
- Pruritus is a symptom of many dermatoses.
- In the absence of skin findings, pruritus may indicate occult malignancy.
- Pruritus is more common in gastrointestinal and lymphoreticular malignancies, especially Hodgkin's disease.

Skin Findings
- Pruritus or itching is non-specific and may not be associated with obvious skin changes.
- Patients may scratch during the examination or may show linear erosions or excoriations distributed in reachable areas of the body.

Non-skin Findings
- Pruritus associated with gastrointestinal symptoms, lethargy, weight loss, night sweats or anemia may alert one to look for malignancy-associated pruritus.

Laboratory and Pathology
- Blood evaluation for liver, biliary, pancreatic and renal disease may be helpful. Routine complete blood count, and erythrocyte sedimentation rate may yield clues to a systemic process.

Course and Prognosis
- The clinical course and prognosis usually depend on the associated internal malignancy.

Differential Diagnosis
- Pruritus has numerous causes. Atopic dermatitis, scabies, renal disease, liver disease, and lymphoreticular disease are a few examples.

Treatment
- Usually, the pruritis improves with treatment of the associated malignancy.
- Antihistamines, topical steroids, emollients (vaseline) and antipruritic lotions (Sarna) are helpful.
- Phototherapy (UVB/PUVA) may help.

Sign of Leser-Trélat
History
- The sudden, eruptive appearance of numerous seborrheic keratoses may indicate internal malignancy.
- This exceedingly rare and ominous entity is known as the sign of Leser–Trélat.
- Adenocarcinoma of the gastrointestinal tract is the most common associated type of malignancy.

Skin Findings
- Widespread seborrheic keratoses are seen in the sign of Leser–Trélat. Lesions are small, monomorphic and widespread.

Laboratory

- The histology of seborrheic keratoses in the sign of Leser–Trélat are similar to other seborrheic keratoses.

Course and Prognosis

- The clinical course and prognosis usually depend on the associated internal malignancy.

Differential Diagnosis

- Widespread seborrheic keratosis not associated with malignancy.

Treatment

- The underlying malignancy is treated.
- Inflamed keratosis can be removed with cryotherapy or light electrodesiccation and curettage.

Dermatomyositis

History

- Adults with dermatomyositis are more likely to have an internal malignancy than age-matched controls.
- The prevalence has been estimated at 5–50% with the greatest prevalence among older patients.
- The prevalence of occult malignancy does not appear to be increased in children with dermatomyositis.
- Many malignancies are diagnosed when the dermatomyositis is diagnosed.
- The most common associated malignancies are cancers of the breast, ovary, lung and gastrointestinal tract.

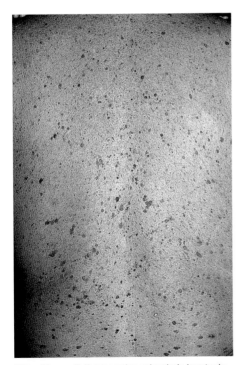

Sign of Leser–Trélat (eruptive seborrheic keratosis as a sign of internal malignancy). The sudden appearance of or sudden increase in the number and size of seborrheic keratosis on non-inflamed skin has been reported to be a sign of internal malignancy.

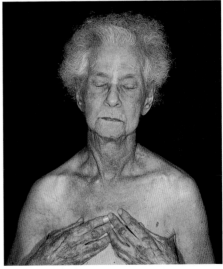

Dermatomyositis. Heliotrope erythema of the eyelids (heliotrope: violet), Gottron's papules (violaceous to red-colored, flat-topped papules that occur over the knuckles and along the sides of the fingers) and a violet erythema that appears on the knuckles and spares the skin over the phalanges and on the sun-exposed areas of the face, neck, back, and arms.

Skin Findings

- The findings of dermatomyositis include Gottron's papules, periorbital heliotrope coloration, photosensitive violaceous eruption, poikiloderma, and periungual telangiectasia.

Non-skin Findings

- Dermatomyositis may be associated with proximal muscle weakness.

Laboratory

- Skin histology shows an interface dermatitis with increased dermal mucin.
- Patients with cutaneous findings suggestive of internal malignancy, without known malignancy, should be carefully evaluated.
- It is especially important to look for ovarian and breast carcinoma in women.

Course and Prognosis

- The clinical course and prognosis usually depend on the associated internal malignancy.

Differential Diagnosis

- Dermatomyositis frequently is confused with lupus and polymorphous light eruption.

Treatment

- Treatment is based on the type of malignancy present.
- Patients with dermatomyositis should be evaluated first by age-appropriate screening for malignancy.

Sweet's Syndrome
History

- Sweet's syndrome is also called acute febrile neutrophilic dermatosis.
- It is a recurrent painful eruption associated with fever, elevated white blood cell count, and arthralgias.
- Women are affected more often than men.
- Sweet's syndrome may be associated with acute infection or with hematologic malignancy, most often acute myelogenous leukemia.

Skin Findings

- The lesions of Sweet's syndrome are red, edematous, pseudovesicular, succulent plaques and coalescing papules. Lesions vary from 0.5–5.0 cm and can be tender on palpation.

Non-skin Findings

- Sweet's syndrome may be associated with an acute infection, in which case there is usually a prodrome of fever and myalgia.

Laboratory

- Histology shows abundant neutrophils without vasculitis.
- Patients with cutaneous findings suggestive of internal malignancy, without known malignancy, should be carefully evaluated.

Course and Prognosis

- The clinical course and prognosis usually depend on the associated internal malignancy.

Differential Diagnosis

- Cellulitis
- Pyoderma gangrenosum
- Other infections

Treatment

- Treatment is based on the type of malignancy present.
- Sweet's syndrome responds to systemic steroids. Malignancy and infection should be ruled out prior to starting steroids.

Paraneoplastic Pemphigus
History

- Paraneoplastic pemphigus is an immunologic blistering disorder of the mucosa.
- It represents a sign of internal malignancy, most often lymphoreticular in nature.
- Chronic lymphocytic leukemia is the most commonly associated malignancy.
- Most patients die from complications of paraneoplastic pemphigus or the underlying malignancy.

Skin Findings

- Paraneoplastic pemphigus presents as ocular inflammation, oral erosions, generalized erythema multiforme-like bullous lesions, and denuded areas with crusting.

Non-skin Findings

■ Paraneoplastic pemphigus is often associated with a hematologic malignancy.

Laboratory

■ Skin biopsy shows supra-basilar acantholysis similar to pemphigus vulgaris.

■ Antibodies targeted to proteins on the keratinocytes and at the dermoepidermal junction can be found in the skin (direct immunofluorescence) and serum (indirect immunofluorescence).

Course and Prognosis

■ The clinical course and prognosis usually depend on the associated internal malignancy.

Differential Diagnosis

■ Paraneoplastic pemphigus mimics other blistering disorders and mucositis due to chemotherapy.

Treatment

■ Treatment is based on the type of malignancy present.

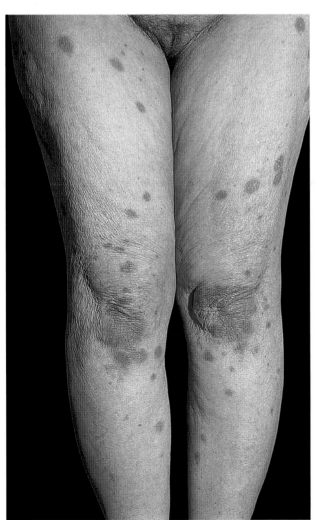

Sweet's syndrome. Acute tender erythematous plaques, pseudovesicles and occasionally blisters with an annular or arciform pattern occur on the head, neck, legs, arms, and particularly the back of the hands and fingers. Careful systemic evaluation is indicated, especially when cutaneous lesions are severe or hematologic values are abnormal. Approximately 20% of cases are associated with malignancy.

Carcinoid Syndrome

History

- Carcinoid syndrome is an episodic, intense flushing of the face, neck, and upper body.
- It is caused by a release of vasoactive mediators from carcinoid tumors into the systemic circulation.
- Most carcinoid tumors arise in the small bowel, usually the appendix.
- Vasoactive mediators released from the tumor are inactivated in the liver before reaching the systemic circulation.
- When carcinoid tumors metastasize to the liver, mediators have access to the systemic circulation.
- Carcinoid tumors also arise in the lung and, as such, release mediators into the systemic circulation.

Skin Findings

- Carcinoid syndrome presents as an acute flushing of the face, neck and chest, that lasts for about 30 minutes. Flushing episodes are often associated with dyspnea, abdominal cramping, and diarrhea.

Non-skin Findings

- Carcinoid syndrome can be associated with an internal bronchial carcinoid tumor or a small bowel carcinoid tumor with hepatic metastases.

Laboratory

- Increased levels of urinary 5-hydroxyindoleacetic acid after 24-hour collection.
- Patients with cutaneous findings suggestive of internal malignancy, without known malignancy, should be carefully evaluated.

Course and Prognosis

- The clinical course and prognosis usually depend on the associated internal malignancy.

Differential Diagnosis

- Carcinoid syndrome can be confused with rosacea, erysipelas and pellagra.

Treatment

- Treatment is based on the type of malignancy present.

Glucagonoma Syndrome

History

- A rare, clinically distinctive syndrome consisting of a dynamic generalized cutaneous eruption associated with a glucagon-secreting tumor of pancreatic α cells.

Skin Findings

- Necrolytic migratory erythema describes the eruption of the glucagonoma syndrome.
- The eruption is generalized but it favors the groin, buttocks and thighs.
- Bright dermal erythema is polycyclic and is followed by flaccid bullae that desquamate, leaving denuded areas and a collarette of scale.
- The process is dynamic, changing and extending each day.

Non-skin Findings

- Glucagonoma syndrome is associated with a tumor of the pancreatic α cells.

Laboratory

- In necrolytic migratory erythema, histology shows characteristic hydropic degeneration of the superficial epidermis along with intracellular edema.

Course and Prognosis

- The clinical course and prognosis usually depend on the associated internal malignancy.

Differential Diagnosis

- Necrolytic migratory erythema may resemble candidiasis or acrodermatitis enteropathica.

Treatment

■ Patients with cutaneous findings suggestive of internal malignancy, without known malignancy, should be carefully evaluated.

■ Treatment is based on the type of malignancy present.

Pearls

■ The importance of recognizing the cutaneous findings associated with internal malignancy lies in the fact that the earliest possible detection of tumor usually offers the best prognosis.

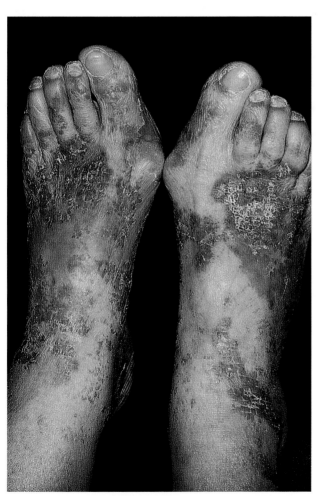

Glucagonoma syndrome (necrolytic migratory erythema). The dermatitis begins as an erythematous area, progresses to superficial blisters, and gradually spreads ("migrates") with central crusting and then healing, followed by hyperpigmentation 7–14 days after the initial erythema.

Inherited Cutaneous Paraneoplastic Syndromes

Description
- Inherited cutaneous paraneoplastic syndromes involve cutaneous findings associated with heritable or genetically related conditions that carry an increased risk of internal malignancy.
- This chapter will discuss Cowden syndrome, Gardner syndrome and Muir–Torre syndrome.

History
- A variety of cutaneous lesions may be associated with internal malignancy.
- Recognition of such signs is only of value if it leads to the prevention, early detection, or treatment of internal malignancy.
- Several genodermatoses carry an increased risk of malignancy.
- Patients with such an inherited disorder may benefit from increased surveillance.
- Genetic testing and counseling may be important to patients and their families.

Cowden Syndrome
Description
- Cowden syndrome—or multiple hamartoma syndrome—is a rare disorder, affecting multiple organ systems.
- Affected people will develop benign and malignant tumors.
- Ductal carcinoma of the breast occurs in more than 30% of female patients with Cowden syndrome. Thyroid carcinoma is also common.

Skin Findings
- In Cowden syndrome characteristic varieties of facial and oral papules develop during early adulthood.
- The facial papules (most often trichilemmomas) are 1–3 mm, smooth and skin-colored, and are concentrated around the eyes, nose, malar cheeks and mouth.
- Biopsy usually confirms the papule as a trichilemmoma, which is characteristic of Cowden syndrome.

- The oral mucosal papules are 1 mm, smooth and white, coalescing into a cobblestone pattern on the tongue and gingiva.
- Punctate keratoses of the palms and soles occur in roughly half of patients.

Non-skin Findings
- A variety of benign and malignant neoplasms have been reported in people with Cowden syndrome.
- Females have a significantly increased risk of ductal carcinoma of the breast.
- Macrocephaly is also commonly seen in Cowden syndrome.

Laboratory and Pathology
- Skin biopsy of the facial papules seen in Cowden syndrome most often confirms the lesion as a trichilemmoma—a benign adnexal tumor.

Course and Prognosis
- The prognosis depends on the malignancy, the stage at the time of diagnosis, and the treatment.

Treatment
- Screening of family members and genetic counseling are indicated for genodermatoses with an increased risk of malignancy.
- Females suspected of having Cowden syndrome should have regular breast examinations, mammograms and very close follow-up.
- Prophylactic bilateral mastectomy has been suggested by some.

Gardner Syndrome
Description
- Gardner syndrome is an autosomal dominant condition consisting of multiple epidermal cysts, fibrous tumors of the skin and subcutaneous tissue, and associated intestinal polyposis.
- Intestinal polyps are usually limited to the colon.
- Malignant degeneration of polyps occurs in 50% of patients.
- There is usually a family history of colon cancer.

FAMILIAL MULTIPLE CANCER SYNDROMES
AUTOSOMAL DOMINANT 'CANCER FAMILY SYNDROMES'

Cowden's disease	**Muir–Torre syndrome**	**Gardener's syndrome**
(Multiple hamartoma syndrome)		(familial adenomatous polyposis with extraintestinal manifestations)

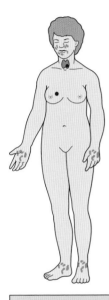 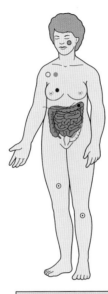 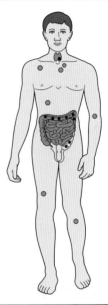

Females

Mucocutaneous lesions
– facial papules
– oral papules
– hand keratosis

Breast lesions
– cancer
– fibrocystic

Thyroid
– goiter
– carcinoma

Males = females

Skin tumors
– sebaceous gland
  (at least one)

Keratoacanthomas

Internal tumors
– colorectal
– genitourinary
– breast

• Solid tumors

Males = females

Skin signs
– epidermal cysts

Osteomas (palpable)
– skull
– jaw

Pigmented ocular fundus
  lesions

Colon
– polyps > 100
– adenocarcinoma

Thyroid carcinoma

Skin Findings

- People with Gardner syndrome develop multiple epidermal cysts, most commonly on the face and scalp.
- Discrete fibrous tumors of the skin are rarely symptomatic.
- Multiple pilar cysts of the scalp are not associated with Gardner syndrome.

Non-skin Findings

- People with Gardner syndrome develop osteomas of the membranous bones of the head, which are visible on x-ray films.
- Pigmented lesions of the retinal fundus are found in 90% of patients.
- Fundal lesions are usually present in infancy and are useful as a screening finding.

Laboratory

- In Gardner syndrome, histologic testing confirms the scalp cysts as epidermal cysts, rather than pilar cysts.

Course and Prognosis

- The prognosis depends on the malignancy, stage at the time of diagnosis, and the treatment.

Treatment

- Screening of family members and genetic counseling are indicated for genodermatoses with an increased risk of malignancy.
- People suspected of having Gardner syndrome should undergo colonoscopy.
- Prophylactic colectomy is usually recommended for patients with Gardner syndrome.

Muir–Torre Syndrome

Description

- Muir-Torre syndrome is an autosomal dominant condition of multiple benign cutaneous sebaceous tumors and colonic polyps with increased risk of malignant degeneration.

Skin Findings

- Muir-Torre syndrome is suggested by the presence of multiple benign tumors of the sebaceous glands, including sebaceous adenoma, sebaceous epithelioma, and or sebaceous carcinoma.
- Of these tumors, the most specific for Muir-Torre is the sebaceous adenoma.
- Patients with Muir-Torre syndrome also develop keratoacanthomas with distinctive sebaceous differentiation.
- Sebaceous hyperplasia is a common condition in otherwise healthy people and is not considered part of the Muir-Torre syndrome.

Non-skin Findings

- A variety of genitourinary malignancies have been described in the Muir-Torre syndrome—all with low incidence.
- The most common malignancy is colon carcinoma, which is usually proximal to the splenic flexure.
- Individuals suspected of having the Muir-Torre syndrome should be screened by colonoscopy.

Laboratory

- Sebaceous adenoma is the most characteristic lesion of Muir-Torre syndrome. Such lesions may have architecture reminiscent of keratoacanthoma.

Course and Prognosis

- The prognosis depends on the malignancy, the stage at the time of diagnosis, and the treatment.

Treatment

- Patients suspected of having Muir-Torre syndrome should undergo colonoscopy.

Discussion

- Screening of family members and genetic counseling are indicated for genodermatoses with an increased risk of malignancy.
- Patients with genodermatoses may benefit from increased surveillance for likely cutaneous and internal tumors.
- Families of affected people may benefit from screening examination and from genetic counseling.

Pearls

- Patients with multiple trichilemmoma should raise the possibility of Cowden syndrome.
- A patient with multiple epidermal cysts of the face and scalp should raise suspicion of Gardner syndrome.
- A skin biopsy showing sebaceous adenoma or keratoacanthoma with sebaceous differentiation should suggest Muir-Torre syndrome.

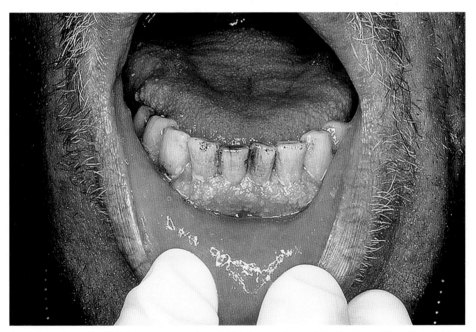

Cowden syndrome (multiple hamartoma syndrome). This is an autosomal dominant condition with variable expression. Hamartomata of the skin and mucosa occur in over 90% of cases. There is an increase in the incidence of breast cancer in women and thyroid cancer in men and women. Other malignancies are reported. Oral mucosal papillomatosus, seen here, are 1–3 mm smooth surfaced, white papules. They are present in the gingival, labial, and palatal surfaces of the mouth. Numerous confluent lesions have a cobblestone appearance. Acral keratoses, and palmoplantar keratoses are commonly seen.

Acanthosis Nigricans

Description

- Acanthosis nigricans is a thickened, velvety hyperpigmentation of the flexural skin.
- It is most commonly associated with obesity and diabetes.
- Less common associations are other endocrine disorders, medications and occult malignancy.

History

- Patients usually complain of an asymptomatic, dirty appearance to the skinfolds that cannot be removed by vigorous washing.
- Usually there is a gradual onset when it is associated with diabetes and obesity.
- Malignancy-associated acanthosis nigricans develops more rapidly and suddenly.
- Attempts to rub, scrub or remove the skin changes are futile.
- There may be a family history of the eruption.

Skin Findings

- There is a symmetric, velvety brown thickening of the skin.
- The surface is rough, warty, or papillomatous.
- The axillae and neck are most commonly involved.
- The crural folds, the belt line, the dorsal fingers, umbilicus, mouth and areolae of the breast may also be involved.
- The severity is variable from mild to extensive.
- Acanthosis nigricans is usually asymptomatic.

Non-skin Findings

- Acanthosis nigricans is a cutaneous marker of tissue insulin resistance.
- Patients without diabetes have high levels of circulating insulin or an impaired response to exogenous insulin.
- The vulva is commonly affected in obese, hirsute, hyperandrogenic, or insulin-resistant women.
- HAIR-AN syndrome is **h**yperandrogenism, **i**nsulin **r**esistance, and **a**canthosis nigricans.

Laboratory

- Glucose levels may be elevated. Other studies are not routinely done.
- There are high levels of circulating insulin.
- There is an impaired response to exogenous insulin.

Discussion and Treatment

- Acanthosis nigricans can be caused by medications such as estrogens and nicotinic acid.
- Other endocrinologic disorders, such as pineal gland tumors, are possible etiologies.
- The eruption is usually asymptomatic and does not require treatment.
- Reducing thick lesions in areas of maceration may decrease the odor and promote comfort.
- Lac-Hydrin, a 12% lactic acid cream, is applied twice a day.
- Retinoic acid (Retin-A cream or gel) applied each day, or less often if irritation occurs, can be helpful.
- There is no treatment that is uniformly effective at completely eradicating the skin changes.

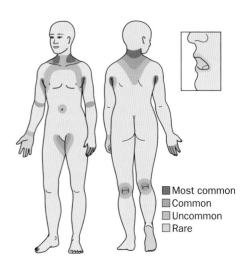

- Most common
- Common
- Uncommon
- Rare

Pearls

- The most common areas involved are the axillae and neck.
- Patients who have this during puberty and into adulthood, usually have insulin resistance.

- A sudden onset and extensive acanthosis nigricans should prompt an evaluation for internal malignancy, such as stomach adenocarcinoma, or new medications such as nicotinic acid.

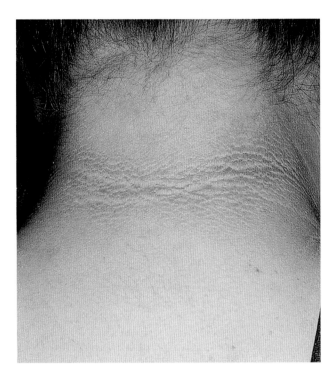

The most common site of involvement is the axilla, but the changes may be observed in the flexural areas of the neck and groin, at the belt line, over the dorsal surfaces of the fingers, in the mouth, and around the areolae of the breasts and umbilicus.

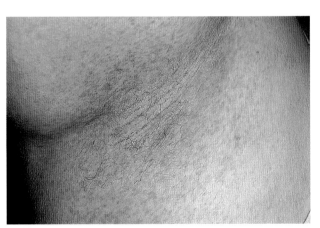

There is a symmetric brown thickening of the skin in the axillae. In time the skin may becomes thickened as the lesion develops a leathery, warty, or papillomatous surface.

Neurofibromatosis

Description

■ Neurofibromatosis is an inherited disorder of the skin and central nervous system made up of at least seven clinical variants.

■ Neurofibromatosis type I is the most common variant.

■ It is also called von Recklinghausen disease.

History

■ The inheritance is autosomal dominant, however 50% of cases arise from a new mutation.

■ The incidence is estimated at 1 in 3000. It affects males and females equally.

■ The pathogenesis is believed to be a defect in the neurofibromin gene.

■ Neurofibromin is a suppressor of products of *ras* proto-oncogenes, and its loss leads to tumor progression.

■ Neurofibromatosis is characterized clinically by café-au-lait macules, neurofibromas, axillary and groin freckling, Lisch nodules in the iris, and body defects.

Skin Findings

■ Neurofibromas are pink or flesh-colored, soft, pedunculated papules, that may be tender. The number varies from a few to hundreds or thousands.

■ Dermal and subcutaneous neurofibromas can be present at around 5 years of age, but typically start appearing around puberty and increase in number with age and with pregnancy.

■ Café-au-lait macules are randomly distributed, tan to brown patches which increase in number and size in the first 5 years of life; more than six café-au-lait macules over 5 mm in diameter suggests the presence of neurofibromatosis 1.

■ Axillary or inguinal freckling (the Crowe sign) is specific for the disease.

■ Plexiform neurofibromas occur along the course of peripheral nerves, creating large, tender nodules, or poorly demarcated masses, often with overlying hyperpigmentation and hypertrichosis.

About 20% of neurofibromatosis patients have plexiform neurofibromas. When present, these tumors are highly diagnostic of neurofibromatosis.

■ Malignant degeneration of cutaneous neural tumors occurs in 2% of patients but is rare before the age of 40.

Non-skin Findings

■ Lisch nodules are asymptomatic iris hamartomas and occur in more than 90% of neurofibromatosis patients over age 6. A slit-lamp examination is needed for Lisch nodules.

■ Optic gliomas occur in two-thirds of patients; they are usually asymptomatic but may lead to blindness.

■ Other tumors of the central nervous system that are seen with increased frequency include astrocytomas, meningioma, vestibular schwannoma (acoustic neuroma), and ependymomas.

■ Patient may have seizures, learning disabilities, poor coordination, and hydrocephalus.

■ Non-central nervous system tumors occurring in neurofibromatosis 1 include neurofibrosarcoma, rhabdomyosarcoma, pheochromocytoma, and Wilms tumor.

■ Renovascular abnormalities may include renal artery stenosis.

■ Skeletal abnormalities include short stature, scoliosis, sphenoid wing dysplasia, and macrocephaly.

■ Peer relationships and psychosocial adjustment are often major issues during adolescence.

Laboratory, Radiology and Pathology

■ Magnetic resonance imaging of the brain and spinal cord may show various central nervous system tumors.

■ Histologically, neurofibromas are well-circumscribed, unencapsulated aggregations of small nerve fibers and spindle cells, with wavy nuclei in the dermis.

■ Genetic testing is available.

Course and Prognosis

■ There is great variation in the severity of the disorder.

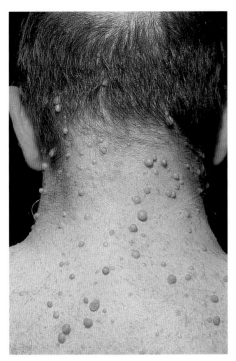

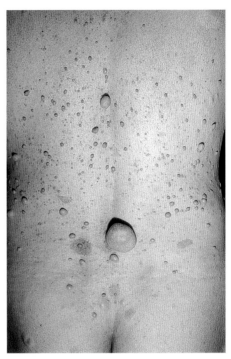

Tumors are usually not present in childhood, but they begin to appear at puberty. Tumors increase in both number and size as the patient ages.

Tumors. The most common is sessile or pedunculated. Early tumors are soft dome-shaped papules or nodules that have a distinctive violaceous hue. Most are benign.

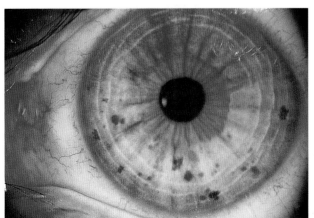

Lisch nodules are pigmented, melanocytic, iris hamartomas. They increase in number with age and are asymptomatic. All adults with neurofibromatosis who are 21 years of age or older have Lisch nodules. Slit-lamp examination is essential for differentiation from iris freckles or nevi.

- Vision and cognitive function may be impaired by central nervous system tumors.
- Central nervous system tumors are usually not present in childhood, but they begin to appear at puberty.
- Tumors increase in both number and size as the patient ages.
- Life-threatening complications may include seizures, increased intracranial pressure, vascular complications from hypertension, and malignancy.

Discussion

- The differential diagnosis includes McCune–Albright syndrome, Noonan syndrome, and Proteus syndrome.
- Consensus criteria for diagnosis were adopted in 1987 by the National Institutes of Health. These criteria require two or more of the following features:
  - Six or more café-au-lait macules over 5 mm in greatest diameter in prepubertal children and over 15 mm in greatest diameter in postpubertal people
  - Two or more neurofibromas of any type, or one plexiform neurofibroma
  - Freckling in the axillary or inguinal regions
  - Optic glioma
  - Two or more Lisch nodules
  - A distinctive osseous lesion such as sphenoid dysplasia or thinning of long-bone cortex, with or without pseudoarthrosis
  - A first-degree relative (parent or sibling) with neurofibromatosis 1
- Lisch nodules are rare in the general population, so their presence in people aged more than 6 years—suspected of having neurofibromatosis—is virtually diagnostic.

Treatment

- Care is best performed via a multidisciplinary approach, with regular follow-up by the primary care physician, ophthalmologist, neurologist, and dermatologist.
- Head circumference and blood pressure should be monitored closely in children.
- Hypertension in a child may indicate renal artery stenosis. In an adult, it may suggest pheochromocytoma.
- The patient should be referred to an orthopedist, a psychiatrist, and a neurosurgeon, as indicated.
- First-degree relatives should be screened for cutaneous and ophthalmologic signs of neurofibromatosis.
- Genetic counseling of patients and their families is recommended.
- There is a 50% chance of inheritance with nearly 100% penetrance. Patients who inherit the gene show clinical signs of NF-1.

Pearls

- An ophthalmologist should perform a slit-lamp examination looking for Lisch nodules. These lesions are highly specific findings for neurofibromatosis 1.
- Patients and their families should be encouraged to contact local neurofibromatosis support groups. The Neurofibromatosis Foundation (http://www.nf.org; Tel: 800 323 7938) has many resources.

Pediatric Considerations

- Definitive diagnosis may not be possible until the pubertal years.
- Café-au-lait macules and neurofibromas are not necessarily diagnostic of neurofibromatosis, unless they are associated with other signs and meet the criteria above.
- Neuroimaging the asymptomatic neurofibromatosis patient is controversial. Seizures, hypertension, and musculoskeletal changes may warrant radiologic work-up early in the disease process.
- Children with multiple café-au-lait macules, but who do not fulfill clinical diagnostic criteria for neurofibromatosis 1, should have the following annual examinations:
  - Eye examination in first decade of life (looking for optic gliomas)
  - Developmental assessment
  - Scoliosis monitoring
  - Complete neurologic examination
  - Blood pressure screening

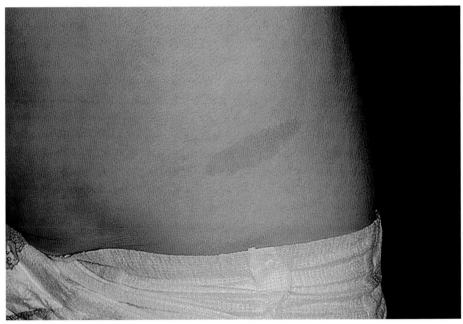

Café-au-lait spots are the earliest manifestation of neurofibromatosis. The brown macules can appear in infancy. They enlarge in size after age 2. They show marked variation in size. Some have smooth borders, others are irregular. Many small lesions occurring in the axillae are referred to as axillary freckling. This is a pathognomic sign of neurofibromatosis. Patients may have café-au-lait spots as an isolated finding. They are also found in tuberous sclerosis, Fanconi anemia and McCune-Albright syndrome.

Tuberous Sclerosis

Description

■ Tuberous sclerosis is an uncommon genodermatosis with characteristic features of the skin and central nervous system, as well as multiple other organs.

■ Tuberous sclerosis is also called Bourneville's disease and epiloia.

History

■ The incidence is estimated at 1 to 10,000, with an equal male and female ratio.

■ Spontaneous mutations account for 75% of cases and autosomal dominant transmission the other 25%.

■ Two separate genes have been implicated.

Skin Findings

■ The disorder typically presents at or just after birth.

■ The earliest sign is "ash leaf" hypopigmented macules, usually found on the trunk or extremities.

■ Hypopigmented macules are also found in 0.2–0.3% of normal neonates but are present in at least half of those with tuberous sclerosis.

■ Polygonal, hypopigmented "confetti" macules are also common, especially in the pretibial area.

■ Wood's light examination accentuates the appearance of ash-leaf macules.

■ Facial angiofibromas, also named adenoma sebaceum, appear in early childhood and increase in number throughout adolescence. These benign hamartomas are smooth and firm, pink papules measuring 1–5 mm, that appear on the nasolabial folds, cheeks, and chin.

■ The shagreen patch is a connective tissue nevus seen in roughly 80% of patients with tuberous sclerosis. Typically located in the lumbosacral area, the shagreen patch is a 1–5-cm, white to yellow plaque, with a pebbled surface.

■ Periungual fibromas are conical, pink, firm projections from the posterior nail folds of the fingers and toes. They appear around the time of puberty and persist indefinitely. Histologically, these are angiofibromas.

■ Fibrous, flesh-colored, discrete plaques on the forehead are sometimes seen and, if present, are considered to be virtually pathognomonic of tuberous sclerosis.

Non-skin Findings

■ Cortical tubers consisting of astrocytes and giant cells, paraventricular calcification, subependymal hamartomas, and astrocytomas may be seen via imaging studies of the head.

■ Seizures occur in 75% of patients with central nervous system lesions.

■ Infantile spasms and mental retardation are also part of the syndrome.

■ Retinal hamartomas (phakomas) may be seen on funduscopic examination.

■ Angiomyolipoma and multiple cysts may be seen on renal ultrasound.

■ Cardiac rhabdomyoma may be visualized by echocardiogram.

■ Careful examination of the oral cavity may reveal enamel pits and gingival fibromas.

■ Phalangeal cysts and periosteal thickening may be seen on plain films of the hands.

■ Pulmonary cysts may be seen on chest x-ray film and may occasionally result in spontaneous pneumothorax.

Laboratory and Pathology

■ Skin biopsy of ash-leaf macules shows the presence of melanocytes but a decrease in melanin, which is different from vitiligo in which all melanocytes are destroyed.

■ Histology of a shagreen patch shows an increased number of collagen bundles, which is consistent with connective tissue nevus.

■ Transfontanelle ultrasound, computed tomography, and magnetic resonance imaging may demonstrate both benign and malignant central nervous system lesions.

■ An electroencephalogram may reveal areas of seizure activity.

■ Funduscopic examination confirms the presence of retinal hamartomas.

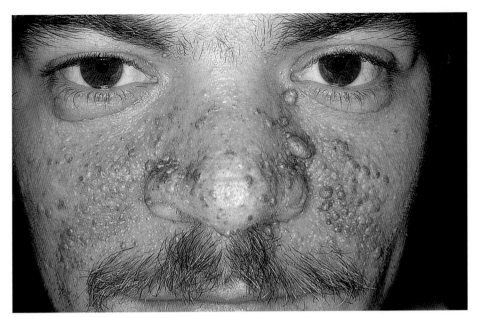

Adenoma sebaceum is the most common cutaneous manifestation of tuberous sclerosis. The lesions consist of smooth and firm 1–5-mm, yellow-pink papules with fine telangiectasia.

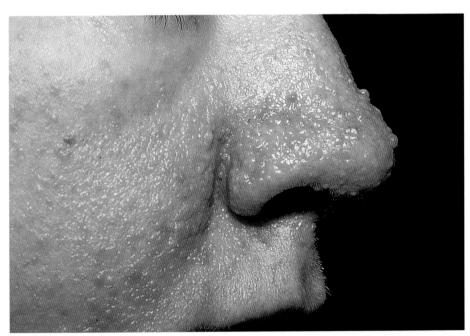

Adenoma sebaceum. The angiofibromas are located on the nasolabial folds, the cheeks and chin, and occasionally the forehead, scalp and ears. The number varies from a few inconspicuous lesions to dense clusters of papules. They are rare at birth but may begin to appear by ages 2–3 years and proliferate during puberty.

- Renal ultrasound and echocardiogram should be performed in neonates when the diagnosis of tuberous sclerosis is suspected.

Course and Prognosis
- About 40% of affected people have normal intelligence; the remainder have subtle or mild mental retardation.
- Cutaneous manifestations may not correlate with mental ability.
- Premature death occurs rarely, most often from status epilepticus or malignant brain tumor.

Differential Diagnosis
- Hypopigmented macules
  - Nevus anemicus
  - Vitiligo
  - Hypomelanosis of Ito
  - Idiopathic guttate hypomelanosis
- Shagreen patch
  - Congenital nevus
  - Hamartoma
- Adenoma sebaceum
  - Acne
  - Cowden syndrome
  - Multiple endocrine neoplasia
  - Multiple trichoepitheliomas
  - Birt–Hogg–Dube syndrome

Treatment
- Complete physical examination with routine follow-up by the primary care physician.
- Imaging studies should be performed to look for cardiac, renal and central nervous system tumors.
- Referral to a pediatric neurologist, including long-term follow-up, should be considered for seizure management.
- Baseline ophthalmologic evaluation should be performed.

- Carbon dioxide laser ablation of facial angiofibromas can significantly improve the cosmetic appearance and self-image.
- If needed, special educational planning should help the patient reach maximal potential.
- Careful cutaneous and general examination of first-degree relatives, as well as genetic counseling, is recommended.

Pediatric Considerations
- Adenoma sebaceum lesions or facial angiofibromas are common in tuberous sclerosus patients and may be misdiagnosed as acne. Cosmetic removal may be indicated.
- Hypomelanotic macules are the earliest sign of tuberous sclerosis and can be missed unless examined with a Wood's lamp.
- Imaging studies of the cranium should be obtained once the diagnosis is confirmed to look for subependymal nodules. These may be difficult to distinguish from astrocytomas.
- Local and national support groups (e.g. Tuberous Sclerosis Alliance; http://www.tsalliance.org) can be valuable sources of information and comfort to affected families.

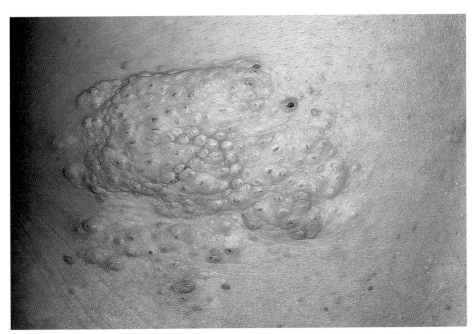

The shagreen patch. There is usually one lesion, but several may be present. They are soft flesh-colored to yellow plaques with an irregular surface that has been likened to pig skin. The lesion consists of dermal connective tissue and appears most commonly in the lumbosacral region.

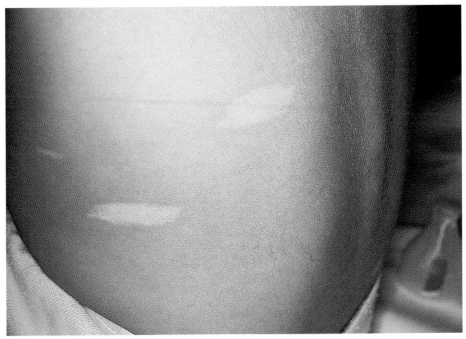

Hypomelanotic macules (oval or ash-leaf shaped, stippled, or confetti-shaped) are randomly distributed with a concentration on the arms, legs, and trunk. They are the earliest sign of tuberous sclerosis.

Granuloma Annulare

Description

■ Granuloma annulare is a slowly progressive, self-limited, granulomatous-like dermal skin disease.

■ It is characterized by round or annular plaques that may initially resemble tinea and spontaneously disappear after a number of years.

■ There is a localized form and a more rare generalized form.

History

■ The female to male ratio is 2 to 1.

■ About 70% of patients are younger than 30 years of age, and 40% are younger than 15 years.

■ The duration is highly variable.

■ 50% of patients are clear in 2 years, but 40% experience recurrence in the same site.

■ Lesions tend to be asymptomatic.

■ Patients become concerned when multiple lesions in multiple areas develop and expand.

Skin Findings

■ The disease begins with an asymptomatic, flesh-colored papule that undergoes central involution.

■ Small firm flesh-colored or violaceous papules then develop in a ring-like fashion.

■ Over months the ring of papules coalesce into a concentric annular plaque that slowly increases in diameter to 0.5–10 cm.

■ The localized form, most common in young women, is usually found on the lateral or dorsal surfaces of the hands and feet, and the extensor aspects of the arms and legs.

■ Individual lesions may persist for many years, then vanish, only to appear later in life at the same or different locations.

■ Disseminated or generalized granuloma annulare occurs in adults and appears with numerous flesh-colored or violaceous papules, some of which form annular rings. The papules may be accentuated in sun-exposed areas. The course is variable, but may persist for many years.

Non-skin Findings

■ There are conflicting reports about the association of granuloma annulare with diabetes mellitus.

■ Most patients with the localized form do not have clinical or laboratory evidence of diabetes.

■ The association between disseminated granuloma annulare and diabetes has been established, but the frequency is unknown.

Laboratory and Pathology

■ The clinical presentation is characteristic, and biopsy may not be required.

■ Histologic testing shows characteristic collagen degeneration, chronic inflammation, and fibrosis.

Differential Diagnosis

■ Tinea

■ Necrobiosis lipoidica

■ Nummular eczema

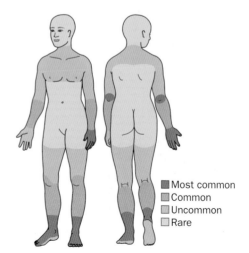

■ Most common
■ Common
■ Uncommon
□ Rare

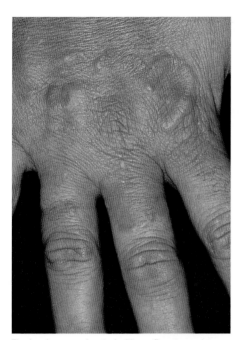

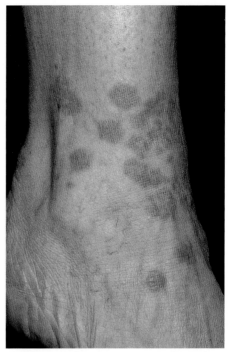

The borders are elevated with confluent papules. Patients might think they have "ring worm". The eruption extends peripherally for months and usually resolves spontaneously in 2–3 years.

Granuloma annulare. The disease begins with an asymptomatic flesh-colored papule that undergoes central involution. The ankle is a common site.

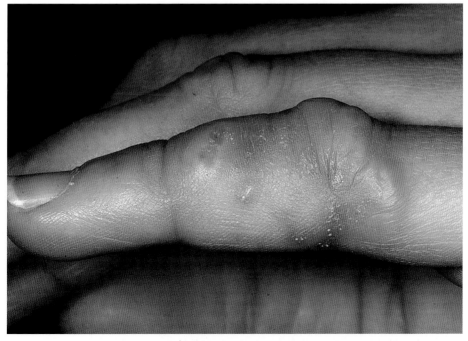

This lesion was dense enough to restrict range of motion of the finger.

567

Treatment

- Localized lesions are asymptomatic and are usually left untreated.
- Superpotent topical steroids used daily at intervals of 2–3 weeks are sometimes effective.
- Lower-potency topical steroids can be occluded for shorter periods of time.
- Intralesional triamcinolone acetonide 2.5–5 mg/ml should be injected only into the elevated border. This is predictably effective and induces long periods of remission. Local atrophy is the potential side effect.
- Disseminated granuloma annulare has been reported occasionally to respond to dapsone 100–200 mg daily, to isotretinoin, hydroxychloroquine, and niacinamide 1.5 g daily.

Pearls

- Granuloma annulare is often diagnosed as tinea because of the round pattern. The border of granuloma annulare does not scale, whereas the border of tinea usually does.
- Unlike necrobiosis lipoidica, granuloma annulare is rarely associated with diabetes.

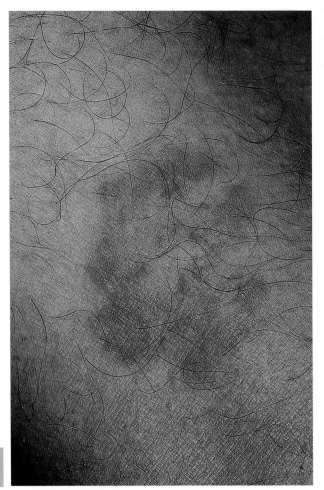

This plaque has been present for months. The borders are not elevated and a biopsy was necessary to confirm the diagnosis of granuloma annulare.

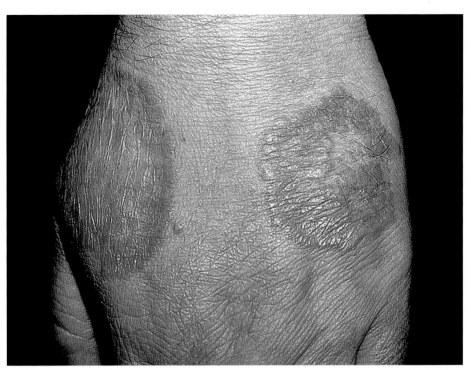

Granuloma annulare. Granuloma annulare is characterized by a ring of small and firm flesh-colored or red papules.

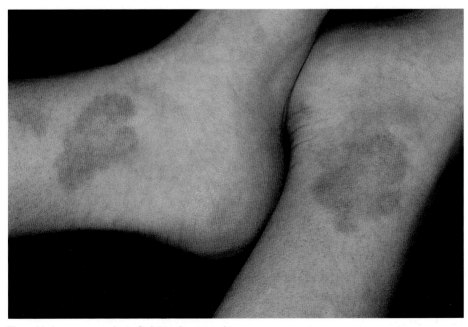

The ankle is a common site to find granuloma annulare.

Necrobiosis Lipoidica

Description
- Necrobiosis lipoidica is an inflammatory condition characterized by collagen degeneration.
- When present, necrobiosis lipoidica is often associated with diabetes; therefore it is called necrobiosis lipoidica diabeticorum.
- However, only 1% of patients with diabetes develop necrobiosis lipoidica.

History
- More than 50% of people with necrobiosis lipoidica also have insulin-dependent diabetes.
- Lesions may appear years before the onset of diabetes.
- Lesions usually develop slowly and are often asymptomatic.
- The onset may occur at any age but the disease most commonly starts in the third and fourth decades.
- About 75% of those affected are women.

Skin Findings
- Lesions are usually limited to the anterior shins but may be seen on the calves, thighs, arms, hands, feet, and scalp.
- They begin as round, violaceous patches and slowly expand.
- The advancing border is red, and the central area turns a characteristic orange-yellow to brown.
- The central area atrophies and shows a shiny, waxy surface with prominent telangiectasias.
- Ulceration may occur, particularly after trauma, in about 15% of cases. These ulcers are exquisitely tender.

Non-skin Findings
- The term necrobiosis lipoidica diabeticorum has fallen out of favor because a significant minority of affected people do not have diabetes.

Laboratory
- Clinical features are often so characteristic that biopsy is not required, although in some cases it can be helpful.
- Since necrobiosis lipoidica diabeticorum may be the presenting sign of diabetes, a glucose tolerance test may be considered.

Course and Prognosis
- The number or severity of lesions or ulcerations has not been correlated with the degree of diabetic control.
- The course is unpredictable.
- Lesions usually heal with atrophic scarring or can be chronic and recurrent.

Treatment
- Topical and intralesional steroids arrest inflammation but promote further atrophy.
- Mid-potency to high-potency corticosteroids can be used under occlusion.
- Intralesional injections can be helpful; the concentration of triamcinolone acetonide (Kenalog) 10 mg/ml should be diluted with saline or Xylocaine, up to 2.5 mg/ml, to avoid atrophy.
- A short course (5–6 weeks) of oral corticosteroids can be considered if disease activity and symptoms are severe, but this is rarely the case.
- Pentoxifylline (Trental) 400 mg three times a day is helpful in some, and has been used in combination with low-dose aspirin for ulcerating necrobiosis lipoidica.
- Skin grafting can be effective for extensive disease.

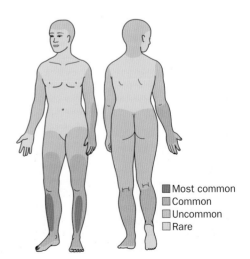

■ Most common
□ Common
□ Uncommon
□ Rare

Pearls

■ Patients with necrobiosis lipoidica, without overt diabetes, should be evaluated periodically for the development of diabetes.

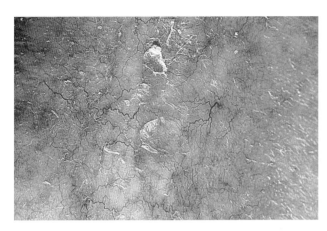

The eruption begins as an oval violaceous patch and expands slowly. The advancing border is red and the central area turns yellow-brown. The central area atrophies and has a waxy surface. Telangiectasias become prominent.

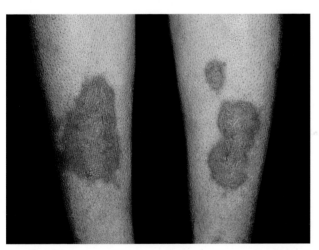

More than 50% of patients with this condition are generally insulin dependent. Most are females, and in most cases the lesions are confined to the anterior surfaces of the lower legs.

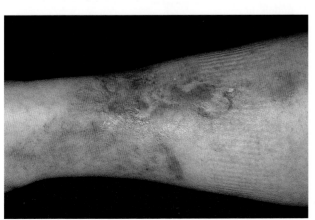

Chronic inflammation and ulceration healed with bound down scars. Treatment with intralesional corticosteroids helped to control the disease activity.

Pyoderma Gangrenosum

Description
- Pyoderma gangrenosum is a necrotizing, non-infectious, inflammatory skin disease characterized by a rapidly enlarging, painful ulceration, usually on the legs.

History
- Lesions may begin spontaneously or at the site of trauma.
- The majority of cases occur in people aged between 25 and 55 years.
- Pyoderma gangrenosum is rare in children.
- The disease is commonly associated with inflammatory bowel disease (Crohn's disease, ulcerative colitis) and rheumatoid arthritis.
- Less commonly it is associated with chronic active hepatitis, immunoglobulin G monoclonal gammopathy, myelodysplasia, paraproteinemia, myeloid leukemias, myeloma and various solid tumors.
- Pathergy (enlargement of the lesion) with trauma is a characteristic of pyoderma gangrenosum.
- Postsurgical pyoderma gangrenosum may masquerade as wound dehiscence or infection.

Skin Findings
- The most common sites are the lower legs, buttocks, and abdomen; it is rare to see pyoderma gangrenosum on the face.
- The lesion begins as a tender red or dusky macule, papule, pustule, nodule, or bulla.
- The initial lesion is often described as a pustule or inflamed red nodule that ulcerates, forming a painful, sharply marginated, violaceously bordered ulcer with a purulent base.
- The edge of the ulcer is characteristically elevated (undermined) and violaceous and may have tiny pustules along the border.
- Expansion of the ulceration can occur rapidly.
- The fully evolved, classic ulcerated lesion is generally smaller than 10 cm.
- Multiple lesions are usually present.
- Eventually lesions may coalesce into larger ulcers with crater-like holes and with small fistula tracks. This is a highly characteristic feature.
- Lesions gradually heal, with irregular, cribiform or stellate scarring.
- Historically, pyoderma gangrenosum is divided into four variants, including pustular, bullous, ulcerative and vegetative forms, but each of these types may coexist in the same patient and one lesion may evolve from one variant to another.

Non-skin Findings
- Pyoderma gangrenosum without a history of inflammatory bowel disease may exist, but this is the most common association and newly diagnosed patients should be evaluated even if there are no gastrointestinal symptoms.
- Arthritis may also accompany the ulcers of pyoderma gangrenosum.
- Most cases of an internal malignancy-associated pyoderma gangrenosum are due to a known cancer, but one should look for internal malignancy if not initially evident.

Laboratory
- The histology of pyoderma gangrenosum is not always diagnostic.
- There are characteristic changes, such as hemorrhage, necrosis, vasculitis and coagulation, at the advancing border.

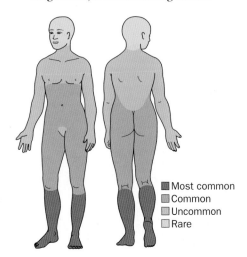

- Most common
- Common
- Uncommon
- Rare

There is a massive inflammatory cell infiltrate with neutrophils and other cell types. Therefore, pyoderma gangrenosum is considered to be a neutrophilic dermatosis.
- Serum protein electrophoresis looks for an underlying gammopathy.
- Associated conditions should be sought and infections excluded.

Differential Diagnosis
- Infected ulcer (*Mycobacteria*, syphilis, deep fungus, *Clostridium*)
- Sweet's syndrome
- Behçet's disease
- Systemic vasculitis (especially Wegener's granulomatosis)
- Spider bite

Treatment
Systemic Therapy
- Hospitalization may be necessary for severe cases.
- Analgesia is often required.
- Most patients require combination therapy with multiple immunosuppressants to obtain control.
- High-dose systemic oral steroids (1–3 mg/kg) or intravenous steroids (1 g/day) for 3–10 days should be administered initially to try to quickly suppress the immune response.
- Cyclosporin 3–5 mg/kg may be the best non-steroidal immunosuppressant for pyoderma gangrenosum, and can be used in combination with systemic steroids in appropriate patients.

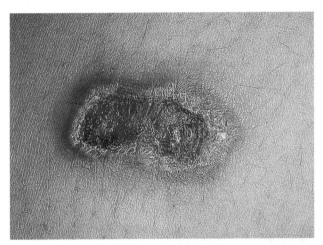

The initiating lesion consists of discrete pustules surrounded by an inflammatory areola. The lesion then degenerates into an ulcer.

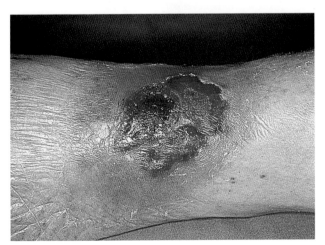

Differentiation from other diseases causing ulcers is sometimes very difficult. Malignancies may present as ulcers with exactly the same appearance. Therefore, a biopsy is justified.

- Dapsone, minocycline, clofazimine and thalidomide have been used anecdotally with variable results.
- Intravenous immunoglobulin is another drug used for pyoderma gangrenosum, which has been poorly studied, but has been successful in some patients. The high cost of this drug limits its use.

Topical Therapy

- Intralesional steroids (Kenalog) 10–40 mg/ml can be used for small or single lesions, but care must be taken not to injure the skin.

- Local wet dressings with Burrow's solution or silver nitrate two or three times daily.
- Superpotent topical steroids and Protopic 0.1% ointment have been used with some success.

Course and Prognosis

- In general, many patients with pyoderma gangrenosum have a chronic relapsing course, even with adequate treatment.
- Although eradication of the disease is the ultimate treatment goal, most regimens are aimed at reducing or removing steroid therapy all together.

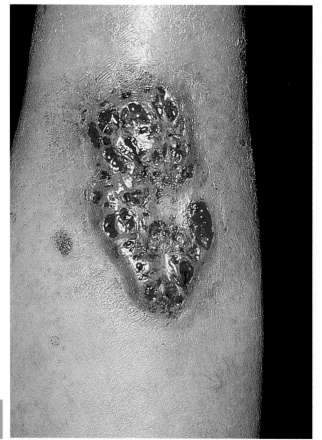

The legs are the most common site. New lesions form at sites of injury in a phenomenon called "pathergy". The new lesions become much larger than the lesion created by the initial injury.

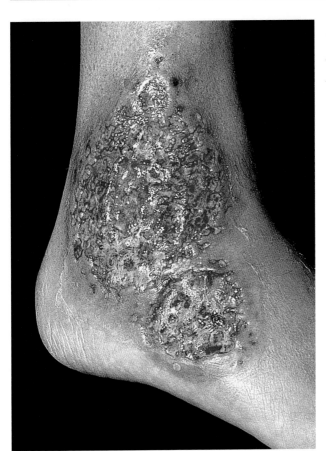

Eventually a lesion forms with multiple ulcers with crater-like holes. This is a highly characteristic feature. The lesions consist of small fistula tracks from which pus can be obtained with pressure.

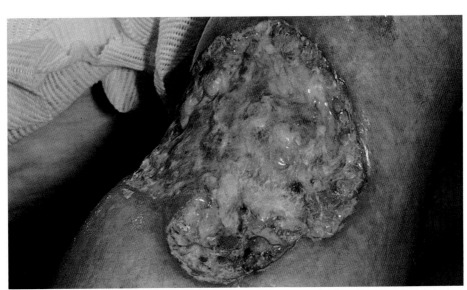

A huge ulcer with the characteristic violaceous border. Lesions are most often found on the legs but they can occur on any skin surface.

A Skin Wellness

- Wellness or health may be defined as a state of normal form and function.
- The skin performs many functions, both simple and complex, as described below.
- Various disease states may alter skin form, often also disrupting skin function.
- The skin has an amazing capacity to adapt and to repair insult and injury.
- Successful treatment of skin disease requires restoration of normal skin form and function and return to a state of skin wellness.

The Skin is a Physical Barrier

- The outermost epidermal layer, the stratum corneum, represents the end stage of keratinization.
- Keratinocytes arise from basal layer cells, which mature while migrating upward.
- The stratum granulosum and stratum spinosum represent generations of similarly maturing, upwardly migrating keratinocytes, which—on terminal keratinization—are members of the stratum corneum.
- The stratum corneum resists water loss through a physical barrier of cornified keratinocytes, intracellular proteins and lipids, and extruded surface sebum.
- A disruption in these components results in increased water loss and increased penetration of topically applied materials, including medicaments and potential allergens.
- The skin recovers in days to weeks to a loss of stratum corneum.
- Repeated physical injury will result in a thickened stratum corneum and callosities as the skin adjusts to added physical stress.
- The stratum corneum resists polar and non-polar chemical insults due to its inherently dual hydrophilic and lipophilic nature.
- The stratum corneum is able to buffer against pH insults over a fairly wide range, though strong enough acids and bases will denature and coagulate surface proteins resulting in chemical burn and sloughing.
- Similarly, excessive applied heat will cause burning and sloughing.
- The depth of the injury determines the time to regenerate the epidermis.
- Full-thickness loss of skin will recover if the area is kept clean, moist and free of infection with topical antibiotic ointment and dressing.
- A dressing assumes the role of skin until enough skin cells have migrated in to resume their role.
- An injury which extends into the dermis will result in some degree of scarring.

The Skin is a Thermostat

- The stratum corneum helps to retain heat by resisting water loss and evaporation.
- The superficial and deep dermal plexuses retain heat by shunting warm blood from the colder superficial vessels to deeper tissues.
- The subcutaneous fat provides an insulating effect, as well as cushioning.
- Prolonged cold exposure results in anoxic tissues, including skin, and is equivalent to a burn injury.
- The eccrine glands produce sweat which, when released onto the skin surface, evaporates to release excess heat in warm weather.
- Light breathable fabrics facilitate air circulation and cooling.

- Occlusion traps sweat, resulting in miliaria.

The Skin is a Parasol

- Melanin produced by melanocytes is packaged into melanosomes and distributed to surrounding keratinocytes.
- Melanosomes are arranged around cell nuclei, shielding DNA from ultraviolet light exposure.
- Ultraviolet light B affects the epidermis and ultraviolet light A affects the dermis.
- Excessive ultraviolet B light exposure results in sunburn, and painful dermal erythema with or without blister formation, and ultimately to lentigines and epidermal thinning.
- Excessive ultraviolet A leads to loss of dermal elasticity and wrinkles.
- Despite the melanin, some ultraviolet light does interact with nuclear DNA and mutations occur.
- Ultraviolet light-induced mutations are usually repaired with remarkable accuracy, but not always correctly.
- Over a lifetime of sun exposure, mutations may accumulate, which may result in cell death or cell autonomy, or skin cancer.
- Regular use of sun-protective clothing and avoidance of the midday sun greatly reduce one's cumulative exposure to ultraviolet light.
- As a final line of defense, a broad-spectrum blocking sunscreen (against ultraviolet A and B) with a sun-protective factor of 30 or more reduces incidental ultraviolet exposure.
- Sunscreens must be applied liberally and frequently throughout outdoor activities.
- Sun damage may be slowed and possibly reversed with topical tretinoin, alpha-hydroxy acid products, and possibly co-enzyme q10.

- Various cosmetic procedures are available to improve skin appearance including laser surgery, cosmetic surgery, and chemical peels.
- These are best reviewed in consultation with a qualified dermatologist.
- There is no substitute for prevention of skin aging with sun protection.

The Skin is an Immune Barrier

- Skin keratinocytes produce antimicrobial peptides that are important in innate immunity.
- Bone-marrow derived immune cells are found residing in normal skin including T and B lymphocytes, plasma cells, monocytes, and Langerhans cells.
- These cells provide an immune surveillance system for infection, cancers, and toxins.
- Ultraviolet light greatly diminishes immune cell surveillance effectiveness.

The Skin is a Habitat

- The skin is home to a variety of commensal bacterial and yeast species.
- Such species colonize skin shortly after birth and maintain a fairly stable population.
- These normal flora may protect from colonization by potentially harmful bacteria.
- Washing removes some surface bacteria, keratinocytes and debris, although the skin flora quickly recover.
- Disrupted or diseased skin may allow harmful bacteria to infect.
- Antibiotics do cause some shifts in populations of normal flora and may impede the ability of harmless flora to compete against antibiotic-resistant invaders (e.g. *Candidiasis*).

Promoting Skin Wellness

■ In general terms, hygienic washing is encouraged; over-washing is often harmful to the skin.

■ Emollients that augment the skin's barrier function are useful in drier, colder climates.

■ Sensible clothing—including gloves, hats, and footwear—should be chosen to maintain comfort for a given climate and season and for the chosen activity.

■ Breathable loose-fitting clothing facilitates cooling in a hot, humid environment.

■ Clothing that blocks the wind, retains heat and wicks away perspiration during activity is best in colder climates.

■ Make good decisions about limiting ultraviolet light exposure—prevent both today's sunburn and tomorrow's skin cancer.

B Primary, Secondary, and Special Lesions

Primary Lesions

Most skin diseases begin with a basic lesion that is referred to as a *primary* lesion. Identification of the primary lesion is the key to accurate interpretation and description of cutaneous disease. Its presence provides the initial orientation and allows the formulation of a differential diagnosis. Definitions of the primary lesions and their differential diagnoses follow.

Secondary Lesions

Secondary lesions develop during the evolutionary process of skin disease, or they are created by scratching or infection. They may be the only type of lesion present, in which case the primary disease process must be inferred. The differential diagnoses of secondary lesions follow.

Special Lesions

A certain number of unique structures and changes called *special* lesions occur. The lesions and their definitions follow.

Primary Skin Lesions

Macule and Patch

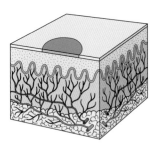

A circumscribed, flat discoloration. A macule is 0.5 cm or smaller, and a patch is larger than 0.5 cm. They may be brown, blue, red, or hypopigmented.

Brown
- Becker's nevus
- Café-au-lait spot
- Erythrasma
- Fixed drug eruption
- Freckle
- Junction nevus
- Lentigo
- Lentigo maligna
- Melasma
- Photoallergic drug eruption
- Phototoxic drug eruption
- Stasis dermatitis
- Tinea nigra palmaris

Blue
- Ink (tattoo)
- Maculae ceruleae (lice)
- Mongolian spot

Red
- Drug eruptions
- Juvenile rheumatoid arthritis
- Rheumatic fever
- Secondary syphilis
- Viral exanthems

Hypopigmented
- Idiopathic guttate hypomelanosis
- Nevus anemicus
- Piebaldism
- Post-inflammatory psoriasis
- Radiation dermatitis
- Tinea versicolor
- Tuberous sclerosis
- Vitiligo

Papule

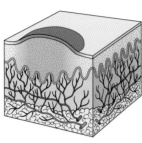

A palpable lesion up to 0.5 cm in diameter. The color varies. Papules may become confluent and form plaques.

Flesh Colored, Yellow, or White
- Acrochordon (skin tag)
- Adenoma sebaceum
- Basal cell epithelioma
- Closed comedo (acne)
- Flat warts
- Granuloma annulare
- Lichen nitidus
- Lichen sclerosis et atrophicus
- Milium
- Molluscum contagiosum
- Neurofibroma
- Nevi (dermal)
- Pearly penile papules
- Pseudoxanthoma elasticum
- Sebaceous hyperplasia
- Skin tags
- Syringoma

Brown
- Dermatofibroma
- Keratosis follicularis
- Melanoma
- Nevi
- Seborrheic keratosis
- Urticaria pigmentosa
- Wart

Red
- Acne
- Atopic dermatitis
- Cat-scratch disease
- Cherry angioma
- Cholinergic urticaria
- Chondrodermatitis helicis
- Eczema
- Folliculitis
- Insect bites
- Keratosis pilaris
- Leukocytoclastic vasculitis
- Miliaria
- Polymorphous light eruption
- Psoriasis
- Pyogenic granuloma
- Scabies
- Urticaria

Blue or Violaceous
- Angiokeratoma
- Blue nevus
- Lichen planus
- Lymphoma
- Kaposi sarcoma
- Melanoma
- Mycosis fungoides
- Venous lake

Plaque

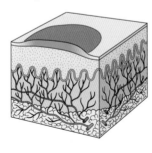

A circumscribed, palpable, solid lesion more than 0.5 cm in diameter, often formed by the confluence of papules.

- Eczema
- Cutaneous T cell lymphoma
- Discoid lupus erythematosus
- Lichen planus
- Paget's disease
- Papulosquamous (papular and scaling lesions)
- Pityriasis rosea
- Psoriasis
- Seborrheic dermatitis
- Sweet syndrome
- Syphilis (secondary)
- Tinea corporis
- Tinea versicolor

Nodule

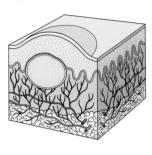

A circumscribed, often round, solid lesion more than 0.5 cm in diameter. A large nodule is referred to as a *tumor*.

- Basal cell carcinoma
- Cutaneous T cell lymphoma
- Erythema nodosum
- Furuncle
- Hemangioma

- Kaposi sarcoma
- Keratoacanthoma
- Lipoma
- Lymphoma
- Melanoma
- Metastatic carcinoma
- Neurofibromatosis
- Prurigo nodularis
- Sporotrichosis
- Squamous cell carcinoma
- Wart
- Xanthoma

Pustule

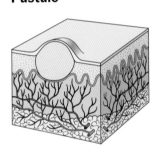

A circumscribed collection of leukocytes and free fluid that varies in size.

- Acne
- Candidiasis
- Chicken pox
- Dermatophyte infection
- Dyshidrosis
- Folliculitis
- Gonococcemia

- Hidradenitis suppurativa
- Herpes simplex
- Herpes zoster
- Impetigo
- Keratosis pilaris
- Pseudomonas folliculitis
- Psoriasis
- Pyoderma gangrenosum
- Rosacea
- Scabies
- Varicella

Vesicle

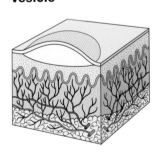

A circumscribed collection of free fluid up to 0.5 cm in diameter.

- Benign familial chronic pemphigus
- Cat-scratch disease
- Chicken pox
- Dermatitis herpetiformis

- Eczema (acute)
- Erythema multiforme
- Herpes simplex
- Herpes zoster
- Impetigo
- Lichen planus
- Pemphigus foliaceus
- Porphyria cutanea tarda
- Scabies

Bulla

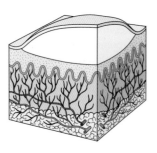

A circumscribed collection of free fluid more than 0.5 cm in diameter.

- Bullae in diabetics
- Bullous pemphigoid
- Cicatricial pemphigoid

- Epidermolysis bullosa acquisita
- Fixed drug eruption
- Herpes gestationis
- Lupus erythematosus
- Pemphigus

Wheal (Hive)

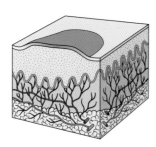

A firm edematous papule or plaque, resulting from infiltration of the dermis with fluid. Wheals are transient and may last only a few hours.

- Angioedema
- Cholinergic urticaria
- Dermographism
- Hives
- Urticaria pigmentosa (mastocytosis)

Secondary Skin Lesions

Scales

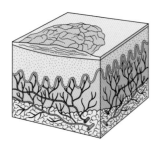

Excess dead epidermal cells that are produced by abnormal keratinization and shedding.

Fine to Stratified
- Erythema craquelé
- Ichthyosis, dominant (quadrangular)
- Ichthyosis, X-linked (quadrangular)
- Lupus erythematosus (carpet tack)
- Pityriasis rosea (collarette)
- Psoriasis (silvery)
- Scarlet fever (fine; on trunk)
- Seborrheic dermatitis

- Syphilis (secondary)
- Tinea (dermatophytes)
- Tinea versicolor
- Xerosis (dry skin)

Scaling in Sheets (Desquamation)
- Kawasaki syndrome
- Scarlet fever (hands and feet)
- Staphylococcal scalded skin syndrome
- Toxic shock syndrome

Crust

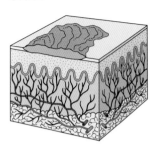

A collection of dried serum and cellular debris; a scab.

- Acute eczematous inflammation
- Atopic (face)

- Impetigo (honey colored)
- Pemphigus foliaceus
- Tinea capitis

Erosion

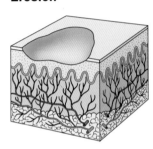

A focal loss of epidermis. Erosions do not penetrate below the dermoepidermal junction and therefore heal without scarring.

- Candidiasis
- Dermatophyte infection
- Eczematous diseases

- Herpes simplex
- Intertrigo
- Neurotic excoriations
- Perlèche
- Senile skin
- Toxic epidermal necrolysis
- Vesiculobullous diseases

Ulcer

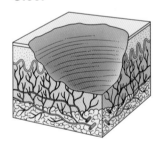

A focal loss of epidermis and dermis. Ulcers heal with scarring.

- Aphthae
- Chancroid
- Decubitus
- Factitial ulcer

- Ischemic ulcer
- Necrobiosis lipoidica
- Neoplasms
- Pyoderma gangrenosum
- Radiation dermatitis
- Stasis ulcer
- Syphilis (chancre)

Fissure

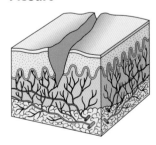

A linear loss of epidermis and dermis with sharply defined, nearly vertical walls.

- Chapping (hands, feet)
- Eczema (fingertip)
- Intertrigo
- Perlèche

Atrophy

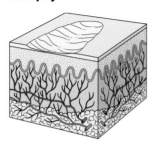

A depression in the skin, resulting from thinning of the epidermis or dermis.

- Aging
- Dermatomyositis
- Discoid lupus erythematosus
- Lichen sclerosis et atrophicus
- Morphea
- Necrobiosis lipoidica diabeticorum
- Radiation dermatitis
- Striae
- Drug-induced reaction (from topical and intralesional steroids)

Scar

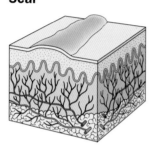

An abnormal formation of connective tissue, implying dermal damage. After injury or surgery, scars are initially thick and pink, but with time become white and atrophic.

- Acne
- Burns
- Herpes zoster
- Hidradenitis suppurativa
- Keloid
- Porphyria
- Varicella

Special Skin Lesions	
Description	**Differential Diagnosis**
Excoriation An erosion caused by scratching; excoriations are often linear	Scabies Atopic dermatitis Primary pruritus Dermatitis herpetiformis Prurigo Acne excorieé Dry skin
Comedo A plug of sebaceous and keratinous material lodged in the opening of a hair follicle; the follicular orifice may be dilated (blackhead) or narrowed (whitehead or closed comedo)	Acne Epidermal cyst Discoid lupus erythematosus Solar comedones
Milia A small, superficial keratin cyst with no visible opening	Chronic solar damage Porphyria cutanea tarda Inherited blistering disorders
Cyst A circumscribed lesion with a wall and a lumen; the lumen may contain fluid or solid matter	Epidermal Pilar

Special Skin Lesions—*continued*	
Description	**Differential Diagnosis**
Burrow A narrow, elevated, tortuous channel produced by a parasite	Scabies Creeping eruption
Lichenification An area of thickened epidermis induced by scratching; the skin lines are accentuated so that the surface looks like a washboard	Atopic dermatitis Lichen simplex chronicus Chronic eczematous dermatitis

Telangiectasia
Dilated superficial blood vessels
	Actinically damaged skin
	Adenoma sebaceum
	Ataxia–telangiectasia
	Basal cell carcinoma
	Bloom syndrome
	CREST syndrome
	Hereditary hemorrhagic
	   telangiectasia
	Keloid
	Lupus erythematosus
	Necrobiosis lipoidica
	   diabeticorum
	Poikiloderma
	Radiation dermatitis
	Rosacea
	Scleroderma
	Vascular spiders
	Pregnancy
	Cirrhosis
	Xeroderma pigmentosum
	Of the proximal nail fold:
	   Dermatomyositis
	   Lupus erythematosus
	   Scleroderma

Petechiae A circumscribed deposit of blood less than 0.5 cm in diameter	Gonococcemia Leukocytoclastic vasculitis Meningococcemia
Purpura A circumscribed deposit of blood greater than 0.5 cm in diameter	Platelet abnormalities Progressive pigmentary purpura Rocky Mountain spotted fever Scurvy Senile traumatic purpura Vascular spider

C Differential Diagnoses by Body Region

Common and important diseases are included. Body regions and then diseases are listed alphabetically. Some common diseases that are obvious to most practitioners are not included.

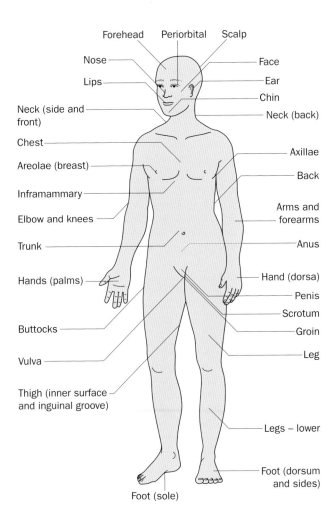

Anus

- Hidradenitis suppurativa
- Lichen sclerosis et atrophicus
- Lichen simplex chronicus
- Psoriasis (gluteal pinking)
- Streptococcal cellulitis
- Vitiligo
- Wart

Areola (Breast)

- Eczema
- Paget's disease
- Seborrheic keratosis

Arm and Forearm

- Acne
- Atopic dermatitis
- Dermatitis herpetiformis (elbows)
- Dermatomyositis
- Erythema multiforme
- Granuloma annulare
- Insect bite
- Keratoacanthoma
- Keratosis pilaris
- Lichen planus
- Neurotic excoriations
- Nummular eczema
- Pityriasis alba (white spots)
- Polymorphic light eruption
- Prurigo nodularis
- Purpura (in sun damaged skin)
- Scabies
- Seborrheic keratosis (flat)
- Squamous cell carcinoma
- Stellate pseudo scars
- Sweet syndrome
- Tinea

Axilla

- Acanthosis nigricans
- Acrochordons
- Candidiasis
- Contact dermatitis
- Erythrasma
- Freckling: Crowe's sign

(von Recklinghausen's disease)
- Furunculosis
- Hailey-Hailey disease
- Hidradenitis suppurativa
- Impetigo
- Lice
- Trichomycosis axillaris

Back

- Acne
- Becker's nevus
- Cutaneous T cell lymphoma
- Dermatographism
- Keloids (acne scars)
- Melanoma
- Nevus anemicus
- Seborrheic keratosis
- Tinea versicolor

Buttock

- Cutaneous T cell lymphoma
- Furunculosis
- Herpes simplex (females)
- Hidradenitis suppurativa
- Psoriasis
- Tinea

Chest

- Acne
- Actinic keratosis
- Darier's disease
- Eruptive syringoma
- Keloids
- Seborrheic dermatitis
- Steatocystoma multiplex
- Tinea versicolor
- Transient acantholytic dermatitis (Grover's disease)

Chin

- Acne
- Atopic dermatitis
- Impetigo
- Perioral dermatitis
- Wart (flat)

Ear

- Actinic keratosis
- Basal cell carcinoma

- Cellulitis
- Chondrodermatitis nodularis chronica helicis
- Eczema (infected)
- Epidermal cyst
- Keloid (lobe)
- Lupus erythematosus (discoid)
- Psoriasis
- Ramsay-Hunt syndrome (herpes zoster)
- Seborrheic dermatitis
- Squamous cell carcinoma
- Venous lake

Elbow and Knee

- Dermatitis herpetiformis
- Lichen simplex chronicus
- Psoriasis

Face

- Actinic keratosis
- Adenoma sebaceum
- Angioedema
- Atopic dermatitis
- Basal cell carcinoma
- Cowden's disease
- Eczema
- Erysipelas
- Favre-Racouchot (solar comedones)
- Herpes zoster
- Impetigo
- Lentigo maligna
- Lupus erythematosus (discoid)
- Lupus erythematosus (systemic)
- Melasma
- Molluscum contagiosum
- Nevus sebaceus
- Perioral dermatitis
- Pityriasis alba (white spots)
- Psoriasis
- Sebaceous hyperplasia
- Seborrheic dermatitis
- Seborrheic keratosis
- Spitz nevus
- Squamous cell carcinoma
- Steroid rosacea

- Sycosis barbae (folliculitis (beard))
- Tinea
- Wart (flat)

Foot (Dorsum and Side)
- Contact dermatitis
- Cutaneus larva migrans
- Erythema multiforme
- Granuloma annulare
- Hand, foot, and mouth disease
- Lichen simplex chronicus
- Stucco keratosis
- Tinea

Foot (Sole)
- Cutaneus larva migrans
- Dyshidrotic eczema
- Erythema multiforme
- Hand, foot, and mouth disease
- Hyperkeratosis
- Juvenile plantar dermatosis
- Melanoma
- Nevi
- Pitted keratolysis
- Psoriasis (pustular)
- Scabies (infants)
- Syphilis (secondary)
- Tinea
- Wart

Forehead
- Actinic keratosis
- Basal cell carcinoma
- Flat warts
- Herpes zoster
- Psoriasis
- Sebaceous hyperplasia
- Seborrheic dermatitis
- Seborrheic keratosis

Groin
- Acrochordons (skin tags)
- Candidiasis
- Condyloma
- Erythrasma
- Extramammary Paget's disease
- Hidradenitis suppurativa

- Intertrigo
- Lichen simplex chronicus
- Molluscum contagiosum
- Psoriasis (without scale)
- Seborrheic keratosis
- Striae (topical steroids)
- Tinea

Hand (Dorsum)
- Actinic keratosis
- Atopic dermatitis
- Contact dermatitis
- Cowden's disease
- Erythema multiforme
- Granuloma annulare
- Keratoacanthoma
- Lentigo
- Paronychia (acute; chronic)
- Polymorphous light eruption
- Porphyria cutanea tarda
- Psoriasis
- Scabies
- Seborrheic keratosis
- Squamous cell carcinoma
- Stucco keratosis
- Tinea
- Vesicular "id reaction"

Hand (Palm)
- Basal cell nevus syndrome (pits)
- Calluses; corns
- Contact dermatitis
- Cowden's disease
- Dyshidrotic eczema
- Eczema
- Erythema multiforme
- Hand, foot, and mouth disease
- Keratolysis exfoliativa
- Pompholyx
- Psoriasis
- Pyogenic granuloma
- Rocky Mountain spotted fever
- Scabies (infants)
- Syphilis (secondary)
- Tinea
- Vesicular "id reaction"
- Wart

Inframammary
- Acrochordon (skin tags)
- Candidiasis
- Contact dermatitis
- Intertrigo
- Psoriasis (without scale)
- Seborrheic keratoses
- Tinea versicolor

Leg (Thigh)
- Basal cell carcinoma
- Bowen's disease
- Eruptive xanthomas
- Kaposi sarcoma
- Livedo reticularis
- Melanoma
- Nummular eczema
- Panniculitis
- Pyoderma gangrenosum
- Squamous cell carcinoma

Leg (Lower)
- Bites
- Cellulitis
- Dermatofibroma
- Diabetic bullae
- Diabetic dermopathy (shin spots)
- Erysipelas
- Erythema nodosum
- Flat warts
- Folliculitis
- Granuloma annulare
- Henoch–Schönlein purpura
- Ichthyosis vulgaris
- Idiopathic guttate hypomelanosis
- Leukocytoclastic vasculitis
- Lichen planus
- Lichen simplex chronicus
- Majocchi's granuloma (tinea)
- Necrobiosis lipoidica
- Prurigo nodularis
- Schamberg's purpura
- Stasis dermatitis
- Vasculitis (nodular lesions)
- Xerosis

591

Lip

- Actinic cheilitis
- Allergic contact dermatitis
- Angioedema
- Aphthous ulcer
- Fordyce's spots (upper lips)
- Herpes simplex
- Labial melanotic macule
- Leukoplakia
- Mucous cyst
- Perlèche
- Pyogenic granuloma
- Squamous cell carcinoma
- Venous lake
- Wart

Neck (Back)

- Acanthosis nigricans
- Acne
- Acne keloidalis
- Epidermal cyst
- Folliculitis
- Furunculosis
- Lichen simplex chronicus
- Neurotic excoriations
- Salmon patch
- Tinea

Neck (Side and Front)

- Acanthosis nigricans
- Acne
- Acrochordon (skin tags)
- Atopic dermatitis
- Berloque dermatitis
- Contact dermatitis
- Epidermal cyst
- Folliculitis
- Poikiloderma of Civatte
- Pseudofolliculitis
- Pseudoxanthoma elasticum
- Sycosis barbae (fungal, bacterial)
- Tinea
- Wart

Nose

- Acne
- Actinic keratosis

- Basal cell carcinoma
- Lupus erythematosus (discoid)
- Herpes simplex
- Impetigo
- Nevus
- Rhinophyma
- Rosacea
- Seborrheic dermatitis
- Squamous cell carcinoma
- Telangiectasia

Penis

- Candidiasis (under foreskin)
- Chancroid
- Condyloma (wart)
- Contact dermatitis (from condoms)
- Erythroplasia of Queyrat (Bowen's disease)
- Fixed drug eruption
- Herpes simplex
- Herpes zoster
- Lichen planus
- Lichen sclerosis et atrophicus (balanitis xerotica obliterans)
- Molluscum contagiosum
- Nevus
- Pearly penile papule
- Penile melanosis
- Psoriasis
- Scabies
- Sclerosing lymphangitis (non-venereal)
- Seborrheic keratosis
- Squamous cell carcinoma
- Syphilis (chancre)

Periorbital Area

- Acrochordons (skin tags)
- Angioedema
- Atopic dermatitis
- Contact dermatitis
- Dermatomyositis
- Milia
- Molluscum contagiosum
- Seborrheic dermatitis
- Senile comedones
- Syringoma
- Xanthelasma

Scalp

- Actinic keratosis
- Alopecia neoplastica (metastases)
- Basal cell carcinoma
- Contact dermatitis
- Folliculitis
- Kerion (inflammatory tinea)
- Lichen planopilaris
- Lupus erythematosus (discoid)
- Neurotic excoriations
- Nevi
- Nevus sebaceus
- Pediculosis capitis
- Pilar cyst (wen)
- Psoriasis
- Seborrheic dermatitis
- Seborrheic keratosis
- Tinea

Scrotum

- Angiokeratoma of Fordyce
- Condyloma
- Epidermal cyst
- Extramammary Paget's disease
- Lichen simplex chronicus
- Nevus
- Scabies
- Seborrheic keratosis

Thigh (Inner Surface and Inguinal Groove)

- Acrochordons (skin tags)
- Candidiasis
- Cutaneous T-cell lymphoma
- Erythrasma
- Extramammary Paget's disease
- Fissures
- Hidradenitis suppurativa
- Intertrigo
- Tinea

Trunk (Chest, Back, Abdomen)

- Accessory nipple
- Ash leaf spot

- Atopic dermatitis
- Capillary hemangiomas
- Chickenpox
- Cutaneous T cell lymphoma (mycosis fungoides)
- Drug eruption (maculopapular)
- Epidermal cyst
- Familial atypical mole syndrome
- Fixed drug eruption
- Folliculitis (classic and hot tub)
- Granuloma annulare (generalized)
- Halo nevus
- Herpes zoster
- Keloids
- Lichen planus (generalized)
- Lichen sclerosis et atrophicus
- Lupus erythematosus (subacute cutaneous)

- Miliaria
- Nevus anemicus
- Pediculosis (lice)
- Pemphigus foliaceous
- Pityriasis rosea
- Pityrosporum folliculitis
- Poikiloderma vasculare atrophicans
- Psoriasis (guttate)
- Scabies
- Seborrheic dermatitis
- Steatocystoma multiplex
- Syphilis (secondary)
- Tinea
- Tinea versicolor
- Transient acantholytic dermatosis (Grover's disease)
- Urticaria pigmentosa
- Viral exanthem
- von Recklinghausen's neurofibromatosis

Vulva

- Allergic contact dermatitis
- Angiokeratoma of Fordyce
- Candidiasis
- Chancroid
- Epidermal cyst
- Erythrasma
- Extramammary Paget's disease
- Fibroepithelial polyp
- Furunculosis
- Hidradenitis suppurativa
- Intertrigo
- Leukoplakia
- Lichen planus
- Lichen sclerosis et atrophicus
- Lichen simplex chronicus
- Molluscum contagiosum
- Nevus
- Pediculosis
- Psoriasis
- Wart

D Quantity of Cream to Apply and Dispense

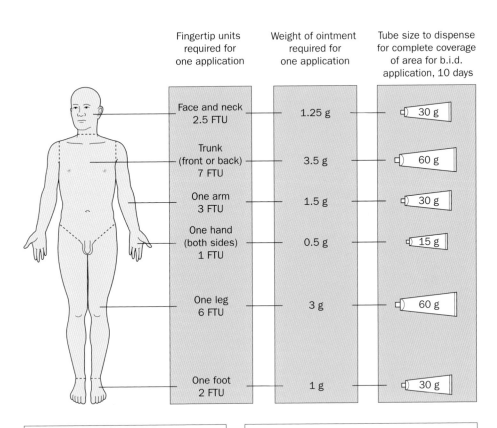

	Fingertip units required for one application	Weight of ointment required for one application	Tube size to dispense for complete coverage of area for b.i.d. application, 10 days
Face and neck	2.5 FTU	1.25 g	30 g
Trunk (front or back)	7 FTU	3.5 g	60 g
One arm	3 FTU	1.5 g	30 g
One hand (both sides)	1 FTU	0.5 g	15 g
One leg	6 FTU	3 g	60 g
One foot	2 FTU	1 g	30 g

Fingertip unit (FTU)

The amount of ointment expressed from tube applied to the fingertip

One FTU weighs about 0.5 g

Hand unit (one side of the hand)

1/2 FTU covers 1 side of the hand
1/2 FTU weighs 0.25 g

0.25 g × Number of hand units = Weight of cream required for one application

Modified from Long CC, Finlay AY (1991) *Clinical and Experimental Dermatology* 16:444-447.

Dermatologic Formulary

Acne medications

Retinoids			
Product	**Base**	**Concentration**	**Packaging**
Retin-A (Tretinoin)	Cream	0.025%	20 g 45 g
		0.05%	20 g 45 g
		0.1%	20 g 45 g
	Gel	0.01%	15 g 45 g
		0.025%	15 g 45 g
	Liquid	0.05%	28 ml
Retin-A Micro (Tretinoin)	Gel	0.1%	20 g 45 g
		0.04%	20 g 45 g
Tazorac (Tazarotene)	Gel	0.1%	30 g 100 g
		0.05%	30 g 100 g
	Cream	0.1%	15 g 30 g 60 g
		0.5%	15 g 30 g 60 g
Differin (Adapalene)	Gel	0.1%	45 g
	Cream	0.1%	45 g
	Pledgets	0.1%	1 box
	Solution	0.1%	30 ml
Azelex (Azelaic acid)	20% cream	20% acid	30, 50 g
Finacea (Azelaic acid)	Gel	15% acid	30 g

Benzoyl Peroxide Cleansers		
Product	**Formulation**	**Packaging**
Benzac AC wash 2.5%	Liquid 2.5%	8 oz
Benzac AC wash 5%	Liquid 5%	8 oz
Benzac AC wash 10%	Liquid 10%	8 oz
Benzac W wash (Rx)	Liquid 5%	4, 8 oz
Benzac W wash (Rx)	Liquid 10%	8 oz
Brevoxyl Cleansing Lotion (Rx)	Liquid 4%	10.5 oz
Brevoxyl Cleansing Lotion (Rx)	Liquid 8%	10.5 oz
Brevoxyl Creamy Wash	Liquid 4%	6 oz tube
Brevoxyl Creamy Wash	Liquid 8%	6 oz tube
Desquam-X 5% wash (Rx)	Liquid 5%	150 ml
Desquam-X 10% wash (Rx)	Liquid 10%	150 ml
Desquam-X 10% bar (Rx)	Bar 10%	4 oz bar
Panoxyl 5 bar (OTC)	Bar 5%	4 oz bar
Panoxyl 10 bar (OTC)	Bar 10%	4 oz bar
Triaz 3%	Liquid 3%	6, 12 oz
Triaz 6%	Liquid 6%	6, 12 oz
Triaz 9 %	Liquid 9%	6, 12 oz
ZoDerm Cleanser	Liquid 4.5%, 10% urea	400 ml
ZoDerm Cleanser	Liquid 8.5%, 10% urea	400 ml

OTC, over the counter; Rx, prescription only.

Benzoyl Peroxide Gels (2.5% to 3.0%)		
Product	**Base**	**Packaging**
Benzac W 2.5	Water	60, 90 g
Benzac AC 2.5%	Water	60, 90 g
Clear By Design (OTC)	Water	45, 90 g
Desquam-X 2.5%	Water	1.5 oz
Desquam-E 2.5	Water	1.5 oz
Panoxyl AQ 2.5	Water	60, 120 g
Triaz 3%	Water	42.5 g and pads #30/box

OTC, over the counter

Benzoyl Peroxide Gels (4% to 8%)

Product	Base	Packaging
Benoxyl 5 (OTC)	Water	1, 2 oz
Benzac 5	12% alcohol	60 g
Benzac AC 5%	Water	60, 90 g
Benzac W 5	Water	60, 90 g
Brevoxyl 4% (Rx)	Water	42.5, 90 g
Brevoxyl 8% (Rx)	Water	42.5, 90 g
5-Benzagel	14% alcohol	42.5, 85 g
Clinac BPO	7%	45 g
Desquam-X 5	Water	45, 90 g
Desquam-E 5	Water	1.5 oz
Panoxyl 5	20% alcohol	60, 120 g
Panoxyl AQ 5	Water	60, 120 g
Sulfoxyl Regular 5 (contains 2.5% sulfur)	Water	30 ml
Triaz 6%	Water	42.5 g and pads #30/box
ZoDerm Cream 4.5%	Urea	125 ml
ZoDerm Gel 4.5%	Urea	125 ml

OTC, over the counter; Rx, prescription only.

Benzoyl Peroxide Gels (8.5% to 10%)

Product	Base	Packaging
Benoxyl 10 (OTC)	Water	1, 2 oz
Benzac 10	12% alcohol	60 g
Benzac AC 10%	Water	60, 90 g
Benzac W 10	Water	60, 90 g
10-Benzagel	14% alcohol	42.5, 85 g
Desquam-X 10	Water	42.5, 85 g
Desquam-E 10	Water	1.5 oz
Panoxyl Aqua Gel 10	Water	42.5 g
Sulfoxyl Strong 10 (contains 5% sulfur)	Water	2 oz
Triaz 9%	Water	42.5 g and pads #30/box
ZoDerm Cream 8.5%	Urea	125 ml
ZoDerm Gel 8.5%	Urea	125 ml

OTC, over the counter

Topical Antibiotics for Acne

Product	Antibiotic ingredients	Packaging
Akne-Mycin	2% erythromycin	25 g ointment
A/T/S	2% erythromycin	60 ml liquid
A/T/S gel	2% erythromycin	60 ml liquid
Azelex	20% azelaic acid	30, 50 g cream
Benzaclin	1% clindamycin 5% benzoyl peroxide	25, 50 g gel
Benzamycin	3% erythromycin 5% benzoyl peroxide	23.3, 46.6 g gel
Benzamycin Pak	3% erythromycin 5% benzoyl peroxide	60 packets
Cleocin T	1% clindamycin	30 g; 60 ml liquid 30 g; 60 ml gel 60 ml lotion #60 pledgets
Clindagel	1% clindamycin	42, 77 g gel
Clindets	1% clindamycin	#69 pledgets
Duac gel	1% clindamycin 5% benzoyl peroxide	45 g gel
Emgel	2% erythromycin	27, 50 g gel
Erycette	2% erythromycin	#60 swabs
EryDerm	2% erythromycin	60 ml liquid
Erygel	2% erythromycin	30, 60 g gel
Erymax	2% erythromycin	2, 4 oz liquid
Finacea	15% azelaic acid	30 g gel
Klaron 10%	10% sodium sulfacetamide	4 oz bottle
Plexion TS (topical suspension)	5% sulfur, 10% sodium sulfacetamide	30 g tube
Plexion Cleanser	5% sulfur, 10% sodium sulfacetamide	6 oz tube, 12 oz
Staticin	1.5% erythromycin	60 ml liquid
Theramycin Z	2% erythromycin	60 ml liquid

Topical Anti-inflammatory Agents for Acne

Product	Active ingredient	Packaging
Nicomide-T Gel	4% nicotinamide	30 g
Nicomide-T Cream	4% nicotinamide	30 g

Drying–Keratolytic Antibiotic Preparations

Product	Sulfur	Other ingredients	Packaging
Avar	5%	10% sodium sulfacetamide	45 g aqueous gel, emollient cream
Avar Green	5%	10% sodium sulfacetamide	45 g aqueous gel, emollient cream with green pigment to mask redness
Clenia	5%	10% sodium sulfacetamide	1 oz emollient cream
Plexion TS (topical suspension)	5%	10% sodium sulfacetamide	30 g tube
Plexion SCT	5%	10% sodium sulfacetamide	4 oz
Rosac cream with sunscreen	5%	10% sodium sulfacetamide	45 g
Rosula	5%	10% sodium sulfacetamide	45 ml aqueous gel with 10% urea
Sulfacet-R lotion (Rx)	5%	10% sodium sulfacetamide	25 ml
Sulfacet-R lotion TF (tint free)	5%	10% sodium sulfacetamide	25 ml
Sulfoxyl lotion regular (Rx)	2%	5% benzoyl peroxide	59 ml
Sulfoxyl lotion strong (Rx)	5%	10% benzoyl peroxide	59 ml

Rx, prescription only.

Medicated Bar Cleansers for Acne

Product	Active ingredient	Packaging
Acne-Aid Cleansing Bar	6.3% surfactant	4, 5.8 oz bar
Panoxyl Bar 5%, 10%	Benzoyl peroxide	4 oz bar
Salicylic acid soap	2% salicylic acid	4 oz bar
Sulfur soap	10% sulfur	116 g bar

Medicated Cleansers for Acne

Product	Active ingredient	Packaging
AVAR Cleanser	5% sulfur, 10% sodium sulfacetamide	8 oz pump
Clenia	5% sulfur, 10% sodium sulfacetamide	6, 12 oz foaming wash
Neutrogena Oil-Free Acne Wash	2% salicylic acid	6 oz pump
Ovace Wash	10% sodium sulfacetamide	6, 12 oz
Plexion Cleanser	5% sulfur, 10% sodium sulfacetamide	6, 12 oz
Rosanil	5% sulfur, 10% sodium sulfacetamide	6 oz
Rosula Aqueous Cleanser	5% sulfur, 10% sodium sulfacetamide	355 ml
SalAc Foam	2% salicylic acid	100 g canister
SalAc	2% salicylic acid	6 oz bottle

Isotretinoin (Accutane, Amnesteen, Claravis, Sotret)

Product	Packaging
Capsules	10, 20, 40 mg (30 mg Sotret only)

Dosing Isotretinoin by Body Weight

Body weight		Total mg/day		
Kilograms	Pounds	0.5 mg/kg	1 mg/kg	2 mg/kg
40	88	20	40	80
50	110	25	50	100
60	132	30	60	120
70	154	35	70	140
80	176	40	80	160
90	198	45	90	180
100	220	50	100	200

Anti-wrinkle Cream

Product	Active ingredient	Packaging
Renova 0.02% emollient	Tretinoin	40 g
Renova 0.05% emollient	Tretinoin	40 g
Avage 0.1 cream	Tazarotene	30 g

Vitamins for Acne

Product	Ingredients	Dosage
Nicomide tablet	Nicotinamide 750 mg, zinc 25 mg, folic acid 500 mg	Usual dose is 1 tablet twice daily

Antibiotics (Oral)

Generic	Brand name	Preparation*	Adult dosage (in mg unless noted)
Cephalosporins			
Cephradine	Velosef	250, 500 mg	1–2 g/24 h bid or qid
Cephalexin	Keflex	250, 500 mg	250–1000 qid
Cefdinir	Omnicef	300 tablet, oral suspension	300 bid
Cefadroxil	Duricef	500, 1000 mg	1 g/24 h bid or once daily
Second generation			
Cefaclor	Ceclor	250, 500 mg	250–500 tid
Cefuroxime	Ceftin	125, 250, 500 mg	250–500 bid
Cefprozil	Cefzil	250, 500 mg 125 mg/5 ml 250 mg/5 ml	250 bid or 500 once daily
Cefixime	Suprax	200, 400 mg	200 bid or 400 once daily
Fluoroquinolones			
Ofloxacin	Floxin	200, 300, 400 mg	200–400 every 12 h
Ciprofloxacin	Cipro	500, 750 mg	500–750 bid
Levofloxacin	Levaquin	250, 500, 750 mg	250–750 mg
Macrolides			
Erythromycin (ethylstearate)	EES, E-Mycin, Pediamycin	250, 400 mg	250–800 qid*
Erythromycin (enteric coated)	ERYC, Ery-Tab, E-Mycin	125, 250, 330, 500 mg	250–500 every 6 h*
Clarithromycin	Biaxin	250, 500 mg	250–500 bid
Azithromycin	Zithromax	250 mg 200 mg oral suspension	500 on first day 250 once daily for 3–4 days
Penicillins			
Ampicillin	Amcill	250, 500 mg	250–500 qid
Penicillin V	Pen-Vee K, etc.	250, 500 mg	250–500 qid
Dicloxacillin	Dynapen	125, 250, 500 mg	125–500 every 6 h
Cloxacillin	Generic	250, 500 mg	500 qid
Amoxicillin	Generic	250, 500 mg	250–500 tid
Amoxicillin clavulanate	Augmentin	250, 500, 875 mg	250–500 every 8 h or 875 bid

Generic	Brand name	Preparation*	Adult dosage
Sulfonamides, sulfones			
Sulfamethoxazole-trimethoprim	Bactrim DS, Septra DS	800 mg/160 mg	1 tablet bid
Dapsone	Generic	25, 100 mg	50–300 qid
Clindamycin	Cleocin	75, 150, 300 mg	150–300 every 6 h
Tetracyclines			
Demeclocycline	Declomycin	150 mg	150 qid or 300 bid
Doxycycline	Monodox, Vibramycin, Doryx, Adoxa	50, 75, 100 mg	100–200/24 h qid or bid
Minocycline	Dynacin tablets	50, 75, 100 mg	100–200/24 h qid or bid

*Many preparations available in liquid form.
bid, twice daily; qid, four times daily; tid, three times daily.

Antibiotics (Topical)*

Generic name	Brand name	Preparation*
Bacitracin	Baciguent ointment	15, 30, 120 g
Chloramphenicol	Chloromycetin cream	30 g
Clioquinol and 1% HC	Vioform cream	20 g
Gentamycin	Garamycin cream, ointment, solution	15 g; 5 ml solution
Iodoquinol and 0.5% or 1% HC	Vytone	1 oz tube
Mafenide acetate	Sulfamylon cream	60, 120, 480 g
Metronidazole	MetroGel cream, lotion	45 g; 1 oz lotion
	Noritate 30 g	
Mupirocin 2%	Bactroban cream, ointment	15, 30 g
	Centany ointment	15, 30 g
Neomycin	Many brands	7.5–60 g
Nitrofurazone	Furacin cream	28 g
Polymyxin and bacitracin	Polysporin ointment (many brands)	15, 30 g (ointment)
	Neosporin powder	10 g (powder)
Polymyxin, neomycin, and bacitracin	Neosporin (many brands)	15, 30 g
Povidone-iodine	Betadine ointment	30 g
Silver sulfadiazine	Silvadene cream	20, 50, 85, 400 g

*Topical antibiotics for acne are listed in the Acne Medications section.

Antifungal agents (oral)

Brand name	Generic name	Packaging
Diflucan	Fluconazole	50, 100, 150, 200 mg
Fulvicin P/G	Griseofulvin ultramicrosize	125, 165, 250, 330 mg
Fulvicin U/F	Griseofulvin microsize	250, 500 mg; 125 mg/ml suspension
Grifulvin V	Griseofulvin microsize	250, 500 mg; 125 mg/5 ml in 4 oz bottle
Gris-PEG	Griseofulvin ultramicrosize	125, 250 mg
Mycosatin	Mystatin	500 000 U, 1 000 000 U capsules
		100 000 U/ml suspension
Nizoral	Ketoconazole	200 mg
Lamisil	Terbinafine	250 mg
Sporanox	Itraconazole	100 mg
Mycelex troches for oral *Candida*		10 mg troche; bottle of 70 or 140. Dissolve 5 per day in mouth for 14 days

Antifungal agents (topical)

Topical Agents Active Against Dermatophytes and Candida		
Brand name	**Generic name**	**Packaging**
Ertaczo	Sertaconazole	30 g
Exelderm	Sulconazole	15, 30, 60 g cream
		30 ml solution
Keralac Nail Gel (50% urea)	Urea	18 ml
Lamisil (not for *Candida*)	Terbinafine hydrochloride cream	12, 24 g cream
		30 ml dropper or spray
Loprox	Ciclopirox olamine	15, 30, 90 g cream
		30, 100 g gel
		30, 60 ml topical suspension
Lotrimin	Clotrimazole	Several creams and solutions
		15, 30, 45, 90 g cream
		10, 30 ml solution
Lotrisone*	Clotrimazole and betamethasone	15, 45 g cream
	Dipropionate	30 ml lotion
Micatin	Miconazole	0.5 oz cream
		3.5 oz spray liquid
		3.5 oz spray powder
Naftin	Naftifine	15, 30, 60 g cream
		20, 40, 60 g gel
Nizoral	Ketoconazole	15, 30, 60 g cream
Oxistat	Oxiconazole	15, 30, 60 g cream
		30 ml lotion
Penlac	Ciclopirox	6.6 ml nail lacquer solution
Spectazole	Econazole	15, 30, 85 g cream
Zeasorb-AF lotion/powder	miconazole	2 oz
Zeasorb-AF powder	miconazole	2.5 oz

*A preparation containing an antifungal agent and potent topical steroid; it is useful for inflamed fungal infections. Potent topical steroids should be used only for short durations in intertriginous areas such as the groin. Change to an antifungal agent once inflammation is controlled.

Topical Agents Active Against *Candida*		
Brand name	**Generic name**	**Packaging**
Fungizone	Amphotericin B	20 g cream
		30 ml lotion
Fungoid tincture	Miconazole	2 oz bottle liquid
Mycostatin	Nystatin	30 g cream
Mycolog II*	Nystatin and triamcinolone	15, 30, 60 g cream or ointment
Mycelex troches†	Clotrimazole	10 mg troche; bottle of 70

*A preparation containing an anti-*Candida* agent and topical steroid; it is useful for inflamed yeast infections. Topical steroids should be used only for short durations in intertriginous areas such as the groin. Change to an anti-*Candida* agent once inflammation is controlled.
†Dissolve in mouth 5 per day for 14 days.

Agents Effective for Treating Tinea Versicolor

Brand name	Generic name	Packaging*	Directions
DHS Zinc (or any other zinc shampoo)	2% pyrithione zinc	6, 12 oz	Apply to trunk, arms, and thighs for 10 min; shower off; repeat for 14 days
Exelderm	Sulconazole	15, 30, 60 g	Every day for 14 days
		30 ml bottle	
Lamisil	Terbinafine hydrochloride	24 g pump	Every day for 14 days
Loprox	Ciclopirox olamine	15, 30, 60 g cream	Every day for 14 days
Lotrimin	Clotrimazole	15, 30, 45, 90 g cream	Every day for 14 days
Micatin	Miconazole	0.5 oz cream	Apply bid for 3 weeks
Sebulex	2% sulfur, 2% salicylic acid	240 ml lotion	Apply at bedtime, wash off in morning, for 7 days
Selsun lotion	2.5% selenium sulfide	Generic lotion	Apply daily for 10 minutes for 7 consecutive days
Spectazole	Econazole	15, 30, 85 g cream	Every day for 14 days
Nizoral	Ketoconazole	200 mg tablet	400 mg single dose each month or 200 mg every day for 5 days
		15, 30, 60 g cream	
		120 ml shampoo	Apply once and rinse off
Diflucan	Fluconazole	50, 100, 150, 200 mg	300 mg single dose
Sporanox	Itraconazole	100 mg	200 mg for 7 days

*Many sizes of these preparations are available. Generally it is most economical to prescribe the largest-sized container because a large area must be treated.
bid, twice daily.

Antihistamines

Medications for Urticaria				
Drug	**Initial dose (adult)**	**Maximal dose* (adult)**	**Liquid formulation**	**Tablet formulation**
H₁-receptor antagonists				
Non-sedating*				
Fexofenadine (Allegra)	180 mg every day	180 mg bid	—	30, 60, 180 mg
Desloratadine (Clarinex)	5 mg every day	10 mg	—	5 mg
Loratadine (Claritin)	10 mg every day	20 mg bid	5 mg/5 ml	10 mg
Cetirizine (Zyrtec)	10 mg every day	10 mg bid	5 mg/5 ml	5, 10 mg
Sedating				
Hydroxyzine (Atarax)	10 mg qid	50 mg qid	10 mg/5 ml Suspension 25 mg/5 ml	10, 25, 50, 100 mg
Diphenhydramine (Benadryl)	25 mg bid	50 mg qid	Elixir 12.5 mg/ 5 ml Syrup 6.25 mg/ 5 ml	25, 50 mg 12.5 mg chewable
Cyproheptadine (Periactin)	4 mg qid	8 mg qid	2 mg/5 ml	8 mg
H₂-receptor antagonists				
Cimetidine (Tagamet)	400 mg bid	800 mg bid	300 mg/5 ml	200, 300, 400, 800 mg
Ranitidine (Zantac)	150 mg bid	300 mg bid	75 mg/5 ml	150, 300 mg
Famotidine Pepcid)	20 mg bid	40 mg bid	40 mg/5 ml	20, 40 mg
H₁- and H₂-receptor antagonists				
Doxepin (Sinequan)	10 mg qid	50 mg qid	10 mg/ml	10, 25, 50, 75, 100, 150 mg
Corticosteroid				
Prednisone	20 mg every other day with gradual tapering	Many other dose schedules	5 mg/5 ml	2.5, 5, 10, 20, 50 mg
Methyl-prednisolone (Medrol)	16 mg every other day with gradual tapering	Many other dose schedules	—	2, 4, 8, 16, 24, 32 mg

Medications for Urticaria—*continued*				
Drug	**Initial dose (adult)**	**Maximal dose* (adult)**	**Liquid formulation**	**Tablet formulation**
Leukotriene antagonists				
Zafirlukast (Accolate)	20 mg bid	—	—	10, 20 mg
Montelukast (Singulair)	10 mg every day	—	—	4 mg, 5 mg chewable 10 mg
Epinephrine Injection				
·	Ana-Guard (1 : 1000)	0.3 ml/dose SC		
·	EpiPen (1 : 1000)	0.3 mg/dose		
·	EpiPen Jr (1 : 2000)	Children <12 years 0.15 mg/dose		
Immunotherapy				
Cyclosporin	2–3 mg/kg daily	4–6 mg/kg daily	100 mg/ml	25, 50, 100 mg
Methotrexate	2.5 mg PO bid for 3 days a week	5 mg PO bid for 3 days a week	25 mg/ml	2.5 mg

*Higher dosages than recommended by the manufacturer may be required for maximum therapeutic effect.
bid, twice daily; PO, orally; qid, four times daily; SC, subcutaneous.

Antineoplastic agents (topical)

	Product	**Packaging**
Aldara	5% imiquimod	Box of 12 packets
Carac	0.5% fluorouracil	30 g tube
Fluoroplex	1% fluorouracil	30 ml solution
	1% fluorouracil	30 g cream
Efudex	2% fluorouracil	10 ml liquid
	5% fluorouracil	10 ml liquid
	5% fluorouracil	25 g cream
Solaraze	3% diclofenac sodium	50, 100 g gel

Antiperspirants

Brand name	Active ingredient	Packaging
Certain-Dri (OTC)	Aluminum chloride (hexahydrate)	1, 2 oz roll-on Pump spray (non-aerosol)
Drysol (Rx)	20% aluminum chloride (hexahydrate) in 93% anhydrous ethyl alcohol	35 ml bottle with Dab-O-Matic applicator 37.5 ml bottle
Hypercare	20% aluminum chloride (hexahydrate) in 93% anhydrous ethyl alcohol	37.5 ml bottle 35, 60 ml bottles with Dab-O-Matic applicator
Lazerformalyde solution* (Rx)	10% formaldehyde	3 oz roll-on
Formaldehyde-10 spray*	10% formaldehyde	2 oz spray bottle
Xerac AC (Rx)	6.25% aluminum chloride (hexahydrate) in 96% anhydrous ethyl alcohol	35, 60 ml bottles with Dab-O-Matic applicator

OTC, over the counter; Rx, prescription only.
*Used to dry excessive moisture of the feet.

Drionic Therapy for Hyperhidrosis (Iontophoresis)

Iontophoresis (the application of low-level electric current to the surface of the skin) results in reduced production of sweat at that site. A battery-operated device conforming to the shape of the treated area—using tap-water wetted pads in contact with the skin of the palms, soles, or axillae—is available for patient self-use. Four to 15 treatments of 20 minutes' duration inhibit sweat for up to 6 weeks; 95% of patients showed improvement in 2 weeks, and 86% remained improved at 6 weeks. Minor re-treatment every 6 weeks is needed to sustain inhibition. Biopsies reveal hyperkeratotic plugs within sweat ducts following treatment.

Three devices (Drionic Hands; Drionic Axillae; Drionic Feet) are available each at US $125.00 per pair. They may be ordered by the patient from General Medical Co., Department DM-8, 1935 Armacost Avenue, Los Angeles, CA 90025 (http://www.drionic.com).

More complicated devices are available from other manufacturers.

Antipruritic creams and lotions

Brand name	Active ingredient	Packaging
Eucerin itch relief	Menthol 0.15%	6.8 oz spray
Neutrogena anti-itch	Camphor 0.1%, dimethicone 0.1%	10.1 oz moisturizer
PrameGel	1% pramoxine, 0.5% menthol	4 oz
Pramosone cream 1%, 2.5%	Hydrocortisone and pramoxine HCL	1, 2 oz
Pramosone lotion 1%	Hydrocortisone and pramoxine HCL	2, 4, 8 oz
Pramosone lotion 2.5%	Hydrocortisone and pramoxine HCL	2, 4 oz
Pramosone ointment 1%, .5%	Hydrocortisone and pramoxine HCL	1 oz
Sarna lotion	0.5% each of camphor, menthol	7.5 oz bottle
Sarnol-HC	1% hydrocortisone, 0.5% each of camphor, menthol	2.0 bottle
Zonalon	5% doxepin	45 g

Antiviral agents

Brand name	Packaging
Abreva (docosanol) (OTC)	2 g
Denavir (penciclovir)	1.5 g ointment
Famvir (famciclovir)	125, 250, 500 mg tablets
Valtrex (valacyclovir)	500 mg, 1 g capsules
Zovirax (acyclovir)	200, 400, 800 mg capsules
Zovirax ointment 5%	3, 15 g tubes

OTC, over the counter.

Topical therapy for Postherpetic Neuralgia	
Brand name	Packaging
Zostrix (capsaicin 0.075% cream)(OTC)	1 oz tube

OTC, over the counter.

Contraceptives (oral)

Drug	Progestin (mg)	Estrogen (ethinyl estradiol) (mg)
Desogen	Desogestrel 0.15	30
Ortho-Cept	Desogestrel 0.15	30
Ortho-Cyclen	Norgestimate 0.25	35
Ortho Tri-Cyclen	Norgestimate 0.25	35
Ovcon-35	Norethindrone 0.4	35
Brevicon 21, 28	Norethindrone 0.5	35
Modicon 21, 28	Norethindrone 0.5	35
Ortho-Novum 7/7/7*	Norethindrone 0.5, 0.75, 1.0	35
Ortho-Novum 10–11*	Norethindrone 0.5, 1.0	35
NEE 10/11 21, 28	Norethindrone 0.5, 1.0	5
Tri-Norinyl*	Norethindrone 0.5, 1.0, 0.5	35
Norinyl 1 1 35 21, 28	Norethindrone 1.0	35
Ortho 1/35 21	Norethindrone 1.0	35
Demulen 1/50 21, 28	Ethynodiol diacetate 1.0	50
Demulen 1/35 21, 28	Ethynodiol diacetate 1.0	35
Triphasil 21, 28	Levonorgestrel 0.05, 0.075, 0.125	30, 40, 30
Tri-Levlen 21, 28	Levonorgestrel 0.05, 0.075, 0.125	30, 40, 30
Levlen 21, 28	Levonorgestrel 0.15	30
Nordette 21, 28	Levonorgestrel 0.15	30
Lo/Ovral 21, 28	Norgestrel 0.3	30
Ovral	Norgestrel 0.5	50
Loestrin 1/20	Norethindrone 1.0	20
Loestrin 1.5/30	Norethindrone 1.5	30

*Many oral contraceptives are available for both 21-day and 28-day regimens. The total androgenic effect of a pill depends on the balance between the estrogen and progestin agents. Pills with low androgenicity are better for acne, alopecia, and hirsutism. Individual response to pills varies. Some women with acne improve with pills with high androgenicity.

Corticosteroids (topical)*

Group	Brand name	%	Generic name	Tube size (in gm unless noted)
I (super)	Clobex lotion	0.05	Clobetasol propionate	30 ml, 59 ml
	Cordran tape		Flurandrenolide	Small roll, large roll, patches
	Cormax cream	0.05	Clobetasol propionate	15, 30, 45
	Cormax ointment	0.05		15, 30, 45
	Cormax scalp solution	0.05		25 ml, 50 ml
	Ultravate cream	0.05	Halobetasol propionate	15, 50
	Ultravate ointment	0.05		15, 50
	Diprolene lotion	0.05	Augmented betamethasone	30 ml, 60 ml
	Diprolene ointment	0.05		15, 50
	Diprolene gel	0.05		15, 50
	Olux foam	0.05	Clobetasol propionate	50 g, 100 g can
	Psorcon ointment	0.05	Diflorasone diacetate	15, 30, 60
	Temovate-E cream	0.05	Clobetasol propionate	15, 30, 45, 60
	Temovate ointment	0.05	Clobetasol propionate	15, 30, 45, 60
	Temovate gel	0.05	Clobetasol propionate	15, 30, 60
II (high)	Cyclocort ointment	0.1	Amcinonide	15, 30, 60
	Diprolene AF cream	0.05	Augmented betamethasone dipropionate	15, 50
	Diprosone ointment	0.05	Betamethasone dipropionate	15, 45
	Diprosone aerosol	0.1	Betamethasone dipropionate	85 g can
	Elocon ointment	0.1	Mometasone furoate	15, 50
	Halog cream	0.1	Halcinonide	15, 30, 60
	Halog ointment	0.1		15, 30, 60
	Halog solution	0.1		20, 60 ml
	Halog-E cream	0.1		30, 60
	Lidex cream	0.05	Fluocinonide	15, 30, 60, 120
	Lidex -E	0.05	Fluocinonide	15, 30, 60
	Lidex gel	0.05		15, 30, 60
	Lidex ointment	0.05		30, 60
	Lidex solution	0.05		20, 60 ml
	Psorcon-E cream	0.05	Diflorasone diacetate	15, 30, 60
	Psorcon-E ointment	0.05		15, 30, 60
	Topicort cream	0.25	Desoximetasone	15, 60
	Topicort gel	0.05		15, 60
	Topicort ointment	0.25		15, 60

Group	Brand name	%	Generic name	Tube size (in gm unless noted)
III (medium)	Alphatrex cream	0.05	Betamethasone dipropionate	45
	Alphatrex ointment	0.05		45
	Aristocort A cream	0.5	Triamcinolone acetonide	15
	Betatrex ointment	0.1	Betamethasone valerate	45
	Cutivate ointment	0.005	Fluticasone propionate	15, 30, 60
	Cyclocort lotion	0.1	Amcinonide	20, 60 ml
	Cyclocort cream	0.1	Amcinonide	15, 30, 60
	Diprosone cream	0.05	Betamethasone dipropionate	15, 45
	Diprosone lotion	0.05	Betamethasone dipropionate	20, 60 ml
	Elocon ointment	0.1	Mometasone furoate	15, 45
	Kenalog cream	0.5	Triamcinolone acetonide	20
IV (medium)	Aristocort A ointment	0.1	Triamcinolone acetonide	15, 60
	Cordran ointment	0.05	Flurandrenolide	15, 30, 60
	Cyclocort cream	0.1	Amcinonide	15, 30, 60
	Dermatop-E ointment	0.1	Prednicarbate	15, 60
	Elocon cream	0.1	Mometasone furoate	15, 45
	Elocon lotion	0.1		30, 60 ml
	Kenalog ointment	0.1	Triamcinolone acetonide	15, 60
	Luxig foam	0.12	Betamethasone valerate	50 g, 100 g can
	Synalar ointment	0.025	Fluocinolone acetonide	15, 60
	Westcort ointment	0.2	Hydrocortisone	15, 45, 60
V (medium)	Aristocort cream	0.1	Triamcinolone acetonide	15
	Betatrex cream	0.1	Betamethasone valerate	45
	Cloderm cream	0.1	Clocortolone pivalate	15, 45
	Cordran SP cream	0.05	Flurandrenolide	15, 30, 60
	Cordran lotion	0.5		15, 60 ml
	Cordran ointment	0.025		5, 30, 60
	Cutivate cream	0.05	Fluticasone propionate	15, 30, 60
	Dermatop-E cream	0.1	Prednicarbate	15, 60
	DesOwen ointment	0.05	Desonide	15, 60
	Kenalog cream	0.1	Triamcinolone acetonide	15, 60, 80
	Kenalog lotion	0.1		60 ml
	Locoid lipocream	0.1	Hydrocortisone butyrate	15, 45
	Locoid cream	0.1	Hydrocortisone butyrate	15, 45
	Locoid ointment	0.1		15, 45

Group	Brand name	%	Generic name	Tube size (in gm unless noted)
	Locoid solution			20, 60 ml
	Synalar cream	0.025	Fluocinolone acetonide	15, 60
	Synemol cream	0.025	Fluocinolone acetonide	60
	Tridesilon ointment	0.05	Desonide	15, 60
	Westcort cream	0.2	Hydrocortisone valerate	15, 45, 60
VI (low)	Aclovate cream	0.05	Prednicarbate	15, 45, 60
	Aclovate ointment	0.05	Prednicarbate	15, 45, 60
	Aristocort A cream	0.025	Triamcinolone acetonide	15, 60
	Capex shampoo	0.01	Fluocinolone acetonide	120 ml
	Dermasmooth	0.01	Fluocinolone acetonide	4 oz
	Cordran SP cream	0.025	Flurandrenolide	30, 60
	DesOwen cream	0.05	Desonide	15, 60, 90
	DesOwen lotion	0.05		2, 4 oz
	Kenalog lotion	0.025	Triamcinolone acetonide	60 ml
	Synalar solution	0.01		20, 60 ml
VII (low)	Epifoam	1.0	Hydrocortisone acetate	10 g can
	Hytone cream	2.5	Hydrocortisone	1, 2 oz
	Hytone lotion	2.5		2 oz
	Hytone ointment	2.5		1 oz
	LactiCare HC lotion	1.0	Hydrocortisone	4 oz
		2.5		2 oz
	Pramosone	1.0	Hydrocortisone acetate	2, 4, 8 oz lotion
			1 pramoxine	1, 2 oz cream
				1 oz ointment
		2.5		2, 4, oz lotion
				1, 2 oz cream
				1 oz ointment
		1.0	Hydrocortisone	Many brands

*Listed by potency of group. Group I is the most potent.

Corticosteroids (oral)

Generic name	Brand name	Preparation	Equivalent dose (mg)
Betamethasone	Celestone	0.6 mg, 0.6 mg/5 ml	0.6
Cortisol (hydrocortisone)	Cortef	5, 10, 20 mg	20
	Hydrocortone	10, 20 mg	20
Cortisone	Cortone	25 mg	25
Dexamethasone	Decadron	0.25, 0.5, 0.75, 1.5, 4, 6 mg	0.75
Dexamethasone	Hexadrol	0.5, 0.75, 1.5, 4 mg, 5 mg/5 ml	0.75
Methylprednisolone	Medrol	2, 4, 8, 16, 24, 32 mg	4
Prednisolone	Delta-Cortef	5 mg	5
	Prelone	15 mg/5 ml	5
Prednisone	Deltasone	1, 2.5, 5, 10, 20, 50 mg 5	
	Liquid Pred	5 mg/5 ml	5
	Metricorten	1, 5 mg	5
	Orasone	1, 5, 10, 20, 50 mg	5
Triamcinolone	Aristocort	1, 2, 4, 8, 16 mg, 2 mg/5 ml	4
	Kenacort	1, 2, 4, 8 mg, 4 mg/5 ml	4

Depigmenting and cosmetic covering agents

Skin Bleaches and Depigmenting Agents

Brand name	Active ingredient	Sun protectant	Packaging
Benoquin cream (Rx)*	20% monobenzone	None	1.25 oz tube
Claripel	4% hydroquinone	Sunscreen	28, 45 g tube
Eldopaque Forte 4% cream (Rx)†	4% hydroquinone	Sunblock	1 oz tube
Eldoquin Forte 4% cream (Rx)	4% hydroquinone	None	1 oz tube
Glyquin	4% hydroquinone	Sunscreen	1 oz jar
Glyquin XM	4% hydroquinone Vitamins C and E Hyaluronic acid	Sunscreen	1 oz jar
Lustra	4% hydroquinone	None	1, 2 oz jar
Lustra AF	4% hydroquinone	Sunscreen	1, 2 oz jar
Alustra	4% hydroquinone Retinol	None	1 oz jar
Melanex topical solution†	3% hydroquinone	None	1 oz bottle
Solaquin Forte 4% cream (Rx)	4% hydroquinone	Sunscreen	1 oz tube
Solaquin Forte 4% gel (Rx)	4% hydroquinone	Sunscreen	1 oz tube
Solage	2% mequinol 0.01% tretinoin	None	30 ml bottle
TriLuma	4% hydroquinone 0.01% fluocinolone acetonide 0.05% tretinoin	None	30 g tube
Ultraquin	Hydroquinone crystals for compounding		

*Indicated for extensive vitiligo to depigment entire body.
†Flesh-tinted cream base.
†Packaged with a narrow plastic and broad-tipped sponge applicator.
Rx, prescription only.

Masking Agents (Cosmetic Covering Agents)

Brand name	Base	Packaging	Shades
Covermark*	Cream	Many products	9–10
Dermablend cover cream*	Cream	Many products	21
Dy-O-Derm†	Liquid	4 oz	
Vitady†	Liquid	15 ml	

*Waterproof concealing makeup.
†A solution to mask vitiligo; transmits most ultraviolet A radiation, so it can be used concurrently with psoralens in vitiligo therapy.

Hair restoration products

Brand name	Ingredient	Packaging
Rogaine	Minoxidil solution	60 ml bottle
	2% for women	
	5% for men	

Immunomodulators (topical)

Steroid-Free Topical Anti-inflammatory Agents		
Elidel cream 1%	Pimecrolimus	30, 60, 100 g
Protopic ointment 0.1 %	Tacrolimus	30, 60, 100 g
Protopic ointment 0.03 %	Tacrolimus	30, 60, 100 g

Lubricating agents

Emollients
Emollients are complex mixtures containing many ingredients. They are listed under their primary ingredient.

Emollients Containing Urea		
Urea promotes hydration and removal of excess keratin.		
Product	Active ingredients	Packaging
Carmol 10 lotion	10% urea	6 oz
Carmol 20 cream	20% urea	3 oz
Keralac gel	50% urea	5, 9 oz
Keralac lotion (Rx)	35% urea	7, 11 oz
Ultra Mide lotion	25% urea	8 oz
Vanamide urea cream	40% urea	85, 199 g

Rx, prescription only.

Emollients Containing Lactic Acid

Lactic acid promotes hydration and removal of excess keratin.

Product	Active ingredients	Packaging
Amlactin cream	12%	4.9 oz
Amlactin AP cream	12% + 1% pramoxine	4.9 oz anti-itch cream
Amlactin lotion	12%	8, 14 oz
Epilyt lotion	5%	4 oz
Lac-Hydrin cream (Rx)	12%	385 g bottle
Lac-Hydrin lotion (Rx)	12%	400 g
LactiCare lotion	5%	7.5, 11.5 oz bottles
Lactinol lotion	10%	8 oz
U-Lactin lotion	—	8 oz

Rx, prescription only.

Ointments

Ointments containing petrolatum

Aquaphor

DML Forté

Elta

Eucerin

Moisturel

Greaseless ointments

Acid Mantle

Unibase

Creams and Gels That Remove Excess Keratin

Product	Active ingredients	Packaging
Keralyt gel	6% salicylic acid and propylene glycol	1 oz
Salex cream	6% salicylic acid	400 g

Protecting Barrier Creams

Brand/generic name	Size	Use
Derma-Guard	2, 12 oz	Industrial (protects against acids)
Desitin ointment	30, 60, 120, 240, 480 g	Protective ointment
Ivy Shield	1.25, 4, 16 oz	Helps prevent poison ivy and oak dermatitis
Kerodex 51	120, 480 g	Protective cream for dry, oily work
Kerodex 71	120, 480 g	Protective cream (water repellent)
pH-Stabil	60, 240 g	Protective cream
SBR-Lipocream	30, 100 g	Protective cream
TheraSeal	6 oz	Protective cream
Zinc oxide 20% ointment	60 g	Protective ointment
Zinc oxide 25% paste	30, 60, 480 g	Protective paste

Psoriasis and seborrheic dermatitis (shampoos)

Antimicrobial Antiseborrheic Shampoos (Pyrithione Zinc and Others)		
Brand name	Active ingredient	Packaging
Capitrol (Rx)	2% chloroxine	85 g
Carmol Deep Cleansing Antibacterial Shampoo	10% urea	8 oz
DHS Zinc	2% pyrithione zinc	8, 12 oz
Head & Shoulders	2% pyrithione zinc	400 ml
Loprox	1% ciclopirox	120 ml
Nizoral	2% ketoconazole	4 oz
ZNP Bar	2% pyrithione zinc	4.2 oz bar

Rx, prescription only.

Selenium Sulfide Shampoos		
Brand name	Concentration	Packaging
Selsun	2.5%	120
Selsun Blue	1%	120, 210, 330 ml
Head & Shoulders Intensive Treatment	1%	400 ml

Tar and Tar-Combination Shampoos

Brand name	Concentration	Packaging
Ala Seb T	5% coal tar solution 2% colloidal sulfur 2% salicylic acid	4, 12 oz
Denorex	2% coal tar gel	60, 120 ml
	2% coal tar lotion	120, 240 ml
DHS Tar	0.5% coal tar	4, 8, 16 oz
DHS Tar gel	0.5% coal tar	8 oz
Ionil T	1.0 % coal tar	16 oz
Liquor carbonis detergens	10–15% coal tar	Any amount in Green soap*
Neutrogena T/gel	2% Newtar	4.4, 8.5, 16 oz
Neutrogena T/gel extra strength	4% Newtar	(1% coal tar) 6 oz
Neutrogena T/sal	3% salicylic acid	4.5 oz
Packer's pine tar	0.82% pine tar	180 ml
Pentrax tar	5% crude coal tar	8 oz
Pentrax Gold	2% crude coal tar	5.7 oz
Polytar	mixture of tars	6 oz
Sebutone	0.5% coal tar, 2% salicylic acid, 2% sulfur	120, 240 g lotion
Tarsum	2% coal tar	4, 8 oz
Tegrin Medicated	5% coal tar extract	60, 132 ml cream 112.5, 198 ml lotion
Theraplex T shampoo	1% coal tar	8 oz
Tiseb-T	0.5% coal tar	
Vanseb-T	5% coal tar	120 ml lotion
Xseb-T plus	10% crude coal tar	4, 8 oz
Zetar	1% whole coal tar	180 ml

*Pharmacist compounded.

Sulfur and Salicylic Acid Shampoos

Product	Sulfur	Salicylic acid	Packaging
Ala-Seb	2%	2% 4, 12 oz	
Ionil Plus		2%	240 ml
DHS Sal		3% 4 oz	
Meted	5%	3%	120 ml
SAStid	5%	3%	3.5 oz bar
Sebulex	2%	2% 7 oz	
Tiseb	—	2%	8 oz
Vanseb	2%	1%	90 g cream 120 ml lotion
Xseb	—	4%	4, 8 oz
P & S	—	2%	4, 8 oz

Antiseborrheic Preparations

Brand name	Active ingredient	Packaging
DermaZinc Therapy spray/drops	(0.25%) zinc pyrithione	4 oz
Loprox gel	Ciclopirox	45 g
Nizoral cream	Ketoconazole	15, 30, 60 g
Ovace wash	10% sulfacetamide sodium	6, 12 oz
Ovace foam	10% sulfacetamide sodium	50 g, 100 g can
Carmol scalp treatment lotion, kit	10% sulfacetamide sodium, 10% urea	90 g, kit

Corticosteroid, Tar, and Other Medicated Scalp Preparations and Shampoos

Brand name	Active ingredient	Base	Packaging
Derma-smoothe/FS (Rx)	Fluocinolone acetonide 0.01%	Peanut oil	120 ml
P & S liquid	Less than 1% phenol, NaCl	Paraffin oil	120, 240 ml
Estar Therapeutic Tar Gel	5% coal tar	Water	3 oz
10% liquor carbonis detergens in Nivea oil*	Liquor carbonis detergens	Nivea oil	8, 16 oz
Capex shampoo (Rx)	0.01% fluocinolone acetonide		120 ml
Overnight scalp treatment	2% salicylic acid	Spray	6 oz

*Pharmacist compounded.
Rx, prescription only.

Psoriasis medications (oral)

Psoralens		
Brand name	**Active ingredient**	**Packaging**
Oxsoralen lotion	Methoxsalen 1% lotion	1 oz bottle
Oxsoralen-Ultra	Methoxsalen (liquid form)	10 mg capsules (green); bottle of 50
8-MOP	Methoxsalen (crystalline form)	10 mg capsules (pink); bottle of 30
Trisoralen tablets	Trioxsalen	5 mg tablets; bottles of 28, 100

Recommended Oxsoralen-Ultra Dosage According to Weight			
Patient's weight		**Dose**	
kg	*lbs*	*Low*	*High*
< 30	< 65	10	10
30–50	65–100	10	20
51–65	101–145	20	30
66–80	146–175	20	40
81–90	176–200	30	50
91–115	200–250	30	60
> 115	> 250	40	70

Acitretin (Soriatane)	
Capsules	10, 25 mg

Methotrexate		
Tablets	2.5, 5, 7.5, 10, 15 mg	
Preservative-free injection	25 mg/ml	2, 4, 8 ml vials
Powder for injection	20 mg, 1 g	20 ml vials or single-use vials

Psoriasis medications (topical)

Anthralin (Dithranol)			
Brand name	**Concentration (%)**	**Base**	**Packaging**
Drithocreme	0.1	Cream	50 g tube
Drithocreme HP 1%	1	Cream	50 g tube
Dritho-Scalp	0.5	Cream	50 g tube*
Psoriatec	1.0	Cream	50 g tube

*With special applicator.

Anthralin Stain-Prevention Treatment			
Brand name	**Active ingredient**	**Packaging**	**Use**
CuraStain	Triethanolamine	4 oz cream or spray	Dermatologic stain remover; apply to surrounding skin and lesions before wash-off; apply to lesions after wash-off

Topical Retinoids		
	Tazorac (tazarotene)	
Gel	0.05%, 0.1%	30 g
		100 g
Cream	0.05%, 0.1%	15 g
		30 g
		60 g

Topical Vitamin D3 Analogs		
Brand name	**Active ingredient**	**Packaging**
Dovonex ointment	Calcipotriene .05	30, 60, 100 g tubes
Dovonex cream	Calcipotriene .05	30, 60, 100 g tubes

Tar-Containing Bath Oil		
Brand name	**Size**	**Packaging**
Balnetar	2.5% coal tar	240 ml
Doak Oil	2% tar distillate	240 ml
Doak Oil Forte	5% tar distillate	120 ml
Lavatar	33.3% tar distillate	120, 480 ml
Polytar Bath	25% polytar	240 ml
Zetar emulsion (Rx)	30% whole coal tar	177 ml (6 oz)

Rx, prescription only.

Tar Creams and Solutions

Brand name	Concentration	Other ingredient(s)	Base Packaging
Aqua Tar	2.5% coal tar extract	—	Gel (water base) 90 g
Cutar	7.5% liquor carbonis detergens		Emulsion 6 oz, 1 gallon
Doak Tar Lotion	5% tar distillate	—	Lotion 4 oz
Elta lite tar	10% LCD		Lotion 8 oz
Elta tar	10% coal tar		Cream 3.8, 16 oz
Estar	5% coal tar	13.8% alcohol	Gel 90 g
Fototar Fototar Stik	2% coal tar 5% coal tar	— —	Cream 85 g, 1 lb jar Wax 15 g
Ichthyol	10% ichthammol	—	Ointment 30 g
Mazon cream	0.18% coal tar	1% salicylic acid, 1% resorcinol, 0.5% benzoic acid	Cream
Oxipor VHC	48.5% coal tar solution	1% salicylic acid	Lotion 2, 4 oz
P & S Plus	8% coal tar solution	2% salicylic acid	Gel 105 g
Packer's	5.87% pine tar		Soap
PolyTar Soap	Blend of tars		Soap Bar
Pragmatar	4% coal tar distillate	3% salicylic acid, 3% sulfur	Ointment
PsoriGel	7.5% coal tar solution	1% alcohol	Gel 4 oz
T/Derm	5% coal tar extract	Alcohol free	Oil 4 oz
Tegrin Medicated	5% crude coal tar extract		Lotion 6 oz Cream 60, 132 g
Unguentum Bossi	5% tar distillate	5% ammoniated mercury	Ointment 60, 480 g

Creams and Gels That Remove Excess Keratin

Brand name	Active ingredients	Packaging
Keralyt gel	6% salicylic acid and propylene glycol	1 oz
Salex cream	6% salicylic acid	400 g

Rosacea medications (topical)

Brand name	Generic name	Packaging
Avar	5% sulfur, 10% sodium sulfacetamide	45 g aqueous gel, emollient cream
Avar Green	5% sulfur, 10% sodium sulfacetamide	45 g aqueous gel, emollient cream with green pigment to mask redness
Clenia	5% sulfur, 10% sodium sulfacetamide	1 oz emollient cream (alcohol free) 6, 12 oz foaming wash
Finacea 15%	Azelaic acid	30 g gel
Klaron 10%	10% sodium sulfacetamide	2 oz bottle
Metro Gel 0.75%	Metronidazole	45 g tube
Metro Cream 0.75%	Metronidazole	45 g tube
Metro Lotion 0.75%	Metronidazole	2 oz bottle
Noritate Cream 1%	Metronidazole	30 g tube
Rosac cream with sunscreens	5% sulfur, 10% sodium sulfacetamide	45 g tube
Sulfacet-R lotion	5% sulfur, 10% sodium sulfacetamide	25 g bottle
Sulfacet-R lotion (tint free)	5% sulfur, 10% sodium sulfacetamide	25 g bottle
Plexion TS (topical suspension)	5% sulfur, 10% sodium sulfacetamide	30 g tube
Plexion Cleanser	5% sulfur, 10% sodium sulfacetamide	6 oz tube
Rosula	5% sulfur, 10% sodium sulfacetamide with 10% urea	45 ml aqueous gel

Vitamins for Rosacea		
Product	Ingredients	Dosage
Nicomide tablet	Nicotinamide 750 mg, zinc 25 mg, folic acid 500 mg	Usual dose is 1 tablet twice daily

Scabicides and Pediculicides

Scabicides		
Brand name	**Generic name**	**Packaging**
Acticin	Permethrin	5% cream: 60 g
Elimite	Permethrin	5% cream: 60 g
Eurax*	Crotamiton	10% cream: 60 g 10% lotion: 2 oz, 1 pint
Kwell	Lindane	1% cream: 2, 16 oz 1% lotion: 2, 16 oz
Kwell shampoo	Lindane	1% lotion: 2, 16 oz
5%–10% precipitated [odd brand name]	Sulfur	Sulfur in petrolatum†
Stromectol	Ivermectin	6 mg tablets

*Eurax has been reported to be less effective than lindane.
†Pharmacist compounded.

Pediculicides		
Brand name	**Generic name**	**Packaging**
A-200 (OTC)	0.33% pyrethrins	30 g gel
A-200 Pyrinate Gel shampoo (OTC)	0.17% pyrethrins	2, 4 oz shampoo
NIX cream rinse	Permethrin	2 oz
Ovide	0.5% malathion	2 oz lotion
R & C shampoo (OTC)	0.3% pyrethrins	2, 4 oz shampoo
RID (OTC)	0.3% pyrethrins	2, 4 oz, 1 gallon liquid

*For removal of lice eggs (nits)—does not kill lice.
OTC, over the counter.

Shampoo—Fragrance free, dye free

Brand name	**Packaging**
DHS Clear	16 oz
Free & Clear	8 oz

Soap-free cleansers

Often used for routine bathing in the management of atopic dermatitis	
Brand name	**Packaging**
Aquanil lotion	8, 16 oz
Cetaphil lotion	4, 8, 16 oz
Cetaphil Daily Facial Cleanser	8 oz
Moisturel sensitive skin cleanser	8.75 oz
Oilatum-AD	8 oz
SFC lotion	8, 16 oz

Soaps—Bar (mild, non-irritating)

Alpha-Keri	Dove	Oilatum (scented, unscented)
Basis glycerin	Neutrogena dry skin	Purpose
Basis superfatted	Nivea Creme	Shepard's moisturizing
Cetaphil	Cetaphil anti-Bacterial	

Sun-protective clothing

Coolibar; Tel: 952 922 1445; http://www.coolibar.com	A full line of sun-protective clothing and glasses
Radicool Australia; Tel: 714 220 4900 (ext. 224); http://www.radicoolaustralia.com	A full line of 100 SPF+ swim wear
Sunday Afternoons; Tel: 888 874 2642; http://www.Sundayafternoons.com	Sun-protective hats and clothing
SunPrecautions; Tel: 800 882 7860; http://www.sunprecautions.com	A full line of sun-protective clothing
Tilley Endurables; Tel: 800 338 2797; http://www.tilley.com	Sun-protective clothing and hats
Tuga Sun Protective Sunwear; Tel: 800 428 TUGA; http://www.plangea.com	SPF 50+ children's swim wear
Wallaroo Hat Company; Tel: 888 925 2766; http://www.wallaroohats.com	SPF 50+ hats

Vaginal anti-*Candida* agents

Topical Therapy for Acute *Candida* Vaginitis		
Drug	**Formulation**	**Dosage**
Butoconazole	Cream	5 g at bedtime for 3 days
Clotrimazole Cream, 1%	5 g at bedtime for 7–14 days	
	Cream, 10%	5 g single application
	Vaginal tablet, 100 mg	1 tablet at bedtime for 7 days or 2 tablets at bedtime for 7 days
	Vaginal tablet, 500 mg	1 tablet once
Miconazole	Cream, 2%	5 g at bedtime for 7 days
	Vaginal suppository, 100 mg	1 suppository at bedtime for 7 days
	Vaginal suppository, 200 mg	1 suppository at bedtime for 3 days
	Vaginal suppository, 1200 mg	1 suppository once
Econazole	Vaginal tablet, 150 mg	1 tablet at bedtime for 3 days
Fenticonazole	Cream, 2%	5 g at bedtime for 7 days
Tioconazole	Cream, 2%	5 g at bedtime for 3 days
	Cream, 6.5%	5 g at bedtime in a single dose
Terconazole	Cream, 0.4%	5 g at bedtime for 7 days
	Cream, 0.8%	5 g at bedtime for 3 days
	Vaginal suppository	80 mg at bedtime for 3 days
Nystatin	Vaginal tablet, 100 000 U	1 tablet at bedtime for 14 days

Preparation for Restoration and Maintenance of Vaginal Acidity			
Drug	**Formulation**	**Packaging**	**Dosage**
Aci-Jel therapeutic vaginal jelly	0.921% acetic acid	85 g tube	85 g tube morning and evening

Dietary Supplements	
Drug	**Formulation**
Derma Vite Dietary Supplement	Vitamins for health skin
Nicomide	Vitamins for acne and rosacea

Wart medications

Cantharidin		
Brand name	**Contents**	**Packaging**
Cantharone	0.7% cantharidin	7.5 ml
Cantharone Plus	30% sal acid, 5% podophyllin, 1% cantharidin	7.5 ml

Order these products from Dormer Laboratories Inc., Tel: 416 242 6167, http://www.dormer.com

Silver Nitrate		
Product	**% Silver nitrate**	**Packaging**
Silver nitrate	10%	30 ml solution
Silver nitrate	10%	30 g ointment
Silver nitrate sticks	Coated tip	Packages of 12

Salicylic Acid Preparations for Treating Warts, Calluses, and Hyperkeratotic Skin (All OTC)		
Brand name*	**% Salicylic acid**	**Packaging**
Compound W Liquid	17	9.3 ml liquid
Compound W Gel	17	7.5 g gel
Duofilm	17	15 g gel
Duofilm patch	40	18 in box
Keralyt	6	30 g gel
Mediplast	40	Plaster
Trans-Plantar	15	Cartons of 20-mm 25 patches, securing tapes, and cleaning file
Trans-Ver-Sal 6mm	15	40 pack + tape + file
Trans-Ver-Sal 12 mm	15	40 pack + tape + file
Trans-Ver-Sal 20 mm	15	25 pack + tape + file

*Many other brands available.
OTC, over the counter.

Podophyllin/Podofilox		
Brand name	**% Podophyllin**	**Packaging**
Condylox gel	0.5% podofilox (podophyllotoxin)	3.5 g
Condylox solution	0.5% podofilox (podophyllotoxin)	3.5 ml
Podocon-25	25% in benzoin tincture	15 ml
Pododerm	25% in benzoin tincture	5 ml

Interferon	
Generic/brand name	**Packaging**
Intron-A (interferon alfa-2b)	10,000,000 IU vial
Alferon N injection (interferon alfa-N3)	1 ml

Dichloroacetic Acid—Keratolytic and Cauterizing	
Generic/brand name	**Packaging**
Dichloroacetic acid*	1, 2 oz

*Order from Delasco, Tel: 800 831 6273; http://www.delasco.com.

Wet dressings

Generic/brand name	Active ingredient
Acetic acid	Vinegar is 5% acetic acid (dilute with water 4:1 or weaker)
AluWets crystals	Aluminum chloride hexahydrate
Buro-Sol powder	Aluminum acetate
Burrow's solution (Domeboro, Bluboro, Pedi-Boro, Buro-Sol)	Aluminum acetate
Domeboro otic solution	2% acetic acid (60 ml)
Domeboro powder, Bluboro, Pedi-Boro	Aluminum sulfate, calcium acetate (boxes of 12, 100 packets)
Domeboro tablets, Bluboro, Pedi-Boro	Aluminum sulfate, calcium acetate (boxes of 2, 100 tablets)
Potassium permanganate	0.025–0.1%, stains skin purple
Silver nitrate	0.1–0.5%, stains skin black (prepared by pharmacist)

Pharmacists that will compound medications

Custom Scripts, Tel: 800 226 7094, http://www.custom-rx.com

Index